Mental Health Care

of Children and Adolescents

A Guide for Primary Care Clinicians

Editor

Jane Meschan Foy, MD, FAAP

American Academy of Pediatrics

DEDICATED TO THE HEALTH OF ALL CHILDREN®

American Academy of Pediatrics Publishing Staff

Mary Lou White, *Chief Product and Services Officer/SVP, Membership, Marketing, and Publishing*

Mark Grimes, *Vice President, Publishing*

Carrie Peters, *Editor, Professional/Clinical Publishing*

Theresa Wiener, *Production Manager, Clinical and Professional Publications*

Amanda Helmholz, *Medical Copy Editor*

Linda Diamond, *Manager, Art Direction and Production*

Linda Smessaert, MSIMC, *Senior Marketing Manager, Professional Resources*

Mary Louise Carr, MBA, *Marketing Manager, Clinical Publications*

Published by the American Academy of Pediatrics
345 Park Blvd
Itasca, IL 60143
Telephone: 630/626-6000
Facsimile: 847/434-8000

www.aap.org

The American Academy of Pediatrics is an organization of 66,000 primary care pediatricians, pediatric medical subspecialists, and pediatric surgical specialists dedicated to the health, safety, and well-being of infants, children, adolescents, and young adults.

The recommendations in this publication do not indicate an exclusive course of treatment or serve as a standard of care. Variations, taking into account individual circumstances, may be appropriate.

Every effort has been made to ensure that the drug selection and dosages set forth in this text are in accordance with the current recommendations and practice at the time of publication. It is the responsibility of the health care professional to check the package insert of each drug for any change in indications and dosages and for added warnings and precautions.

The American Academy of Pediatrics is not responsible for the content of any of the resources mentioned in this publication. Web site addresses are as current as possible but may change at any time.

Brand names are furnished for identification purposes only. No endorsement of the manufacturers or products mentioned is implied.

The publishers have made every effort to trace the copyright holders for borrowed materials. If they have inadvertently overlooked any, they will be pleased to make the necessary arrangements at the first opportunity.

This publication has been developed by the American Academy of Pediatrics. The authors, editors, and contributors are expert authorities in the field of pediatrics. No commercial involvement of any kind has been solicited or accepted in the development of the content of this publication.

Every effort is made to keep *Mental Health Care of Children and Adolescents: A Guide for Primary Care Clinicians* consistent with the most recent advice and information available from the American Academy of Pediatrics.

Special discounts are available for bulk purchases of this publication. E-mail Special Sales at aapsales@aap.org for more information.

Printed in the United States of America

9-388/0518   1 2 3 4 5 6 7 8 9 10

MA0860

ISBN: 978-1-61002-150-0
eBook: 978-1-61002-151-7
EPUB: 978-1-61002-233-0
Kindle: 978-1-61002-234-7

Library of Congress Control Number: 2017940501

Contributors

Sarah Bagley, MD, MSc, FAAP
Assistant Professor of Medicine and
Pediatrics
Director, CATALYST Program
Boston University School of Medicine/
Boston Medical Center
Boston, Massachusetts
31: *Substance Use 2: Use of Other
Substances*
32: *Substance Use 3: Specialty Referral
and Comanagement*

Rebecca Baum, MD, FAAP
Chief, Developmental and Behavioral
Pediatrics
Nationwide Children's Hospital
Department of Pediatrics
The Ohio State University
Columbus, Ohio
10: *Adapting Psychosocial Interventions
to Primary Care*
24: *Medically Unexplained Symptoms*

Robert J. Bidwell, MD
Associate Clinical Professor of Pediatrics
John A. Burns School of Medicine
University of Hawaii
Honolulu, Hawaii
19: *Gender Expression and Identity*

Denise Bothe, MD
Associate Professor of Pediatrics
Division of Developmental and
Behavioral Pediatrics and Psychology
Rainbow Babies and Children's Hospital
Case Western Reserve University
Cleveland, Ohio
8: *Self-regulation Therapies and
Biofeedback*

John Campo, MD
Professor of Psychiatry and Behavioral
Health
The Ohio State University
Columbus, Ohio
24: *Medically Unexplained Symptoms*

David R. DeMaso, MD
Psychiatrist-in-Chief and Leon
Eisenberg Chair in Psychiatry,
Boston Children's Hospital

George P. Gardner and Olga E. Monks
Professor of Child Psychiatry and
Professor of Pediatrics
Harvard Medical School
Boston, Massachusetts
13: *Agitation, Suicidality, and Other
Psychiatric Emergencies*

Mary Iftner Dobbins, MD, FAAP
Associate Professor of Pediatrics and
Psychiatry
Director, Integrated Care Initiatives
Department of Family and Community
Medicine
Southern Illinois University School of
Medicine
Springfield, Illinois
18: *Family Dysfunction*

Susan dosReis, PhD
Professor
University of Maryland School of
Pharmacy
Baltimore, Maryland
11: *Psychotropic Medications in Primary
Care*

Marian Earls, MD, MTS, FAAP
Clinical Professor of Pediatrics
University of North Carolina Medical
School
Chapel Hill, North Carolina
Director of Pediatric Programs
Deputy Chief Medical Officer
Community Care of North Carolina
Raleigh, North Carolina
23: *Maternal Depression*

Robin S. Everhart, PhD
Assistant Professor
Department of Psychology
Virginia Commonwealth University
Richmond, Virginia
25: *Nonadherence to Medical Treatment*

Barbara H. Fiese, PhD
Professor and Director, Family
Resiliency Center
University of Illinois at
Urbana-Champaign
Urbana, Illinois
25: *Nonadherence to Medical Treatment*

Martin Fisher, MD, FAAP
Chief, Division of Adolescent Medicine
Cohen Children's Medical Center
Northwell Health
Professor of Pediatrics
Donald and Barbara Zucker School of
    Medicine at Hofstra/Northwell
Hempstead, New York
16: *Eating Abnormalities*

Jane Meschan Foy, MD, FAAP
Professor of Pediatrics
Wake Forest School of Medicine
Winston-Salem, North Carolina
1: *Integrating Preventive Mental Health
    Care Into Pediatric Practice*
2: *Pediatric Care of Children and
    Adolescents With Mental Health
    Problems*
3: *Office and Network Systems to Support
    Mental Health Care*
4: *Partnering to Improve Community
    Mental Health Systems*
11: *Psychotropic Medications in Primary
    Care*

**Barbara L. Frankowski, MD, MPH,
FAAP**
Professor of Pediatrics
University of Vermont Children's
    Hospital
Burlington, Vermont
21: *Learning Difficulty*

Mary Margaret Gleason, MD, FAAP
Associate Professor, Psychiatry and
    Behavioral Sciences
Clinical Assistant Professor, Pediatrics
Tulane University School of Medicine
New Orleans, Louisiana
17: *Emotional or Behavioral Disturbance
    in Children Younger Than 5 Years*

Laura Hart, MD, MPH, FAAP
Primary Care Research Fellow
The Cecil G. Sheps Center for Health
    Services Research
University of North Carolina at Chapel
    Hill
Chapel Hill, North Carolina
12: *Transitioning Adolescents With
    Mental Health Conditions to
    Adult Care*

Nancy Heath, PhD
James McGill Professor
Department of Educational and
    Counselling Psychology
McGill University
Montreal, Quebec, Canada
27: *Self-injury*

Nicole Heilbron, PhD
Co-Chief, Division of Child and Family
    Mental Health and Developmental
    Neuroscience
Associate Professor, Department of
    Psychiatry and Behavioral Sciences
Duke University School of Medicine
Durham, North Carolina
12: *Transitioning Adolescents With
    Mental Health Conditions to Adult
    Care*

Jane R. Hull, MD, FAAP
Pediatrician, Preferred Pediatrics
Pediatric Hospitalist, Children's National
    Pediatric Hospitalist Program at Mary
    Washington Healthcare
Assistant Professor, Pediatrics, Edward
    Via College of Osteopathic Medicine
Fredericksburg, Virginia
9: *Complementary and Integrative
    Medical Therapies*

Kelly J. Kelleher, MD, MPH, FAAP
ADS/Chlapaty Endowed Chair for Inno-
    vation in Pediatric Practice
Vice President for Community Health
    and Services Research
Director, Center for Innovation in Pedi-
    atric Practice
The Research Institute at Nationwide
    Children's Hospital
Distinguished Professor
Colleges of Medicine and Public Health
The Ohio State University
Columbus, Ohio
3: *Office and Network Systems to Support
    Mental Health Care*

Penelope Knapp, MD, FAAP
Professor Emeritus
Departments of Pediatrics and
    Psychiatry and Behavioral Sciences
University of California, Davis
Davis, California
6: *Iterative Mental Health Assessment*

Danielle Laraque-Arena, MD, FAAP
Professor of Pediatrics, Psychiatry and
 Behavioral Sciences and Public Health
 and Preventive Medicine
President and Health System CEO,
 SUNY Upstate Medical University
Syracuse, New York
3: *Office and Network Systems to Support
 Mental Health Care*
6: *Iterative Mental Health Assessment*

Sharon Levy, MD, MPH, FAAP
Director, Adolescent Substance Abuse
 and Addiction Program
Boston Children's Hospital
Associate Professor of Pediatrics
Harvard Medical School
Boston, Massachusetts
31: *Substance Use 2: Use of Other
 Substances*
32: *Substance Use 3: Specialty Referral
 and Comanagement*

Meghan McAuliffe Lines, PhD
Clinical Director of Integrated Primary
 Care Psychology
Nemours/Alfred I. duPont Hospital for
 Children
Wilmington, Delaware
Assistant Professor of Pediatrics
Sidney Kimmel Medical College of
 Thomas Jefferson University
Philadelphia, Pennsylvania
7: *Psychosocial Therapies*

Ronald V. Marino, DO, MPH, FAAP
Associate Chair, Department of
 Pediatrics
NYU Winthrop University Hospital
Mineola, New York
Professor of Clinical Pediatrics
Stony Brook Medical School
Stony Brook, New York
NYIT College of Osteopathic Medicine
Old Westbury, New York
26: *School Absenteeism and School
 Refusal*

Gary Maslow, MD, MPH, FAAP
Assistant Professor of Pediatrics and
 Psychiatry and Behavioral Sciences
Duke University School of Medicine
Durham, North Carolina
12: *Transitioning Adolescents With
 Mental Health Conditions to
 Adult Care*

Anne May, MD, FAAP
Assistant Professor of Clinical Pediatrics
The Ohio State University School of
 Medicine
Columbus, Ohio
28: *Sleep Disturbances*

Timothy R. Moore, PhD, LP, BCBA-D
Director of Positive Behavior Support
Minnesota Department of Human
 Services
St Paul, Minnesota
27: *Self-injury*

Karen N. Olness, MD, FAAP
Professor Emerita of Pediatrics, Global
 Health and Diseases
Case Western Reserve University
Cleveland, Ohio
8: *Self-regulation Therapies and
 Biofeedback*

James M. Perrin, MD, FAAP
Professor of Pediatrics, Harvard Medical
 School
John C. Robinson Chair in Pediatrics
Associate Chair, MassGeneral Hospital
 for Children
Boston, Massachusetts
4: *Partnering to Improve Community
 Mental Health Systems*

David Pruitt, MD
Professor of Psychiatry and Pediatrics
Director, Division of Child and
 Adolescent Psychiatry
University of Maryland School of
 Medicine
Baltimore, Maryland
11: *Psychotropic Medications in Primary
 Care*

Gloria Reeves, MD
Associate Professor
Division of Child and Adolescent
 Psychiatry
University of Maryland School of
 Medicine
Baltimore, Maryland
11: *Psychotropic Medications in Primary
 Care*

Mark A. Riddle, MD
Professor of Psychiatry and Pediatrics
Johns Hopkins University School of
 Medicine

Baltimore, Maryland
11: *Psychotropic Medications in Primary Care*

Maris Rosenberg, MD
Children's Evaluation and Rehabilitation Center
Department of Pediatrics
Albert Einstein College of Medicine
The Children's Hospital at Montefiore
Bronx, New York
29: *Speech and Language Concerns*

Marcie Schneider, MD, FAAP
Greenwich Adolescent Medicine
Greenwich, Connecticut
16: *Eating Abnormalities*

Mark L. Splaingard, MD
Director of Pediatric Sleep Medicine
Nationwide Children's Hospital
Professor of Pediatrics
The Ohio State University School of Medicine
Columbus, Ohio
28: *Sleep Disturbances*

Jack T. Swanson, MD, FAAP
Pediatrician
Ames, Iowa
1: *Integrating Preventive Mental Health Care Into Pediatric Practice*

Frank Symons, PhD
Department of Educational Psychology
College of Education and Human Development
University of Minnesota
Minneapolis, Minnesota
27: *Self-injury*

Susanne E. Tanski, MD, MPH, FAAP
Associate Professor of Pediatrics
Section Chief, General Academic Pediatrics
Geisel School of Medicine at Dartmouth College
Lebanon, New Hampshire
30: *Substance Use 1: Use of Tobacco and Nicotine*

Nancy Tarshis, MA, MS, CCC-SLP
Supervisor of Speech and Language Services
Children's Evaluation and Rehabilitation

Center
Montefiore Medical Center
Bronx, New York
29: *Speech and Language Concerns*

Jessica R. Toste, PhD
Assistant Professor
Department of Special Education
The University of Texas at Austin
Austin, Texas
27: *Self-injury*

W. Douglas Tynan, PhD
Professor of Pediatrics
Sidney Kimmel Medical College of Thomas Jefferson University
Philadelphia, Pennsylvania
7: *Psychosocial Therapies*
10: *Adapting Psychosocial Interventions to Primary Care*

Sandra Vicari, PhD, LCPC
Associate Professor, Department of Psychiatry
Southern Illinois University School of Medicine
Springfield, Illinois
18: *Family Dysfunction*

Heather J. Walter, MD, MPH
Professor, Psychiatry and Pediatrics
Boston University School of Medicine
Senior Lecturer on Psychiatry
Harvard Medical School
Boston, Massachusetts
13: *Agitation, Suicidality, and Other Psychiatric Emergencies*

Lawrence S. Wissow, MD, MPH, FAAP
James P. Connaughton Professor of Community Psychiatry
Division of Child and Adolescent Psychiatry
Johns Hopkins School of Medicine
Baltimore, Maryland
5: *Effective Communication Methods: Common Factors Skills*
6: *Iterative Mental Health Assessment*
11: *Psychotropic Medications in Primary Care*
14: *Anxiety and Trauma-Related Distress*
15: *Disruptive Behavior and Aggression*
20: *Inattention and Impulsivity*
22: *Low Mood*

American Academy of Pediatrics Reviewers

Committee on Communications and Media

Committee on Nutrition

Committee on Psychosocial Aspects of Child and Family Health

Committee on School Health

Medical Home Implementation Project Advisory Committee

Mental Health Leadership Workgroup

Poverty and Child Health Leadership Workgroup

Provisional Section on Minority Health, Equity, and Inclusion

Section on Pediatric Pulmonology and Sleep Medicine

Task Force on Diversity and Inclusion

Acknowledgments

I am grateful to the many authors and mentors who have contributed to this work, to the colleagues who served with me on the American Academy of Pediatrics (AAP) Task Force on Mental Health and the AAP Mental Health Leadership Work Group, to the AAP staff who supported and inspired the work of those 2 groups, and to the staff and my fellow coeditors of the *American Academy of Pediatrics Textbook of Pediatric Care,* 2nd Edition, who recognized the need for *Mental Health Care of Children and Adolescents: A Guide for Primary Care Clinicians.* I am indebted to Carrie Peters for her patient and diligent collaboration in bringing the book to publication.

In the spirit of this book, I also want to acknowledge the contributions of my family: Isadore and Rachel Farrer Meschan, who were physician-educators as well as loving parents; my husband, Miles Foy, whose support and encouragement made this book and all my life's work possible; and my children and grandchildren, who have been my inspiration to make the world a kinder, better place for children.

Jane Meschan Foy, MD, FAAP

Contents

Introduction

Jane Meschan Foy, MD

> "The book aims to boost reader confidence and capacity
> through reinforcement of sound, intuitive pediatric
> approaches and full realization of the prime pediatric
> advantage: a trusting therapeutic relationship
> with patients and their families."

During the past 2 decades, the mental health specialty system has focused its efforts and resources on children and adolescents with severely impairing mental disorders. Pediatric clinicians often comanage or complement the mental health specialty care of these patients while independently managing the care of others with common less impairing mental disorders. Many excellent psychiatry textbooks provide guidance to clinicians on the assessment and treatment of children and adolescents with diagnosable mental disorders.

This book, by contrast, aims to help pediatric clinicians provide mental health care, not just for the 13% to 20% of children and adolescents with diagnosable disorders[1] but also for those who may not, and hopefully will not, cross any diagnostic threshold for a mental disorder. They include the estimated 19% of children who have impairment caused by mental health symptoms in the absence of a diagnosable condition.[2] Some of these children and adolescents may become adults before their symptoms reach the threshold for a diagnosis; in fact, of people diagnosed as having a mental disorder as adults, approximately half began experiencing symptoms by the age of 14 years.[3] A longitudinal study has shown that adults who, as children, had a subthreshold mental health condition (ie, impairment without a diagnosable disorder) have 3 times the odds of 1 adverse outcome in health, legal, financial, or social functioning, compared with peers without any mental health condition during childhood, and 5 times higher odds of 2 or more adverse outcomes, even after controlling for childhood psychosocial hardships and adult-onset psychiatric conditions.[4] Clearly, children and adolescents with subthreshold symptoms deserve attention and care.

Children and adolescents without symptoms or functional impairment may also benefit from mental health care. Parents or teachers (or both) may believe a child has a behavioral disturbance, even when the child exhibits behavior that is typical for his or her developmental stage, a situation likely to produce conflict and distress. In addition, many children and adolescents without perceived or actual current problems are at increased risk for mental health problems by virtue of their social circumstances or their exposure to trauma and adversity. They and, in fact, all other children and adolescents can potentially benefit from efforts to enhance their emotional resilience: any of them may encounter toxic stress, trauma, or loss, with the risk of untoward mental health effects.

The term *mental health care* in this book encompasses care of children and adolescents who are experiencing the full range of social-emotional and behavioral health challenges, including substance use. This broad definition is not to suggest that pediatric clinicians are themselves responsible for the full range of mental health care but rather that pediatric clinicians provide a medical home and, often, medical subspecialty care to children and adolescents who may experience the full range of mental health challenges. Authors use the term *primary care clinicians* (PCCs) in the book to encompass pediatricians, family physicians, internists, nurse practitioners, and physician assistants who provide a medical home to children and adolescents. Authors use the term *pediatric clinicians* in the book to encompass not just PCCs but also pediatric subspecialists, who may have a consultative role in mental health care (eg, developmental-behavioral pediatricians, adolescent specialists), and subspecialists who have a primary care role in circumstances that require frequent, close supervision (eg, pediatric hematologists/oncologists who care for children with cancer, pulmonologists who care for children with cystic fibrosis, endocrinologists who care for children with type 1 diabetes mellitus).

Pediatric PCCs have frequent contact with patients and their families, often beginning prenatally or early in the child's life. This longitudinal relationship is at the heart of "the pediatric advantage," outlined in Box 1. Pediatric subspecialists also enjoy this advantage through long-term relationships with patients and families in the care of their patients' chronic medical conditions or developmental disabilities. The book informs pediatric clinicians about the opportunities for mental health care that are inherent in this advantage.

Box 1. The Pediatric Advantage

- Longitudinal, trusting, and empowering therapeutic relationships with children and family members
- Patient and family centeredness of pediatric practice
- Unique opportunities to prevent future mental health problems through promoting healthy lifestyles, "purposeful" and positive parenting, and play; identifying and addressing toxic stress and social adversities; anticipatory guidance; and timely intervention for common behavioral, emotional, educational, and social problems encountered in pediatric practice
- Understanding of common social, emotional, and educational problems in the context of a child's or an adolescent's development and environment
- Comfort and capacity to care for children and adolescents with uncertain diagnoses
- Experience coordinating general care and specialty care
- Familiarity with chronic care principles and practice-improvement methods
- Greater accessibility to children, adolescents, and families than that of mental health specialty care
- Potential effectiveness in countering stigma and mental health racial and ethnic disparities

Adapted from Foy JM; for the American Academy of Pediatrics Task Force on Mental Health. Enhancing pediatric mental health care: report from the American Academy of Pediatrics Task Force on Mental Health. Introduction. *Pediatrics.* 2010;125(suppl 3):S71. http://pediatrics. aappublications.org/content/125/Supplement_3/S69. Accessed March 8, 2018.

In a policy statement published in 2009, the American Academy of Pediatrics (AAP) articulated the knowledge and skills that PCCs need to provide children and adolescents with mental health care: "The Future of Pediatrics: Mental Health Competencies for Pediatric Primary Care."[5] These competencies include, for example, the capacity to develop office routines for identifying occult mental health problems; to apply evidence-based communication methods and therapies to the care of children, adolescents, and their families; and to access current data about the safety and efficacy of common pharmacological and psychosocial interventions in children and adolescents. This book includes information, tools, and resources that will contribute to achievement of these and other pediatric mental health competencies.

The book has 4 parts.

Part 1, The Pediatric Advantage, algorithmically describes a process for integrating mental health care into the flow of pediatric practice. Chapters in Part 2, Enhancing Pediatric Mental Health Care, offer guidance for implementing practice- and network-level enhancements to mental health care, strategies for improving community mental health systems to complement those in the practice and network, and a description of "common factors" communication skills, which are foundational competencies for effective mental health practice. Chapters in Part 3, Elements of Care, begin with a description of the iterative mental health assessment characteristic of primary care, followed by an overview of available nonpharmacological interventions: psychosocial therapies, self-regulation therapies and biofeedback, and complementary and integrative medical therapies. Other chapters in Part 3 provide guidance for adapting selected evidence-based nonpharmacological interventions to primary care, offer a framework for using psychotropic medications in primary care, and describe methods for transitioning adolescents with mental health conditions to adult care.

Chapter topics in Part 4, Pediatric Care of Children With Common Mental Health Concerns, Signs, and Symptoms, include, for example, psychiatric emergencies, family dysfunction, symptoms of emotional disturbance in young children, nonadherence to medical treatment, medically unexplained symptoms, sleep disturbances, gender expression and identity issues, trauma-related distress, disruptive behavior, eating abnormalities, inattention, and substance use. In each case, the authors describe findings that suggest the need for intervention, initial interventions appropriate to pediatric practice (and not dependent on a diagnosis), and indications for further diagnostic assessment and mental health specialty involvement. A robust index includes additional signs and symptoms and guides the reader to the relevant chapters.

The book contains additional resources: Within chapter narratives are URLs of Web resources. A section following each chapter lists any AAP policies relevant to the topic. The book's appendixes contain selected tables and figures that are helpful across multiple chapters.

This book complements 2 other AAP publications developed to assist pediatric clinicians in achieving the AAP-recommended mental health competencies: *Promoting Mental Health in Children and Adolescents: Primary Care Practice and Advocacy* (in press)[6] and *Pediatric Psychopharmacology for Primary Care* by Mark A. Riddle, MD,[7] a guide to prescribing medications for children and adolescents in the primary care setting.

People whose lifework involves caring for children and families are typically compassionate people who know more than they think they know about mental health care. For this reason, readers of this book will undoubtedly recognize their own thought processes, instincts, and practices in the book's clinical guidance. This sense of familiarity is as it should be. The book aims to boost reader confidence and capacity through reinforcement of sound, intuitive pediatric approaches and full realization of the prime pediatric advantage: a trusting therapeutic relationship with patients and their families—the most effective of all mental health interventions.

References

1. Perou R, Bitsko RH, Blumberg SJ, et al; Centers for Disease Control and Prevention. Mental health surveillance among children—United States, 2005-2011. *MMWR Suppl.* 2013;62(2):1–35
2. Burns BJ, Costello EJ, Angold A, et al. Children's mental health service use across service sectors. *Health Aff (Millwood).* 1995;14(3):147–159
3. Kessler RC, Berglund P, Demler O, Jin R, Merikangas KR, Walters EE. Lifetime prevalence and age-of-onset distributions of *DSM-IV* disorders in the National Comorbidity Survey Replication. *Arch Gen Psychiatry.* 2005;62(6):593–602
4. Copeland WE, Wolke D, Shanahan L, Costello EJ. Adult functional outcomes of common childhood psychiatric problems: a prospective, longitudinal study. *JAMA Psychiatry.* 2015;72(9):892–899
5. American Academy of Pediatrics Committee on Psychosocial Aspects of Child and Family Health and Task Force on Mental Health. The future of pediatrics: mental health competencies for pediatric primary care. *Pediatrics.* 2009;124(1):410–421
6. Foy JM, ed. *Promoting Mental Health in Children and Adolescents: Primary Care Practice and Advocacy.* Itasca, IL: American Academy of Pediatrics. In press
7. Riddle MA, ed. *Pediatric Psychopharmacology for Primary Care.* Elk Grove Village, IL: American Academy of Pediatrics; 2016

Integrating Preventive Mental Health Care Into Pediatric Practice

Jack T. Swanson, MD, and Jane Meschan Foy, MD

"Pediatric primary care clinicians...have an important role to play in influencing the intentional pursuit of optimal mental health as part of each child's or adolescent's development."

Introduction

Mental health (MH), including all its psychosocial and emotional aspects, is an intrinsic part of overall health and well-being. Pediatric primary care clinicians (PCCs) (pediatricians, family physicians, internists, nurse practitioners, and physician assistants who provide frontline, longitudinal health care to children and adolescents) have an important role to play in influencing the intentional pursuit of optimal MH as part of each child's or adolescent's development. Good MH has been described as "the reasonable, regular experience and effective practice of

- ► Confidence and courage
- ► Adaptability
- ► Cheerfulness
- ► Attention/concentration
- ► Harmony
- ► Hardiness
- ► Social connectedness"[1]

The foundation of MH begins before birth, with the parents' and caregivers' own well-being and with preparations they make for the physical and emotional care of the child. Caregivers continue to build on this foundation after the child's birth by providing their attention and love in a safe and nurturing environment. Interaction between the child's biological makeup and his or her environment—particularly the relational experiences—affect the architecture of the child's brain. The environment expands from the child's home to include the child care setting, school, and community, ultimately affecting his or her biological reactivity to stress, psychological resilience, and immunologic resistance throughout life. Box 1-1 provides examples of the skills needed by caregivers in all settings to nurture social-emotional competence in a young child.

Each stage of childhood provides PCCs and other members of the medical home team with unique opportunities to promote MH during regular contacts with the child or adolescent and his or her caregivers. These

---

Box 1-1. Examples of Caregiver Skills to Promote Social-Emotional Competence

- Engage infants in frequent face-to-face social interactions each day (verbal and nonverbal behaviors).

- Quickly respond to infants' and toddlers' cries or other signs of distress by providing physical comfort and needed care.

- Support children's development of friendships and provide opportunities for children to play with and learn from each other.

- Help children practice social skills and build friendships by helping them enter into, sustain, and enhance play.

- Help children resolve conflicts by helping them identify feelings, describe problems, and try alternative solutions.

- Help children talk about their own and others' emotions; provide opportunities for them to explore a wide range of feelings and the different ways to express them.

- Actively teach children social communication and emotional regulation.

- Help children manage their behavior by guiding and supporting them to (1) persist when frustrated; (2) play cooperatively with other children; (3) use language to communicate needs; (4) learn turn-taking; (5) gain control of physical impulses; (6) express negative emotions in ways that do not harm others or themselves; (7) use problem-solving techniques; and (8) learn about themselves and others.

From National Association for the Education of Young Children (NAEYC). NAEYC Early Childhood Program Standards and Accreditation Criteria & Guidance for Assessment. NAEYC Web site. https://www.naeyc.org/sites/default/files/globally-shared/downloads/PDFs/accreditation/early-learning/Standards%20and%20Accreditation%20Criteria%20%26%20Guidance%20for%20Assessment_April%202017_3.pdf. Updated November 8, 2017. Accessed November 8, 2017. Copyright © 2017 National Association for the Education of Young Children.

unique opportunities, described by the American Academy of Pediatrics (AAP) Task Force on Mental Health (TFMH) as "the primary care advantage," have been adapted by the AAP Mental Health Leadership Work Group (MHLWG) to describe more broadly "the pediatric advantage." (See Introduction, Box 1.) This concept applies also to pediatric subspecialists, who often have longitudinal relationships with children, adolescents, and their families and many opportunities to promote MH and to offer primary and secondary preventive services.

Mental health problems occur often during childhood and adolescence. In the United States, between 9.5% and 14.2% of children from birth to 5 years of age experience social-emotional problems that cause harm to the child and family and interfere with functioning.[2,3] Among children and adolescents aged 8 to 15, approximately 13% have had a diagnosable mental disorder during the previous year,[4] and more than 20% of adolescents aged 13 to 18 years either have a seriously debilitating mental disorder currently or had one at some point in their lives.[5] Furthermore, as many as 19% or more of children and adolescents have impaired MH functioning without a diagnosable mental disorder,[6] and half of adults with mental disorders experienced the onset of symptoms by age 14 years.[7] Mental health problems are more common among children and adolescents with chronic medical or developmental conditions and among those who have experienced abuse or neglect, foster care, poverty, racism, homophobia, separation or divorce of parents, domestic violence, school failure, parental or family mental illness or substance use, natural disasters, military deployment of a family member, and grief accompanying the illness or death of a family member.

Unfortunately, children, adolescents, and their parents may be reluctant to discuss their MH or substance use concerns with their PCC because of embarrassment, because they do not understand that their concerns may be MH issues, because they do not see the PCC as an MH resource, or because past experiences with trauma make them guarded and defensive. Primary care clinicians can address these barriers by preparing their practices in the ways described in Chapter 3 of this book, Office and Network Systems to Support Mental Health Care—for example, by posting information about MH-related topics and events and offering MH brochures and handouts in the physical practice, by including MH content on the practice Web site and in newsletters. They can ensure that all members of the practice respect the privacy of children, adolescents, and families and that their language and attitudes reflect that mental illnesses are treatable, that they are no one's fault, and that they do not define the person (eg, a person has schizophrenia; he or she is not a schizophrenic). Primary care clinicians can also promote MH through the practice of family-centered, culturally effective communication and through the choice of topics discussed at each visit, whether providing routine health supervision (RHS), acute care, or management of a chronic illness. By integrating MH care into all contacts with the patient and family, the PCC and office staff demonstrate the importance of MH, normalize the process of providing MH care in the medical home, and help reduce the stigma of mental illness.[8]

Primary care clinicians can also prepare for their role as MH providers by working at the community level to effect system changes supportive of MH services in primary care. Chapter 4 of this book, Partnering to Improve Community Mental Health Systems, highlights opportunities to collaborate with other MH advocates and specialists in these efforts.

Identifying Psychosocial Strengths and Problems at Routine Health Supervision Visits and Visits for Mental Health Concerns

The TFMH developed 2 algorithms to describe a process for incorporating MH services into primary care visits.[9] In 2017 the MHLWG revised them to a single algorithm, A Process for Integrating Mental Health Care Into Pediatric Practice (Appendix 1). The discussion that follows describes steps 1 through 10 and introduces step 11 of this algorithm; see Figure 1-1, subtitled "Health Promotion, Identification of Strengths and Concerns, Initial Intervention." Chapter 2, Pediatric Care of Children and Adolescents With Mental Health Problems, describes the remainder of the algorithm, subtitled "Addressing Identified Concerns."

In the discussion that follows, numbers in brackets beside each subheading refer to the algorithm steps. Chapters cited within the text offer readers opportunities to gain more in-depth knowledge of a particular topic.

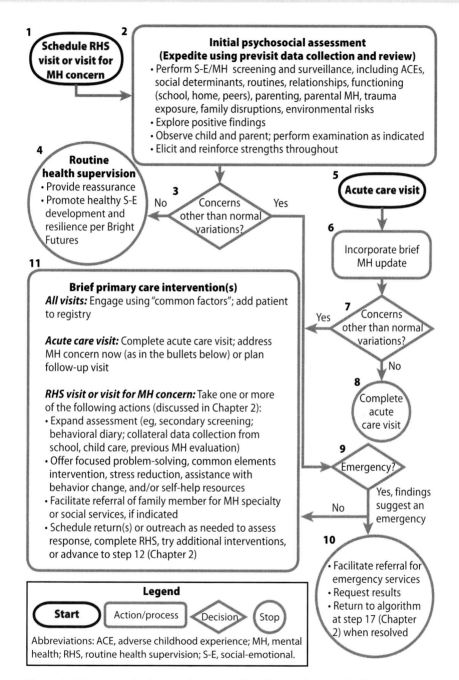

Figure 1-1. A process for integrating mental health care into pediatric practice: health promotion, identification of strengths and concerns, initial intervention.

Adapted with permission from Foy JM; American Academy of Pediatrics Task Force on Mental Health. Enhancing pediatric mental health care: algorithms for primary care. *Pediatrics.* 2010;125(suppl 3):S109–S125.

Initial psychosocial assessment [2]

Perform S-E/MH screening and surveillance, including ACEs, social determinants, routines, relationships, functioning (school, home, peers), parenting, parental MH, trauma exposure, family disruptions, environmental risks

Whether scheduled for an RHS visit or an MH concern, the process of MH care begins by systematically gathering psychosocial information about the patient and family. Use of a previsit questionnaire, either paper or electronic, filled out at home or in the waiting area and reviewed by the clinician in advance of the visit, enables the clinician to focus on building rapport and on exploring findings, rather than on rote data gathering, while still being systematic in obtaining information.

When an MH concern has prompted the visit, it is helpful to collect additional information in advance, such as

▶ Questionnaires or behavior checklists completed by other key adults, such as teachers, child care providers, or a noncustodial parent

▶ Transfer of records of prior psychological assessment or previous MH care

▶ Acquisition of report cards or other school records

Studies demonstrate the feasibility of using brief, psychometrically sound MH screening tools in the primary care setting.[10,11] Validated screening tools may be incorporated into previsit data collection or into the visit itself. In the Tools for Practice section in this chapter, Boxes 1-8 and 1-9 summarize psychosocial surveillance and screening guidance compatible with *Bright Futures: Guidelines for Health Supervision of Infants, Children, and Adolescents,* 4th Edition.[12]

Appendix 2, Mental Health Tools for Pediatrics, is a compendium of psychosocial tools appropriate for use in primary care, organized according to the algorithm steps. A number of these instruments include parent, teacher, and youth reporting formats. Electronic tools have the advantage of greater acceptability to adolescents.[13,14] Furthermore, electronic questionnaires provide an opportunity for the use of "item responses." For example, the computer asks the respondent 2 or 3 basic questions. If the answer is no to those, the respondent moves on; if the answer is yes, the computer asks more questions.

Clinicians may encounter some limitations to the use of screening tools, including their use with populations that have low literacy levels, those for whom English is a second language, and those for whom the cultural context of a patient's behavior or family's parenting may vary from that of the population with which the screening tool was validated. It is important to remember that screening is not an end in itself: the screening leads to further exploration of any findings and becomes "a discussion template for anticipatory guidance and asset building."

If previsit data collection is not feasible, the PCC will need to incorporate data collection into the clinical encounter. Table 1-1 lists common MH problems of childhood and adolescence and the questions a clinician can use to elicit these concerns as part of an interview.

Whatever questionnaires, screening instruments, or interview questions are used, a structured process, developed by the practice in advance, should ensure that the following content is covered:

▶ Family's priorities for the visit

▶ Family and social history, including adverse childhood experiences (ACEs); social stressors such as poverty, food insecurity, racism, and homophobia; support system; and environmental risk assessment, including MH of family members, trauma, separation, and loss

▶ Identification of the patient's and family's strengths

▶ Functional assessment of the patient

▶ Temperament and risk behaviors

▶ Bedtime routines, family meals, physical activity, and media use patterns

▶ Sleep

▶ Concerns of school or child care providers

▶ Symptoms of psychosocial problems

Table 1-1. Eliciting Common Mental Health Concerns

Mental Health Concern	Possible Prompts
Newborn Period and Infancy (Birth–11 Months)	
Poor attachment	(Observe parent-child interactions.) Since the baby was born, have you been feeling down, depressed, irritable, or hopeless? Who is helping/supporting you?
Difficult temperament (eg, irritable, hard to console, unpredictable needs, difficulty feeding)	Are you able to comfort and care for your baby? Do you have people to call if you feel frustrated?
Child abuse/domestic violence or substance use	Do you feel safe in your home? Has your partner ever hurt you or your baby? Have you ever experienced abuse? Have you ever been afraid you might hurt your baby?
Delayed development	Do you have any concerns about your child's development, learning, or behavior?
Poor attachment	Do you have any difficulty understanding or responding to your child's needs? What kinds of activities do you do with your child and as a family?
Difficulty forming relationships	How comfortable is your child around other people?
Behavioral problem (impulsivity/tantrums/aggression)	Do you reward your child for good behavior? What circumstances tend to lead to your child's misbehavior? How do you correct your child for misbehavior? Has your child ever had a very frightening or painful experience or an extended separation from you or another loved one?
Middle Childhood (5–10 Years)	
Poor success at school, learning difficulties, inattention	How is your child learning and doing in school?
Bullying/violence at school	Does your child feel safe and happy at school?
Anxiety, worries	How does your child sleep? Does your child have more fears or worries than most children his or her age? Has your child ever had a very frightening or painful experience or an extended separation from you or another loved one?

Table 1-1. Eliciting Common Mental Health Concerns (*continued*)	
Mental Health Concern	**Possible Prompts**
Middle Childhood (5–10 Years)	
Behavioral problems (impulsivity/tantrums/aggression/oppositional behavior)	Do you reward your child for good behavior? What circumstances tend to lead to your child's misbehavior? How do you correct your child for misbehavior? Has your child ever had a very frightening or painful experience or an extended separation from you or another loved one?
Depression	Does your child often seem irritable, sad, or depressed?
Late Childhood and Adolescence (11–18 Years)	
School problems	How are you doing in school? What do you plan to do after high school?
Depression/suicide	During the past 2 wk, how often have you felt down, depressed, irritable, or hopeless? How often have you felt little interest or pleasure in doing things? Have you had trouble falling asleep, staying asleep, or sleeping too much? Have you ever tried to kill yourself or thought about trying to kill yourself?
Anxiety	Do you worry a lot or feel overly stressed? How do you sleep?
Substance use or substance use disorder	During the past 12 mo, have you drunk any alcohol (more than a few sips), smoked any marijuana or hashish, or used anything else to get high? Have you ever ridden in a car driven by someone (including yourself) who was high or had been using alcohol or drugs? Have you talked with your adolescent about alcohol, drugs, and misuse of medications?
Sexual abuse/dating violence	Have you ever felt forced to touch someone or be touched by someone in ways that made you uncomfortable?

Two topics deserve emphasis in the context of the psychosocial assessment.

Adolescents

The increasing independence of adolescents and the likelihood that parents and guardians may not be fully aware of their adolescents' activities or feelings reinforce the need for private, confidential discussions between clinicians and their adolescent patients. These discussions should augment, not replace, discussions with parents. Adolescents and parents differ in their abilities to report on various MH conditions: for example, a parent may have a more accurate picture of the effect of externalizing symptoms (eg, hyperactivity, inattention, oppositional behavior), while an adolescent may be better able to articulate the toll of internalizing symptoms or conditions (eg, anxiety, depression). Or the adolescent and parents may disagree about the nature or importance of symptoms. As part of these discussions, clinicians are obliged to address confidentiality and its limits with both adolescents and their parents.

Adolescents caution that questions on substance use and other sensitive topics may seem intrusive and unlikely to yield a candid response. A framing statement, such as "Many young people I'm seeing feel lots of stress this time of year" or "…lots of pressure to use drugs," or a circular question, such as "Do any of your friends smoke, drink, or use other drugs?" may be better received than direct questions about the adolescent's behaviors. Assurance that the clinician asks all adolescents these questions may be helpful to rapport.

Sleep

Because of the association between sleep difficulties and MH conditions, questions regarding sleep are helpful throughout childhood and adolescence (and fit well with other RHS activities). The wording of such questions is important to adolescents, who may have conflict with their parents around sleep issues. Clinicians may find that questions requiring only yes or no answers are less useful than open-ended questions such as "How hard is it for you to fall asleep when you want to?" (See Chapter 28, Sleep Disturbances.)

Explore positive findings

During the face-to-face encounter, the clinician can complete the following steps (expanded in Chapter 6, Iterative Mental Health Assessment):

▶ Review previsit questionnaire, screening tools, and other data collected (or complete data collection) and update information about adjustment and progress in child care, preschool, or school.

▶ Identify, elicit, or review the patient's and family's priorities for the visit.

▶ Broaden the agenda by indicating openness to MH issues. For example, elicit further information about any current concerns, the patient's or family's past or current sources of care for the concerns, and progress on previous concerns. If screening tools have been completed, use any positive responses as a springboard to further discussion and clarification. Ask broad, open-ended questions such as "What has been the hardest part about taking care of Jonah?" followed by "What has been the best part?" Such questions convey the clinician's interest in family functioning and invite vexing questions that may have been posed to relatives and friends but may have not been felt appropriate for this medical setting. Whatever methods are used to gather information, include inquiry about parental well-being (looking particularly for problems with parental mood, affect, or attachment to the child) and any developmentally specific symptoms of emotional disturbance in the patient. Also, consider the family's cultural context.

When findings from a questionnaire, a screening, or the interview point to traumatic events or losses in the life of the patient and family, it is important to explore their impact. Examples of such events or losses include the death of a loved one or pet; a move; homelessness; conflict, separation, or divorce of parents; military deployment of a parent or other loved ones; incarceration of the child or a loved one; breakup of a relationship; abuse or bullying by the child or targeting the child; racism; homophobia; exposure to violence (either directly or emotionally, through death or injury of a loved one); or a natural disaster. It is necessary to inquire separately of patients and their parents, because some events that affect children and adolescents may go unrecognized by the parent or be confidential from the parent, and some parents may be reluctant to discuss some events or losses in front of their children and adolescents. When interviewing children or adolescents about trauma exposure, the clinician should allow them to share their own narrative of the experience but not lead them into reliving the incident, which may result in further trauma.

Observe child and parent; perform examination as indicated

This step includes several components.

▶ Observe parent-child interaction and assess attachment between parent and child or adolescent, a critical component of healthy development at every stage of childhood. See Box 1-2.

Box 1-2. Attachment Patterns

Secure Attachment

- Parent: Is sensitive, responsive, and available.

- Child: Feels valued and worthwhile; has a secure base; feels effective; feels able to explore and master, knowing that parent is available; and becomes autonomous. During visit, engages with health care professional and seeks and receives reassurance and comfort from parent.

Insecure and Avoidant Attachment

- Parent: Is insensitive to child's cues, avoids contact, and rejects.

- Child: Feels no one is there for him, cannot rely on adults to get needs met, feels he will be rejected if needs for attachment and closeness are shown and therefore asks for little to maintain some connection, and learns not to recognize his own need for closeness and connectedness. During visit, may act fearful but also angry with the parent, may seek contact but then arch away and struggle, and also may act extremely helpful or sad but not seek comfort and protection.

Insecure Attachment Characterized by Ambivalence and Resistance

- Parent: Shows inconsistent patterns or care, is unpredictable, maybe excessively close or intrusive but then push away. This pattern is seen frequently with depressed caregiver.

- Child: Feels he should keep adult engaged because he never knows when he will get attention back and is anxious, dependent, and clingy.

Reprinted with permission from Hagan JF, Shaw JS, Duncan PM, eds. *Bright Futures.* 3rd ed. Elk Grove Village, IL: American Academy of Pediatrics; 2007.

▶ Interact with the patient.

▶ Examine your own reactions to the parent and patient.

▶ Perform a physical examination (including vision and hearing screening, because a sensory deficit may cause academic or behavioral difficulties), with particular emphasis on areas of the body associated with any physical symptoms and signs (Box 1-3).

Elicit and reinforce strengths throughout

Effective MH care requires that clinicians move from a medical model focused on problems to a more comprehensive view of the patient's and family's capacities. There are 8 empirically determined independent "intelligences": linguistic, logical-mathematical, spatial, bodily kinesthetic, musical, interpersonal, intrapersonal, and naturalistic.[15] Acknowledging strengths—one or more of these intelligences; talents; qualities such as resilience, generosity, courage, tenacity, goal orientation, and focus; social supports such as strong family bonds, extended family support, and good peer relations; healthy behaviors such as regular exercise/sleep routines and participation in extracurricular or spiritual/ religious activities; or attitudes such as hope, optimism, and motivation

---

Box 1-3. Physical Symptoms and Signs Suggestive of Mental Health and Substance Abuse Concerns

Sleep Problems
- Excessive sleep
- Significant change in sleep pattern
- Difficulty falling or staying asleep
- Nightmares

Somatic Concerns
- Chronic, recurrent, or unexplained physical symptoms
- Abdominal pain
- Joint pain
- Headache
- Fatigue or low energy
- Loss of appetite
- Epigastric pain or gastritis (suggesting alcohol use)
- Chest pain or difficulty breathing (panic/anxiety attacks)
- Menstrual irregularities, especially in girls of low or high weight (anorexia, bulimia, teen pregnancy)

Neurological Symptoms
- Leg weakness
- Limb paralysis (conversion reaction)
- Pseudoseizures
- Non-physiologic neurological symptoms
- Difficulty concentrating, inattention in school
- Irritability, restlessness

> **Box 1-3. Physical Symptoms and Signs Suggestive of Mental Health and Substance Abuse Concerns (*continued*)**
>
> Physical Findings
>
> - Excess weight gain or loss
>
> - Parotid gland enlargement, dental enamel erosion, calluses or erosions on knuckles (purging)
>
> - Cigarette burns, multiple linear cuts or patterns (self-harm, maltreatment)
>
> - Metabolic abnormalities such as hypochloremic metabolic alkalosis, low potassium, or elevated amylase (purging)
>
> - Recurrent injuries (maltreatment, self-harm)
>
> - Isolated systolic hypertension (alcohol use)
>
> - Chronic nasal congestion (cocaine use)
>
> - Chronic red eyes (marijuana use)
>
> Other
>
> - Worsening symptoms of previously well-managed chronic illness
>
> - School absences
>
> Adapted with permission from Foy JM; American Academy of Pediatrics Task Force on Mental Health. Appendix S13: symptoms and signs suggestive of mental health and substance abuse concerns. *Pediatrics*. 2010;125(suppl 3):S193–S194.

to seek help—can build rapport, provide groundwork for an intervention plan, and facilitate accomplishment of subsequent steps. Diagnosing strengths may also stimulate the family to provide further opportunities for the child's or adolescent's development of competence, serving as a buffer for the challenges and peer pressures of adolescence and offering alternatives to risky activities.[16]

Concerns other than normal variations? [3]

At this point, the PCC need not feel pressed to make a diagnosis, but simply to determine whether there may be threats to the patient's healthy development or an MH concern about the patient (eg, symptoms, weak attachment to parent, functional impairment, ACEs, risk behavior) or family (eg, social-economic stressors, parental MH problems, ineffective parenting, negative perception of the child). Box 1-4 outlines common symptoms of emotional and behavioral disturbance by age, and Box 1-3 lists examples of physical symptoms and signs that may, in some instances, point to MH or substance use problems. If the family has concerns about behaviors that are in fact developmentally appropriate for the child or adolescent, it is important to differentiate the patient's behaviors from behaviors that may suggest an emotional or behavioral disturbance.

Box 1-4. Behavioral or Emotional Symptoms of Mental Health Concerns by Age-group

Infants and Young Children
- Excessive crying
- Feeding problems or poor weight gain
- Dysregulation (difficulty organizing feelings and emotions, difficulty being soothed or comforted, difficulty falling or staying asleep)
- Irritability, lacking in joy
- Extreme aggression, severe tantrums, difficulty adjusting to child care or preschool
- Excessive clinginess or fearfulness for developmental stage
- Excessive activity level or impulsivity for developmental age
- Absence of age-appropriate stranger anxiety
- Rigid behavioral patterns or habits interfering with functioning
- Poor eye contact or engagement with caregiver, lack of social reciprocity
- Concerning caregiver behaviors: very negative about child, does not soothe or comfort child, excessively protective or controlling of child, does not allow normal exploration

School-aged Children
- Anger
- Bullying
- Fighting
- Irritability
- Fear of separation
- Fluctuating moods
- Sleep disturbance
- Academic decline
- Sadness
- Isolation

Box 1-4. Behavioral or Emotional Symptoms of Mental Health Concerns by Age-group (*continued*)

Adolescents

- Numbness or avoidance of feelings

- Anger

- Fearfulness

- Aggression, fighting, rule- or lawbreaking

- Self-injury

- Poor school attendance; disciplinary problems; suspension or expulsion

- Appetite change, weight loss or gain

- Difficulty sleeping or excessive sleeping

- Exaggerated mood swings

- Academic decline

- Isolation, withdrawal from friends, loss of interest in usual activities

- Substance use, sexual promiscuity, or other risky behaviors

All Age-groups

- Chronic, recurrent, or unexplained physical symptoms

- Very disruptive or persistent nightmares

- Regression to earlier behavior

- Change in sleep pattern

- Exacerbation of chronic mental condition

Adapted with permission from Foy JM; American Academy of Pediatrics Task Force on Mental Health. Appendix S13: symptoms and signs suggestive of mental health and substance abuse concerns. *Pediatrics*. 2010;125(suppl 3):S193–S194.

Routine health supervision [4]

When there are no concerns other than normal developmental variations, the path leads to algorithm step 4, "Routine health supervision."

Provide reassurance

If the family is worried about behaviors that are developmentally appropriate, the clinician's first role is to provide education and reassurance that the behaviors are normal. If the family resists reassurance or persists in negative perceptions about the child or adolescent, the clinician will need to reframe the family's worry as a significant concern and follow the algorithm accordingly.

Promote healthy S-E development and resilience per Bright Futures

If no significant concerns are identified, the PCC can move on, following *Bright Futures*, 4th Edition, guidelines.[12] These guidelines recommend that PCCs incorporate psychosocial topics and promote healthy social-emotional development and resilience at every contact, from the prenatal visit through adolescence.

On the other hand, if there are concerns—that is, functional impairment; symptoms concerning to the patient, family, or clinician; family distress; exposure to ACEs or to significant environmental risks, such as adverse social determinants or a family member with mental illness; risky behaviors; or perceived problems not amenable to reassurance—the clinician will proceed to step 9, discussed after the following section.

Identifying Psychosocial Concerns at Acute Care Visits

Because families sometimes miss RHS visits and because stress and other MH issues may be the cause of symptoms presenting as acute problems (eg, fatigue, headache, gastrointestinal symptoms, recurrent somatic concerns, injuries), acute care visits present an opportunity to elicit MH concerns.

Incorporate brief MH update [6]

The TFMH drew from the expertise of its professional members, opinions of its adolescent members and their parents, and informal trials in primary care practices to develop a brief MH update.[8,9] (See Box 1-5.)

Responses to these questions may alert clinicians to the need for more extensive assessment. In the absence of any concern, 3 to 5 general questions can be completed in a brief time.

Alternatively, PCCs can use the context of the acute care visit, for example, an injury, to lead naturally into MH topics: "Had you or your friends been drinking when this happened?" or "Has this person (the perpetrator of the injury) ever threatened you or injured you before?"

Box 1-5. Using an Acute Care Visit for a Brief Mental Health Update: Suggested Questions by Age

Ages 0-5 Years

- How have things been going since our last visit?
- How are you coping with [the presenting acute illness]?
- How is [the illness] affecting your child, other than primary symptoms?
- (If an injury) How did it happen?
- How is your child sleeping, in general and in light of the condition?
- How are things going at home in general?
- Is there anything else that's worrying you about parenting your child?

Ages 5-12 Years

- How have things been going since our last visit?
- How are you coping with [the presenting acute illness]?
- How is [the illness] affecting your child, other than primary symptoms?
- (If an injury) How did it happen?
- How is your child sleeping, in general and in light of the condition?
- How is everyone getting along at home?
- Has your child been enjoying school? (To the child) How's school going?
- What is the best part of parenting this child? What is the most difficult part?
- Do you have any worries or concerns about your child's mental health, emotions, or behaviors?

Ages 12-21 Years (Parent/Child Separately)

- How have things been going since our last visit?
- How are you/how is your child coping with [the acute presenting illness]?
- How is [the illness] affecting you/your child, other than primary symptoms?
- (If an injury) How did it happen? Had anyone been drinking or using drugs?
- How are you/how is your child sleeping, in general and in light of the condition?
- How are you/how is your child getting along at home? At school?
- [Parents of] teenagers often mention that they are having difficulties with stress, worries, or changes in mood—has this been a problem for you/your child?

Select questions as appropriate to the clinical circumstances and time available.

Reprinted with permission from American Academy of Pediatrics Task Force on Mental Health algorithm teams, group discussion, fall 2005; and Foy JM; American Academy of Pediatrics Task Force on Mental Health. Appendix S8: brief mental health update. *Pediatrics.* 2010;125(suppl 3):S159–S160.

Concerns other than normal variations? [7]

If no concerns are raised, clinicians can acknowledge the patient's and family's strengths and return to addressing the acute concern that prompted the visit. Office procedures can ensure that children and adolescents not up-to-date on their RHS visits are scheduled for return (algorithm step 1).

Addressing Identified Concerns

Emergency? [9]

Identification of an MH, substance use, or social-emotional concern triggers the triage process. Psychiatric and social emergencies include sexual or physical abuse, suicidality, marked agitation, threat of violence to or by the patient, psychosis, heavy use of or withdrawal from substances, acute intoxication, and family dysfunction or social circumstances that threaten the safety of the patient (eg, domestic violence). Inadequate family resources (eg, homelessness, hunger) may also pose urgent health and safety risks.

Clinicians will need to ask key questions regarding suicidal or homicidal thoughts, presence of a plan, access to lethal weapons such as firearms, and support systems. On the basis of responses, the clinician can assess the level of risk and determine if immediate intervention is indicated. (See Chapter 13, Agitation, Suicidality, and Other Psychiatric Emergencies.) Appendix 2, Mental Health Tools for Pediatrics, lists tools to assist in emergency triage. It is critically important to have a system in place to ensure immediate MH specialty evaluation of children and adolescents with suicidal or homicidal thoughts or other symptoms of a psychosocial emergency and to ensure that the patient receives emergency services, as outlined below.

Yes, findings suggest an emergency [10]

Facilitate referral for emergency services

The presence of certain psychiatric or social emergencies (eg, suspicion of abuse or neglect, risk of homicide) may require immediate action mandated by state law (eg, reporting to social services or legal authorities) and steps to protect the safety of anyone threatened by the emergency, as well as referral of the patient for psychiatric care. Ideally, procedures would have been established in advance with MH specialty and social service providers in the community or region. (For guidance, see Chapter 3, Office and Network Systems to Support Mental Health Care, and Chapter 4, Partnering to Improve Community Mental Health Systems.) The PCC should provide acute medical care as indicated, follow procedures for notification of authorities, and provide reassurance to the patient and family about the clinician's ongoing interest in them. Information about the patient's and the family's progress in MH specialty treatment or social services is critical to primary care follow-up. The PCC can facilitate sharing of information with MH specialty or social service providers by obtaining written permission from the family in advance of the referral.

Request results

Patients referred for an MH emergency will receive an MH specialty assessment and, if indicated, treatment. Ideally, the PCC stays abreast of findings and disposition through contacts with the MH specialists involved, as well as contacts with the family. Critically important communications include notification when the patient is discharged from a psychiatric facility or treatment program, transfer from MH specialty to primary care follow-up, and transition of responsibility for prescribing or monitoring psychopharmacological treatment from MH specialists to the PCC.

Return to algorithm at step 17 (Chapter 2) when resolved

For those patients who have received an assessment in the MH specialty system, the care process picks up at step 17, development of a family-centered care plan, which is covered in Chapter 2, Pediatric Care of Children and Adolescents With Mental Health Problems. Among its other elements, this plan delineates treatment goals of the patient and family and roles of clinicians and agencies involved in the patient's care.

Patients who are not up-to-date on RHS can be scheduled for a visit. Other visits should be scheduled in accordance with the monitoring requirements of the patient's condition.

Brief primary care intervention(s) [11]

All visits: Engage using "common factors"; add patient to registry

If one or more concerns are identified and no findings suggest an emergency, the PCC's most important role is to convey his or her commitment to help the patient and family address the concern(s). Using the patient's and family's own words to describe the concern and keeping in mind that unsolicited advice is implied criticism, clinicians can apply "common factors" techniques to engage the patient and family in a therapeutic alliance. This type of intervention can be done efficiently and effectively in primary care settings. These techniques are summarized by the HELP mnemonic (Box 1-6) and described in Chapter 5, Effective Communication Methods: Common Factors Skills.

The aim is to achieve agreement with the family on a plan of action, whether primary care intervention (either at the current visit or later) or referral for MH specialty care. Whatever action is taken, the PCC can take the additional step of adding the patient to a practice registry that will trigger mechanisms for tracking and monitoring the patient until the issue is resolved.

Acute care visit: Complete acute care visit; address MH concern now (as in the bullets below) or plan follow-up visit

RHS visit or visit for MH concern: Choose one or more of the following (discussed in Chapter 2):

► Expand assessment (eg, secondary screening; behavioral diary; collateral data collection from school, child care, records of previous MH evaluation)

Box 1-6. Common Factors Mnemonic: HELP Build a Therapeutic Alliance

H = Hope

E = Empathy

L² = Language, Loyalty

P³ = Permission, Partnership, Plan

Adapted with permission from American Academy of Pediatrics. *Addressing Mental Health Concerns in Primary Care: A Clinician's Toolkit*. Elk Grove Village, IL: American Academy of Pediatrics; 2010. For the fully annotated mnemonic, please refer to Appendix 5.

▶ Offer focused problem-solving, common elements intervention, stress reduction, assistance with behavior change, and/or self-help resources

▶ Facilitate referral of family member for MH specialty or social services, if indicated

▶ Schedule return(s) or outreach as needed to assess response, complete RHS, try additional interventions, or advance to step 12 (Chapter 2)

Chapter 2, Pediatric Care of Children and Adolescents With Mental Health Problems, discusses in detail the range of options listed in algorithm step 11 for responding to an MH concern in the context of an acute care or RHS visit and a visit for MH concerns. Regardless of context, the PCC can offer suggestions for promoting the patient's MH. Several natural strategies have been identified by the AAP Section on Complementary, Holistic, and Integrative Medicine and the TFMH. (See Box 1-7.) These are universally applicable, safe interventions that can potentially enhance any child's or adolescent's well-being.

Common factors approaches include techniques for closing a visit supportively, while conveying the clinician's ongoing commitment to the patient and family.

Box 1-7. Natural Strategies for Promoting Mental Health

- Outdoor time (with appropriate skin protection)
- Special one-on-one time for child or adolescent with caregiver
- Sufficient sleep
- Social connections
- Good nutrition
- Expressions of appreciation and kindness
- Physical activity
- Limited screen time
- Stress management through self-regulation techniques

Preventive Mental Health Care of Children and Adolescents With Chronic Medical Conditions

A chronic medical problem or disability places a child or an adolescent at greater risk for MH problems. Furthermore, he or she may have experienced medical trauma (eg, painful procedures, disfigurement, separation from loved ones during hospitalization) in the course of receiving necessary care. Unidentified MH problems—particularly anxiety and depression—in children and adolescents with special health care needs may contribute to poor adherence to prescribed therapy, somatization, and overuse of medical services by both the patient and the parents.[17] Efforts to identify MH concerns are important at each contact with a chronically ill patient, especially if the patient has experienced frequent emergency department visits, hospitalizations, or poor adherence to treatment. Parents and siblings may also experience stress and need support, respite, or MH care. The process for providing MH care to these families in the medical home can flow from either step 1 or step 5 of the algorithm, depending on the reason for the PCC's encounter with the patient.

Summary

Pediatric PCCs have unique opportunities to promote MH in children, adolescents, and their families and to identify and address emerging MH and substance use problems. These opportunities may present themselves in the course of RHS visits, acute care visits, or the monitoring of patients with chronic medical conditions. This chapter describes a process for incorporating preventive psychosocial services into primary care settings. This process is represented by steps 1 through 11 of the algorithm depicted in Figure 1-1. Tools and resources developed by the AAP may be helpful in implementing a systematic approach to promotion of MH and early identification of MH and substance use problems.

Acknowledgments: The authors acknowledge the American Academy of Pediatrics Task Force on Mental Health for authoring the original algorithm and the article that described it: Enhancing pediatric mental health care: algorithms for primary care. *Pediatrics.* 2010;125(suppl 3):S109–S125.

The task force included Jane Meschan Foy, MD (chairperson and lead author); Paula Duncan, MD; Barbara Frankowski, MD, MPH; Kelly Kelleher, MD, MPH (lead author); Penelope K. Knapp, MD; Danielle Laraque, MD (lead author); Gary Peck, MD; Michael Regalado, MD; Jack Swanson, MD; and Mark Wolraich, MD; the consultants were Margaret Dolan, MD; Alain Joffe, MD, MPH; Patricia O'Malley, MD; James Perrin, MD; Thomas K. McInerny, MD; and Lynn Wegner, MD; the liaisons were Terry Carmichael, MSW (National Association of Social Workers); Darcy Gruttadaro, JD (National Alliance on Mental Illness); Garry Sigman, MD (Society for Adolescent Medicine); Myrtis Sullivan, MD, MPH (National Medical Association); and L. Read Sulik, MD (American Academy of Child and Adolescent Psychiatry); and the staff members were Linda Paul and Aldina Hovde.

Tools for Practice

Box 1-8. Surveillance and Screening of Family and Social Environment for Strengths and Risk Factors

1. Use questionnaires or prompts to systematically update family psychosocial history (including family mental health, social adversities, disruptions, strengths, and protective factors) at each health supervision visit and when symptoms or signs suggest possible psychosocial issues in the child.

2. Use a validated instrument to screen for maternal depression at ages 1, 2, 4, and 6 mo and when psychosocial history indicates.

3. If maternal depression or any other risk factors are identified, flag child's health record and proceed to Box 1-9, step 5.

Box 1-9. Mental Health Screening and Surveillance of Children and Adolescents in Primary Care

1. Perform family-centered psychosocial and behavioral assessment (including child social-emotional health, caregiver depression, and social determinants of health) at every health supervision visit to identify both risks and strengths.

Box 1-9. Mental Health Screening and Surveillance of Children and Adolescents in Primary Care (*continued*)

2 Use validated instruments to screen for social-emotional development in newborns, infants, and children 0–5 years of age as part of routine developmental screening (typically performed at 9 mo, 18 mo, and 24 or 30 mo) and in the following circumstances:

- Abnormal developmental screening test results
- Abnormal ASD screening test results (typically performed at 18 mo and 24 mo)
- Poor growth
- Poor attachment
- Symptoms such as excessive crying, irritability, clinginess, or fearfulness for developmental stage
- Regression to earlier behavior
- Psychosocial concerns of family

3 Use a validated instrument to screen child for psychosocial symptoms and impaired psychosocial functioning in the following circumstances, at any age:

- Risk factors are identified in family history (Box 1-8), psychosocial and behavioral assessment, or developmental surveillance of child
- Exposure to violence, racism, homophobia, or bullying
- Family disruption
- Poor functioning in child care or school
- Behavioral difficulties reported by parent, school, or other authorities
- Symptoms or signs of mental health problems
- Recurrent somatic concerns
- Involvement of a social service or juvenile justice agency
- Psychosocial concerns of child or family or both

4 Use a validated instrument to screen all adolescents for substance use (including tobacco) at each health supervision visit and whenever circumstances such as an injury, a car crash, or a decrease in school performance suggest the possibility of substance use. If an adolescent reports using one or more substances, assess extent of use.

5 Use a validated instrument to screen all adolescents for depression at routine health supervision visits and whenever symptoms suggest the possibility of depression.

Abbreviation: ASD, autism spectrum disorder.

AAP Policy

American Academy of Pediatrics Committee on Psychosocial Aspects of Child and Family Health and Task Force on Mental Health. The future of pediatrics: mental health competencies for pediatric primary care. *Pediatrics.* 2009;124(1):410–421. Reaffirmed August 2013 (pediatrics.aappublications.org/content/124/1/410)

Cohen GJ; American Academy of Pediatrics Committee on Psychosocial Aspects of Child and Family Health. The prenatal visit. *Pediatrics.* 2009;124(4):1227–1232. Reaffirmed May 2014 (pediatrics.aappublications.org/content/124/4/1227)

Earls MF; American Academy of Pediatrics Committee on Psychosocial Aspects of Child and Family Health. Incorporating perinatal and postpartum depression recognition and management into pediatric practice. *Pediatrics.* 2010;126(5):1032–1039. Reaffirmed December 2014 (pediatrics.aappublications.org/content/126/5/1032)

Shonkoff JP, Garner AS; American Academy of Pediatrics Committee on Psychosocial Aspects of Child and Family Health; Committee on Early Childhood, Adoption, and Dependent Care; and Section on Developmental and Behavioral Pediatrics. The lifelong effects of early childhood adversity and toxic stress. *Pediatrics.* 2012;129(1):e232–e246. Reaffirmed July 2016 (pediatrics.aappublications.org/content/129/1/e232)

Weitzman C, Wegner L; American Academy of Pediatrics Section on Developmental and Behavioral Pediatrics, Committee on Psychosocial Aspects of Child and Family Health, and Council on Early Childhood; Society for Developmental and Behavioral Pediatrics. Promoting optimal development: screening for behavioral and emotional problems. *Pediatrics.* 2015;135(2):384–395 (pediatrics.aappublications.org/content/135/2/384)

References

1. Kemper KJ. *Mental Health, Naturally: The Family Guide to Holistic Care for a Healthy Mind and Body.* Elk Grove Village, IL: American Academy of Pediatrics; 2010
2. Egger HL, Angold A. Common emotional and behavioral disorders in preschool children: presentation, nosology, and epidemiology. *J Child Psychol Psychiatry.* 2006;47(3–4):313–337
3. Brauner CB, Stephens CB. Estimating the prevalence of early childhood serious emotional/behavioral disorders: challenges and recommendations. *Public Health Rep.* 2006;121(3):303–310
4. Any disorder among children. National Institute of Mental Health Web site. https://www.nimh.nih.gov/health/statistics/prevalence/any-disorder-among-children.shtml. Accessed October 6, 2017
5. Merikangas KR, He J, Burstein M, et al. Lifetime prevalence of mental disorders in U.S. adolescents: results from the National Comorbidity Study Adolescent Supplement (NCS-A). *J Am Acad Child Adolesc Psychiatry.* 2010;49(10):980–989
6. Burns BJ, Costello EJ, Angold A, et al. Children's mental health service use across service sectors. *Health Aff (Millwood).* 1995;14(3):147–159

7. Kessler RC, Berglund P, Demler O, Jin R, Merikangas KR, Walters EE. Lifetime prevalence and age-of-onset distributions of *DSM-IV* disorders in the National Comorbidity Survey Replication. *Arch Gen Psychiatry.* 2005;62(6):593–602

8. Foy JM, Kelleher KJ, Laraque D; American Academy of Pediatrics Task Force on Mental Health. Enhancing pediatric mental health care: strategies for preparing a primary care practice. *Pediatrics.* 2010;125(suppl 3):S87–S108

9. Foy JM; American Academy of Pediatrics Task Force on Mental Health. Enhancing pediatric mental health care: algorithms for primary care. *Pediatrics.* 2010;125(suppl 3):S109–S125

10. Hacker KA, Myagmarjav E, Harris V, Suglia SF, Weidner D, Link D. Mental health screening in pediatric practice: factors related to positive screens and the contribution of parental/personal concern. *Pediatrics.* 2006;118(5):1896–1906

11. Zuckerbrot RA, Maxon L, Pagar D, Davies M, Fisher PW, Shaffer D. Adolescent depression screening in primary care: feasibility and acceptability. *Pediatrics.* 2007;119(1):101–108

12. Hagan JF Jr, Shaw JS, Duncan PM, eds. *Bright Futures: Guidelines for Health Supervision of Infants, Children, and Adolescents.* 4th ed. Elk Grove Village, IL: American Academy of Pediatrics; 2017

13. Paperny DM, Aono JY, Lehman RM, Hammar SL, Risser J. Computer-assisted detection and intervention in adolescent high-risk health behaviors. *J Pediatr.* 1990;116(3):456–462

14. Olson AL, Gaffney CA, Hedberg VA, Gladstone GR. Use of inexpensive technology to enhance adolescent health screening and counseling. *Arch Pediatr Adolesc Med.* 2009;163(2):172–177

15. Gardner H. *Intelligence Reframed: Multiple Intelligences for the 21st Century.* New York, NY: Basic Books; 2000

16. Duncan PM, Garcia AC, Frankowski BL, et al. Inspiring healthy adolescent choices: a rationale for and guide to strength promotion in primary care. *J Adolesc Health.* 2007;41(6):525–535

17. Bernal P. Hidden morbidity in pediatric primary care. *Pediatr Ann.* 2003;32(6):413–418

CHAPTER 2

Pediatric Care of Children and Adolescents With Mental Health Problems

Jane Meschan Foy, MD

"Pediatric clinicians can be effective in reducing the patient's and family's distress and improving the patient's functioning, even in the absence of a specific diagnosis."

Introduction

Increasingly, families and communities across the United States are looking to primary care clinicians (PCCs)—that is, pediatricians, family physicians, internists, nurse practitioners, and physician assistants providing frontline care to children and adolescents—as a source of mental health (MH) care, a gateway to specialty MH care, and a source of primary care that is coordinated with specialty MH care. The opportunity and urgency for PCCs to fulfill these roles was articulated in the President's New Freedom Commission on Mental Health final report,[1] *Mental Health: A Report of the Surgeon General,*[2] and the Future of Pediatric Education II (commonly known as FOPE II) Project.[3] In 2004, in response to these reports and requests from its members, the American Academy of Pediatrics (AAP) formed the Task Force on Mental Health (TFMH) to assist pediatric PCCs in meeting these challenges. The TFMH recognized "the primary care advantage," that is, the unique skills and experience of PCCs and their opportunity for longitudinal, trusting relationships with families. Building on this advantage, the TFMH issued guidance for the care of children and adolescents with MH problems in the pediatric medical home. This chapter and many other chapters in this book draw from the publications of the TFMH.[4-10]

Pediatric subspecialists also have many opportunities to support the MH of their patients and families and to recognize MH problems that may affect a child or adolescent's medical condition and general well-being. In fact, the AAP Mental Health Leadership Workgroup (MHLWG) has expanded the concept of the primary care advantage to "the pediatric advantage," as articulated in the introduction to this book; this formulation recognizes the bond of trust that pediatric subspecialists develop with their patients and families through longitudinal relationships and care of their patients during medical crises. This chapter and Chapters 13 through 32, which offer guidance in caring for children and adolescents presenting with common concerns, signs, and symptoms, may be useful to both PCCs and pediatric subspecialists (collectively called *pediatric clinicians* in this chapter) who want to play a role in addressing their patients' MH needs.

The term *mental health*, as used in this chapter, incorporates the full range of social-emotional, substance use (SU), behavioral, and psychosocial issues. This definition is not to suggest that pediatric clinicians are solely responsible for this full spectrum of care but rather that children and adolescents with the full range of MH conditions need a medical home and, often, pediatric subspecialty care, as do others with special health care needs. Pediatric clinicians play a critical role in identifying their patients' needs, engaging them in care, coordinating their care with other professionals, and monitoring their progress in care.

General Principles of Pediatric Mental Health Care

Certain principles apply universally to the pediatric MH care of children and adolescents.

▶ Pediatric clinicians can be effective in reducing the patient's and family's distress and improving the patient's functioning, even in the absence of a specific diagnosis.

▶ Mental health problems occur within a social context that can either buffer their effects or exacerbate them; pediatric clinicians should identify and reinforce the patient's and family's strengths, as well as identify and address social factors that may be affecting the patient adversely.

▶ Mental health problems can impair a child or adolescent's functioning, even in the absence of a diagnosable disorder; thus, the assessment and monitoring of MH functioning is basic to caring for a child or adolescent with MH problems.

▶ Mental health problems often coexist with developmental and physical health problems.

▶ Although physical health conditions can cause MH symptoms and should always be considered as a possible source, the pediatric clinician need not exclude physical health problems before considering and caring for a child or adolescent's MH problems.

▶ All children and adolescents with MH problems should be triaged for psychiatric emergencies, including the potential to do harm to themselves or others.

▶ Children, adolescents, and their families may not be ready to take action on an MH or a social problem once it is identified; ensuring the patient and family's engagement in care is a fundamental role of pediatric clinicians. This role involves assessing the patient and family's state of readiness to take action and identifying any barriers to moving forward, such as conflict within the family, a sense of hopelessness, or prior adverse experiences with seeking help, and then addressing barriers and moving the patient and family toward a greater state of readiness.

▶ A therapeutic alliance, that is, a bond of trust between the clinician and the patient and family, is the most effective of all MH interventions; using communication techniques that convey hopefulness and loyalty, the pediatric clinician can enhance the likelihood of good outcomes.

▶ The patient's and family's strengths, perceived needs, and preferences are central to developing a plan for the patient's care.

▶ The chronic care model, used in organizing the care of children and adolescents with medical conditions such as asthma and diabetes, is applicable to the care of children and adolescents with MH problems.

The Primary Care Clinician's Role in Addressing Mental Health Problems

Mental health problems may come to the attention of PCCs in a variety of ways: for example, referral by school or child care personnel, expression of concern by a patient or parent directly to the PCC, or findings by the PCC through surveillance or formal psychosocial screening. Frequently, patients and families have not framed these visits as MH related. They may be seeking routine health supervision, acute care for a physical concern, help with a challenging behavior, or simply reassurance. Often, the patient's problem is undifferentiated (eg, a child who is not functioning well in child care or school, parents who are frustrated and angry with an adolescent's rebelliousness, a child or adolescent who is not fitting in well with peers).

Thus, the role of the PCC often begins with eliciting psychosocial and MH concerns and differentiating normal developmental variations from MH problems that adversely affect the child's or adolescent's functioning. The PCC's priority is to recognize emergent situations that compel an immediate intervention. In their absence, the PCC's role may be providing reassurance when that is appropriate, engaging the patient and family to seek care for significant problems, addressing any barriers to their seeking and receiving care, assessing and treating the patient in the primary care setting, or guiding the family toward appropriate referral sources and comanaging the patient's care with any involved MH specialists.

Whether providing MH services alone or collaboratively, the PCC can also monitor the patient's and family's functioning and progress in care, apply chronic care principles as for other children and adolescents with special health care needs, and provide and coordinate care of their comorbid medical conditions. Primary care clinicians have the challenge of fulfilling these roles within the constraints of a busy practice without compromising the efficiency and financial viability of the practice. The AAP has issued a policy statement describing the MH competencies requisite to these roles.[5]

The Mental Health Practice Readiness Inventory (introduced in Chapter 3, Office and Network Systems to Support Mental Health Care, and reproduced in Appendix 3, Mental Health Practice Readiness Inventory), developed by the TFMH and revised in 2017 by the AAP MHLWG, enables PCCs to assess their practice's strengths and needs in providing and comanaging the care of children and adolescents with MH problems and to focus quality improvement efforts on enhancing their office systems in support of that care.

Mental health care is not confined to the traditional pediatric primary care visit. Care begins when the family schedules an appointment for an MH concern. A pediatric practice ideally establishes the following routines, triggered by an MH-related appointment:

▶ Completion of parent and youth psychosocial questionnaires and behavior checklists in advance of the visit, either electronically or by paper and pencil

▶ Completion of behavior checklists by other key adults, such as teachers, child care providers, or a noncustodial parent

▶ Transfer of records of prior psychological assessment or previous MH care

▶ Acquisition of report cards or other school records

During a single extended visit or multiple brief visits that fit the pace of primary care, the PCC can observe the patient and family, as well as their interactions; explore significant responses in the data previously gathered (separate conversations with parents and adolescents); and perform a psychosocial and physical assessment. Each contact with the patient and family incorporates engagement techniques that express the clinician's commitment to the patient and family, address any barriers to care, and find common ground for future action steps. A process for incorporating these activities into primary care visits is introduced in Chapter 1, Integrating Preventive Mental Health Care Into Pediatric Practice, and continues in the current chapter.

The Pediatric Subspecialist's Role in Addressing Mental Health Problems

Children and adolescents may self-refer or be referred by their PCC to pediatric subspecialists, often after multiple primary care visits, seeking a second opinion for concerns such as

▶ Chronic, recurrent, or unexplained physical symptoms (eg, abdominal pain, joint pain, headache)

▶ Fatigue or low energy

▶ Loss of appetite

▶ Acute episodes of chest pain or difficulty breathing

▶ Menstrual irregularities, especially in girls of low and high weights

▶ Psychogenic pseudoseizures

▶ Non-physiologic neurological symptoms

These patients are at risk for unnecessary, costly, and potentially dangerous evaluations and procedures. The pediatric subspecialist's role in the care of these patients is to include somatic symptom disorders, anxiety, and depression in the patient's differential diagnosis, rather than relegating them to diagnoses of exclusion. (See Chapter 24, Medically Unexplained Symptoms.)

Pediatric subspecialists also provide care to children with chronic medical conditions, who have an increased risk for MH problems.[11-13] In addition to the common comorbidities of anxiety and depression, these children may have experienced medical trauma (eg, painful procedures, disfigurement, separation from families during hospitalization), which is an adverse childhood experience in its own right. The parents and siblings of children and adolescents with a chronic illness may also experience sleep deprivation, poor MH, financial pressures, diversion of attention and resources to the sick child, and family disruption. These MH issues in the patient and family may complicate the patient's medical care by affecting adherence to medical treatment, use of emergency facilities, frequency of hospitalization, and outcomes.

Some subspecialty clinics incorporate an MH professional as a team member to participate in patients' assessments, to assess families' support systems and coping mechanisms, and to provide MH services or referrals. For some subspecialties (eg, hematology-oncology and endocrinology), inclusion of an MH professional on the care team is held up as a standard of care.[14,15] However, these MH professionals are often stretched thin, and their positions may be difficult to sustain economically. Pediatric subspecialists would be well served to achieve core MH competencies, particularly "common factors" communication techniques (see Chapter 5, Effective Communication Methods: Common Factors Skills), and to collaborate with the patient's PCC and any involved MH specialists to address their patients' MH problems. They may also follow the steps described in the next section of this chapter, Addressing Identified Mental Health Concerns in Pediatrics: Key Concepts.

Many of the practice enhancements that support MH care in primary care settings can be applied to subspecialty practice (eg, routines for collecting psychosocial history; screening for MH symptoms and impaired psychosocial functioning; exchange of information with the PCC and school; referral to accessible sources of social and MH services, when needed; family-centered care planning). As bundled payment and pay-for-value methods replace fee-for-service payment, the capacity to address MH and social needs in subspecialty settings may become increasingly important from the business, as well as the health, perspective.

Addressing Identified Mental Health Concerns in Pediatrics: Key Concepts

Other chapters in the book discuss many topics that bear on the subject of addressing identified MH concerns in pediatrics. Highlights are summarized herein, with reference to chapters that provide more detailed discussion.

Psychosocial Assessment in Primary Care

[C] Iterative Nature of the Assessment (Chapter 1, Integrating Preventive Mental Health Care Into Pediatric Practice, and Chapter 6, Iterative Mental Health Assessment)

Unlike a diagnostic evaluation performed in the MH specialty system, which is often a discrete formal process, psychosocial assessment in pediatrics typically happens iteratively and consists of multiple elements:

▶ Previsit health surveillance questionnaires (patient's and family's psychosocial history, risks, and strengths)

▶ Screening (for symptoms, functional impairment, and caregiver's MH problem)

▶ Interview in the context of routine health supervision, acute care, or chronic illness care

▶ Observations of the child, the parent(s), and their interactions

▶ Response to primary care interventions

▶ Periodic functional assessment (using brief pediatric tools)

▶ Collateral information (from schools, child care, noncustodial parent, and other caregivers; MH specialty evaluation, if any)

Global Functional Assessment (Chapter 1, Integrating Preventive Mental Health Care Into Pediatric Practice; Chapter 3, Office and Network Systems to Support Mental Health Care; and Chapter 6, Iterative Mental Health Assessment)

A global functional assessment can serve as a baseline for monitoring the impact of the child's or adolescent's problem over time and can contribute to decision-making about resources he or she will require. Children and adolescents whose functioning is severely impaired will require care in the MH specialty system; for those with lesser degrees of impairment, the pediatric clinician and family can decide together whether to involve an MH specialist in the assessment, the treatment, or both, according to their preferences and other factors, discussed later. Primary care–friendly (and potentially subspecialty clinic–friendly) tools, such as the Impact Scale of the Strengths and Difficulties Questionnaires and the Columbia Impairment Scale, are available to measure functional impairment and can become a routine element in assessing and monitoring children and adolescents with MH problems, much like a vital sign. (See Appendix 2, Mental Health Tools for Pediatrics.)

Social Determinants (Chapter 6, Iterative Mental Health Assessment)

Mental health problems are more common among children who experience such stresses as poverty, parental unemployment, immigration, racism, and homophobia. Addressing their social needs in concert with the child's MH care is critical to favorable outcomes.

Sleep Pattern (Chapter 28, Sleep Disturbances)

Poor sleep can cause MH symptoms. Poor sleep can result from a child or adolescent's physical or mental illness, treatments of that illness, or breakdown in the child or adolescent's routine sleep patterns when families are disrupted by parental illness, social problems, or environmental problems. Parents of older children and adolescents presenting with MH problems often report that the young person gets insufficient sleep. The clinician should determine whether she is unable to sleep *even when she wants to sleep* (potentially a presenting sign of serious mental illness, such as a bipolar disorder, depression, or schizophrenia), whether she is missing sleep because of a physiologic sleep problem such as obstructive sleep apnea or an environmental problem such as a noisy household or upsetting media exposure, or whether she is communicating with peers at all hours, doing homework, or losing sleep for other reasons associated with unclear boundaries, adolescent-parent conflict, procrastination, learning difficulties, or other factors. These are important distinctions that influence care. Sleep deprivation can exacerbate symptoms, increase irritability, and decrease resilience of the child or adolescent (and the parents, if their sleep is also disrupted); as such, addressing it appropriately is an important component of management.

Use of Complementary and Integrative Medicine Therapies (Chapter 8, Self-regulation Therapies and Biofeedback, and Chapter 9, Complementary and Integrative Medical Therapies)

Because parents and adolescents commonly try complementary and integrative medicine approaches before or while seeking help from health care professionals for psychosocial problems, and because some medicinal therapies may interact with prescription medications, it is important to inquire about them as part of the psychosocial assessment. It is also important to be aware of research on effectiveness of a number of mind-body therapies and practices that may be beneficial to children and adolescents.[16,17] If asked directly, adolescents and parents may report interest in these approaches.

Strength-Based Approach (Chapter 1, Integrating Preventive Mental Health Care Into Pediatric Practice, and Chapter 6, Iterative Mental Health Assessment)

Throughout the assessment, the clinician can point out findings that suggest strengths and assets in the patient and family: for example, one or more of the 8 empirically determined independent "intelligences"; talents; qualities such as resilience, generosity, courage, tenacity, goal orientation, and focus; social supports such as strong family bonds, extended family support, and good peer relations; healthy behaviors such as regular exercise/sleep routines and participation in extracurricular or spiritual/religious activities; or attitudes such as hope, optimism, and motivation to seek help. A focus on strengths can build rapport, provide groundwork for an intervention plan, and facilitate accomplishment of subsequent steps.

Addressing Mental Health Problems in Primary Care: An Algorithm to Guide the Process

In 2010 the AAP published algorithms to guide the process of incorporating MH services into primary care pediatric practice.[9] In 2017 the AAP MHLWG revised them into a single algorithm, A Process for Integrating

Mental Health Care Into Pediatric Practice (Appendix 1). Chapter 1, Integrating Preventive Mental Health Care Into Pediatric Practice, describes the first segment of the algorithm, steps 1 through 10, and introduces step 11. The discussion herein reiterates the important steps of emergency triage and referral (steps 9 and 10) and describes steps 11 through 21. This second segment of the algorithm is represented in Figure 2-1, on pages 42 and 43, subtitled "Addressing Mental Health Concerns."

Triage [9] and referral [10] for psychiatric and social emergencies

Triage

The presence of an MH concern triggers the triage process. Psychiatric and social emergencies include sexual or physical abuse, suicidality, threat of violence to or by the child, psychosis, heavy use of or withdrawal from substances, acute intoxication, and family dysfunction or social circumstances that threaten the safety of the child or adolescent (eg, domestic violence). Inadequate family resources (eg, homelessness, hunger) may also pose urgent health and safety risks.

Clinicians should ask key questions regarding suicidal or homicidal thoughts, presence of a plan, access to lethal weapons such as firearms, and support systems. Clinicians will need a system in place to ensure immediate psychiatric evaluation of children and adolescents at risk for suicide. (See also Chapter 13, Agitation, Suicidality, and Other Psychiatric Emergencies.)

Referral for emergency services

The presence of certain psychiatric or social emergencies (eg, suspicion of abuse or neglect, risk of homicide) may require immediate action mandated by state law (eg, reporting to social services or legal authorities) and steps to protect the safety of anyone threatened by the emergency, as well as referral for psychiatric care. Ideally, the practice would have procedures in place and a community-wide understanding of optimal care for children and adolescents experiencing a psychiatric or social emergency.[7,8] The clinician's role is to provide medical care as indicated, follow procedures for notification of authorities, ensure that the patient receives needed emergency psychiatric services, provide reassurance to the patient and family about the clinician's ongoing commitment to them, and put into place a plan to follow up and provide other pediatric services.

The clinician can facilitate sharing of information with MH specialty or social service providers by obtaining written permission from the family for exchange of information about the patient's or family's progress in MH specialty treatment or social services. While the Health Insurance Portability and Accountability Act (HIPAA) allows this exchange among providers of health care to a mutual patient, some MH providers and virtually all agencies require explicit consent. Exchange of information is critical to pediatric follow-up.

Brief primary care intervention(s) [11]

All visits: Engage using "common factors"; add patient to registry

Whether MH concerns are identified in the course of routine health supervision, acute care, assessment of recurrent somatic concerns, or visits to monitor a chronic medical condition, pediatric clinicians can and should initiate care. Studies have shown that common factors interventions provided by a trusted clinician can reduce distress and improve the child's functioning.[18]

Common factors skills can be represented by the HELP mnemonic, described in Box 2-1.

These skills are core competencies in the care of children and adolescents with MH problems.[5] They are drawn from evidence-based therapeutic approaches, including motivational interviewing, cognitive behavioral therapy, and family therapy. Application of these skills has been effective in decreasing parents' distress and improving children's functioning across a range of MH problems.

The purposes of this initial generic intervention are to develop a therapeutic alliance with the patient and family, to involve the patient and family in developing a plan for addressing the problem, and to identify and address any barriers to carrying out that plan. At times, especially if symptoms are just emerging and functional impairment is minimal, this intervention may be all that is needed. When referring to an MH specialist, common factors methods can be applied to readying the patient and family for referral and increasing their sense of hopefulness about receiving help.

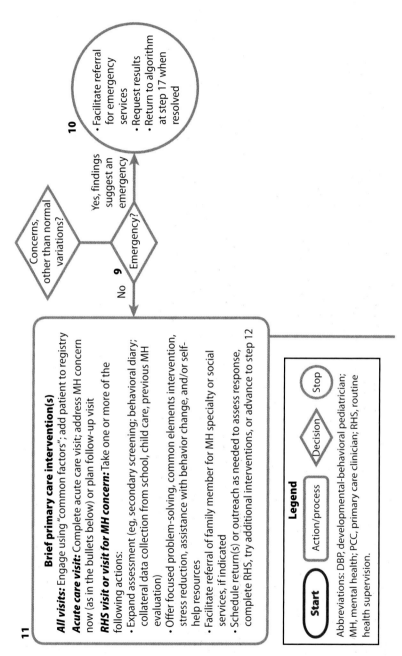

Figure 2-1. A process for integrating mental health care into pediatric practice: addressing mental health concerns.

Adapted from Foy JM; American Academy of Pediatrics Task Force on Mental Health. Enhancing pediatric mental health care: algorithms for primary care. *Pediatrics*. 2010;125(suppl 3):S109–S125.

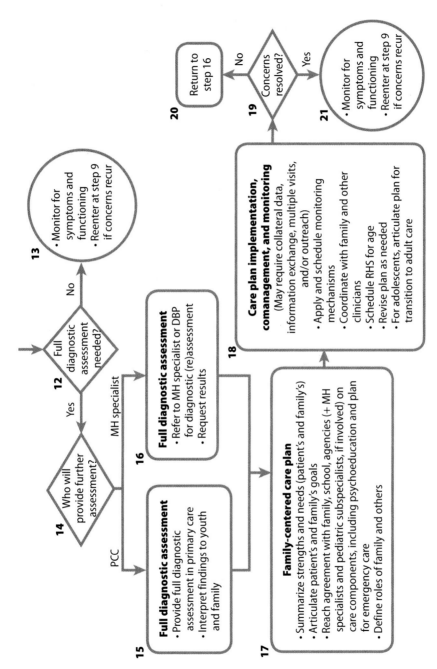

Figure 2-1. A process for integrating mental health care into pediatric practice: addressing mental health concerns. (*continued*)

Box 2-1. Common Factors Mnemonic: HELP Build a Therapeutic Alliance

H = Hope

E = Empathy

L^2 = Language, Loyalty

P^3 = Permission, Partnership, Plan

Adapted with permission from American Academy of Pediatrics. *Addressing Mental Health Concerns in Primary Care: A Clinician's Toolkit.* Elk Grove Village, IL: American Academy of Pediatrics; 2010. For the fully annotated mnemonic, please refer to Appendix 5.

If one or more concerns are identified at a pediatric visit and no findings suggest an emergency, the clinician's most important role is to convey his or her commitment to help the patient and family address the concern(s). Using the patient's and family's own words to describe the concern and keeping in mind that unsolicited advice is implied criticism, clinicians can apply common factors techniques, described earlier, to build a therapeutic alliance with the patient and family. This type of intervention can be done efficiently and effectively in primary care settings. It can be applied in brief sessions of 15 minutes or less, allowing for the rapid pace of pediatric practice. It includes techniques helpful in managing conflict between family members during the visit (eg, avoiding taking sides, acknowledging the legitimacy of feelings, reminding that strong feelings often occur when people care about each other, offering to have separate conversations with adolescents and parents to give both a chance to be fully heard). Importantly, a common factors intervention can also be applied to bringing the conversation to a supportive close in the event circumstances (eg, the patient's need to complete an acute care visit, the clinician's time limitations) require that further MH intervention be deferred. The aim is to achieve agreement with the family on a plan of action, whether a primary care intervention (either at the current visit or later) or referral for MH subspecialty care. Whatever agreement is reached, the clinician can take the important step of adding the patient to the practice registry, which triggers follow-up procedures that prevent the patient from being lost to care.

Acute care visit: Complete acute care visit; address MH concern now or plan follow-up visit

The context and pace of an acute care visit may not be conducive to further MH intervention. On the other hand, the context may lead naturally to further MH inquiry: for example, at the time of an injury, "Had you or your friends been drinking when this happened?" or "Has this person (the perpetrator of the injury) ever threatened you or injured you before?" In the absence of responses that suggest an emergency, the clinician, patient, and family can decide together whether to proceed with MH care at the present visit or schedule a return.

RHS visit or visit for MH concern

A number of options are available as a next step at the current visit, at subsequent visit(s), or, in some cases, in the interval between visits.

Expand assessment

When primary psychosocial screens have identified concerns, secondary screening may be useful in corroborating the finding or increasing the clinician's understanding of the patient's problem. Appendix 2, Mental Health Tools for Pediatrics, includes examples.

The patient and family may be amenable to gathering additional information between visits. In some circumstances, it may be helpful to ask the patient or family to keep a diary of symptoms or behaviors, their antecedents, and consequences. The clinician can also seek information about the patient from collateral sources. If primary care findings point to academic or behavioral problems in school, the PCC will need details about the child or adolescent's functioning in the school setting and any discrepancy between cognitive ability and academic achievement that would suggest a learning disability. The clinician can also request information about preschool-aged children from their child care providers. If the patient or family has been involved with a social service agency, information about that experience will also be important. For children or adolescents in foster care, it is essential to work through caseworkers to collect information from biological and foster parents if adults who are unfamiliar with the patient's history accompanied him to the visit. If the patient has undergone an MH specialty assessment or treatment, this information is also important. When collateral information is needed, office procedures can ensure that parents complete a form authorizing exchange of information.

If parents are separated, divorced, or in conflict and that parent is involved in the child's or adolescent's life, it is important to gather information from the parent who is not represented at the visit. If a grandparent, a foster parent, or another guardian is involved in the care of the child, information from this individual is also important. Several validated tools have parent versions that can be used for this purpose. (See Appendix 2, Mental Health Tools for Pediatrics.) Use of a tool does not substitute for including this caregiver in future discussions involving the patient.

If the patient or family has experienced trauma (death of a loved one or pet; a move; homelessness; conflict, separation, or divorce of parents; military deployment of a family member; incarceration of the patient or a loved one; breakup of a relationship; abuse or bullying by the patient or targeting the patient; racism; homophobia; or exposure to violence or a natural disaster), it is important to explore its impact. It is necessary to inquire separately of the patient and her parents, because some events that affect children and adolescents may go unrecognized by the parent or be confidential from the parent, and some parents may be reluctant to discuss some events or losses in front of their son or daughter. When interviewing children or adolescents about trauma exposure, the clinician should allow them to share their own narrative of the experience but not lead them into reliving the incident, which may result in further trauma. See Chapter 14, Anxiety and Trauma-Related Distress, for more discussion about approaching these issues.

Offer focused problem-solving, common elements intervention, stress reduction, assistance with behavior change, and/or self-help resources

Focused problem-solving. This might include advice on parenting techniques to address acute problems (eg, toileting, homework, sibling conflicts, anger outbursts) or other strategies that motivated parents can learn during brief primary care encounters or from well-vetted resources. Even when plans may involve referral of the patient for further MH specialty assessment or treatment, parents will want advice to tide them over the often long waiting period until the referral is complete. Table 2-1 offers advice for parents whose child or adolescent is experiencing one of the problems listed.

Table 2-1. Advice for Parents Regarding Common Mental Health Concerns

Mental Health Concern	Advice for Parents
Infancy (Birth–11 Months)	
Infant-parent attachment	Hold, cuddle, talk to, and sing to your baby often. Respond promptly to your baby's needs. Ask for help from family and friends. Explore and address any sources of stress inside or outside the family that might be affecting your ability to respond to your child.
Difficult temperament (irritable, hard to console, unpredictable needs, difficulty feeding)	Take time for yourself and your partner. Ask for help from family and friends. Explore and address any sources of stress inside or outside the family that might be affecting your own resilience and ability to attend to your child's needs. If you find you are losing patience or control with your child, let your pediatrician know right away.
Delayed development	Read to your child often. Enroll your child in pre-school or Head Start. Review developmental screening results with your pediatrician in order to identify strengths, as well as weaknesses. Your pediatrician can help you with referral to Early Intervention services.
Weak attachment	Be alert for your child's spoken and unspoken messages and feelings; respond promptly to needs. Set aside "special time" one-on-one with your child. Play and eat together as a family.
Difficulty forming relationships	Make sure your child has the chance to play with other children. Model kindness to others, taking turns, sharing, and empathy.
Behavioral problem (impulsivity/tantrums/ aggression)	Notice and praise your child's good behavior. Do not hit, spank, or yell at your child. Set age-appropriate limits on your child's behavior, and ensure all caregivers use the same rules. Help your child develop vocabulary to describe his or her feelings. Use positive messages whenever possible (eg, "Please use your inside voice" instead of "Don't yell"). Consider a parenting class. Encourage healthy habits: good diet, sufficient sleep, physical activity, limited screen time, and outdoor play.

Table 2-1. Advice for Parents Regarding Common Mental Health Concerns (*continued*)

Mental Health Concern	Advice for Parents
Middle Childhood (5–10 Years)	
Poor success at school, learning difficulties, inattention	Attend parent-teacher meetings and school events. Limit screen time. Show interest in your child's school experiences and homework. If your child is struggling academically, request testing by the school psychologist and convey results to your pediatrician. Avoid battles over homework.
Bullying/violence at school	Talk with your child about bullies and bullying. Discuss bullying concerns with school personnel.
Anxiety, worries	Talk about what worries your child. Show your child techniques for relaxing. Instead of avoiding feared activities or objects, reward small steps toward managing fears/brave behavior. If you learn that your child's worries began after a frightening or painful experience, let your pediatrician know.
Behavioral problems (impulsivity/tantrums/ aggression/ oppositionality)	Notice and praise your child's good behavior. Do not hit, spank, or yell at your child. Set age-appropriate limits on your child's behavior and ensure all caregivers use the same rules. Help your child talk about his or her feelings. Consider a parenting class. Encourage healthy habits: good diet, sufficient sleep, physical activity, limited screen time, and outdoor play. Discuss your concerns with your child's teacher.
Depression	Help your child talk about his or her feelings. Encourage activities that make your child feel happy, confident, and generous. Encourage healthy habits: good diet, sufficient sleep, physical activity, limited screen time, and outdoor play.
Late Childhood and Adolescence (11–18 Years)	
School problems	Attend parent-teacher conferences and school events. Monitor and limit screen time and use of social media. Show interest in your child's school experiences and homework. Praise your child's positive accomplishments in school and involvement in extracurricular activities. Check in with your child's teacher about academic progress and relationships with peers. If your child is struggling academically, request testing by the school psychologist and convey results to your pediatrician. Avoid battles over homework.

Table 2-1. Advice for Parents Regarding Common Mental Health Concerns (*continued*)	
Mental Health Concern	**Advice for Parents**
Late Childhood and Adolescence (11–18 Years)	
Depression/suicide	Listen to your adolescent's hopes and concerns. Encourage activities that make your adolescent feel happy, confident, and generous and those that promote his or her sense of belonging (eg, sports team, extracurricular program, group music or arts activities, volunteer project, youth group, boys' or girls' club). Encourage healthy habits: good diet, sleep, physical activity, and limited screen time. Be sure your child does not have access to weapons or medications. With your pediatrician create a plan for emergency care in case your adolescent experiences thoughts of self-harm or harming others.
Anxiety	Set aside time to listen to your teen's hopes and concerns. Encourage healthy habits: good diet, sleep, physical activity, and limited screen time. Support your adolescent as he or she figures out healthy ways other than avoidance to relax and deal with the stress of participating in activities important to his or her development. Monitor and limit screen time and use of social media.
Substance use or abuse	Make sure your son or daughter knows how you feel about alcohol and drugs. Know his or her friends and whereabouts. Be a positive role model. Have a safety plan in case your son or daughter finds himself or herself in a car driven by someone who is high.
Sexual abuse/dating violence	Know your son or daughter's friends and whereabouts. Model and talk with him or her about healthy, respectful relationships.

Common elements interventions. Common elements of evidence-based psychosocial therapies may be amenable to use in primary care. See Chapter 10, Adapting Psychosocial Interventions to Primary Care, for further discussion and Appendix 7, Common Elements of Evidence-Based Practice Amenable to Primary Care: Indications and Sources, for a synopsis. If screening results, completed behavior checklists, findings from clinical assessment, or observations over the course of visits suggest that the patient's problem predominantly involves the common concerns, signs, or symptoms included as titles in Chapters 13 through 32 of this book, readers can find evidence-informed guidance for further assessment of the patient and initial management. This guidance can be applied even when the patient's symptoms do not reach the threshold for a disorder. In addition, many signs and symptoms not named in the chapter titles, but mentioned within those chapters, are listed in the index.

Inter-visit activities for these children might include an evidence-based electronic treatment program (Internet or software applications).

Several natural strategies for promoting mentally healthy lifestyles have been identified by the AAP Section on Complementary, Holistic, and Integrative Medicine and the TFMH (Box 2-2). These are universally applicable, safe interventions that can potentially enhance any child's well-being.

Stress reduction. A number of mind-body therapies can be helpful to children, adolescents, and family members who are experiencing stress. These include breathing techniques, relaxation (eg, progressive muscle relaxation), mental imagery, and self-hypnosis. Adjunctive use of biofeedback may also be useful. See Chapter 8, Self-regulation Therapies and Biofeedback, for more discussion about these approaches.

Assistance with behavior change. For patients engaged in unhealthy behaviors or families whose routines (or lack thereof) are contributing to MH problems in their child or adolescent, motivational interviewing can be effective in overcoming barriers to behavior change. See Chapter 5,

---

Box 2-2. Natural Strategies for Promoting Mental Health

- Outdoor time (with appropriate skin protection)
- Special one-on-one time for child with caregiver
- Sufficient sleep
- Social connections
- Good nutrition
- Expressions of appreciation and kindness
- Physical activity
- Limited screen time
- Stress management through self-regulation techniques

Effective Communication Methods: Common Factors Skills, for further guidance in applying these techniques.

Self-help resources. These resources can include books, pamphlets, and important websites (Box 2-3).

Facilitate referral of family member for MH specialty or social services, if indicated

In some circumstances, a family member may need assistance with his or her socioeconomic problems, MH needs, or parenting. The clinician can explore this person's readiness to seek and accept help and initiate referrals accordingly, taking care to avoid "blaming" language. The clinician can also offer community resources and educational materials that may aid family members in understanding the child's or adolescent's MH concern(s).

Schedule return(s) or outreach as needed to assess response, complete RHS, try additional interventions, or advance to step 12

It is important to leave the patient and family with reassurance about their ongoing relationship with the clinician and the medical home. This may involve scheduling a return to assess response to initial interventions, try additional interventions, or advance to the next step of the algorithm. The clinician can monitor the child's progress by enlisting the parents to

---

Box 2-3. Helpful Web Sites for Families of Children With Behavioral Problems

- Healthy Children (www.healthychildren.org)
- Zero to Three (www.zerotothree.org)
- National Alliance on Mental Illness (www.nami.org)
- American Psychological Association (www.apa.org)
- Children and Adults with Attention-Deficit/Hyperactivity Disorder (www.chadd.org)
- National Federation of Families for Children's Mental Health (www.ffcmh.org)
- Substance Abuse and Mental Health Services Administration (www.samhsa.gov)
- American Academy of Child and Adolescent Psychiatry (www.aacap.org)

observe for persistence or worsening of symptoms in the interim. In some circumstances, the clinician or another member of the primary care team may check in with the family periodically by telephone, text, or e-mail, depending on privacy considerations and the family's preferences. If addressing the MH concern has distracted from completing the routine health supervision visit, it is important to reschedule the patient to complete that process. Inclusion of the patient on the practice registry and application of monitoring mechanisms will assure that he is not lost to follow-up and that any member of the primary care team can inquire about his progress at the time of return visits. At the close of every visit, the clinician can return to the HELP mnemonic (see Box 2-1) to ensure that all components have been completed.

Full diagnostic assessment needed? [12]

In the absence of functional impairment or indications of a specific, treatable condition, further assessment may not be necessary. Examples include a 10-year-old who is attending a new school and experiencing decreased sociability, an adolescent mother with mild anxiety, sleeplessness in a toddler whose parent just deployed for military service, increased parent-child conflict at a time of family stress, and flare-ups of chronic but relatively mild problems related to temperament or delayed social skills. In each of these examples and other circumstances involving mild, manageable symptoms, the clinician can proceed to step 13.

Monitor for symptoms and functioning [13]

Indications for further diagnostic assessment include impaired functioning, screening results that suggest the probability of a disorder, symptoms that worsen or persist despite initial primary care interventions, a parent or patient who manifests distress out of proportion to findings, and clinician concern or discomfort. In any of these instances, the process continues at step 14.

Who will provide further assessment? [14]

The decision about whether and when to involve an MH specialist is pivotal. Multiple factors must be taken into account, including the family's preferences; the pediatric clinician's comfort; and the availability, accessibility, and appropriateness of MH, substance use disorder, and developmental specialty resources. Clinicians should consider MH specialty involvement for any child or adolescent whose functioning does not improve with primary care interventions, for one whose symptoms worsened or persisted despite initial interventions, and for a parent, a child, or an adolescent who manifests distress out of proportion to findings.

General guidance for involving a subspecialist can be summarized by age-group.

Newborns, infants, and children from birth to age 5 years

Newborns, infants, and children from birth to 5 years of age with significant symptoms of social-emotional problems (see Chapter 17, Emotional or Behavioral Disturbance in Children Younger Than 5 Years) should ideally receive evaluation and management by specialists. Examples of problems requiring specialty care of young children include poor attachment, disordered parent-child relationship, parental mental illness, language or communication delay (often associated with social-emotional concerns), disruptive behavior with aggression, abuse or neglect of the child, and self-injury.

For this age-group, the clinician can consider referring the child for assessment by a developmental-behavioral pediatrician (DBP), an MH specialist with expertise in early childhood, a therapist for the parent or the parent-child dyad, or a specific professional (eg, speech pathologist, developmental evaluation team, or another community resource).

The federal law known as the Individuals with Disabilities Education Act (IDEA) mandates that states have an Early Intervention (EI) agency to identify newborns, infants, and children 0 to 3 years of age (Part C of IDEA) with developmental delays. States receiving certain categories of federal funding must provide assessment (not necessarily including general or subspecialty pediatric assessment) and an Individualized Family Service Plan (commonly known as IFSP) to all 0- to 3-year-olds who are substantiated as abused or neglected or who are identified as affected by illegal SU or withdrawal symptoms that result from prenatal drug exposure. Newborns, infants, and children 0 to 3 years of age who qualify for services (ie, occupational, physical, or speech therapy; education) must receive them in the least restrictive environment (commonly known as LRE), usually their homes, on the basis of their respective documented delays in language, motor, personal social, and adaptive domains.[19] Some states provide EI services free of charge or charge on a sliding fee scale according to families' incomes; others do not provide financial assistance. Some states go beyond the IDEA mandates to screen for developmental risk factors and social-emotional problems and extend EI services to children with these concerns. Primary care clinicians will need specific knowledge about the range of EI services provided in their own states and the process for gaining access to them.

Developmental and educational services for children aged 3 to 5 years are mandated and regulated by the IDEA Part B. In most states, the public school system is responsible for developmental assessment and education of children with significant delays, whereas in other states, the EI programs continue to provide assessment and services for this age-group.

See Chapter 17, Emotional or Behavioral Disturbance in Children Younger Than 5 Years, for examples of evidence-based interventions for newborns, infants, and young children and their parents or caregivers. High-quality child care and preschool have a long-lasting protective bene-fit, especially for children at high developmental and behavioral risk; clinicians may also refer to these programs.

Children, adolescents, and young adults aged 5 to 21 years

For patients in this age-group, the pediatric clinician may provide further assessment or the clinician may decide to involve a specialist. One or more of the following circumstances typically constitute an indication for specialty referral:

- ▶ Suicidal or homicidal intent
- ▶ Severe functional impairment, regardless of symptoms or diagnosis
- ▶ Rapid cycling mood
- ▶ Depressive symptoms in a preadolescent
- ▶ Extreme outbursts and problems with conduct
- ▶ Severe eating problems
- ▶ Psychotic thoughts or behavior
- ▶ Self-injury

► Comorbidity of SU and MH problems

► Loss of control or compulsive drug use

► Attention-deficit/hyperactivity disorder (ADHD) with comorbidities

► Behavioral or emotional symptoms in a child with a history of abuse, neglect, or other trauma or loss

► Behavioral or emotional symptoms in a child with a developmental disability or physical condition

► Any other problem that the pediatric clinician does not feel prepared to address

Provide full diagnostic assessment in primary care; interpret findings to youth and family [15]

If the decision has been made to provide the full diagnostic assessment in primary care, the PCC can review all the data gathered during previous primary care contacts (previsit health surveillance questionnaires [patient's and family's psychosocial history, risks, and strengths], screening [symptoms, functional impairment, and caregiver's MH], interview [in the context of routine health supervision, acute care, or chronic illness care], observations of the child and parents, response to primary care interventions, functional assessment, and collateral information [from schools, child care, noncustodial parent, and other caregivers; MH specialty evaluation, if any]. Chapter 6, Iterative Mental Health Assessment, includes suggestions for organizing this information and incorporating it into a formulation of specific diagnoses in accordance with the *Diagnostic and Statistical Manual of Mental Disorders* or *Zero to Three: Diagnostic Classification of Mental Health and Developmental Disorders of Infancy and Early Childhood* (www.zerotothree.org/resources/services/dc-0-3r).

Whether or not the patient meets criteria for a disorder, both patient and parents will need an explanation of the clinician's findings, definition of any terms used to describe his condition, and reassurance that the condition is treatable. An explanation of the care planning process can also provide reassurance that the clinician remains committed to help with both care and coordination and that the goals and preferences of the patient and family will be central to that process.

Refer to MH specialist for diagnostic (re)assessment; request results [16]

Specialists in a wide range of disciplines can provide diagnostic (and therapeutic) assistance in these situations, including DBPs, neurodevelopmental pediatricians, adolescent medicine specialists, pediatric neurologists, psychiatrists, clinical psychologists, school psychologists, clinical social workers, licensed professional counselors, licensed marriage and family therapists, advanced practice nurses with specialized psychiatric training, and SU specialists. (See Appendix 4, Sources of Key Mental Health Services.) These professionals may practice in public MH or developmental clinics, in schools, in private practice, or in university settings. Ideally, the referring clinician would have a directory of referral resources. (See Chapter 3, Office and Network Systems to Support Mental Health Care.) It is important to know whether MH specialists that are accessible and affordable to the family have expertise in the care of children and adolescents.

If an MH referral will require authorization by the family's health insurance plan, entry into a "carved-out" or parallel private behavioral health insurance plan, or entry into the public MH system, the family will likely need guidance and time to research the options. The Mental Health Parity and Addiction Equity Act of 2008 may ultimately have the effect of diminishing administrative and financial barriers that have historically impeded access to MH services.[20] Because stigma and administrative, financial, and logistical barriers often prevent children from seeking or receiving MH specialty care, referring clinicians will need to provide support to families in the referral process and in navigating the MH specialty system. (See Chapter 3, Office and Network Systems to Support Mental Health Care.) This support might include telephone or personal contact with staff members, caseworkers, family advocates, or paid providers of peer support services. Written materials that demystify the referral process and the types of MH specialty resources available in the community will reinforce information shared verbally with the patient and family.

As with any other specialty referral, the process is enhanced by clear and efficient communication from the referring clinician to the specialist, stating the primary concern and reason for the referral, and then providing a succinct synopsis of the clinical situation. A structured tool may be useful in this process. For example, Harrison et al have developed a tool called the Five S's to create a common language and structure for PCCs and child psychiatrists participating in a consultation model. Its framework is summarized in Box 2-4.

Although HIPAA allows exchange of information among professionals who are involved in the care of a mutual patient,[21] many MH professionals are reluctant to share information without express consent of the patient and family. By obtaining written consent and providing it to the MH professional along with the referral, the referring clinician can convey interest and facilitate 2-way communication.

It is important that clinicians (or another member of the care team) track patients referred for MH specialty care because many will fail to complete the referral. If the family is unsuccessful in acquiring timely assessment or treatment of the child, the clinician can offer generic interventions as described earlier, further assessment and management strategies, or periodic telephone contacts to monitor for worsening or emergent problems. Unfortunately, it may be necessary in some instances to use emergency procedures to obtain needed services.

Once the diagnostic assessment is complete and the pediatric team has gathered reports and recommendations, the process moves to care planning.

Box 2-4. The Five S's: Key Questions for Consultation

Safety: Are there concerns about safety?

Specific behaviors: What are the behaviors that are causing the most problems?

Setting: Where and when are the most problematic behaviors occurring?

Scary: Have any hard or scary things happened?

Screenings/Services: Has the child had any assessments and/or received any treatment or services?

Reproduced with permission from Harrison J, Wasserman K, Steinberg J, Platt R, Coble K, Bower K. The Five S's: a communication tool for child psychiatric access projects. *Current Probl Pediatr Adolesc Health Care.* 2016;46(12):411–419.

Family-centered care plan [17]

The purpose of a family-centered care plan is to seek improvement in the child's overall emotional health and functioning. Participants in developing and maintaining the plan are the patient and family, the PCC, MH specialists and pediatric subspecialists involved in the patient's care, and others involved in the patient's and family's care and support.

A care planning conference is a helpful (some would say essential) mechanism to develop and coordinate a plan of care for a child or adolescent with an MH or SU disorder. Ideally, all participants (or their representatives) would be present for the care planning conference; however, this may not be feasible. The family should not be placed into the position of transmitting information between professionals who are involved in their child's care; if the inclusion of involved specialists or subspecialists in the care planning conference is not feasible, the PCC needs information from them in advance of the conference to ensure understanding of the patient's problems and the options available for further care. Together, the family, the PCC, and other partners can set the timetable of care, determine need for involvement of additional or alternative specialists, and select interventions. Regardless of whether or not he or she is able to attend, each participant should become familiar with the care plan and take responsibility for updating the plan and other participants when circumstances or the patient's status changes.

For children and adolescents previously involved in MH specialty care, a care plan may already be in place and may omit primary care issues, such as healthy lifestyle (eg, nutrition, exercise, sleep, stress management, social support), routine health supervision, or care of chronic medical conditions. In this instance, rather than developing a new or an alternative plan of care, pediatric clinicians can augment the existing plan by pointing to the roles they can play in coordinating and complementing the care of the MH specialists.

Some children with severely impairing emotional disturbance may have an MH or EI care manager, a peer navigator, or both involved in their care; if so, the participation of these individuals is central to the process. The care manager may organize periodic meetings of teachers, social workers, and agency representatives involved with the patient and family.

In the MH specialty system, such processes are sometimes called a *system of care* approach, that is, a coordination system built around the family's strengths and priorities.[22] If such a system exists, the PCC (or staff representative), often inadvertently omitted, can join in that process as an alternative to convening a primary care conference.

Participation in care planning is time-consuming. A primary care–integrated MH specialist can be a tremendous asset to the PCC in the care planning process, representing primary care perspectives and ensuring coordination of medical and MH specialty care. In the absence of an integrated MH specialist, participation by the PCC or another member of the primary care team is valuable to the patient and family and may ultimately produce efficiencies in the care of children and adolescents with complex conditions. In the future, secure electronic methods may be developed to house care plans that are accessible to the family and to all those participating in the patient's care.

The care plan has a number of functions: family engagement, exchange of information, medication reconciliation, coordination, and monitoring of treatment effects. Box 2-5 outlines elements of a family-centered care plan for a child or adolescent with an MH problem.

Several steps in the care planning process deserve emphasis:

Summarize strengths and needs (patient's and family's)

This component of the planning process draws from psychosocial assessment of the patient and family to develop a shared understanding of protective factors and the patient's and family's needs, which may include psychoeducation; social services; educational assistance; psychosocial therapy, pharmacological therapy, or both; primary care; care coordination; and social support.

Articulate patient's and family's goals

This critical component of the care planning process gives voice to the patient's short- and long-term health and educational goals, as well as the family's goals for the patient. They might include, for example, lifestyle changes; goals for improvement in functioning and decrease of symptoms; goals for school attendance and performance; vocational goals;

Box 2-5. Elements of a Family-Centered Care Plan

- The patient's preferences for what he/she would like to be called by members of the care team.
- Family context (eg, demographic information, cultural and religious issues important to the family, list of family members with whom the health system has permission to share information).
- The patient's and family's strengths and needs; patient's baseline functioning at home, school, and with peers; patient's short-term and long-term health and educational goals; and action plan for achieving them.
- A record of shared decision-making processes that have taken place.
- Documentation of conflict resolution strategies between the patient or family and the care team (eg, any actions that may cause conflict and the patient's and family's views on how to resolve conflict most effectively).
- Any further information that the patient and family want the care team to know.
- Documentation of dialogue with the patient and family about the benefits of having a shared record, discussion of any risks or concerns about shared records, and explanation of precautions taken to protect the confidentiality of MH records.
- Patient and family psychoeducation about conditions, treatments, and self-management, including monitoring for adverse treatment effects and signs or symptoms suggesting a psychiatric emergency.
- Team roles and goals—the team members responsible for specific goals or tasks, including a list of other providers in the larger health network who have standing permission to exchange information.
- Names and roles of school- or community-based support and other services outside the health system and the status of permission to exchange information with each of them.
- Medical treatments, including pharmacological treatment (shared problem list and medication list).
- Role of psychotherapy, community groups, or other nonpharmacological behavioral health or substance use disorder therapy or support.
- Counseling or coaching (eg, motivational interviewing, behavioral activation).
- Contingency plan for emergency care, if needed.
- For adolescents, a plan for transition to adult medical and MH services.
- A "sign-out" summary consisting of the care team's brief overview of the patient's health status at each episode of care.

Abbreviation: MH, mental health.

Adapted from Agency for Healthcare Research and Quality. Develop a shared care plan. AHRQ Web site. http://www.integrationacademy.ahrq.gov/products/playbook/develop-shared-care-plan. Accessed February 7, 2018.

goals for self-care or family care; and, ultimately, plans for the transition to adult primary care and specialty health services. Achievement of established goals provides benchmarks for monitoring the patient's and family's progress in care.

Reach agreement with family, school, agencies (+ MH specialists and pediatric subspecialists, if involved) on care components, including psychoeducation and a plan for emergency care

Appendix 4 provides a comprehensive listing of key MH services the patient or family may need. When needed services are unavailable or inaccessible within the community, participants in the patient's care will need to accommodate as well as possible through the care planning process.

Critically important elements of care are the psychoeducation of the patient and family—demystification of symptoms, explanation of terms they are likely to encounter in seeking care, description of effective therapies and the professionals who provide them, and anticipated course—and symptoms and signs that indicate adverse treatment effects, worsening of the condition, or the need for emergency care. The family and all team members should have a common understanding of a contingency plan for emergency care, if it should be needed.

Define roles of family and others

The care plan should indicate who is responsible for each element of care, including psychoeducation of the patient and family.

Responsibility for collecting reports from referral sources can be assigned to the PCC's staff members, in accordance with office protocols, or to a care coordinator or navigator external to the practice. Fax-back forms, developed collaboratively by PCCs and MH professionals in a community, have been successfully used for this purpose.[10] Telephone and e-mail contacts may be helpful in some instances, if privacy can be assured.

For children in the foster care system, the assigned social service agency must authorize exchange of information. It is important to collect information from caseworkers and to convey information back to the worker. If the child changes placement and the caregivers are unaware of previous health assessment, plan of care, and sources of care, the child experiences discontinuity of health care as well as placement. In some situations, the pediatric clinician may need to be the primary advocate for the MH of a child in the foster system, expressing concerns and recommendations clearly and repeatedly to the appropriate social service agency.

The decision about which clinicians to involve depends on the types of therapy the patient needs.

Evidence-based psychosocial therapies

There are many effective evidence-based psychosocial therapies (often simply called *therapy* in MH parlance) for children and adolescents with MH and SU disorders, including a growing number of electronic, interactive programs to address specific concerns. See Chapter 7, Psychosocial Therapies, for a synopsis of these treatments and Appendix 6 for a table summarizing the level of evidence supporting them. In deciding on a referral source, it is important to know which evidence-based treatments a therapist provides.

Psychotropic medications

A number of childhood mental disorders are responsive to psychotropic medications. Chapter 11, Psychotropic Medications in Primary Care, describes these medications and provides a rationale that the PCC can apply in determining which medications she can safely and effectively prescribe. *Any child who is diagnosed as having a mental disorder and who is a candidate for psychotropic medication should be offered concomitant evidence-based psychosocial therapy.* See Chapter 7, Psychosocial Therapies, for further information about these therapies.

Responsibility for prescribing medication depends on a number of factors. For children or adolescents with ADHD, major depressive disorder, or generalized anxiety disorder (which fall within MH patient care competencies proposed by the AAP[5]), PCCs may choose to prescribe and monitor a psychotropic medication themselves. For children or adolescents with multiple conditions or other conditions, a child psychiatrist, a DBP, a neurologist, an adolescent specialist, or another licensed PCC with specialized MH training would ideally participate in the patient's care, either by prescribing the psychotropic medication or by consulting with the PCC in the use of medication.

Whichever physician prescribes the psychotropic medication, responsibility may fall to the PCC to ensure that the patient is monitored for adverse effects, either by the prescribing physician or by the PCC, and that care of the patient's medical conditions is coordinated with the MH care.

Care plan implementation, comanagement, and monitoring [18]

This step may require collection of collateral data; information exchange between the PCC and other participants in care, including schools, MH specialists, and agencies; multiple primary care visits; multiple visits to MH specialists; outreach from the primary care practice to the patient, the family, and other involved professionals; or some combination of these actions. The following activities contribute to successful implementation of the care plan.

Apply and schedule monitoring mechanisms

To assess the patient's current status, clinicians may rely on progress reports from other professionals involved in the patient's care; functional assessment scales completed by the parent, teacher, and youth; and their own clinical assessments. When pharmacological agents are part of the treatment plan, laboratory tests may be necessary to monitor levels and adverse effects.

Office systems used to organize and monitor the care of children and adolescents with chronic medical conditions such as asthma and diabetes can be applied to the care of patients with MH and SU conditions. (See Chapter 3, Office and Network Systems to Support Mental Health Care.) Elements important to monitoring care of children with MH and SU problems include

▶ *Registries* (lists of children with MH problems that require monitoring): Registries can be developed within the practice for children and adolescents with positive psychosocial screening results, those with concerns that do not rise to the level of a diagnosis, those whose families are not yet ready to seek or accept care for MH problems, those with social concerns that pose a risk to the patient (eg, infants whose mothers have a positive screening result for postpartum depression, children exposed to trauma), children and adolescents with disorders, and those who have been prescribed psychotropic medication.

▶ *Assignment of staff roles* in care of children on the MH and SU registry. Examples might include

- Obtaining parental permission for information exchange with the MH or SU professional and school or child care

- Tracking referral completion

- Scheduling return to the primary care practice

- Gathering collateral data (eg, school or child care progress reports, functional assessment scale)

- Reaching out to patient and family between visits

- Monitoring medication positive and adverse effects

▶ *Forms and tools* to facilitate these office processes.

▶ *Educational tools and resources* for patients and families. (See Box 2-3.)

▶ *Directory of community resources,* including providers of evidence-based psychosocial therapies and parenting programs. (See Appendix 4 for a listing of key services.)

▶ *Resources to support PCCs* in decision-making.

▶ *Coding and billing strategies* to optimize payment.

The interval between primary care contacts will be determined by the acuity and severity of the patient's condition; the patient's and family's strengths, needs, and preferences; adverse effects and monitoring requirements of any treatments; the role of other professionals in monitoring the patient; and the level of the patient's impairment. Just as spirometry measures pulmonary function and assists the clinician in monitoring children with asthma, global functional assessment scales assist the clinician in monitoring children and adolescents with mental illness. See Appendix 2 for a description of these tools.

Coordinate with family and other clinicians

Primary care clinicians can follow the process laid out in the care plan for systematic 2-way communication with the family and other team members.

Schedule RHS for age

Studies show that adults with a mental illness die, on average, a decade or more before their peers, largely from acute and chronic comorbid medical conditions—including cardiovascular and pulmonary diseases, the major causes of mortality in the rest of the population.[23] This suggests that the excessive mortality of people with mental illness may be reduced by preventively addressing their unhealthy behaviors such as smoking, physical inactivity, and poor diet. For this reason it is important to establish routines for providing preventive services to children and adolescents with mental disorders and to include specific plans for their preventive medical care in transitioning them to adulthood.

Primary care within the mental health specialty system

Some MH specialty facilities offer primary care services. These may or may not be oriented toward children and adolescents and may or may not be linked to the patient's pediatric medical home. Primary care clinicians can problem-solve with families about primary care issues and assure that immunizations, age-appropriate anticipatory guidance, other pediatric preventive services, and transition planning are available and accessible to the patient.

Mental health specialty care within pediatric settings

In some parts of the United States, payment structures have the potential to support an MH professional on-site in the primary care practice. Ideally, this professional is fully integrated within the primary care team, accepting "warm handoffs" from the PCC (ie, face-to-face introductions, transfer of trust), participating in real-time decision-making with the family and primary care team, providing MH care, using a common health record, expediting consultation with school- and other community-based MH specialists when indicated, and enhancing communication among the primary care team, family, and involved MH specialists. Such an arrangement has many advantages, including convenience and de-stigmatization for the patient and family, increased adherence to treatment, high PCC and patient satisfaction, and "cross-fertilization" and mutual support of the professionals involved.[24–26] Pediatric subspecialty clinics may also have the opportunity to include MH professionals (eg, a licensed social worker or psychologist) as on-site members of the care team. In these settings, the MH professional can play a role similar to the one described previously. Lacking such an arrangement, pediatric clinicians can build relationships with community-based MH and SU professionals to collaborate in the treatment of children and adolescents with MH and SU problems.

Child psychiatry consultation programs, currently offering support to pediatric PCCs in at least 27 states, have been well received and show promise in expanding pediatric clinicians' comfort and capacity to provide MH services.[27]

Revise plan as needed

All team members should revisit the plan periodically to determine the patient's status, new circumstances that influence treatment or recovery, and new psychoeducational needs that have emerged. They should also affirm the family's role in monitoring for potential emergencies. Inevitably, the care plan will require periodic revision, repeating the process described above for assuring input from the family and all involved providers. Again, communication among all providers is necessary to assure continuity of care and mutual accountability. The PCC can use each contact with the patient and family to convey hopefulness about treatment and recovery.

For adolescents, articulate plan for transition to adult care

Transition planning is an iterative process that begins in adolescence and continues until transition to adult care is complete. Chapter 12, Transitioning Adolescents With Mental Health Conditions to Adult Care, discusses this process in detail.

Concerns resolved? [19]

Applying chronic care principles to the patient's care does not mean that the patient's condition is permanent. Children and families can and do recover from mental illnesses. The clinician can periodically repeat functional assessment and clinical evaluation, collect collateral reports, and reconvene a conference with the family (and adolescent) to determine whether concerns are persisting and whether further assessment or a change of plan is indicated.

Return to step 16: refer to MH specialist for diagnostic (re)assessment; request results [20]

If the patient's problems worsen or do not resolve, reassessment is necessary, typically by an MH specialist.

Monitor for symptoms and functioning [21]

If the patient's problems have resolved, he can return to a schedule of routine health supervision that includes close monitoring for further MH issues. If concerns recur, the clinician can return to algorithm step 9 for guidance.

Summary

Increasingly, PCCs are expected to be a source of MH care, a gateway to specialty MH care, and a source of primary care that is coordinated with specialty MH care. They can recognize emergent situations that compel an immediate intervention, find ways to support and help the family that is resistant to seeking psychosocial care, assess and treat the patient in the primary care setting, or comanage the patient's care with MH professionals. Pediatric subspecialists frequently care for children and adolescents with chronic medical conditions complicated by MH comorbidities. With the requisite competencies and with office systems in place to organize and monitor the care of patients with MH problems, pediatric clinicians are positioned to fulfill these roles. By applying evidence-based communication techniques, the clinician can reduce distress of the patient and family and improve the patient's functioning across a variety of MH problems, even in the absence of a diagnosis and while awaiting MH specialty assessment and treatment.

Factors determining the role of the pediatric clinician in a particular patient's care include the type and severity of problem the patient is experiencing, the family's preferences, the clinician's comfort, and accessibility of MH specialists with pediatric expertise. For children and adolescents with a chronic mental disorder, both PCCs and pediatric subspecialists have a critical role to play in facilitating development of a family-centered plan that coordinates the patient's care and defines roles for the family members and MH specialists involved.

Acknowledgments: The author acknowledges the American Academy of Pediatrics Task Force on Mental Health for authoring Algorithm B and the article that originally described it: Enhancing pediatric mental health care: algorithms for primary care. *Pediatrics.* 2010;125(suppl 3):S109–S125.

The task force included Jane Meschan Foy, MD (chairperson and lead author); Paula Duncan, MD; Barbara Frankowski, MD, MPH; Kelly Kelleher, MD, MPH (lead author); Penelope K. Knapp, MD; Danielle Laraque, MD (lead author); Gary Peck, MD; Michael Regalado, MD; Jack Swanson, MD; and Mark Wolraich, MD; the consultants were Margaret Dolan, MD; Alain Joffe, MD, MPH; Patricia O'Malley, MD; James Perrin, MD; Thomas K. McInerny, MD; and Lynn Wegner, MD; the liaisons were Terry Carmichael, MSW (National Association of Social Workers); Darcy Gruttadaro, JD (National Alliance on Mental Illness); Garry Sigman, MD (Society for Adolescent Medicine); Myrtis Sullivan, MD, MPH (National Medical Association); and L. Read Sulik, MD (American Academy of Child and Adolescent Psychiatry); and the staff members were Linda Paul and Aldina Hovde.

AAP Policy

Adams RC, Tapia C; American Academy of Pediatrics Council on Children With Disabilities. Early intervention, IDEA Part C services, and the medical home: collaboration for best practice and best outcomes. *Pediatrics.* 2013;132(4):e1073–e1088. Reaffirmed May 2017 (pediatrics.aappublications.org/content/132/4/e1073)

American Academy of Pediatrics Committee on Hospital Care and Institute for Patient- and Family-Centered Care. Patient- and family-centered care and the pediatrician's role. *Pediatrics.* 2012;129(2):394–404 (pediatrics.aappublications.org/content/129/2/394)

American Academy of Pediatrics Committee on Psychosocial Aspects of Child and Family Health and Task Force on Mental Health. The future of pediatrics: mental health competencies for pediatric primary care. *Pediatrics.* 2009;124(1):410–421. Reaffirmed August 2013 (pediatrics.aappublications.org/content/124/1/410)

American Academy of Pediatrics Section on Integrative Medicine. Mind-body therapies in children and youth. *Pediatrics.* 2016;138(3):e20161896 (pediatrics.aappublications.org/content/138/3/e20161896)

Chun TH, Mace SE, Katz ER; American Academy of Pediatrics Committee on Pediatrics Emergency Medicine, American College of Emergency Physicians Pediatric Emergency Medicine Committee. Evaluation and management of children and adolescents with acute mental health or behavioral problems. Part I: common clinical challenges of patients with mental health and/or behavioral emergencies. *Pediatrics.* 2016;138(3):e20161570 (pediatrics.aappublications.org/content/138/3/e20161570)

Chun TH, Mace SE, Katz ER; American Academy of Pediatrics Committee on Pediatrics Emergency Medicine, American College of Emergency Physicians Pediatric Emergency Medicine Committee. Evaluation and management of children with acute mental health or behavioral problems. Part II: recognition of clinically challenging mental health related conditions presenting with medical or uncertain symptoms. *Pediatrics.* 2016;138(3):e20161573 (pediatrics.aappublications.org/content/138/3/e20161573)

References

1. President's New Freedom Commission on Mental Health. *Achieving the Promise: Transforming Mental Health Care in America; Final Report.* Rockville, MD: Substance Abuse and Mental Health Services Administration; 2003. DHHS publication SNA-03-3832. http://govinfo.library.unt.edu/mentalhealthcommission/reports/FinalReport/downloads/downloads.html. Accessed February 7, 2018

2. Center for Mental Health Services, National Institute of Mental Health. *Mental Health: A Report of the Surgeon General.* Bethesda, MD: National Institutes of Health; 1999. https://profiles.nlm.nih.gov/ps/access/NNBBHT.pdf. Accessed February 7, 2018

3. American Academy of Pediatrics Task Force on the Future of Pediatric Education. The future of pediatric education II. Organizing pediatric education to meet the needs of infants, children, adolescents, and young adults in the 21st century. A collaborative project of the pediatric community. *Pediatrics.* 2000;105(1, pt 2):157–212

4. American Academy of Child and Adolescent Psychiatry Committee on Health Care Access and Economics, American Academy of Pediatrics Task Force on Mental Health. Improving mental health services in primary care: reducing administrative and financial barriers to access and collaboration. *Pediatrics.* 2009;123(4):1248–1251

5. American Academy of Pediatrics Committee on Psychosocial Aspects of Child and Family Health and Task Force on Mental Health. The future of pediatrics: mental health competencies for pediatric primary care. *Pediatrics.* 2009;124(1):410–421

6. Foy JM; American Academy of Pediatrics Task Force on Mental Health. Enhancing pediatric mental health care: report from the American Academy of Pediatrics Task Force on Mental Health. Introduction. *Pediatrics.* 2010;125(suppl 3):S69–S74

7. Foy JM, Perrin J; American Academy of Pediatrics Task Force on Mental Health. Enhancing pediatric mental health care: strategies for preparing a community. *Pediatrics.* 2010;125(suppl 3):S75–S86

8. Foy JM, Kelleher KJ, Laraque D; American Academy of Pediatrics Task Force on Mental Health. Enhancing pediatric mental health care: strategies for preparing a primary care practice. *Pediatrics.* 2010;125(suppl 3):S87–S108

9. Foy JM; American Academy of Pediatrics Task Force on Mental Health. Enhancing pediatric mental health care: algorithms for primary care. *Pediatrics.* 2010; 125(suppl 3):S109–S125

10. American Academy of Pediatrics Task Force on Mental Health. *Addressing Mental Health Concerns in Primary Care: A Clinician's Toolkit.* Elk Grove Village, IL: American Academy of Pediatrics; 2010

11. Perrin JM, Gnanasekaran S, Delahaye J. Psychological aspects of chronic health conditions. *Pediatr Rev.* 2012;33(3):99–109

12. Barlow JH, Ellard DR. The psychosocial well-being of children with chronic disease, their parents and siblings: an overview of the research evidence base. *Child Care Health Dev.* 2006;32(1):19–31

13. Roy-Byrne PP, Davidson KW, Kessler RC, et al. Anxiety disorders and comorbid medical illness. *Gen Hosp Psychiatry.* 2008;30(3):208–225

14. Delamater AM, de Wit M, McDarby V, Malik J, Acerini CL; International Society for Pediatric and Adolescent Diabetes. ISPAD clinical practice consensus guidelines 2014. Psychological care of children and adolescents with type 1 diabetes. *Pediatr Diabetes.* 2014;15(suppl 20):232–244

15. Weiner L, Kazak AE, Noll RB, Patenaude AF, Kupst MJ. Standards for the psychosocial care of children with cancer and their families: an introduction to the special issue. *Pediatr Blood Cancer.* 2015;62(suppl 5):S419–S424

16. American Academy of Pediatrics Section on Integrative Medicine. Mind-body therapies in children and youth. *Pediatrics.* 2016;138(3):e20161896

17. Resources for health care providers. National Center for Complementary and Integrative Health Web site. https://nccih.nih.gov/health/providers. Updated September 24, 2017. Accessed February 7, 2018

18. Wissow LS, Gadomski A, Roter D, et al. Improving child and parent mental health in primary care: a cluster-randomized trial of communication skills training. *Pediatrics.* 2008;121(2):266–275

19. IDEA 2004: building the legacy; Part C (birth–2 years old). Department of Education Web site. http://idea.ed.gov/part-c/search/new.html. Accessed February 7, 2018

20. Implementation of the Mental Health Parity and Addiction Equity Act. Substance Abuse and Mental Health Administration Web site. https://www.samhsa.gov/health-financing/implementation-mental-health-parity-addiction-equity-act. Updated January 24, 2017. Accessed February 7, 2018

21. Office for Civil Rights. Summary of the HIPAA privacy rule. US Department of Health and Human Services Web site. https://www.hhs.gov/hipaa/for-professionals/privacy/laws-regulations/index.html. Reviewed July 26, 2013. Accessed February 7, 2018

22. SAMHSA: increasing access to behavioral health services and supports through systems of care. Substance Abuse and Mental Health Services Administration Web site. https://www.samhsa.gov/sites/default/files/programs_campaigns/childrens_mental_health/awareness-day-2016-short-report.pdf. Accessed February 7, 2018

23. Walker ER, McGee RE, Druss BG. *JAMA Psychiatry.* 2015;72(4):334–341

24. Williams J, Shore SE, Foy JM. Co-location of mental health professionals in primary care settings: three North Carolina models. *Clin Pediatr (Phila).* 2006;45(6):537–543

25. Butler M, Kane RL, McAlpine D, et al. Integration of mental health/substance abuse and primary care. *Evid Rep Technol Assess (Full Rep).* 2008;(173):1–362

26. Guevara JP, Greenbaum PE, Shera D, Bauer L, Schwarz DF. Survey of mental health consultation and referral among primary care pediatricians. *Acad Pediatr.* 2009;9(2):123–127

27. Straus JH, Sarvet B. Behavioral health care for children: The Massachusetts Child Psychiatry Access Project. *Health Aff (Millwood).* 2014;33(12):2153–5161

Enhancing Pediatric Mental Health Care

Office and Network Systems to Support Mental Health Care

Jane Meschan Foy, MD; Kelly J. Kelleher, MD, MPH;
and Danielle Laraque-Arena, MD

"Pediatric practices are typically child- and family-friendly places and can readily take additional steps to normalize and destigmatize mental health concerns."

Introduction

Promotion of mental health and prevention of mental health problems will involve broad community-level strategies such as decreasing exposure to violence, eliminating adverse social determinants of health (eg, poverty, food insecurity), and enhancing community and school programs that protect and support children and families. Promoting mental health in individual children and families, preventing them from developing mental health problems if possible, and caring for those who develop mental health problems are all part of the continuum of services provided in pediatrics. This chapter will focus specifically on office- and network-level efforts to enhance the effectiveness of these services. Recognizing that pediatricians share the front lines of pediatrics with family physicians, internists, nurse practitioners, and physician assistants, this chapter will encompass all these groups by using the term *primary care clinicians* (PCCs). Pediatric subspecialists may also have longitudinal relationships with children and adolescents and many opportunities to recognize and address their mental health problems; while not explicitly called out in this chapter, subspecialty pediatric practices can potentially benefit from many of the same practice improvement strategies as PCCs.

The authors acknowledge that multisite, multispecialty groups; Federally Qualified Health Centers; and practices integrated within schools and other nonmedical settings are changing the organizational structure of pediatric health care delivery in many parts of the United States. Clinicians working in these settings will need to adapt this chapter's guidance to their respective situations.

Applying the Chronic Care Model to Children With Mental Health Problems

Children with mental health problems are children with special health care needs because most mental health problems have a recurring or relapsing nature. Although many people can and do recover from their mental health problems, they may chronically experience symptoms or some level of impaired functioning or both. Although much of the literature on the chronic care model focuses on medical rather than mental health conditions and on adults rather than children with mental illness,[1,2] the American Academy of Pediatrics (AAP) Task Force on Mental Health (TFMH) (2004–2010) recognized the applicability of chronic care methods to children with mental health problems and the potential importance of these methods in creating a "medical home" and "medical neighborhood" for children who experience mental health problems.

The payoff at the network and practice levels can be substantial. For example, most studies on adults with depression treated with chronic care methods in primary care settings have documented significant improvement in quality and outcomes,[3] as have 3 studies on adolescent collaborative care.[4-6] Moreover, a number of studies have shown decreases in the cost of care or reductions in the use of health services.[3]

Many practices and health systems will not be able to implement quickly all the elements of the chronic care model. Practice change is a slow and incremental process that requires learning and modification at the practice level along with supportive infrastructure and payment mechanisms at the network level. Primary care clinicians and managers can consider which strategies seem most feasible and are most consistent with other aspects of their practice and gradually plan the enhancements they choose in collaboration with specialty partners and larger health systems.

The Mental Health Practice Readiness Inventory (Appendix 3), developed by the TFMH as a portal into its toolkit[7] and revised in April 2017, can assist PCCs and managers in assessing the strengths and needs of the practice and in setting its priorities. The inventory is organized in accordance with key elements of the chronic care model: community resources, health care financing, support for children and families, clinical information systems and delivery system redesign, and decision support for clinicians. While initially developed for PCCs, the inventory has many aspects that may also apply to pediatric subspecialty practices wishing to enhance the mental health care they provide; such efforts should be closely coordinated with PCCs wherever possible. Individual clinicians and practices may have limited influence over some of these elements at the system level, but there are steps that any practice can take to improve mental health service delivery. Segments of the inventory precede each section of the narrative that follows.

Primary care clinicians may find changes more manageable if they gain experience first by addressing needs of children and adolescents in their practice with identified mental disorders. Discussions with mental health specialists about these patients will enhance the collaborative and clinical skills of PCCs, and experience with scheduling, coding, and billing will build a business infrastructure for the practice's mental health services. Primary care clinicians can next apply the chronic care principles to children whose mental health problems do not meet the criteria for a diagnosable disorder but require care and monitoring nevertheless; finally they can move to prevention and mental health promotion activities.

Critically important to the care of children with mental health problems are a community protocol and resources for triaging and managing psychiatric emergencies; see the Clinical Information Systems and Delivery System Redesign section later in this chapter and Chapter 13, Agitation, Suicidality, and Other Psychiatric Emergencies, for guidance in these efforts. Each practice site should be prepared to identify those who need emergency services and to facilitate the child's or adolescent's access to them.

Mental Health Practice Readiness Inventory

To use the guidance in this chapter, apply the following rating system to evaluate your practice:

1 = We do this well; that is, substantial improvement is not currently needed.

2 = We do this to some extent; that is, improvement is needed.

3 = We do not do this well; that is, significant practice change is needed.

For areas with scores of 2 or 3, determine which ones align with strong interest of the practice team and are feasible in the broader context of the health system. These can become the priority for practice change.

Community Resources

Building resilience and promoting mental health in children and adolescents will require the participation of many organizations and individuals throughout the community. (See Chapter 4 for a full discussion.) Prevention and treatment of childhood mental illness will require strong collaborative relationships between PCCs and the agencies and individuals providing social services to families and between PCCs and mental health specialists. These collaborations will function in ways that will improve the PCC's practice and improve patient care. See Table 3-1 for prompts related to community resources.

Create an inventory of community mental health and substance use disorder resources (and the types of payment accepted) and community sources of social support

The guide might include developmental-behavioral pediatricians, adolescent specialists, mental health and substance abuse specialists; family support groups; Early Intervention (EI) services; human service agencies; nonprofit and faith-based sources of social, legal, and spiritual support; child care consultants; parenting education programs; key school contacts; youth organizations; recreation programs; and others who are involved in supporting or serving children, adolescents, and families.

Appendix 4 summarizes key mental health services necessary to care for children with mental health problems. A variety of specialists may be

Table 3-1. Mental Health Practice Readiness Inventory: Community Resources			
Topic	**Score**		**Target**
Inventory of referral resources	1 2 3		Practice has an up-to-date inventory of accessible developmental-behavioral pediatricians, adolescent medicine specialists, or child psychiatrists (or any combination thereof); community- and school-based mental health and substance use professionals trained in evidence-based therapies, including trauma-focused care; Early Intervention program; special education programs; evidence-based parenting education programs; child protection agencies; youth recreational programs; family and peer support programs; evidence-based home visiting programs; and mental health care coordinators.
Core services	1 2 3		Practice team is knowledgeable about eligibility requirements, contact points, and services of the programs and providers listed previously and type or types of payment they accept.
Collaborative relationships	1 2 3		Practice team has collaborative relationships with school- and community-based providers of key services.

qualified and paid to offer evidence-based services, depending on state licensing policies and insurers' credentialing decisions. The selection of service providers depends on current information about the safety and efficacy of various treatments for the common childhood mental disorders. See Appendix 6 for sources of this information.

Methods to use in creating or adapting a resource guide for the practice are detailed in a kit developed by the AAP. (See www.aap.org/en-us/advocacy-and-policy/aap-health-initiatives/Mental-Health/Pages/Chapter-Action-Kit.aspx.) Organizations in the community (eg, the public mental health agency; the department of public health; the local mental health association; local branches of consumer organizations such as the National Alliance on Mental Illness and the Federation of Families for Children's Mental Health; support groups for families of children with specific disabilities, such as autism spectrum disorder and attention-deficit/hyperactivity disorder [ADHD]) typically benefit from such an inventory and are willing to participate in developing it or in building on one that is already in place.

It is important to note the type or types of third-party payment that each specialist or resource accepts and the types of assessment or therapies (or both) they provide. Early Intervention services are critical for young children who are experiencing social-emotional or developmental problems.[8] As federally mandated services, they are universally available in the United States but variable in quality and accessibility. Details about EI referral criteria and intake procedures are important to include in the inventory.

The burgeoning body of knowledge about early brain development calls attention to the critical importance of parenting, attachment, and high-quality child care on the emotional, social, and cognitive development of young children.[9] Many communities have begun offering such services as nurse visits to pregnant and parenting women who are at high risk, parenting programs, child care consultation, and therapeutic child care settings. In fact, a growing number of practices are offering evidence-based parenting programs either in the primary care setting or in partnership with community agencies, a practice recommended by individual members of the Collaborative on Healthy Parenting in Primary Care.[10] For children affected by violence or other trauma, a US Task Force on Community Preventive Services review[11] updated in 2017[12] and a summary of evidence created using the PracticeWise Evidence-Based Services Database (see Appendix 6 and updates posted biannually at www.aap.org/en-us/Documents/CRPsychosocialInterventions.pdf) differ from each other in some respects but concur in listing individual cognitive behavioral therapy (CBT) and CBT with parents as having the best supporting evidence. Ideally, these services would be available in every community and accessible to children in the practice.

These resources should be included in the inventory, along with resources to help parents and teachers who are dealing with anxiety, depression, substance use, mental illness, trauma, or other personal challenges that affect the quality or continuity of their relationships with young children.

The AAP is active in raising awareness of powerful social determinants of health, such as food and housing insecurity and poverty.[13-17] It is important to include in the resource inventory agencies and organizations capable of offering financial, legal, and social support to families in need and to note the eligibility criteria for each of these services.

Schools are key partners in providing mental health services to children and in collecting data about children's academic and social functioning. In rural areas of the country, they may, in fact, be the major provider of mental health services to children.[18] Guidance counselors are typically the initial contact for clinicians seeking to establish a connection with the child's school; these counselors, school nurses, or other school-based personnel may be helpful in making classroom observations, gathering behavioral scales from teachers, assisting with implementation of classroom interventions, and pursuing testing for special educational services. They may also assist the PCC in monitoring a child's progress and providing support and education to the family. A school psychologist can provide psychological testing, a school social worker can often provide counseling and linkage to other school and community resources, and the school system's special education officer can assist in determining a child's eligibility for special educational services or respond to questions about those services. School-based health centers may house additional professionals, including mental health specialists; when collaborative relationships exist between school-based health centers and PCCs, these centers augment, rather than fragment, care. In fact, school locations are often extensions of primary care sites for many Federally Qualified Health Centers and other community health programs providing primary care.

Involvement in extracurricular school activities enhances a child's attachment to school and improves his or her resilience.[19,20] Involvement in community service and involvement in a faith community are also protective factors for youths.[18-22] Recreation programs, youth groups, and family support groups may all play significant roles in providing children and adolescents with positive experiences and social skills; for this reason, all are relevant to child and adolescent mental health and warrant inclusion in the practice's resource directory.

Become knowledgeable about the available community resources

Most clinicians are understandably reluctant to refer to sources that are unfamiliar to them. Chapter 4, Partnering to Improve Community Mental Health Systems, suggests some strategies for getting to know mental health specialists and other child advocates through participation in efforts to address community mental health issues and gaps in services. In a policy statement on mental health competencies, the AAP suggests ideas for joint educational efforts, which may serve the additional purpose of fostering interpersonal relationships.[23]

Referred families are also an invaluable source of information about community resources. Primary care practices can annotate their resource directories with the feedback received from patients and families. This information will assist clinicians in creating matches between families and service providers or community programs. Practices might consider adding families affected by mental health problems to their family advisory groups or similar councils. (See the section on Support for Children and Families, later in this chapter.)

Develop collaborative relationships with providers of key services

A priori understanding about respective roles of primary care team members and key mental health service providers can create efficiencies and improve coordination of care before actual cases arise. For example, school personnel and PCCs can meet to determine how they will collaboratively assess and monitor the progress of children with learning and behavioral problems that affect school performance. Together, they can decide what circumstances or symptoms will trigger an evaluation at the school; what tools will be used to measure the child's cognitive ability, academic achievement, and classroom behavior; who will gather the information and relay it to the PCC; and what mechanisms will be used to convey the PCC's assessment and care plan back to the school and monitor the child's progress in the classroom.[24] Similarly, prior understanding with community agencies, such as child protective services or the juvenile justice system, about collecting a psychosocial and medical history from the biological parents before the child's placement in foster care or a juvenile detention facility can greatly improve continuity of care and assessment of the child's or adolescent's mental health needs.

Ultimately, collaborative clinical relationships are built through jointly caring for children and families. Personal contact and conversation are the starting point, yet these can be challenging for busy PCCs and mental health and human service professionals. Mental health professionals often lack "front-office" personnel and instead function with little support and use voice mail to capture messages while they are in therapy sessions. They are also extremely protective of their patients' confidentiality, often exceeding standards of the Health Insurance Portability and Accountability Act (HIPAA). A pediatric practice can develop office procedures to support collaboration (eg, routinely requesting families to sign a consent for exchange of information at the time of a referral; developing a prior understanding with mental health colleagues about a convenient time to chat; providing mental health colleagues with the PCC's direct line; hosting "lunch and learn" sessions for primary care team members and mental health professionals to exchange information, review cases, and coordinate care). See the Clinical Information Systems and Delivery System Redesign section, later in this chapter, for more detail about the types of collaborative relationships that clinicians can nurture and office procedures to support collaboration.

Human service professionals (eg, public health; social services; Women, Infants, and Children [commonly known as WIC] Food and Nutrition Services) are often stretched thin by the many administrative demands of their agencies, high caseloads, and the needs of their clients. Primary care clinicians can develop personal relationships with supervisors and familiarity with intake and communication procedures. Primary care clinicians whose patients generate a high demand for services of a particular agency can consider requesting a designated liaison from the agency to the practice and offering a workstation within the clinic and a scheduled conference time for the liaison to meet with clinicians in the practice.

Health Care Financing

To sustain innovations that improve care, PCCs will require substantial enhancements in payment for their mental health services. See Table 3-2 for prompts related to health care financing.

Provide a realistic business framework for mental health services

Many PCCs in the United States are not adequately paid for the mental health care they provide. In some cases, this inadequate payment is because PCCs are not aware of coding mechanisms that lead to payment. In other cases, it is because insurers do not pay for the mental health

Table 3-2. Mental Health Practice Readiness Inventory: Health Care Financing			
Topic	**Score**		**Target**
Third-party payment	1	2	3	Practice has access to specialty provider lists and authorization procedures of major public and private health plans insuring patients in the practice and has processes for addressing claim denials and gaps in benefits and payment.
Coding	1	2	3	Practice has coding and billing procedures to capture payment for primary care mental health–related services covered by major health plans.

services that PCCs provide (screening, assessment, EI to address emerging problems that do not rise to the level of disorders, interaction with schools and agencies, consultation with mental health specialty providers, care coordination, patient and family education, and family conferences). Furthermore, many insurers do not allow PCCs to serve as mental health providers; instead, their insurance plans have mental health "carve-outs," that is, separate mental health specialty networks with separate gatekeeping or intake procedures that exclude PCCs from participation and disallow payment of PCCs for the mental health treatment services they provide to children and adolescents with mental health diagnoses. All these factors contribute to a lessening of financial support for primary care activities in the treatment and management of children and adolescents with or at risk for mental health problems.

Preparation for enhancements in mental health practice will require advocacy efforts aimed at insurers of their patients and major purchasers of their patients' insurance plans. Strategies applicable to these efforts are detailed in the AAP chapter action kit at www.aap.org/en-us/advocacy-and-policy/aap-health-initiatives/Mental-Health/Pages/Chapter-Action-Kit.aspx. A white paper developed jointly by the TFMH and the American Academy of Child and Adolescent Psychiatry, addressing the administrative and financial barriers to providing collaborative mental health care, was published in April 2009 in *Pediatrics*.[25]

Gain access to mental health and substance use disorder provider lists and authorization procedures of major public and private health insurers

Because mental health benefits and formularies are quite variable and often poorly understood by patients and families, many offices struggle to find out what resources are appropriate for referral, what medications are covered, and what the patient cost sharing for such services is likely to be. Some large insurers are providing online resources for rapid access. American Academy of Pediatrics chapter pediatric councils are forums whereby pediatricians meet with health plan medical directors to discuss carrier policies and administrative practices that affect access to, quality of, coverage of, and payment for pediatric services. (See AAP Practice Transformation Online at www.aap.org/en-us/professional-resources/practice-transformation/Pages/practice-transformation.aspx.) Pediatricians in a region (or perhaps AAP chapter or district) can collaborate or work through their council to acquire or develop portals through which practices can identify appropriate resources and drug formularies for insured patients.

Prepare the practice to code and bill effectively to ensure payment for mental health services

Informed by AAP coding resources (www.aap.org/en-us/professional-resources/practice-transformation/getting-paid/Coding-at-the-AAP/Pages/Resources.aspx), primary care practices can create encounter forms to capture necessary documentation and ensure that the mental health services provided are billed for appropriately and efficiently.

Support for Children and Families

Pediatric practices are typically child- and family-friendly places and can readily take additional steps to normalize and destigmatize mental health concerns. Engagement of children, adolescents, and their families in their own care is one of the best correlates of successful outcomes. Such efforts may focus on patient and family motivation, education, skill building, or emotional support. When mental health specialty care is needed, patients and families need support in the referral process. See Table 3-3 for prompts related to support for children and families.

Table 3-3. Mental Health Practice Readiness Inventory: Support for Children, Adolescents, and Families			
Topic	**Score**		**Target**
First contact	1	2	3	Staff has good "first-contact skills" to help children, adolescents, and families feel welcome and respected.
Culturally effective care	1	2	3	Practice team is supportive of people facing mental health challenges, demonstrating sensitivity to cultural differences and avoiding stigmatizing language.
Mental health promotion	1	2	3	Practice team promotes the importance of mental health through posters, practice Web sites, newsletters, handouts, or brochures and by incorporating conversations about mental health into each office visit.
Confidentiality	1	2	3	Practice team assures children, adolescents, and families of confidentiality in accordance with standard medical ethics and state and federal laws.
Adolescents	1	2	3	Practice team is prepared to address mental health and substance use needs of adolescents.
Engagement	1	2	3	Practice team actively elicits mental health and substance use concerns, assesses patients' and families' readiness to address them, and engages children, adolescents, and families in planning their own mental health care at their own pace.
Self-management and family management	1	2	3	Practice team fosters self-management and family management (eg, provides patient and family educational materials appropriate to literacy level and culture, articulates patient's and family's roles in care plan, stays abreast of online and print self-care resources).
Referral assistance	1	2	3	Practice is prepared to support families through referral assistance and advocacy in the mental health referral process.
Care coordination	1	2	3	Practice routinely seeks to identify children and adolescents in the practice who are involved in the mental health specialty system, ensuring that they receive the full range of preventive medical services and monitoring their mental health or substance use conditions.

Topic	Score			Target
Table 3-3. Mental Health Practice Readiness Inventory: Support for Children, Adolescents, and Families (*continued*)				
Special populations	1	2	3	Practice team is prepared to address mental health needs of special populations within the practice (eg, those with ACEs and other social adversities; those with disrupted families caused by military deployment, separation, divorce, incarceration, or foster care; LGBTQ children and adolescents; those in the juvenile justice system; those whose family members have mental health or substance use problems; those who have experienced immigration, racism, homophobia, homelessness, violence, or natural disasters).
Family centeredness	1	2	3	Practice has family members involved in advising the practice; practice team periodically assesses the family centeredness of the practice.
Trauma-informed care	1	2	3	Practice team is knowledgeable about the impact of trauma; considers impact of adversities and traumatic life events in context of behavioral concerns and pays attention to resilience factors and trauma reminders; offers support, resources, and referral to evidence-based trauma services; monitors patient/family adjustment over time; attends to staff members' psychosocial needs with attention to impact of secondary traumatic stress.
Quality improvement	1	2	3	Practice periodically assesses the quality of care provided to children and adolescents with mental health problems and takes action to improve care, in accordance with findings.

Abbreviations: ACE, adverse childhood experience; LGBTQ, lesbian, gay, bisexual, transgender, or questioning.

Ensure that children and families with mental health concerns have a positive first contact with the practice

Clinical staff, receptionists, and administrative staff may figure importantly in a patient's and family's engagement or continuation in mental health care. McKay et al developed a 1-day training that assists staff of outpatient mental health facilities in developing "first-contact skills" (including telephone engagement skills) and in identifying key barriers to seeking mental health care.[26] Evaluation of sites that implemented engagement strategies suggested that they had significantly higher appointment-keeping rates than did sites not implementing these strategies. Although not developed specifically for pediatrics, the application of evidence-based engagement principles is likely to be beneficial to staff in pediatric settings that provide mental health services.

Address stigma

Creating an environment supportive of children, adolescents, and families facing mental health challenges requires that pediatric practices address stigma. Clinicians can reflect with their staff members on the important role they can all play in making patients and families comfortable to share and address mental health concerns. Staff members can examine their own knowledge and attitudes. They can affirm that mental illnesses are treatable; that children, adolescents, and adults living with these illnesses can achieve recovery and lead full and productive lives; and that mental illness is not a character flaw, a sign of moral weakness, or anyone's fault. They can eliminate language that contributes to stigma through defining people by their conditions (eg, referring to someone as "a schizophrenic" or saying, "he is bipolar," instead of "a person with schizophrenia or a bipolar disorder").

Promote the concept of mental health as integral to the care of children and adolescents in the medical home

Separation of mental health services from medical care contributes to stigma, poor coordination of care, and increased costs.[27] The office environment can speak to the importance of mental health and substance use issues (eg, posters that invite mental health and substance use questions, educational materials about common mental health problems, brochures for crisis lines and support groups, meeting places for evening support and treatment groups). (See www.aap.org/en-us/advocacy-and-policy/aap-health-initiatives/Mental-Health/Pages/Tips-For-Pediatricians.aspx.) By implementing *Bright Futures: Guidelines for Health Supervision of Infants, Children, and Adolescents,* 4th Edition, PCCs can normalize mental health care and incorporate conversation about psychosocial issues into every routine health supervision visit. When given the opportunity during a child health supervision visit, most parents will express some concern about a behavioral or developmental issue.[28]

Many PCCs have concerns about the time and expertise required to address mental health concerns and about poor payment for the mental health services they provide.[29] The use of previsit questionnaires and electronic tools to gather information from patients and families in advance of an office visit can allow clinicians to redirect their time from gathering data to addressing concerns.[30–33] The practice can host educational sessions to assist clinicians in acquiring new skills (eg, improving diagnostic skills, gaining knowledge of treatment strategies, applying effective communication techniques to address concerns during primary care encounters, developing a contingency or crisis plan for urgent mental health problems, closing a visit in a supportive and efficient manner, facilitating coding and billing that are specific to mental health).[22,34]

Assure children and families about confidentiality

People with mental health and substance use concerns are usually deeply concerned about confidentiality. Office procedures should ensure that all interactions between staff and the patients and families they serve are private, including sign-in procedures, discussion of the reason for the visit or primary concern, and each phase of the clinical process, including any referrals made to mental health or substance use disorder (SUD) specialists. In accordance with HIPAA, the practice should post information about its privacy rules and offer families written information about them. Staff members can reinforce their commitment to maintaining confidentiality at the time they request consent for exchange of information with other health care professionals and schools. All faxes should have cover sheets that label the information as confidential. When faxing information to schools or agencies that may have fax machines used by multiple staff members, previous arrangements (eg, a call ahead) may be necessary to ensure that the intended recipient is awaiting the fax and protects its confidentiality. Certain mental health information (eg, psychotherapy notes and information related to SUD treatment) is protected by federal statutes that supersede HIPAA.

In states in which minors are allowed to consent for their own mental health and substance use services, there should be a clear understanding with both adolescents and their parents or guardians about "conditional confidentiality," which is the clinician's right and responsibility to break confidentiality if he or she judges the adolescent or others to be in danger. Office procedures must ensure that adolescents treated for a mental health or substance use problem without their parents' or guardians' knowledge express their preferences in relation to messages left on telephones and mailing of communications such as billing statements, laboratory results, and explanations of benefits.

Prepare to address the mental health and substance use needs of adolescents

Children gradually assume responsibility for their own health care. The timing and pace will depend on the child's or adolescent's maturity and cognitive abilities. By the time they reach adolescence, most of them will want an opportunity to air concerns directly with their health care professionals and, at times, to receive care without knowledge of their parents or guardians. The laws governing the confidentiality of minors' health care in relation to their parents or guardians and minors' legal rights to consent without parental knowledge to various types of care, such as reproductive choice, behavioral health, and others, vary from state to state.[35,36] Keeping these factors in mind, primary care practice staff may choose to mark the occasion of a patient's upcoming adolescent health supervision visit or 12th birthday by sending a letter to the adolescent and parents describing expectations for the adolescent's increasing independence in seeking and receiving health care and their practices in relation to privacy. At every visit with an adolescent, clinicians can reinforce the conditional confidentiality of their relationship. Appointment scheduling for adolescents should take into account the need to speak with both the adolescent and the parent or guardian privately. Both conversations are important, because parents and guardians may not be fully aware of their adolescents' activities or feelings, because adolescents may be reluctant to share some concerns with their parents or guardians, and because adolescents and parents often differ in their abilities to report on various mental health conditions.

Focus effort on engagement of patients and families in help seeking

At the time a PCC identifies a patient with a mental health problem, the patient or family may be resistant to taking action to address the problem, perhaps because of the stigma of mental illness, conflict within the family, lack of resources, distraction by other family priorities, anger, denial, or a sense of hopelessness, possibly rooted in unsuccessful past efforts. Behavior change science has demonstrated that people are in various stages of readiness to address a health problem: some are not even contemplating action, some are contemplating action but are ambivalent, some are ready to act, and some are already acting to create change. Rather than using a prescriptive approach, clinicians are more effective if they assess a family's readiness to address a problem and then help them to move to the next stage of readiness at their own pace.

The practice can collaborate with a mental health specialist to train clinicians in these techniques, which are known as "common factors" skills and encompass motivational interviewing (MI). (See Chapter 5, Effective Communication Methods: Common Factors Skills.) Application of these techniques is quite manageable within the pace of a busy primary care practice, particularly if the clinician is prepared with skills to bring a visit to an efficient and supportive close and to reschedule the family for additional brief sessions, if necessary. However, such primary care interventions are typically briefer and different in content from usual mental health outpatient services. Practice preparations to ensure appropriate scheduling, *Current Procedural Terminology* (commonly known as *CPT*) coding, and billing for these sessions will help make these activities sustainable.

Offer self-help interventions

Although not usually a substitute for specialty care, interactive support services that assist patients and their families in managing, tracking, and working on symptoms seem to be effective in extending the reach and success of mental health care. Results of randomized trials support the efficacy of ADHD-support Web sites, online depression management, telephone case management, MI services, text-messaging reminders for medication adherence, and related services with targeted populations, especially when facilitation is provided.[37-46] In addition, practices can have available a range of written materials and Web resources aimed at promoting mental health, educating the patient and family about particular behavioral challenges, and providing guidance in self-management and family management of problems. Whatever resources are offered, the primary care practice plays a critical role in monitoring to determine the patient's and family's progress in managing problems.

Support families in the referral process

The common factors communication techniques, described earlier in this chapter as part of patient and family engagement, are helpful in preparing a family for referral to mental health specialty services, which is otherwise completed by a family less than 50% of the time.[47,48] Primary care clinicians can also increase the likelihood that families complete referrals and successfully navigate the mental health system by providing referral support services, including telephone or personal contact by staff members, caseworkers, family advocates, or paid providers of peer support services.[49–53] Written materials that describe the referral process and the types of mental health specialty resources available in the community will reinforce information shared verbally. It is critical to implement a tracking mechanism for children who are referred for mental health specialty care.

Identify children involved in the mental health system, and provide them with a medical home

The practice will need to work systematically to identify children and adolescents who have not shared information with their PCC about their existing mental health conditions. Some of them have a severe and impairing mental illness, known to the mental health specialty system but not to the PCC. This situation may arise because the family self-referred into the mental health system or entered the mental health or juvenile justice system after a crisis such as a suicide attempt, group-home placement, arrest, or incarceration. Even a family who has a warm relationship with its child's or adolescent's PCC may feel embarrassed by his or her problems and reluctant to share this information, not recognizing the PCC's potential role in coordinating services or the potential risk of keeping the PCC unaware of psychiatric care, particularly pharmacological treatment.

Primary care practices will need to scrutinize their intake forms and processes to ensure that they include queries about mental health specialty care. They will also need to take general steps to communicate their interest in mental health and substance use issues through integration of these topics into health supervision and acute care visits and through posters and brochures in the waiting area. The PCC or practice manager may also advocate with local agencies and with contracted insurance plans to request notification of the primary care practice when a child seeks services from mental health specialists or prepares for discharge from a hospital or group home.

As these children are identified, they may be added to a registry and incorporated into chronic care protocols, as described in the Clinical Information Systems and Delivery System Redesign section, later in this chapter. Together, PCCs and families can explore eligibility for Supplemental Security Income for children with mental health problems significant enough to cause long-term disability and special education through Individualized Education Programs (IEPs). These 2 services can provide dramatic relief to children, adolescents, and families confronting disabling mental health problems. The practice will need to make a special effort to reassure the families of its support and willingness to partner with them and their son's or daughter's mental health specialty provider or providers. Families of children and adolescents with mental disorders have a range of experiences in mental health specialty and pediatric care and will likely become important sources of education for the PCC about community resources and supportive pediatric practices. They are also potential fellow advocates in the quest for improved insurance benefits and improved payment rates.

Children with severely impairing mental illness often qualify for and receive services of a mental health care manager and may also qualify for special services in education and other sectors. The mental health care manager is responsible for coordinating the agencies involved in the patient's care and for overseeing development and implementation of a "person-centered plan" (abbreviated PCP, which often confuses primary care physicians, who are also known as PCPs) or "family-centered plan," intended to create a system of care (SOC) around the child or adolescent and the family. The SOC philosophy, developed in the 1990s, reflects the influence of *consumers* (preferred term in the mental health advocacy community for people with mental illness) on mental health specialty care and has the following core principles[54]:

► A focus on strengths rather than problems
► "Nothing about us without us"
► Commitment to recovery as a goal
► Consumer choice among treatment options

► Services provided in the least restrictive environment

► A plan of care, developed with the family, built around the family's needs and preferences, and articulating the therapeutic goals and roles of all service providers

Primary care clinicians are often not engaged in the mental health SOC of these patients, and the primary care needs of these patients may be overlooked. There may be a number of possible explanations: PCCs may not feel that they have the expertise to participate in a mental health SOC; PCCs may be unaware of community efforts toward building a SOC; mental health specialists and agencies may not recognize PCCs' potential to contribute to the patients' and families' care; families may resist involvement of PCCs because of stigma; and families and mental health specialists may be overwhelmed with patients' mental illnesses to the neglect of basic pediatric concerns. Whatever the reasons, an expression of interest on the part of a PCC is very likely to be appreciated and valued by families and mental health specialists. A natural entry point for the PCC into a community's mental health SOC efforts is the mutual care of a child or an adolescent. However, to be effective, PCCs and professional organizations that represent them must participate in systemic planning at the regional and state levels.

Increasingly, the essential role of primary care in SOC-planning efforts is being recognized.[55] People with severe mental illness experience dramatically higher rates of morbidity and mortality from medical illnesses than do others.[56] Incorporating primary care into the plan of care for all children and adolescents with mental illness may establish a pattern that has lifelong benefits.

As adolescents with mental illness approach adulthood, they face transition to new primary care and specialty providers, as well as developmental tasks for which they may be inadequately prepared: completing high school or an equivalent course of study, attaining higher education, living independently, building social supports, finding employment and housing, and adhering to their treatment regimens. Although transition services for adolescents with mental illnesses are absent or insufficient in many communities, PCCs can apply medical home principles, as they do for other adolescents with special health care needs: they can ensure that their practice provides education to young people and their families about transition issues and anticipates the health, educational, social, and vocational needs they may encounter. (See Chapter 12, Transitioning Adolescents With Mental Health Conditions to Adult Care.) In communities without adequate transition resources for young people with mental illness, clinicians can partner with others to address deficiencies.

Prepare to address the mental health and substance use needs of special populations within the practice

Some populations of children and adolescents are likely to have greater mental health needs than their peers.

▶ Children exposed to adverse childhood experiences (ACEs)

▶ Families new to the United States

▶ Children in foster or kinship care or involved with child welfare

▶ Adopted children

▶ Children in poverty

▶ Children of divorce

▶ Children in military families

▶ Lesbian, gay, and bisexual youths

▶ Children with gender expression and identity issues

▶ Children in gay- and lesbian-parented families

▶ Children in self-care

▶ Homeless children

▶ Children affected by racism

▶ Children with chronic medical conditions

▶ Adolescents who are pregnant or parenting

▶ Children in the juvenile justice system

There may also be other groups within the community, such as alternative school populations, that have particular needs for mental health and SUD services and social support.

All these are children and adolescents likely to experience unusual levels of stress and to have unrecognized symptoms. Routine use of psychosocial questionnaires and updates of psychosocial information are helpful in identifying these children and adolescents. Office systems can assure that their records are flagged, their names are added to an appropriate registry, and customized protocols are implemented to provide heightened surveillance and mental health screening.

Through partnership with other health care and human service providers who serve these populations, PCCs can determine how the medical home and neighborhood can best serve the mental health needs of these children and adolescents and coordinate services with other providers. Primary care practices benefit from a previous shared understanding about respective responsibilities for collecting a psychosocial history, administering and scoring mental health and substance use screening tools, enlisting support from nonprofit or volunteer agencies, and identifying culturally appropriate and accessible assessment and treatment services.

Ensure the family friendliness of the practice

The Institute of Medicine defined *patient-centered care* as "respectful of and responsive to individual patient preferences, needs, and values, and ensuring that patient values guide all clinical decisions."[57] By extension (and necessity), pediatric practice requires family-centered care.

Involvement of families in clinical care is not sufficient, however. Family centeredness requires that families have a voice in decision-making at the practice level as well. Families, particularly those who have experienced mental health problems and navigated mental health systems, are an invaluable resource to a practice striving to enhance its mental health services. Dayton et al[58] identified many barriers challenging families' involvement (eg, recruitment, sustaining engagement, demographic representation, staff and leadership buy-in, logistics, confidentiality, training, role clarity). However, they also identified strategies to address these barriers. The potential gains are well worth these efforts.

The practice can take general steps to ensure that it is partnering successfully with children, adolescents, and families. The AAP participated with Family Voices, the Maternal and Child Health Bureau, and other partners in developing tools to assess the family centeredness of the care a practice provides.[59] These tools, along with a guide that enables users to apply findings to practice improvements, are available at www.familyvoices.org.

Become a trauma-informed practice

Adverse childhood experiences may affect a person's physical and mental health for a lifetime.[11] Examples include trauma such as abuse or neglect, placement in foster care, death of a loved one, a move, separation and divorce of parents, military deployment of one or both parents or a sibling, incarceration of a parent or sibling, breakup of a relationship, and exposure to violence or a natural disaster (eg, plane crash, tornado, war, crime, flood). The clinician will need to view all future physical and mental health issues in the family through the prism of their traumatic experiences.

Children and adolescents vary widely in their reactions to these events depending on their developmental levels, temperaments, previous states of mental health, coping mechanisms, parental responses, and support systems. Practices should establish office systems that routinely collect information about such stressful experiences in the patient's life and flag them in the health record of the patient and siblings to signal clinicians' interest and support,[60] and they should offer resources such as the AAP *Feelings Need Check Ups Too* and Web site at www.aap.org/en-us/advocacy-and-policy/aap-health-initiatives/Children-and-Disasters/Pages/Feelings-Need-Checkups-Too-Toolkit.aspx to monitor the children's adjustment over time and make appropriate referrals if a patient's functioning is impaired. For referrals, identifying specialists expert in trauma-informed care, especially CBT, is advantageous. Conversely, overlooking such experiences and failing to follow up on the patient's and family's progress after a traumatic event are lost opportunities to connect with the patient and family around important mental health issues.

The anniversary date of a traumatic event or loss can be recorded on the office calendar. Such practices as remembering a deceased loved one through use of his or her name during contacts with the patient and other members of the family and sending them a note on the anniversary of the loved one's death can communicate support; it will also keep the door open to further conversations about the reactions of family members to trauma and loss and their effects.[61]

The experience of seeking health care is itself traumatic for many children, adolescents, and families. They may have undergone medical trauma themselves or accompanied a loved one who experienced pain, illness, or death. Memory of these or nonmedical traumatic experiences may be triggered by activities such as an invasive procedure, removal of clothing, physical touch, embarrassing questions, power dynamics, gender of the health care professional, a vulnerable physical position, and loss of privacy. Staff members should be knowledgeable about trauma effects and respond respectfully and flexibly to ensure that patients and families feel safe in the practice. Staff members should also attend to their own psychosocial needs, including compassion fatigue and burnout, which can potentially prevent them from responding supportively to patients and families.

Children can easily learn self-regulation therapies such as mindfulness or meditation. They can apply them to managing everyday life stressors, solving problems such as acute pain and anxiety, and gaining an increased sense of control and participation in their treatments.[62] Clinicians and staff members can be trained in teaching self-regulation techniques to children and adolescents and in integrating these techniques into primary care practice and into their own self-care.[63,64] The National Pediatric Hypnosis Training Institute (www.nphti.org) offers annual trainings through which clinicians can learn to select language and apply simple techniques that can be used to make a child or an adolescent more comfortable during routine office procedures, such as receiving shots or undergoing throat cultures or just being examined by a stranger. (See Chapter 8, Self-regulation Therapies and Biofeedback.)

Periodically assess the quality of care the practice provides to children and adolescents with mental health problems and take action to improve care

A number of AAP resources are available to help PCCs with their quality-improvement efforts: AAP Practice Transformation Online (www.aap.org/en-us/professional-resources/practice-transformation/Pages/practice-transformation.aspx), EQIPP (Education in Quality Improvement for Pediatric Practice [www.eqipp.org]), and the Improving Chronic Illness Care Web site (www.improvingchroniccare.org). Specific AAP projects also provide resources on particular topics (eg, Bright Futures [https://brightfutures.aap.org/Pages/default.aspx] and "Practicing Safety: A Child Abuse and Neglect Prevention Improvement Project" [www.aap.org/en-us/professional-resources/quality-improvement/Quality-Improvement-Innovation-Networks/Pages/Practicing-Safety-A-Child-Abuse-and-

Neglect-Prevention-Improvement-Project.aspx]). Clinicians may monitor their psychosocial care in maintenance of certification by using such quality-improvement programs as EQIPP and developing relevant pay-for-performance and quality indicators for health plans.

Equally as important, the clinician can take leadership responsibilities in ensuring that psychosocial issues and behavioral health services are included in quality improvement and outcome measures for health systems and practice networks. Mental health problems are often excluded from such initiatives, and quality of mental health care may suffer as a result.

Clinical Information Systems and Delivery System Redesign

Clinical information systems ensure continuity of patient information across settings and time and facilitate collaboration between PCCs and mental health specialists. Collaboration is particularly important in the care of children and adolescents with medical and mental health comorbidities. Local resources and clinical circumstances will dictate the specific model or models of collaboration and the design of delivery systems that are necessary to support them. See Table 3-4 for prompts related to clinical information systems and delivery system redesign.

Table 3-4. Mental Health Practice Readiness Inventory: Clinical Information Systems and Delivery System Redesign			
Topic		Score	**Target**
Registry	1 2 3		Practice has a registry in place identifying children and adolescents with risks (patient or family), positive mental health or substance use screening results, and mental health or substance use problems (including those not yet ready to address problems).
Recall and reminder systems	1 2 3		Recall and reminder systems are in place to identify missed appointments and ensure that children and adolescents with mental health or substance use concerns (including those not ready to take action) receive appropriate follow-up and routine health supervision services.
Medication management	1 2 3		Practice has a system for monitoring medication efficacy, adverse effects, adherence, and renewals.

Table 3-4. Mental Health Practice Readiness Inventory: Clinical Information Systems and Delivery System Redesign (*continued*)

Topic	Score			Target
Emergency	1	2	3	Practice has a crisis plan in place for the handling of psychiatric emergencies, including suicidality.
Information exchange	1	2	3	Practice has office procedures to support collaboration (eg, routines for requesting parental consent to exchange information with specialists and schools, fax-back forms for specialist feedback, psychosocial history accompanying foster children and adolescents).
Tracking systems	1	2	3	Practice has systems in place and staff roles assigned to monitor patients' progress (eg, check on referral completion, periodic telephone contact with family and therapist, periodic functional assessment, periodic behavioral scales from classroom teachers and parents, communications to and from care coordinator), as appropriate to setting.
Care plans	1	2	3	Practice includes patients, family, school, agency personnel, primary care team, and any involved specialists in developing a comprehensive plan of care for a child or an adolescent with one or more mental health problems, including definition of respective roles.
Collaborative models	1	2	3	Practice team is prepared for participation in the full range of collaborative approaches and has explored innovative models (eg, colocated mental health specialist, child psychiatry consultation network, telepsychiatry) to fill service gaps and enhance quality.
Interactive Web-based tools	1	2	3	Practice is current with Web-based treatment options.
Screening and assessment tools	1	2	3	Office systems are in place to collect and score findings from mental health and substance use screening and assessment tools at or prior to scheduled routine health supervision visits and visits scheduled for a mental health concern and to perform a brief mental health update at acute care visits and visits scheduled to monitor chronic conditions, as appropriate to the setting.

Create registries of children and adolescents with mental health risks and problems

Preparing the practice to care for children and adolescents with identified mental health conditions is similar to preparing the practice to care for those with chronic medical conditions such as diabetes and asthma. It depends on registries of patients with mental health problems (including those who are not yet ready to address their problems). Electronic health records (EHRs) have improved dramatically in their capabilities to facilitate this step. Most major vendors now have chronic care registries, population health modules, and screening and tracking reminders structured within their systems. Several of these features support patient portals to allow periodic assessments by parents and sometimes by teachers and patients as well. Practices seeking to apply advanced chronic care methods to the care of patients with mental health problems or other chronic conditions should incorporate an EHR system.

Without an EHR system, options are limited. However, it is possible to create registries using claims data and other approaches. As examples, the AAP toolkit for ADHD[65] contains tracking procedures for patients with ADHD; Community Care of North Carolina, the state's homegrown Medicaid managed care program, successfully used pharmacy and other claims data to identify patients with mental health conditions likely to benefit from application of care protocols and targeted care management services.

Use monitoring, prescribing, and tracking systems for psychosocial therapy and psychotropic drugs

Some patients have mental health problems that resolve quickly; some have mental disorders that require treatment to be administered over extended periods of time and monitored for initial remission and symptoms of recurrence; and some recover from mental disorders and return to normal functioning. Primary care systems cannot act as a medical home for children and adolescents with mental health problems without the capacity to monitor receipt and outcomes of treatment. Monitoring systems can be set up in a variety of ways that ensure that information will be shared, with appropriate consents, among the family, EI specialist, school (or preschool), PCC, and other involved health care professionals. At the core of such a system is a registry of children with certain conditions, as described earlier in this section, and an established protocol that assigns responsibility for communication to a certain team member, who will assist in the monitoring process. Although "tickler" systems, that is, the use of automated or manual reminders entered onto a staff member's calendar or a "record review" entered onto a provider's clinic schedule, can be used for this purpose, electronic systems that are capable of extracting information from records and producing notices, reports, text messages, or appointments (or any combination thereof) are especially useful.

Put into place a plan for managing psychiatric and social emergencies

Primary care clinicians need access to emergency services for children and adolescents with suicidal thoughts and other psychiatric emergencies. Virtually all communities in the United States have some resource and process identified for handling psychiatric emergencies, although capacity varies widely and, in many areas, depends on law enforcement agencies and emergency departments. Some communities have 24 hours per day, 7 days per week emergency psychiatric facilities or mobile response units (or both) staffed by experienced personnel. Primary care clinicians need to be aware of these services, participate in community dialogue about management of psychiatric and social emergencies, and establish office protocols that link pediatric patients and their families immediately to appropriate services. (See www.aap.org/en-us/advocacy-and-policy/aap-health-initiatives/Mental-Health/Pages/Chapter-Action-Kit.aspx and Chapter 13, Agitation, Suicidality, and Other Psychiatric Emergencies, for further discussion of this strategy.)

Put office systems into place to support prevention, screening, assessment, and collaboration

The foundation of preventive services is the iterative psychosocial assessment, discussed in detail in Chapter 6. To expedite the process of gathering data about the patient and family, use of a previsit questionnaire, either paper or electronic, filled out at home or in the waiting area, creates efficiency and consistency and enables the clinician to focus on building rapport and on exploring findings, rather than on rote data gathering during child health supervision visits. The clinician may also choose to incorporate validated screening instruments into the previsit collection of data. (See discussion in the Decision Support section, later in this chapter, about selection of tools.) The clinician may also decide to perform a brief mental health update at acute care visits or visits scheduled to monitor a chronic condition. (See Box 1-5 in Chapter 1, Integrating Preventive Mental Health Care Into Pediatric Practice.) Whatever questionnaires and screening instruments are used, a structured process, developed by the practice in advance, should ensure that the following content is covered:

▶ Family's priorities for the visit

▶ Family and social history, including ACEs; social stressors such as poverty, food insecurity, racism, and homophobia; support system; and environmental risk assessment, including mental health of family members, trauma, separation, and loss

▶ Identification of the patient's and family's strengths

▶ Functional assessment of the patient

▶ Temperament and risk behaviors

▶ Bedtime routines, family meals, physical activity, and media use patterns

▶ Sleep

▶ Concerns of school or child care providers

▶ Symptoms of psychosocial problems

If previsit data collection is not feasible, the PCC will need to incorporate data collection into the clinical encounter and synthesize it with previous findings, current observations, interview of family and patient, and examination results to formulate an assessment of the patient's mental health. Chapter 1, Integrating Preventive Mental Health Care Into Pediatric Practice, and Chapter 2, Pediatric Care of Children and Adolescents With Mental Health Problems, describe a process for integrating components of the assessment into primary care flow. Chapter 6, Iterative Mental Health Assessment, conceptualizes these various components of the assessment (eg, previsit questionnaires, screening tools, observations, responses to primary care interventions, periodic functional assessments, and collateral information) as gauges on a dashboard and describes them in more detail.

Also important to preventive efforts is a registry (described earlier in this section) of children with identified personal or family psychosocial risks and positive screening results, office protocols to guide next steps, referral sources and follow-up procedures, and educational materials, both print and Web, to assist patients and families in pursuing their mental health goals.

When the involvement of a mental health specialist will be necessary, patients and families will need information about the mental health system and providers of mental health services. The AAP has developed a handout, *Your Child's Mental Health: When to Seek Help and Where to Get Help* (https://patiented.solutions.aap.org), to assist in demystifying these elements of care.

Office procedures to ensure exchange of information between the primary care practice and mental health specialists are critical for effective care and coordination. Although HIPAA allows mental health specialists and PCCs involved in the care of the same patient to exchange information (other than psychotherapy notes and SUD treatment records) without the patient's and family's consent, some mental health specialists are very protective of privacy, even from referring physicians. Primary care clinicians may need to collaborate with and educate mental health specialists about the concepts of medical home and medical neighborhood for children and adolescents with special health care needs, the PCC's role and interest in the care of children and adolescents with mental illness, and the PCC's need for information about their patients' mental health treatments, especially as a treatment may affect other elements of a patient's care (including medication interactions).

Many patients and families will readily agree to the exchange of information between their mental health specialist and PCC, if asked. Routine use of forms that document consent for exchange of information will facilitate communication. Use of fax-back forms or other methods to facilitate exchange has been helpful in some communities.[66,67] Telephone calls may be less convenient for mental health specialists, who are typically scheduled with back-to-back 45- to 60-minute appointments and have little administrative support; however, previous understanding about convenient times to talk may be beneficial. E-mail is often convenient, but, as with other uses of e-mail in health care settings, secure communication must be in place and confidentiality must be carefully considered.

Whatever methods are used, primary care practices can demonstrate their commitment to bidirectional communication with mental health specialists. Office procedures can ensure that mental health specialists receive, for example, a summary of the presenting concern, the family's level of engagement in the process, results from tools used to measure symptoms or functioning or both, and the PCC's capacity and preferences in relation to comanagement. The primary care practice can create the expectation that, in return, it will receive from the mental health specialist a summary of diagnostic findings, treatment recommendations, and clarification of respective roles in ongoing comanagement of the identified problem.

Collaboratively develop care plans

Chronic care principles suggest that optimal outcomes are achieved when the family, primary care team, and pediatric and mental health specialists involved in assessment and treatment collaboratively develop a comprehensive plan of care. Key elements of collaborative care plans include identification of family concerns, education of the family about the condition and self-management strategies, listing of all professionals involved in the care of the child, listing of the strengths and resources available to the family and child, a comprehensive account of diagnoses and therapies, therapeutic goals, and a specific plan for monitoring progress toward these goals, including periodic functional assessment. Care-plan development is discussed in more depth in Chapter 2, Pediatric Care of Children and Adolescents With Mental Health Problems. Sample paper-based care plans for chronic conditions in pediatric settings are available at https://medicalhomeinfo.aap.org/Pages/default.aspx.

Prepare for participation in the full range of collaborative models

Previous strategies have addressed the need for a resource directory and for relationships with providers of key mental health services. The model of collaboration between a practice and one or more mental health specialists in a particular clinical situation depends on the needs of the patient, patient and family preferences, availability of the needed resources, and the PCC's comfort with the patient's condition and its severity. A patient may move between models as the mental health condition changes in severity or the patient achieves recovery. In regions in which mental health specialty services are inaccessible or insufficient, including most rural areas of the country, primary care practices may need to plan for collaboration by telephone, Internet, or video with off-site mental health specialists. Innovative systems in several regions of the country have been developed to provide decision support for PCCs.[68–72] Social workers or referral coordinators can help patients navigate public and private mental health specialty systems. In all collaborative models, a system of communication among providers is critically important to prevent clinicians from relying on family members as conduits of clinical information.

A literature review of coordinated/telephonic, colocated, and integrated models[73] found that integration of behavioral health services into pediatric primary care practices can…

▶ Promote family engagement in evidence-based behavioral health services.

▶ Reduce barriers to care.

▶ Enable providers to reach a greater number of families than standard mental health care.

▶ Result in improved patient outcomes.

A meta-analysis of integrated care models, broadly defined to include diverse approaches that aim to unify behavioral health and primary care (eg, consultation by telephone or web, colocation, team-based collaborative care), showed significantly better outcomes for youths receiving an integrated behavioral health intervention than randomly selected youths receiving usual care.[74]

The PCC and family, together, will need to collaborate with school and community resource providers, whether or not other pediatric specialists and mental health specialists are also involved. The following paragraphs describe various relationships between the PCC and his or her collaborators and the family's role in each model.

Primary Care

In this model, the patient can be assessed and treated appropriately and successfully in the primary care practice. The patient's mental health needs are clear (either the patient's condition is uncomplicated by comorbidities or the PCC has received additional training in management of the patient's conditions), the family has confidence in the PCC's capacity to care for the patient, and the patient responds positively to primary care interventions. For example, a child with ADHD who requires medication and behavior management and does not have coexisting conditions may be treated in primary care. The practice is prepared to work directly with the child, family, and school in developing, implementing, and monitoring the child's plan of care. Health promotion and positive parenting training can occur in primary care settings, in partnership with schools or other community agencies.

Primary Care With Mental Health Specialty Consultation

This model is applicable to children and adolescents with chronic medical conditions accompanied by impairing mental health comorbidities such as anxiety or depression, to those with mental disorders that are beyond the comfort or capacity of PCCs, and to those whose families desire specialty involvement. The primary care practice serves as the source of primary care and coordination of school and specialty services, fostering relationships that enable the PCC to consult with one or more of the following professionals:

▶ **A psychologist or another mental health therapist (eg, licensed clinical social worker, licensed marriage and family therapist, licensed professional counselor).** The PCC typically provides the initial assessment and, with the family's support, asks the mental health specialist to help clarify the diagnosis; to provide information about types of psychosocial therapy approaches that may be beneficial; to guide the PCC's management; to review or address complicating developments such as new behavioral problems, family conflicts, and high-risk behaviors; or to perform any combination thereof. If medication is part of the treatment plan, the PCC manages the prescription and monitoring of medication directly with the family. This type of mental health consultation typically involves the patient's participation in one or more face-to-face visits with the mental health specialist and intermittent conversations between the specialist and the PCC. It may occur with or without consultation with a physician specialist, as described in the next bullet.

▶ **A physician specialist, such as a child and adolescent psychiatrist, a developmental-behavioral pediatrician, a neurodevelopmental pediatrician, a pediatric neurologist, or an adolescent specialist.** The PCC (or collaborating mental health specialist, as described in the previous bullet), with involvement of the patient and family, may pose specific questions about diagnosis or management strategies, including medication issues (eg, choice of agent, potential interactions, adverse effects, dosage adjustments), coexisting conditions, and suicide risk or other safety concerns. The consulting physician may provide an initial evaluation with the intention that the patient will return to the PCC (and mental health specialist) for ongoing care. The consultant may also offer advice intermittently when new behavioral problems, medication questions, family conflicts, or high-risk behaviors occur. Examples of this model include the Massachusetts Child Psychiatry Access Project, which provides PCCs with telephonic access to 1 of 6 regional teams that includes a child psychiatrist.[75] The model's success has led to replication in more than 25 states, organized as members of the National Network of Child Psychiatry Access Programs. More information about these models is available at www.nncpap.org.

Shared Care or Comanagement With Mental Health Specialists

In this model, the primary care practice fosters relationships that enable its clinicians to "share" the mental health care of the patient with one or more mental health specialists; that is, both (or all) are jointly responsible for decision-making, monitoring mental health symptoms, response to therapy, and effects of medication, if prescribed. In this model, ongoing communication with and about the patient and family and among the providers is particularly critical.

The PCC may comanage the care of the child with any combination of the following mental health specialists:

▶ Child and adolescent psychiatrist, who provides not only an initial evaluation but also ongoing treatment.

▶ Mental health therapist such as a psychologist or social worker, who provides individual, group, or family psychosocial therapy.

▶ Multidisciplinary team, which may include the child's mental health care manager, an agency representative from the Department of Social Services or juvenile justice system, mental health specialists such as those listed on the previous page, and one or more school representatives such as social workers, school counselors, and special education IEP case managers. In situations that involve children or adolescents with higher levels of complexity, additional multidisciplinary team members may participate: for example, teams that care for patients with mental disorders who require partial hospitalization or day treatment may include representatives of the mental health specialty facility; teams that care for patients with chronic medical conditions such as cancer or chronic pulmonary disease may include the patient's medical subspecialist or specialty clinic coordinator.

Shared-care models include all the following features:

▶ Central role of the patient and family in developing the plan of care

▶ Mutual understanding of the roles of family members, school or child care personnel, and providers, including frequency of and responsibility for follow-up, with mental health specialists assuming relatively more responsibility for patients with safety concerns and those whose mental health conditions are of high severity or acuity

▶ General health supervision by the PCC, including care of medical illnesses, immunizations and other preventive services, and coordination of subspecialty and educational services

▶ A communication protocol, including parental consent for exchange of information, clear understanding of respective responsibilities and mechanisms for monitoring progress toward therapeutic goals, mechanisms for sharing information among providers, and contact persons in each provider's practice and patient's school or child care setting

Mental Health Specialty Care With Primary Care Clinician Involvement

In this model, the mental health specialty system assumes primary responsibility for the patient's care because of the level of severity and complexity of the patient's problems, higher levels of concern regarding safety, or the coexistence of other complicating mental health or social conditions (or any combination of those factors). The primary care practice ideally receives regular communication about progress from both the specialty providers and the family and about any changes in the level of care such as hospitalization or group-home placement. The PCC makes recommendations concerning the patient's ongoing primary medical care and coordination of medical specialty services. Examples include a child or an adolescent with psychosis or major depressive disorder.

On-site (Colocated) Mental Health Specialist

A growing number of primary care practices across the country have successfully brought one or more mental health specialists into their primary care sites.

The events of September 11, 2001; Hurricane Katrina; and other disasters have brought to light the particular need for primary care practices to integrate mental health services in times of disasters. Evidence points to families' preference for these services within primary care settings, as compared with traditional mental health settings.[76] A report describing experience in an inner city primary care pediatric clinic with an integrated behavioral health model showed improved access and outcomes for children and families residing in poverty.[77]

Role of colocated mental health specialist. The role of a colocated mental health specialist is ideally developed in response to the needs of the practice and the population it serves. Collaboration with PCCs may fall within any or all of the collaborative models described previously. In areas with a shortage of child psychiatrists or developmental-behavioral pediatricians, a colocated mental health specialist, such as a licensed clinical social worker or psychologist, can enhance the level of assessment that is shared in advance with consulting physicians, which increases the efficiency and appropriateness of the consultative process and facilitates implementation of a treatment plan and follow-up afterward.[78] This type of arrangement also enriches the involved primary care team members and mental health specialists through informal consultation and shared problem-solving around patients and families in their mutual care.

The colocated mental health specialist may function in a number of ways, depending on practice preferences and business realities. The mental health specialist may function similarly to his or her role in a mental health specialty site, offering traditional mental health assessment and treatment services in 30- to 60-minute blocks, or the mental health specialist may provide services more closely integrated with the PCC's: he or she may off-load certain activities from the PCC, such as collecting an interval history, scoring mental health screening tools, or providing supportive services such as parent education (or any combination of these functions). The colocated mental health specialist can collaborate with the

PCC to assess children with identified problems, communicate with school personnel or other mental health specialists, provide mental health interventions, address barriers to care, monitor progress in care, provide periodic contact and support to the family, or link the child and family to referral sources (or perform any combination of these roles). In one model, a mental health case manager supported by the practice provided many of the non-reimbursed mental health services, such as data collection and care coordination; this case manager created efficiencies and increased PCCs' productivity, more than compensating for the cost of supporting this position.[79]

Another approach to on-site collaboration (sometimes including more than one primary care practice) involves a mental health specialist in carrying out an evidence-based protocol to care for patients with a specific condition. This approach, which has been effective with adults, has also shown promising results in children and adolescents. [4–6,80] One random controlled clinical trial compared 2 approaches to the care of patients aged 8 to 16 years meeting criteria for depression or an anxiety disorder: (1) a series of brief primary care behavioral therapy sessions vs (2) assisted mental health specialty referral. The primary care–treated group showed significantly better outcomes, particularly for Hispanic patients. This finding suggests the possibility that collaborative models of this type may help to address racial and ethnic disparities in mental health care.[81]

In all the models, PCCs and their patients benefit from the "cross-fertilization" of multidisciplinary practice. In fully integrated mental health models, the collaboration with a mental health specialist in primary care is a seamless part of all encounters, team meetings, and practice improvement efforts.

Business arrangements for colocation models. Choice of business arrangements depends importantly on the mental health benefit structure and reimbursement rates of regional public and private insurers, their requirements for authorizing services, and their requirements for credentialing mental health specialists to participate in their plans. Practices that are contemplating colocation should develop a business plan based on their unique needs, resources, payer mixes, and rates of payment. The simplest financial arrangement is one in which the primary care practice rents office space to an independent mental health specialist, who performs his or her own billing and collecting of fees; however, this model may limit the extent to which real integration can occur. Other business models include a mental health specialist employed by the primary care practice and a mental health specialist employed by a mental health agency or hospital and "out-stationed" in the primary care practice. Some states support integrated models by allowing payment of mental health specialists in Article 28 facilities (eg, hospital, primary care settings, school-based health centers). Practices with a high concentration of Medicaid beneficiaries should pay attention to their state's Medicaid "incident to" rules; these rules may allow mental health specialists employed by a physician or by the same entity that employs the physician to bill in a physician's name, incident to that physician's on-site supervision. This arrangement, if available, may allow a higher payment rate, more flexibility, and more genuine integration of the mental health specialist into the practice than do arrangements in which the mental health specialist bills directly for his or her services, adhering to traditional mental health codes and billing processes.

A number of successful colocation models have been sustained with grant dollars during the implementation phase, until reimbursements became sufficient to support the mental health specialist. While in several regions of the country, colocation models have been sustained through third-party payment,[82] others have not found this to be the case but are satisfied with the model nevertheless.[83] The AAP is collecting the experiences of primary care practices that have colocated or integrated a mental health specialist.[84] The AAP places high priority on research to identify best practices in implementing, sustaining, and evaluating these models.

Some practices have also incorporated a child psychiatrist (usually employed by a separate entity such as a mental health agency or an academic institution) who provides periodic consultation on-site or through telephone or telemedicine hookup. A colocated mental health specialist such as a social worker or psychologist can greatly improve the efficiency of psychiatric consultation services by gathering data and performing a psychosocial assessment in advance of the psychiatrist's encounter with the patient and family, by posing specific clinical questions to be answered by the psychiatrist, by spending time with the patient and family after the psychiatric consultation to provide education about the psychiatrist's findings and recommendations, by identifying and addressing any barriers to engaging in further care, and by following up with the family periodically to monitor progress.

Decision Support

Tools that inform diagnosis and management at various stages and for diverse conditions will assist primary care practices in enhancing their mental health care. See Table 3-5 for prompts related to decision support.

Table 3-5. Mental Health Practice Readiness Inventory: Decision Support for Clinicians			
Topic	**Score**		**Target**
Functional assessment	1 2 3		Clinicians use validated functional assessment scales to identify and evaluate children and adolescents with mental health problems and monitor their progress in care.
Clinical guidance	1 2 3		Clinicians have access to reliable, current sources of information concerning diagnostic classification of mental health and substance use problems, evidence about safety and efficacy of psychosocial and psychopharmacological treatments of common mental health and substance use disorders, and information about the safety and efficacy of complementary and integrative therapies often used by children, adolescents, and families.
Psychiatric consultation	1 2 3		Clinicians have access to a psychiatrist with expertise in children and adolescents for consultation and guidance in assessment and management of their patients' mental health problems.
Protocols	1 2 3		Practice has tools and protocols in place to guide assessment and care and to foster self-treatment of children and adolescents with common mental health and substance use conditions.
Screening and surveillance	1 2 3		Clinicians routinely use psychosocial history and validated screening tools at preventive visits and brief mental health updates at acute care visits to elicit mental health and substance use problems and to identify patient and family strengths and risks.

Select one or more validated functional assessment tools for use in identifying mental health problems and in monitoring a patient's and family's progress toward therapeutic goals

Although PCCs are accustomed to using spirometry and hemoglobin A_{1c} levels for assessing and monitoring the clinical status of patients with asthma and those with type 1 diabetes, respectively, they may be unfamiliar with tools used for assessing and monitoring the clinical status of patients with mental health conditions. In mental health specialty practice, tools that measure patient and family functioning are a routine part of the assessment and monitoring process. Such tools can provide clinicians with information about a patient's areas of strength as well as the child's problem areas. The tools may also lead to identification of patients who do not meet diagnostic criteria for a specific mental disorder but have some impairment in functioning at home, at school, or with peers, or they may measure the effects that a patient's mental disorder has on the patient, the family, the patient's interpersonal relationships, and the patient's school performance.

Measuring the global functioning of children, adolescents, and families offers all the following potential benefits to PCCs[85]:

▶ Functional assessments demonstrate better inter-reporter reliability than symptom-based assessments for a number of mental disorders.

▶ Impaired functioning may precede the recognition of specific mental health symptoms and may resolve more slowly than symptoms do.

▶ Identifying areas of functional strength and challenge can guide the development and monitoring of treatment goals.

▶ Improved functional outcome is a measure of the efficacy of mental health services and is important to children, adolescents, and families.

Although many tools used to assess mental health functioning are not applicable to primary care settings, a few have shown promise in assisting PCCs in screening, assessment, and monitoring of children and adolescents for mental health problems, and several are available in the public domain. These are discussed in Appendix 2.

Select instruments for the assessment of children and adolescents whose screening results or clinical findings suggest the presence of a mental health or substance use problem

A number of tools are available to assist the clinician in further assessment of children and adolescents with suspected mental health or substance use problems. Appendix 2 contains a table of those with sound psychometric properties and potential for use in primary care settings.

Identify reliable, current sources of information concerning diagnostic classification of mental health problems and evidence about the safety and efficacy of treatments

A number of AAP publications, including this book, provide guidance to PCCs in the assessment and management of common mental health problems in children and adolescents. Several additional resources are available to assist clinicians in weighing the risks and benefits of mental health and substance use treatments, as well as complementary and integrative therapies, which are commonly used by children, adolescents, and families experiencing mental health difficulties and may have benefit in some situations.

Primary care clinicians are often faced with caring for patients who have been prescribed a psychotropic medication (or multiple medications) by a mental health specialist, sometimes without access to ongoing consultation with that specialist. This circumstance underscores the importance of the strategy that follows.

Establish a relationship with one or more physician specialists (eg, child psychiatrist, developmental-behavioral pediatrician, neurodevelopmental pediatrician, adolescent medicine specialist, pediatric neurologist) who have expertise in prescribing psychopharmacological therapy for children and adolescents

This strategy is a significant challenge in many communities. In a number of areas of the country, PCCs have collaborated with academic institutions to develop models of telepsychiatry, regional psychiatric consultation, or colocation of a child psychiatrist within a primary care practice. Evaluation of several programs has demonstrated their value in enhancing the self-efficacy of primary care pediatricians and decreasing their use of polypharmacy for pediatric mental disorders. See discussion in the Primary Care With Mental Health Specialty Consultation section earlier in this chapter.

Develop and implement evidence-based protocols

Development of office protocols and flow sheets, in accordance with evidence-based guidelines or locally developed standards of care, will routinize the essential elements of the care process. A logical starting point might be children with ADHD, a mental disorder that most PCCs feel comfortable assessing and managing and for which there are established clinical guidelines[86] and extensive experience in quality-improvement efforts.[87–89]

Implementing mental health management protocols within the practice will involve a team-building process and significant participation by staff. These staff members, for instance, may be charged with

► Requesting information or records from schools, the child welfare system, and other care providers when a patient on the registry is scheduled for a visit

► Collecting and scoring assessment tools in advance of the visit

► Clarifying insurance benefit and provider issues

► Scheduling medication checks (eg, adherence, positive and adverse effects, laboratory surveillance, refills)

► Obtaining height and weight measurements and vital signs

► Periodically assessing the functioning of the patient and family (See earlier in this chapter in the Decision Support section.)

► Checking progress toward therapeutic goals

► Calling the patient or the family or both for a structured follow-up or appointment reminder or for a recall after a missed visit

► Assisting with the referral process

These mechanisms can be enhanced through an EHR system that improves access to the chart for all treating clinicians and support staff (at appropriate levels), improves routing of information to appropriate clinicians, supports jointly developed care management plans, automates recall for missed appointments, and embeds the results of automatically scored behavioral and functional scales. Other models include Web-based portals that allow patients or parents to complete previsit questionnaires and send results to an EHR or another electronic tool, which then links the clinician to sources of information about the patient's presenting difficulties. Regardless of the specific tools, PCCs must consider both the content of instruments or tools and how such tools will be administered, recorded, and monitored.

Examples of protocols and tools for ongoing management of chronic medical conditions can be found on the AAP medical home Web site (www.medicalhomeinfo.org). Specific protocols for tracking and monitoring mental health conditions are available for ADHD[86] and adolescent depression.[90]

The mass use of EHRs will eventually automate the use of evidence-based clinician order sets, flow sheets, and tracking reports to assist in improving the quality of care for people with chronic conditions. Electronic reminders, quality reports, and standardized order sets have already been shown to reduce medical errors, improve patient satisfaction, increase guideline-compliant care by physicians, and assist in identifying unmet health care needs in some settings.[91–95] However, several challenges have emerged in routine practice. First, the quality and completeness of data documenting behavioral health visits in EHRs often leaves much to be desired and prevents quality measurement. Second, clinicians seem to use automated screening modules in some EHRs for validation of high-risk cases, rather than universal screening. Finally, improvements in quality of practice have been noted in randomized trials of routine practice,[96,97] but symptom improvements have been modest. It is clear that individual practices are limited in their ability to improve long-term monitoring and tracking of patients; therefore, health systems and coaches will be required to achieve improvements such as those associated with chronic care models applied in cases of adult depression and diabetes.

Consider routine screening for mental health and substance use problems in children, adolescents, and families with identified social risks

Many children with mental health problems or difficulty in their parent-child relationships, families experiencing psychosocial stresses, and parents with mental illness are not identified as needing mental health or social services, although they may frequent primary care settings. This lack of identification is particularly true for children and adolescents with chronic medical conditions. Furthermore, their unrecognized mental health problems may drive their use (and their parents' use) of medical services.[98] The many unmet mental health needs of children, adolescents, and their families warrant enhanced primary care efforts to identify those pediatric patients with occult mental health problems and families in need of mental health or social assistance.

Recognizing these many occult needs, clinicians may be tempted to begin the process of mental health practice improvement by introducing psychosocial screening. However, efforts to implement screening before office systems, collaborative relationships, decision support, and referral supports are in place are unlikely to achieve sustainable benefits. On the other hand, with these practice improvements and business systems in place, clinicians will be prepared to enhance their efforts to identify children and adolescents with occult mental health and substance use problems.

Bright Futures, 4th Edition, affirms the importance of using all routine health supervision visits for psychosocial assessment (surveillance) of a child's and family's psychosocial well-being. *Bright Futures,* 4th Edition, also recommends routinely screening for maternal depression during a child's infancy and for depression and substance use in adolescents. Although not part of the Bright Futures/AAP *Recommendations for Preventive Pediatric Health Care* (periodicity schedule), universal psychosocial screening at additional child and adolescent health supervision visits has been successfully implemented by many primary care practices.

Chapter 1, Integrating Preventive Mental Health Into Pediatric Practice, describes a clinical process for integrating these activities into the work flow of a primary care practice. Boxes 1-8 and 1-9 in that chapter summarize guidance for incorporating validated screening tools.

Routine psychosocial screening typically requires incremental implementation. Depending on the population served by the practice and its health risks and strengths, the clinician may choose to begin by identifying one or more high-needs groups within the practice (eg, children and adolescents in foster care, those with parents who have been deployed in military service, those with identified ACEs, those within a certain zip code or neighborhood known to house low-income families or to experience violence, those who have experienced racism or homophobia) and screening them for mental health problems. In some settings, the practice may seek cooperation of school guidance counselors or nurses, school-based clinics, or community agencies (eg, public health, social services, juvenile justice) to collect previsit data at their intake points and relay the information to the practice.

Appendix 2 contains examples of mental health screening tools that have sound psychometric properties and are accessible to PCCs. In each category are tools that can be feasibly implemented in primary care settings.

Screening tools for consideration should have the following characteristics:

▶ User-friendly for patients.

▶ Do not require special training to administer.

▶ Designed to elicit information from multiple reporters (ie, have versions available that can be completed by youths, parents, and teachers). Multiple data sources offer additional insights in the course of mental health assessment.

▶ Available in multiple platforms. Providing options for patients and families to complete screenings online outside the office or via a computer in the waiting area may have advantages; however, some practices will prefer traditional pen-and-paper screenings.

▶ Relatively brief and easily scored. The TFMH suggested that screenings require no longer than 10 to 15 minutes to complete.

▶ Multilingual. Screenings should be available in the preferred language of each reporter.

▶ Available in the public domain or affordable.

Use of these or other screening tools does not replace the clinical interview needed to confirm findings and expand on identified problems.

Use acute care visits to elicit mental health concerns

Recognizing that many school-aged children and adolescents do not seek routine health supervision, the TFMH urged that primary care practices consider using acute care visits as opportunities for brief mental health updates, especially for children and adolescents who do not receive routine health supervision services. The task force drew from the expertise of its professional members, opinions of its adolescent and family participants, and informal trials in primary care practices to develop sample questions that PCCs can consider using during acute care visits and potentially during subspecialty visits as well. See Chapter 1, Integrating Preventive Mental Health Care Into Pediatric Practice, for a description of this approach and sample questions. Research is necessary to determine outcomes and best practices.

Conclusion

Pediatricians and other PCCs can use a mental health practice readiness inventory to assess their needs and establish priorities for incrementally enhancing their practice's mental health care. The key elements, drawn from the chronic care model and principles of trauma-informed care, are

▶ Community resources

▶ Health care financing

▶ Support for children and families

▶ Clinical information systems and delivery system redesign

▶ Decision support

This chapter describes approaches clinicians can take in response to the practice's identified needs, with the guidance of patients and families. The returns are likely to be substantial: building resilience in children, adolescents, and families served by the practice; enhancing the early identification of those with psychosocial risks, such as exposure to trauma, and those who need care for mental health and substance use problems (including those that may not rise to the level of a diagnosable disorder); increasing the likelihood of engaging in care those who have these needs; and improving the quality of care that is provided to them.

Acknowledgments: The authors acknowledge the American Academy of Pediatrics Task Force on Mental Health for authoring the original article on this topic. The task force included Jane Meschan Foy, MD (chairperson and lead author); Paula Duncan, MD; Barbara Frankowski, MD, MPH;

Kelly Kelleher, MD, MPH (lead author); Penelope K. Knapp, MD; Danielle Laraque, MD (lead author); Gary Peck, MD; Michael Regalado, MD; Jack Swanson, MD; and Mark Wolraich, MD; the consultants were Margaret Dolan, MD; Alain Joffe, MD, MPH; Patricia O'Malley, MD; James Perrin, MD; Thomas K. McInerny, MD; and Lynn Wegner, MD; the liaisons were Terry Carmichael, MSW (National Association of Social Workers); Darcy Gruttadaro, JD (National Alliance on Mental Illness); Garry Sigman, MD (Society for Adolescent Medicine); Myrtis Sullivan, MD, MPH (National Medical Association); and L. Read Sulik, MD (American Academy of Child and Adolescent Psychiatry); and the staff were Linda Paul and Aldina Hovde.

AAP Policy

Adams RC; Levy SE; American Academy of Pediatrics Council on Children With Disabilities. Shared decision-making and children with disabilities: pathways to consensus. *Pediatrics.* 2017;139(6):e20170956 (pediatrics.aappublications.org/content/139/6/e20170956)

American Academy of Pediatrics Committee on Hospital Care, Institute for Patient- and Family-Centered Care. Patient- and family-centered care and the pediatrician's role. *Pediatrics.* 2012;129(2):394–404 (pediatrics.aappublications.org/content/129/2/394)

American Academy of Pediatrics Committee on Psychosocial Aspects of Child and Family Health and Task Force on Mental Health. The future of pediatrics: mental health competencies for the care of children and adolescents in primary care settings. *Pediatrics.* 2009;124:(1):410–421. Reaffirmed August 2013 (pediatrics.aappublications.org/content/124/1/410)

American Academy of Pediatrics Council on Children With Disabilities and Medical Home Implementation Project Advisory Committee. Patient- and family-centered care coordination: a framework for integrating care for children and youth across multiple systems. *Pediatrics.* 2014;133(5):e1451–e1460 (pediatrics.aappublications.org/content/133/5/e1451)

American Academy of Pediatrics Section on Integrative Medicine. Mind-body therapies in children and youth. *Pediatrics.* 2016;138(3):e20161896 (pediatrics.aappublications.org/content/138/3/e20161896)

American College of Obstetricians and Gynecologists. *Collaboration in Practice: Implementing Team-Based Care.* Washington, DC: American College of Obstetricians and Gynecologists; 2016. AAP endorsed (www.acog.org/Resources-And-Publications/Task-Force-and-Work-Group-Reports/Collaboration-in-Practice-Implementing-Team-Based-Care)

References

1. Wagner EH. Chronic disease management: what will it take to improve care for chronic illness? *Eff Clin Pract.* 1998;1(1):2–4

2. Wagner EH, Austin BT, Davis C, Hindmarsh M, Schaefer J, Bonomi A. Improving chronic illness care: translating evidence into action. *Health Aff (Millwood).* 2001;20(6):64–78

3. Bodenheimer T, Wagner EH, Grumbach K. Improving primary care for patients with chronic illness: the chronic care model, part 2. *JAMA.* 2002;288(15):1909–1914

4. Richardson LP, Ludman E, McCauley E, et al. Collaborative care for adolescents with depression in primary care: a randomized clinical trial. *JAMA.* 2014;312(8):809–816

5. Wright DR, Haaland WL, Ludman E, McCauley E, Lindenbaum J, Richardson LP. The costs and cost-effectiveness of collaborative care for adolescents with depression in primary care settings: a randomized clinical trial. *JAMA Pediatr.* 2016;170(11):1048–1054

6. Asarnow JR, Jaycox LH, Duan N, et al. Effectiveness of a quality improvement intervention for adolescent depression in primary care clinics: a randomized controlled trial. *JAMA.* 2005;293(3):311–319

7. Foy JM; American Academy of Pediatrics Task Force on Mental Health. Enhancing pediatric mental health care: report from the American Academy of Pediatrics Task Force on Mental Health. Introduction. *Pediatrics.* 2010;125(suppl 3):S69–S74

8. IDEA 2004: building the legacy; Part C (birth–2 years old). US Department of Education Web site. http://idea.ed.gov/part-c/search/new.html. Accessed January 4, 2018

9. Shonkoff JP, Phillips DA, eds. *From Neurons to Neighborhoods: The Science of Early Childhood Development.* Washington, DC: National Academies Press; 2000

10. Collaborative on Healthy Parenting in Primary Care. *Supporting Healthy Parenting in Primary Care.* Washington, DC: Forum on Promoting Children's Cognitive, Affective, and Behavioral Health at the National Academies of Sciences, Engineering, and Medicine; 2016. http://sites.nationalacademies.org/cs/groups/dbassesite/documents/webpage/dbasse_174781.pdf. Accessed January 4, 2018

11. Wethington HR, Hahn RA, Fuqua-Whitley DS, et al; US Task Force on Community Preventive Services. The effectiveness of interventions to reduce psychological harm from traumatic events among children and adolescents: a systematic review. *Am J Prev Med.* 2008;35(3):287–313

12. Dorsey S, McLaughlin KA, Kerns SEU, et al. Evidence base update for psychosocial treatments for children and adolescents exposed to traumatic events. *J Clin Child Adolesc Psychol.* 2017;46(3):303–330

13. American Academy of Pediatrics Council on Community Pediatrics. Providing care for children and adolescents facing homelessness and housing insecurity. *Pediatrics.* 2013;131(6):1206–1210

14. American Academy of Pediatrics Council on Community Pediatrics and Committee on Nutrition. Promoting food security for all children. *Pediatrics.* 2015;136(5):e1431–e1438

15. American Academy of Pediatrics, Food Research and Action Center. *Addressing Food Insecurity: A Toolkit for Pediatricians.* Washington, DC: Food Research and Action Center; 2017. http://frac.org/aaptoolkit. Accessed January 4, 2018

16. APA Task Force on Childhood Poverty. A strategic road-map: committed to bringing the voice of pediatricians to the most important problem facing children in the US today. Academic Pediatrics Association Web site. http://www.academicpeds.org/public_policy/pdf/APA_Task_Force_Strategic_Road_Mapver3.pdf. Published April 30, 2013. Accessed January 4, 2018

17. Poverty and child health. American Academy of Pediatrics Web site. https://www.aap.org/en-us/advocacy-and-policy/state-advocacy/Pages/Poverty%20and%20Child%20Health%20State%20Advocacy%20Resources.aspx. Accessed January 4, 2018

18. Burns BJ, Costello EJ, Angold A, et al. Children's mental health service use across service sectors. *Health Aff (Millwood).* 1995;14(3):147–159

19. Youngblade LM, Theokas C, Schulenberg J, Curry L, Huang IC, Novak M. Risk and promotive factors in families, schools, and communities: a contextual model of positive youth development in adolescence. *Pediatrics.* 2007;119 (suppl 1):S47–S53

20. Center for Mental Health Services. *Promotion and Prevention in Mental Health: Strengthening Parenting and Enhancing Child Resilience.* Rockville, MD: Substance Abuse and Mental Health Services Administration; 2007. DHHS publication CMHS-SVP-0175. https://store.samhsa.gov/product/Strengthening-Parenting-and-Enhancing-Child-Resilience/SVP07-0186. Accessed January 4, 2018

21. Jessor R, Turbin MS, Costa FM. Protective factors in adolescent health behavior. *J Pers Soc Psychol.* 1998;75(3):788–800

22. Carothers SS, Borkowski JG, Lefever JB, Whitman TL. Religiosity and the socioemotional adjustment of adolescent mothers and their children. *J Fam Psychol.* 2005;19(2):263–275

23. American Academy of Pediatrics Committee on Psychosocial Aspects of Child and Family Health and Task Force on Mental Health. The future of pediatrics: mental health competencies for pediatric primary care. *Pediatrics.* 2009;124(1):410–421

24. Foy JM, Earls MF. A process for developing community consensus regarding the diagnosis and management of attention-deficit/hyperactivity disorder. *Pediatrics.* 2005;115(1):e97–e104

25. American Academy of Child and Adolescent Psychiatry Committee on Health Care Access and Economics, American Academy of Pediatrics Task Force on Mental Health. Improving mental health services in primary care: reducing administrative and financial barriers to access and collaboration. *Pediatrics.* 2009;123(4):1248–1251

26. McKay MM, Hibbert R, Hoagwood K, et al. Integrating evidence-based engagement interventions into "real world" child mental health settings. *Brief Treat Crisis Interv.* 2004;4(2):177–186

27. President's New Freedom Commission on Mental Health. *Achieving the Promise: Transforming Mental Health Care in America; Final Report.* Rockville, MD: Substance Abuse and Mental Health Services Administration; 2003. DHHS publication SMA-03-3831. https://store.samhsa.gov/product/Achieving-the-Promise-Transforming-Mental-Health-Care-in-America-Executive-Summary/SMA03-3831. Accessed January 4, 2018

28. Sturner RA, Granger RH, Klatskin EH, Ferholt JB. The routine "well child" examination: a study of its value in the discovery of significant psychological problems. *Clin Pediatr (Phila)*. 1980;19(4):251–260

29. Horwitz SM, Kelleher KJ, Stein RE, et al. Barriers to the identification and management of psychosocial issues in children and maternal depression. *Pediatrics*. 2007;119(1):e208–e218

30. Julian TW, Kelleher K, Julian DA, Chisolm D. Using technology to enhance prevention services for children in primary care. *J Prim Prev*. 2007;28(2):155–165

31. Chisolm DJ, Gardner W, Julian T, Kelleher KJ. Adolescent satisfaction with computer-assisted behavioural risk screening in primary care. *Child Adolesc Ment Health*. 2008;13(4):163–168

32. Horwitz SM, Hoagwood KE, Garner A, et al. No technological innovation is a panacea: a case series in quality improvement for primary care mental health services. *Clin Pediatr (Phila)*. 2008;47(7):685–692

33. Bergman DA, Beck A, Rahm AK. The use of internet-based technology to tailor well-child care encounters. *Pediatrics*. 2009;124(1):e37–e43

34. Laraque D, Adams R, Steinbaum D, et al. Reported physician skills in the management of children's mental health problems following an educational intervention. *Acad Pediatr*. 2009;9(3):164–171

35. Center for Adolescent Health and the Law. *State Minor Consent Laws: A Summary*. 3rd ed. Chapel Hill, NC: Center for Adolescent Health and the Law. http://www.cahl.org/state-minor-consent-laws-a-summary-third-edition. Accessed January 4, 2018

36. Ho WW, Brandfield J, Retkin R, Laraque D. Complexities in HIV consent in adolescents. *Clin Pediatr (Phila)*. 2005;44(6):473–478

37. Bhatara VS, Vogt HB, Patrick S, Doniparthi L, Ellis R. Acceptability of a Web-based attention-deficit/hyperactivity disorder scale (T-SKAMP) by teachers: a pilot study. *J Am Board Fam Med*. 2006;19(2):195–200

38. Ruwaard J, Schrieken B, Schrijver M, et al. Standardized Web-based cognitive behavioural therapy of mild to moderate depression: a randomized controlled trial with a long-term follow-up. *Cogn Behav Ther*. 2009;38(4):206–221

39. van Straten A, Cuijpers P, Smits N. Effectiveness of a Web-based self-help intervention for symptoms of depression, anxiety, and stress: randomized controlled trial. *J Med Internet Res*. 2008;10(1):e7

40. Wade SL, Walz NC, Carey JC, Williams KM. Preliminary efficacy of a Web-based family problem-solving treatment program for adolescents with traumatic brain injury. *J Head Trauma Rehabil*. 2008;23(6):369–377

41. Cho JH, Lee HC, Lim DJ, Kwon HS, Yoon KH. Mobile communication using a mobile phone with a glucometer for glucose control in type 2 patients with diabetes: as effective as an Internet-based glucose monitoring system. *J Telemed Telecare*. 2009;15(2):77–82

42. Kwon HS, Cho JH, Kim HS, et al. Establishment of blood glucose monitoring system using the internet. *Diabetes Care*. 2004;27(2):478–483

43. Wegner SE, Humble CG, Feaganes J, Stiles AD. Estimated savings from paid telephone consultations between subspecialists and primary care physicians. *Pediatrics*. 2008;122(6):e1136–e1140

44. Stevens J, Kelleher KJ, Gardner W, et al. Trial of computerized screening for adolescent behavioral concerns. *Pediatrics*. 2008;121(6):1099–1105

45. Leung SF, French P, Chui C, Arthur D. Computerized mental health assessment in integrative health clinics: a cross-sectional study using structured interview. *Int J Ment Health Nurs.* 2007;16(6):441–446

46. Olson AL, Gaffney CA, Lee PW, Starr P. Changing adolescent health behaviors: the healthy teens counseling approach. *Am J Prev Med.* 2008;35(5)(suppl):S359–S364

47. Grupp-Phelan J, Mahajan P, Foltin GL, et al; Pediatric Emergency Care Applied Research Network. Referral and resource use patterns for psychiatric-related visits to pediatric emergency departments. *Pediatr Emerg Care.* 2009;25(4):217–220

48. Gardner W, Kelleher KJ, Pajer K, Campo JV. Follow-up care of children identified with ADHD by primary care clinicians: a prospective cohort study. *J Pediatr.* 2004;145(6):767–771

49. Manfredi C, Lacey L, Warnecke R. Results of an intervention to improve compliance with referrals for evaluation of suspected malignancies at neighborhood public health centers. *Am J Public Health.* 1990;80(1):85–87

50. Friman PC, Finney JW, Rapoff MA, Christophersen ER. Improving pediatric appointment keeping with reminders and reduced response requirement. *J Appl Behav Anal.* 1985;18(4):315–321

51. Simon GE, VonKorff M, Rutter C, Wagner E. Randomised trial of monitoring, feedback, and management of care by telephone to improve treatment of depression in primary care. *BMJ.* 2000;320(7234):550–554

52. Oxman TE, Dietrich AJ, Williams JW Jr, Kroenke K. A three-component model for reengineering systems for the treatment of depression in primary care. *Psychosomatics.* 2002;43(6):441–450

53. Sabin JE, Daniels N. Managed care: strengthening the consumer voice in managed care; VII. The Georgia Peer Specialist Program. *Psychiatr Serv.* 2003;54(4):497–498

54. Center for Mental Health Services. *Helping Children and Youth With Serious Mental Health Needs: Systems of Care.* Rockville, MD: Substance Abuse and Mental Health Services Administration; 2006. https://store.samhsa.gov/product/Helping-Children-and-Youth-With-Serious-Mental-Health-Needs-Systems-of-Care/SMA06-4125. Accessed January 4, 2018

55. *The Children's Plan: Improving the Social and Emotional Well Being of New York's Children and Their Families.* Albany, NY: New York State Office of Mental Health; 2008. http://ccf.ny.gov/files/5013/7962/7099/childrens_plan.pdf. Accessed January 4, 2018

56. Parks J, Svendsen D, Singer P, Foti ME, eds. *Morbidity and Mortality in People With Serious Mental Illness.* Alexandria, VA: National Association of State Mental Health Program Directors; 2006. https://www.nasmhpd.org/content/morbidity-and-mortality-people-serious-mental-illness. Accessed January 4, 2018

57. Institute of Medicine Committee on Quality of Health Care in America. *Crossing the Quality Chasm: A New Health System for the 21st Century.* Washington, DC: National Academies Press; 2001

58. Dayton L, Buttress A, Agosti J, et al. Practical steps to integrate family voice in organization, policy, planning, and decision-making for socio-emotional trauma-informed integrated pediatric care. *Curr Probl Pediatr Adolesc Health Care.* 2016;46(12):402–410

59. Family-centered care. Family Voices Web site. http://www.familyvoices.org/work/family_care. Accessed January 4, 2018

60. Dayton L, Agosti J, Bernard-Pearl D, et al. Integrating mental and physical health services using a socio-emotional trauma lens. *Curr Probl Pediatr Adolesc Health Care.* 2016;46(12):391–401

61. Coleman WL, Richmond JB. After the death of a child: helping bereaved parents and brothers and sisters. In: Carey WB, Crocker AC, Coleman WL, Elias ER, Feldman HM, eds. *Developmental-Behavioral Pediatrics.* 4th ed. Philadelphia, PA: Saunders Elsevier; 2008:366–372

62. Kohen DP, Olness K. *Hypnosis and Hypnotherapy With Children.* 4th ed. New York, NY: Routledge; 2011

63. Kohen DP, Kaiser P, Olness K. State-of-the-art pediatric hypnosis training: remodeling curriculum and refining faculty development. *Am J Clin Hypn.* 2017;59(3):292–310

64. American Academy of Pediatrics Section on Integrative Medicine. Mind-body therapies in children and youth. *Pediatrics.* 2016;138(3):e20161896

65. American Academy of Pediatrics. *ADHD: Caring for Children With ADHD; A Resource Toolkit for Clinicians.* 2nd ed. Elk Grove Village, IL: American Academy of Pediatrics; 2011

66. Stille CJ, McLaughlin TJ, Primack WA, Mazor KM, Wasserman RC. Determinants and impact of generalist-specialist communication about pediatric outpatient referrals. *Pediatrics.* 2006;118(4):1341–1349

67. Grimshaw JM, Winkens RA, Shirran L, et al. Interventions to improve outpatient referrals from primary care to secondary care. *Cochrane Database Syst Rev.* 2005;(3):CD005471

68. Connor DF, McLaughlin TJ, Jeffers-Terry M, et al. Targeted child psychiatric services: a new model of pediatric primary clinician—child psychiatry collaborative care. *Clin Pediatr (Phila).* 2006;45(5):423–434

69. Van Cleave J, Le TT, Perrin JM. Point-of-care child psychiatry expertise: the Massachusetts Child Psychiatry Access Project. *Pediatrics.* 2015;135(5):834–841

70. Dela-Cruz M, Steinbaum D, Battista A, Zuckerbrot R, Laraque D. Web-Based Child Psychiatry Access Project (Web-CPAP): a feasibility study. Presented at: 2007 American Public Health Association Meeting; November 5, 2007; Washington, DC

71. Komaromy M, Bartlett J, Manis K, Arora S. Enhanced primary care treatment of behavioral disorders with ECHO case-based learning. *Psychiatr Serv.* 2017;68(9):873–875

72. Guevara JP, Greenbaum PE, Shera D, Bauer L, Schwarz DF. Survey of mental health consultation and referral among primary care pediatricians. *Acad Pediatr.* 2009;9(2):123–127

73. Njoroge WF, Hostutler CA, Schwartz BS, Mautone JA. Integrated behavioral health in pediatric primary care. *Curr Psychiatry Rep.* 2016;18(12):106

74. Asarnow JR, Rozenman M, Wiblin J, Zeltzer L. Integrated medical-behavioral care compared with usual primary care for child and adolescent behavioral health: a meta-analysis. *JAMA Pediatr.* 2015;169(10):929–937

75. Sarvet B, Gold J, Bostic JQ, et al. Improving access to mental health care for children: the Massachusetts Child Psychiatry Access Project. *Pediatrics.* 2010;126(6):1191–1200

76. Chemtob CM, Nakashima JP, Hamada RS. Psychosocial intervention for postdisaster trauma symptoms in elementary school children: a controlled community field study. *Arch Pediatr Adolesc Med.* 2002;156(3):211–216

77. Hodgkinson S, Godoy L, Beers LS, Lewin A. Improving mental health access for low-income children and families in the primary care setting. *Pediatrics*. 2017;139(1):e20151175

78. Williams J, Shore SE, Foy JM. Co-location of mental health professionals in primary care settings: three North Carolina models. *Clin Pediatr (Phila)*. 2006;45(6):537–543

79. Reiss-Brennan B. Can mental health integration in a primary care setting improve quality and lower costs? A case study. *J Manag Care Pharm*. 2006; 12(2)(suppl):14–20

80. Kolko DJ, Campo J, Kilbourne AM, et al. Collaborative care outcomes for pediatric behavioral health problems: a cluster randomized trial. *Pediatrics*. 2014;133(4):e981–e992

81. Weersing VR, Brent DA, Rozenman MA, et al. *JAMA Psychiatry*. 2017;74(6): 571–578

82. American Academy of Pediatrics. Connecting for children's sake: integrating physical and mental health care in the medical home. Plenary presentations at: Pediatrics for the 21st Century (Peds-21) Symposium Series; October 7, 2005; Washington, DC

83. Levy SL, Hill E, Mattern K, McKay K, Sheldrick RC, Perrin EC. Colocated mental health/developmental care. *Clin Pediatr (Phila)*. 2017;56(11):1023–1031

84. Mental health initiatives. American Academy of Pediatrics Web site. https://www.aap.org/en-us/advocacy-and-policy/aap-health-initiatives/Mental-Health/Pages/ProgramSearch.aspx. Accessed January 4, 2018

85. Winters NC, Collett BR, Myers KM. Ten-year review of rating scales, VII: scales assessing functional impairment. *J Am Acad Child Adolesc Psychiatry*. 2005;44(4):309–338

86. Wolraich M, Brown L, Brown RT, et al; American Academy of Pediatrics Subcommittee on Attention-deficit/Hyperactivity Disorder and Steering Committee on Quality Improvement and Management. ADHD: clinical practice guideline for the diagnosis, evaluation, and treatment of attention-deficit/hyperactivity disorder in children and adolescents. *Pediatrics*. 2011;128(5): 1007–1022

87. Epstein JN, Langberg JM, Lichtenstein PK, Mainwaring BA, Luzader CP, Stark LJ. Community-wide intervention to improve the attention-deficit/hyperactivity disorder assessment and treatment practices of community physicians. *Pediatrics*. 2008;122(1):19–27

88. Homer CJ, Horvitz L, Heinrich P, Forbes P, Lesneski C, Phillips J. Improving care for children with attention deficit hyperactivity disorder: assessing the impact of self-assessment and targeted training on practice performance. *Ambul Pediatr*. 2004;4(5):436–441

89. Lannon C, Dolins J, Lazorick S, Crowe VL, Butts-Dion S, Schoettker PJ. Partnerships for Quality project: closing the gap in care of children with ADHD. *Jt Comm J Qual Patient Saf*. 2007;33(12)(suppl):66–74

90. Guidelines for Adolescent Depression in Primary Care (GLAD-PC) Toolkit. The REACH Institute Web site. http://www.gladpc.org. Accessed January 4, 2018

91. Heymann AD, Hoch I, Valinsky L, Shalev V, Silber H, Kokia E. Mandatory computer field for blood pressure measurement improves screening. *Fam Pract*. 2005;22(2):168–169

92. Shekelle PG, Morton SC, Keeler EB. Costs and benefits of health information technology. *Evid Rep Technol Assess (Full Rep)*. 2006;(132):1–71

93. Chaudhry B, Wang J, Wu S, et al. Systematic review: impact of health information technology on quality, efficiency, and costs of medical care. *Ann Intern Med*. 2006;144(10):742–752

94. Adams WG, Mann AM, Bauchner H. Use of an electronic medical record improves the quality of urban pediatric primary care. *Pediatrics*. 2003;111(3): 626–632

95. McAlearney AS, Chisolm D, Veneris S, Rich D, Kelleher K. Utilization of evidence-based computerized order sets in pediatrics. *Int J Med Inform*. 2006;75(7):501–512

96. Epstein JN, Langberg JM, Lichtenstein PK, Kolb R, Simon JO. The myADHDportal.com Improvement Program: an innovative quality improvement intervention for improving the quality of ADHD care among community-based pediatricians. *Clin Pract Pediatr Psychol*. 2013;1(1):55–67

97. Epstein JN, Kelleher KJ, Baum R, et al. Impact of a web-portal intervention on community ADHD care and outcomes. *Pediatrics*. 2016;138(2):e20154240

98. Bernal P. Hidden morbidity in pediatric primary care. *Pediatr Ann*. 2003; 32(6):413–418

Partnering to Improve Community Mental Health Systems

Jane Meschan Foy, MD, and James M. Perrin, MD

"Partnership across disciplines can stimulate fresh and effective approaches to advocacy and policy."

Introduction

Communities very much affect children's health, growth, and well-being, including their mental health. All health conditions reflect the interaction of biological factors with the psychosocial and physical environments, and the environment can affect the manifestations of illness, access to care, and response to treatment. A community's mental health and social services are a critical part of that environment for the growing number of children and families who experience mental health and social problems.

Sources of key mental health and social services are summarized in Appendix 4. Chapter 3, Office and Network Systems to Support Mental Health Care, discusses strategies primary care clinicians can use to identify resources available in a given community and develop relationships with key providers. This chapter complements Chapter 3 by offering strategies for enhancing a community's mental health and social services, using the tools of collaboration and advocacy.

Community systems of care take many forms. Typically, they include programs for early identification and referral of mental health concerns, not only in pediatric practice but also in child care settings, Early Intervention (EI) sites, and schools. They involve an array of community mental health and developmental-behavioral specialists working on both prevention and treatment, as well as other health and human service providers who interact with children, adolescents, and families with mental health concerns. Figure 4-1 describes a system of services for children and adolescents with special health care needs, including those with mental health problems. It not only notes the wide array of services that affect the health

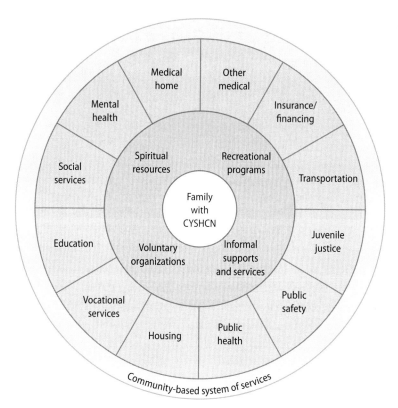

Figure 4-1. Family-centered, community-based system of services for children and youth with special needs.

Abbreviation: CYSHCN, children and youth with special health care needs.

Reproduced with permission from Perrin JM, Romm D, Bloom SR, et al. A family-centered, community-based system of services for children and youth with special health care needs. *Arch Pediatr Adolesc Med.* 2007;161(10):933–936.

and wellness of children, adolescents, and families, including the medical home, but also encompasses such programs as transportation, public health, housing, education, and social services. Box 4-1 points to key community partners who may participate in developing coalitions to improve mental health. Partnerships will help pediatric clinicians (ie, primary care clinicians including family physicians, internists, nurse practitioners, and physician assistants who provide health care to children and adolescents, as well as developmental-behavioral and adolescent specialists) pursue the strategies described in this chapter.

Almost every region of the United States has a public agency responsible for managing or providing mental health and substance use disorder

Box 4-1. Community Partners in a System of Services for Children and Adolescents With Mental Health Concerns

- Pediatricians and other primary care clinicians who serve children
- Pediatric subspecialists (eg, developmental-behavioral pediatricians, adolescent specialists)
- Mental health specialists
  - Psychiatrists (child and other)
  - Psychologists (doctoral and master's trained)
  - Psychiatric social workers
  - Psychiatric nurse practitioners
  - Substance use disorder health care professionals
  - Marriage and family therapists
- School system providers
  - Guidance counselors
  - Social workers
  - Nurses
  - Psychologists
  - School-based health center personnel
  - Special education teachers
  - Drop-out prevention specialists
  - Vocational rehabilitation and training specialists
- Early childhood and EI programs
- Public health personnel
- Child protective services personnel
- Juvenile justice personnel
- Child and family advocacy organizations (eg, NAMI, CHADD, FFCMH)
- Other community service providers
- Peer navigators
- Care coordinators

Abbreviations: CHADD, Children and Adults with Attention-Deficit/Hyperactivity Disorder; EI, Early Intervention; FFCMH, Federation of Families for Children's Mental Health; NAMI, National Alliance on Mental Illness.

(SUD) services to specific populations (often those with severely impairing conditions). The same agency may also manage or provide EI services, or another agency may have this responsibility. Agencies typically organize advisory groups of family members who have been affected by these conditions along with providers of EI, mental health, and SUD services. Groups often inadvertently omit pediatric clinicians from their memberships but usually welcome their involvement if it is offered. Consumer and advocacy groups such as the National Alliance on Mental Illness (NAMI), the Federation of Families for Children's Mental Health (FFCMH), Children and Adults with Attention-Deficit/Hyperactivity Disorder (ADHD) (CHADD), and the local mental health association also welcome pediatricians' interest and involvement in their activities. Increasingly, the public health community has come to view mental health as a public health issue, mirroring the clinical movement toward "reconnecting" the mind and the body. All these organizations are potential partners in an advocacy effort.

A multidiscipline, multiagency group interested in improving mental health services may gather to address a crisis that calls attention to the community's mental health needs, to develop a grant proposal, to reconfigure services after a loss or gain of funding, or simply to accept the invitation of an influential member of the community to begin a conversation. Whatever the reason, the following strategies may provide ideas for their work together.

Strategy 1: Applying a Population Perspective to Understand the Mental Health Needs of Children and Adolescents in the Community

Some factors place children and adolescents at risk for mental health problems later in life, while other protective factors reduce risks (Figure 4-2).[1-3] As indicated in the figure, the community, family, schools, and child care personnel interacting with child-specific factors all influence resilience in children and adolescents.

To identify needs and track progress toward community goals, pediatric clinicians and their partners can review measures of child and adolescent well-being in their communities (eg, child abuse and neglect reports, EI referrals, kindergarten screening results, adolescent suicide and homicide rates, high school drop-out and graduation rates, school suspension and expulsion rates, and substance use and teen pregnancy rates). Analysis of data according to school or zip code may yield additional insights and lead to specific interventions tailored to a particular school or neighborhood.

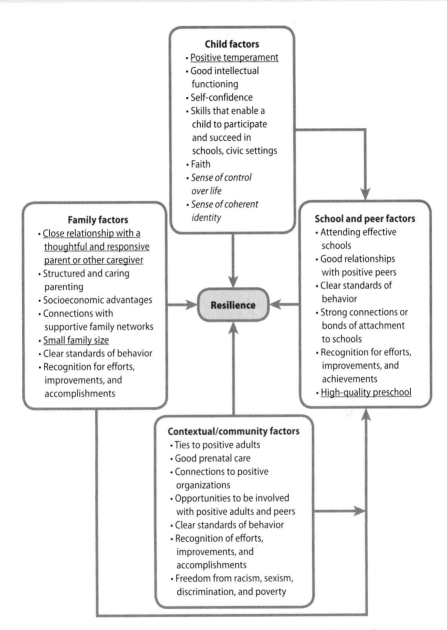

Figure 4-2. Protective, or buffering, factors that promote resilience. The underlined factors apply especially to young children; *italicized* factors apply especially to adolescents.

Adapted from Center for Mental Health Services. *Promotion and Prevention in Mental Health: Strengthening Parenting and Enhancing Child Resilience.* Rockville, MD: Substance Abuse and Mental Health Services Administration; 2007. DHHS publication CMHS-SVP-0175.

An additional source of statistics is the Youth Risk Behavior Surveillance System (commonly known as YRBSS), which monitors health-risk behaviors, including behaviors that contribute to unintentional injuries and violence, alcohol and other drug use, tobacco use, sexual behaviors, dietary behaviors, and physical activity. State, territorial, tribal, and local surveys are conducted in partnership with the Centers for Disease Control and Prevention (commonly known as CDC) and made available to school districts and communities to facilitate program planning.[4]

Pediatric clinicians have increasingly addressed the social determinants of health. Poverty, food insecurity, substandard housing, homelessness, and neighborhoods with high crime rates all powerfully affect health of children, adolescents, and families.[5] Pediatric clinicians and their partners can look at the needs of populations that have higher risk for mental health problems, including those affected by these social adversities, as well as those affected by trauma, toxic stress, and natural disasters; those with parents deployed in military service, developmental disabilities, and other chronic medical conditions; those who experience academic difficulties; or those in foster care. Pervasive racial and ethnic disparities affect children's and adolescents' health and educational outcomes and their access to effective mental health services.[6,7] Other issues such as xenophobia and homophobia may also affect the mental health of groups within the community by contributing to their stress and isolation.

Stigma prevents many people from seeking care for their mental health and substance use concerns. Community coalitions can work together to combat stigma at the community level. Partnerships can employ the following strategies:

▶ Battling stigma with facts. For example, mental illnesses are treatable; children, adolescents, and adults who live with these illnesses can achieve recovery and lead full and productive lives; children and adolescents often have behavioral problems; mental illness is not a character flaw, a sign of moral weakness, or anyone's fault.

▶ Establishing support groups and education programs for families (combating the social isolation that so often accompanies mental illness, for people of all ages).

▶ Eliminating language that contributes to stigma through defining people by their conditions (eg, referring to someone as a "schizophrenic") and instead using "people-first" language (eg, "a person with schizophrenia").

Review of use of local or regional emergency facilities, mental health outpatient and inpatient services, nonprofit and private-sector programs, and the school system's exceptional children's or special educational services can also provide helpful evidence and assist in developing priorities for school-based initiatives and for other community programs as needed.

Just as the public health perspective enlightens a discussion of mental health, the mental health perspective can enlighten discussions of public health issues (physical inactivity, poor diet, environmental toxins [eg, lead, mercury], neighborhood violence, unintended pregnancy, and injuries). Each of these issues has mental health causes or mental health effects or both, and each has implications for the mental, as well as physical, health of children in the community. Partnership across disciplines can stimulate fresh and effective approaches to advocacy and policy. Recent reports demonstrate, for example, the effectiveness of public policy in reducing youth alcohol and marijuana use.[8,9]

Strategy 2: Addressing Gaps in the Community's Mental Health and Social Resources

Service gaps often dominate discussions among child and adolescent mental health advocates, and the goal of coalitions is to identify and repair such gaps. For children and adolescents, mental health resources of all types are almost always insufficient.[10] Public mental health program funding may leave out infants and young children.

Appendix 4 lists key mental health, SUD, and social services for children and adolescents. Efforts to fill gaps or expand capacity should build on available evidence about effective programs and services. The Substance Abuse and Mental Health Services Administration (commonly known as SAMHSA) National Registry of Evidence-based Programs and Practices (www.nrepp.samhsa.gov) is an excellent resource for pediatric clinicians to use with local partners in developing strategies that address community needs. The American Academy of Pediatrics (AAP), in partnership with PracticeWise, provides a table of evidence-based child and adolescent psychosocial interventions; a snapshot of this resource is included as Appendix 6. It is updated biannually at www.aap.org/en-us/documents/crpsychosocialinterventions.pdf. Essential services include interventions that meet criteria for best evidence (levels 1 and 2 in this table).

Previous chapters in this book go into depth on such age-specific services as child care, Head Start, EI, nurse home visiting, and school-based mental health programs and services. Common gaps and opportunities in services include care coordination, community mental health services, transition care, access to mental health consultation, and integrated care. We discuss each in the following paragraphs.

Care Coordination

Care coordination can help children and families meet their needs. Roberts et al[11] delineated 6 central characteristics of care coordination: responsive to family challenges, priorities, and strengths; developed in partnership with constituents; reflective and respectful of the cultural norms and practices of the participating families; accessible to everyone; affordable to those who need assistance; and organized and coordinated through collaboration so resources are equitably distributed in an efficient and effective manner. To these characteristics, Perrin et al[12] added that such a system recognizes and addresses the specific developmental needs of infants, children, and adolescents and their important developmental transitions and is organized to promote cost-effective provision of services. Much evidence exists to support the value of coordination of care, especially with the complex systems of care that may affect the mental health of children, adolescents, and families.

The mental health specialty world calls such coordinated programs of services *systems of care*.[13] Involvement in a system of care improves coordination of care and educational outcomes for children and adolescents with mental illness and other psychosocial challenges. In communities in which such a system is under development, pediatricians can help design systems. A pediatric clinician's involvement in an individual child's system of care planning provides an invaluable opportunity for building professional relationships while enhancing the child's care.

Community Mental Health Services

Although a number of therapies and parenting programs are effective in treating the emotional, behavioral, and relationship problems of children and their families, many barriers limit access to nonpharmacological therapies: shortage and maldistribution of child mental health specialists trained to provide them; third-party payment systems that reward brief medication-focused visits, despite the lower risk of nonpsychopharmaco-logical treatments; and a billing and coding system that does not recognize relationship-focused therapy. Less than 50% of young children with emotional disturbances receive any treatment.[14] In communities in which these services are missing, child and adolescent advocates can rely on evidence to make a strong case for programs serving first-time, pregnant, low-income women; children and adolescents in foster care; infants and parents experiencing relationship disturbances; high-risk parents; and children of all ages exposed to trauma (including sexual abuse and domestic violence). See Chapters 7, 8, and 9 for discussion of evidence-based psychosocial therapy, self-regulation therapies and biofeedback, and complementary and integrative medical therapies, respectively.

Transition Services

As young adults with mental health problems "age out" of pediatric care, insurance plans, and the community resources that supported them during their childhood and adolescence, they must find new providers of their primary and specialty health care and face the stresses experienced by other young adults with special health and developmental needs. They may have limited educational, vocational, or social opportunities; financial hardships; difficulty finding housing; and inadequate services to assist them in overcoming or coping with these problems and in achieving their health, educational, vocational, and social goals. Pediatric clinicians can partner with the mental health community to address deficiencies in transition services for young people who are living with mental illness. Programs in several areas of the country may serve as models.[15,16] See Chapter 12 for more information about mental health transition services.

Mental Health Consultation

Although many communities do not have child psychiatrists, psychologists, or developmental-behavioral pediatricians,[17] some regions of the country have used creative strategies to gain access to mental health consultation for pediatric clinicians. In Massachusetts, a statewide psychiatry telephone consultation service assists pediatricians in assessing and managing the mental health problems of children and adolescents. Evaluation of this program indicated high rates of use and satisfaction among participatants.[18] More than 28 states have now adopted some variation of the Massachusetts program. Several states and communities use telemedicine clinics to provide access to consultation for children and adolescents remote from child psychiatrists and other mental health specialists. The National Network of Child Psychiatry Access Programs (http://web. jhu.edu/pedmentalhealth/nncpap_resources.html) provides examples of consultation models.

In many rural areas, consultation is provided by general psychiatrists and other mental health specialists whose training in child and adolescent mental health may be limited; in such areas, educational programs to enhance the providers' pediatric skills and their access to child and adolescent specialists for consultation may be useful adjuncts.

Project ECHO (Extension for Community Healthcare Outcomes) uses telemedicine technology to engage primary care clinicians in a learning system and link them to specialist mentors at an academic medical center or hub. This approach is already improving comprehensive community care for children with autism spectrum disorder and shows promise in expanding workforce capacity, decreasing costs, and enhancing access to care for underserved patients with other chronic conditions; however, more research will be necessary to affirm its benefits for patients with mental health conditions.[19]

Integrated Care

A number of reports have described the integration of one or more mental health specialists into primary care settings. Studies have focused primarily on adults with depression, but case reports suggest that integrated care may benefit patients with a variety of other conditions, as well as the clinicians and health systems that serve them. (See Chapter 3, Office and Network Systems to Support Mental Health Care.) A report describing an integrated behavioral health model in an inner city primary care clinic showed improved access and outcomes for children and families living in poverty.[20]

Policy recommendations for promoting integration of primary care and behavioral health were put forward by a workgroup of the 2013 Patient-Centered Medical Home Research Conference. These recommendations include building demonstration projects to test integration approaches, developing interdisciplinary training programs for members of the integrated care team, implementing population-based strategies to improve behavioral health, eliminating behavioral health "carve-outs" (separate insurance plans that deliver mental health and SUD benefits), testing innovative payment models, and developing population-based measures to evaluate integration.[21] Other recent reports have described integrated care and mechanisms to implement such care in primary care.[22,23]

Strategy 3: Enhancing Communication Between Pediatric Clinicians and Providers of Mental Health Specialty and Social Services

Enhancing communication among different providers, agencies, and schools is an important priority. Effective communication among pediatric clinicians, mental health specialists, educators, and agency representatives depends in part on an understanding of their different cultures and different priorities. For example, pediatric clinicians may come to a community mental health meeting with a focus on prevention, early identification of mental health problems, and care of children and adolescents with mild to moderate mental health disorders, perhaps only those with specific disorders such as ADHD. Representatives of a chronically underfunded public mental health agency may focus primarily on children with severe mental health conditions, with little capacity to address prevention or early identification or provision of consultative services to pediatric clinicians for their patients with less severe impairment. School representatives may focus primarily on behavioral problems that interfere with students' school attendance, classroom behaviors, and academic success; representatives of social service agencies may focus on the needs of children and adolescents in foster care; and representatives of the juvenile justice system may focus on the unmet mental health needs of adjudicated adolescents. Each group wants to engage the other's time and resources for its priority activities. As with any coalition, progress depends on compromise and finding common ground. Effective communication depends in part on understanding the different vocabularies of the mental health and medical systems. For example, *PCP* in medical terminology means a primary care physician, but *PCP* in mental health terminology means a "person-centered plan."

The care of mutual patients often drives relationships between pediatric clinicians and medical subspecialists. However, privacy concerns and perceived confidentiality barriers keep many mental health specialists and SUD health care professionals from communicating with pediatric clinicians or with other community service providers. Dialogue with local mental health agencies, emergency departments (EDs), and others who provide mental health and SUD services can raise awareness about the importance of communication with pediatric medical home providers. Ideally, routine intake procedures of EDs and mental health specialty facilities would prompt mental health specialists to seek families' consent for exchange of information with pediatric clinicians, and routine procedures in primary care offices would prompt staff to seek information about other sources of health care and request consent for exchange of information. Such routine procedures can become a goal of community-level problem-solving.

Schools are the largest de facto provider of mental health services.[24] The climate of each school, that is, its acceptance of diverse students, disciplinary processes, extracurricular activities, responsiveness to special needs of students, involvement of parents, and attention to students' safety, affects the well-being of its students. School-employed mental health personnel (eg, guidance counselors, social workers, psychologists) typically function in parallel with the mental health system. Although their focus is often on attendance, testing, and, in high schools, course selection and college preparation, these school-employed mental health specialists may play an important role in children's and adolescents' comprehensive mental health care, especially when the school personnel have effective connections with community mental health systems. School social workers and nurses may be more likely than other school personnel to see their roles as communicating with primary care clinicians and mental health specialists; however, school social workers and nurses typically have high caseloads and may travel to multiple schools, limiting their accessibility. Guidance counselors are more often based full-time in an assigned school. One guidance counselor in a school is often assigned the responsibility of chairing a committee that considers students' eligibility for special education and other services; as such, this individual may be the pediatric clinician's best option for communicating with the school around the mental health needs of an individual student. One community documented its success in developing and sustaining a community protocol that established a process for exchanging information between schools and primary care practices and articulated respective roles in assessing students with inattention and behavioral problems; in this process, school guidance counselors played a central role.[25] The principal is the key contact for issues involving the mental health climate of the school and any concerns about its disciplinary approach, which may weigh heavily on students with behavioral problems. Advocacy for enhanced communication between schools and primary care practices requires partnership with the local school board or local school health advisory council and school administrators (or both) as well as mental health specialty partners, other community health and service agencies, adolescents, parents, and teachers.

School-based health centers in many areas of the country provide students with enhanced access to an array of clinical services, including care for mental health and substance use problems; such programs are especially effective when linked to a student's medical home and to the system of care in the community. Procedures for enrollment in the school-based center can routinely document the parent's permission for exchange of information with medical home and other health care professionals.

Strategy 4: Developing a Community Protocol for Managing Psychiatric Emergencies

Deaths from homicide, suicide, and child abuse are tragically common.[26,27] Life-threatening mental health problems, including acute intoxication, delirium, psychosis, mania, severe family dysfunction, acute stress responses, domestic violence, severe mood disorders, and medical crises associated with eating disorders, also occur frequently. Pediatric clinicians may be the source from whom a child, an adolescent, or a family is most comfortable seeking help. Primary care clinicians have a role in preventing crises by identifying children and adolescents with mental health or substance use problems early, developing a relationship when the patient is not in crisis, and collaborating with the family to develop a crisis plan in advance. They also have a role in applying a management strategy to a crisis situation, which involves assessing the level of urgency of the patient's need for care, identifying intervention options, and using appropriate resources.

A natural disaster, an act of violence, war, or industrial disaster may inflict trauma and loss on many children, adolescents, and families simultaneously, those directly exposed and those emotionally exposed through death or injury of loved ones, and may pose even greater threats to children and adolescents with preexisting mental health issues. Pediatric clinicians have a role in planning with their community partners to deal with both short-term and long-term aftermath of these crises.[28]

Many EDs lack resources to address psychiatric emergencies in children and adolescents.[29,30] Through overcrowding, exposure to stressful sights and sounds, and long delays, they may inadvertently increase the distress and trauma experienced by children, adolescents, and their families.[31] Boarding of child and adolescent psychiatric patients in nonpsychiatric settings should be avoided as much as possible. When such boarding is unavoidable, every attempt should be made to ensure that patients are hospitalized in the least restrictive setting possible and transferred to a psychiatric facility as expeditiously as possible. Here, too, pediatric clinicians can participate in community and regional efforts to develop and fund needed services.

Some communities have specific psychiatric emergency services (eg, mobile crisis units that can be deployed to a medical office or school; mental health screening, triage, and referral centers; psychiatric and SUD intake facilities; intensive outpatient treatment programs); however, pediatric clinicians (as well as school and agency personnel with whom pediatric clinicians collaborate) may be unaware of them. As part of an inventory of community mental health resources (see Chapter 3, Office and Network Systems to Support Mental Health Care), pediatric clinicians can identify and prepare to use the emergency mental health services that are most appropriate for children and adolescents, often in the mental health system rather than an ED. Pediatric clinicians can negotiate with providers of emergency mental health services to secure ready access for their patients in "urgent" assessment slots. Primary care clinicians can work with mental health specialists to ensure that the primary care clinicians are informed about children and adolescents served in their systems and that arrangements are made for their continued monitoring and care after discharge from hospital or residential facilities.

Strategy 5: Participating in Community Efforts to Address Payment and Broader System Issues

Pediatric clinicians require adequate payment for the mental health services they provide and a policy environment that supports their involvement in mental health care. In coalitions, all players likely have inadequate funding for their services. A key aspect of community coalitions is to broaden advocacy for adequate financing for the services that children and families need. For pediatric clinicians, payment models require understanding of the additional time and effort needed to address mental health issues in pediatric practice. Many successful AAP chapter advocacy efforts have achieved significant policy changes in private (employer-based) health insurance, state Medicaid programs, and the State Children's Health Insurance Program. American Academy of Pediatrics chapters can be effective leaders in payment and system improvement. See www.aap.org/en-us/advocacy-and-policy/aap-health-initiatives/Mental-Health/Pages/Improve-Financing.aspx for strategies to maximize mental health benefits and financing.

Health care payment arrangements often prohibit children's and adolescents' access to key services. The transient nature of many conditions and the difficulties in assigning specific diagnoses, especially for younger children, complicate payment for early identification and treatment services. Ideally, Medicaid and commercial insurers would incorporate the *DC:0–5; Diagnostic Classification of Mental Health and Developmental Disorders of Infancy and Early Childhood*,[32] which recognizes the transient nature of diagnoses in this age-group and reflects that children and adolescents with significant problems may not fit fifth edition of *Diagnostic and Statistical Manual of Mental Disorders* (*DSM-5*) criteria.[33] Ideally, private insurers would also recognize that children and adolescents can be impaired by mental health symptoms that do not rise to the level of a *DSM-5* disorder. System features that support and foster mental health practice in primary care settings include

▶ Payment of primary care clinicians for mental health services

▶ Payment for multiple mental health visits to primary care before the establishment of a diagnosis (ie, to conduct an iterative assessment or to monitor and address emerging symptoms)

▶ Authorization of mental health referrals by primary care clinicians

▶ Notification of the primary care practice when a child enters the mental health specialty system

▶ Payment structure that supports mental health specialists colocated or integrated within the primary care setting; elimination of carve-outs (See discussion in the next paragraph.)

▶ Payment of both primary care clinicians and mental health specialists for consultation and care planning conferences

▶ An electronic system to access families' mental health benefits and provider panels

Many areas of the country have managed care carve-outs, providing insured households with a limited panel of mental health specialists. Carve-outs limit the numbers and range of mental health specialists, and panels may lack pediatric expertise. They may also limit information available to clinicians or families about participating mental health specialists. Typically, families must access these services directly, effectively preventing the referring clinician from conveying clinical information to the mental health professional or establishing a referral relationship. Names of providers to call may be out-of-date or inaccurate. Pediatric councils and mental health task forces in many AAP chapters have helped pediatricians work with regional directors of ambulatory managed care plans and employers to make them more knowledgeable of pediatric needs. Advocacy around mental health and substance use issues can become agenda items in these meetings (eg, notification of the patient's primary care practice when a family accesses mental health services, routine exchange of information between mental health specialists and primary care clinicians, expansion of mental health panels to include pediatric specialists). The federal law that mandates parity of mental health and physical health insurance benefits has established regulations that should provide incentive for such efforts.[34]

Strategies for System Change in Children's Mental Health: A Chapter Action Kit and the AAP mental health Web site offer strategies for AAP chapters and other medical associations to use in efforts to achieve equity of mental health benefits in insurance plans, fair payment of physicians and mental health specialists for the services they provide, policies that support and promote collaboration, and support of public mental health systems. The AAP Task Force on Mental Health worked with the American Academy of Child and Adolescent Psychiatry to develop a white paper on administrative and financial barriers to children's mental health care, published in *Pediatrics* in April 2009.[35] This paper continues to be valuable in informing advocacy efforts. Consumer groups such as NAMI, CHADD, and FFCMH are invaluable to pediatric clinicians' advocacy efforts.

Conclusion

Pediatric clinicians can play a critical role in building, supporting, and enhancing community programs to promote mental health, reduce the risk of mental illness, and improve mental health services. Strategies should reflect the community's specific needs and the clinician's practice priorities. Forming a group of interested pediatricians, primary care clinicians from other disciplines (family physicians, internists, nurse practitioners, physician assistants), developmental-behavioral and adolescent specialists, advocates, educators, agency representatives, mental health specialists, and SUD health care professionals helps enhance relationships while ensuring coordination and synergy of effort. The resources available on the AAP mental health Web site can provide assistance. Facilitating system changes at the community level will help pediatric clinicians enhance mental health care at the practice level.

Community-level strategies for enhancing children's and adolescents' mental health include

1. Apply a "population" perspective to gain understanding of the mental health needs of children and adolescents in the community, including the positive and negative social determinants of health.

2. Address gaps in the community's mental health and social resources.

3. Enhance communication among pediatric clinicians and other community providers and programs.

4. Develop a community protocol for managing psychiatric emergencies.

5. Participate in community efforts to address payment and broader system issues.

Acknowledgments: The authors acknowledge contributions to this work by the American Academy of Pediatrics (AAP) Task Force on Mental Health (2004–2010).

The AAP Task Force on Mental Health included Jane Meschan Foy, MD (chairperson, lead author); Paula Duncan, MD; Barbara Frankowski, MD, MPH; Kelly Kelleher, MD, MPH; Penelope K. Knapp, MD; Danielle Laraque, MD; Gary Peck, MD; Michael Regalado, MD; Jack Swanson, MD; and Mark Wolraich, MD; the consultants were Margaret Dolan; James Perrin, MD; and Lynn Wegner, MD.

AAP Policy

American Academy of Pediatrics Committee on Pediatric Emergency Medicine. Access to optimal emergency care for children. *Pediatrics.* 2007;119(1):161–164. Reaffirmed July 2014 (pediatrics.aappublications.org/content/119/1/161)

American Academy of Pediatrics Committee on Pediatric Emergency Medicine, American College of Emergency Physicians Pediatric Emergency Medicine Committee. Pediatric mental health emergencies in the emergency medical services system. *Pediatrics.* 2006;118(4):1764–1767. Reaffirmed April 2013 (pediatrics.aappublications. org/content/118/4/1764)

American Academy of Pediatrics Council on Children With Disabilities and Medical Home Implementation Project Advisory Committee. Patient- and family-centered care coordination: a framework for integrating care for children and youth across multiple systems. *Pediatrics.* 2014;133(5):e1451–e1460 (pediatrics.aappublications.org/content/133/5/e1451)

References

1. Webster-Stratton C, Taylor T. Nipping early risk factors in the bud: preventing substance abuse, delinquency, and violence in adolescence through interventions targeted at young children (0-8 years). *Prev Sci.* 2001;2(3):165–192

2. Wille N, Bettge S, Ravens-Sieberer U; BELLA Study Group. Risk and protective factors for children's and adolescents' mental health: results of the BELLA study. *Eur Child Adolesc Psychiatry.* 2008;17(suppl 1):133–147

3. Center for Mental Health Services. *Promotion and Prevention in Mental Health: Strengthening Parenting and Enhancing Child Resilience.* Rockville, MD: Substance Abuse and Mental Health Services Administration; 2007. DHHS publication CMHS-SVP-0175. http://store.samhsa.gov/shin/content/SVP07-0186/SVP07-0186.pdf. Accessed January 4, 2018

4. Centers for Disease Control and Prevention. YRBSS: questionnaires. https://www.cdc.gov/healthyyouth/data/yrbs/questionnaires.htm. Centers for Disease Control and Prevention Web site. Accessed January 4, 2018

5. American Academy of Pediatrics Council on Community Pediatrics. Poverty and child health in the United States. *Pediatrics.* 2016;137(4):e20160339

6. Center for Mental Health Services. *Mental Health: Culture, Race, and Ethnicity—A Supplement to Mental Health: A Report of the Surgeon General.* Rockville, MD: Substance Abuse and Mental Health Services Administration; 2001. https://www.ncbi.nlm.nih.gov/books/NBK44243. Accessed January 4, 2018

7. Alegría M, Green JG, McLaughlin KA, Loder S. *Disparities in Child and Adolescent Mental Health and Mental Health Services in the U.S.* New York, NY: William T. Grant Foundation; 2015. http://wtgrantfoundation.org/library/uploads/2015/09/Disparities-in-Child-and-Adolescent-Mental-Health.pdf. Accessed January 4, 2018

8. Xuan Z, Blanchette JG, Nelson TF, et al. Youth drinking in the United States: relationships with alcohol policies and adult drinking. *Pediatrics.* 2015;136(1):18–27

9. Saloner B, McGinty EE, Barry CL. Policy strategies to reduce youth recreational marijuana use. *Pediatrics.* 2015;135(6):955–957

10. Huang L, Macbeth G, Dodge J, Jacobstein D. Transforming the workforce in children's mental health. *Adm Policy Ment Health.* 2004;32(2):167–187

11. Roberts RN, Behl DD, Akers AL. Building a system of care for children with special healthcare needs. *Infants Young Child.* 2004;17(3):213–222

12. Perrin JM, Romm D, Bloom SR, et al. A family-centered, community-based system of services for children and youth with special health care needs. *Arch Pediatr Adolesc Med.* 2007;161(10):933–936

13. Stroul BA. *Issue Brief—Systems of Care: A Framework for System Reform in Children's Mental Health.* Washington, DC: National Technical Assistance Center for Children's Mental Health, Georgetown University Child Development Center; 2002

14. Gleason MM, Goldson E, Yogman MW; American Academy of Pediatrics Council on Early Childhood, Committee on Psychosocial Aspects of Child and Family Health, and Section on Developmental and Behavioral Pediatrics. Addressing early childhood emotional and behavioral problems. *Pediatrics.* 2016;138(6):e20163025

15. Bloom SR, Kuhlthau K, Van Cleave J, Knapp AA, Newacheck P, Perrin JM. Health care transitions for youth with special health care needs. *J Adolesc Health.* 2012;51(3):213–219

16. Stein REK, Perrin JM, Iezzoni LI. Health care: access and medical support for youth and young adults with chronic health conditions and disabilities. In: Lollar D, ed. *Launching Into Adulthood.* Baltimore, MD: Paul H. Brookes Publishing Co; 2010:77–102

17. Cama S, Malowney M, Smith AJB, et al. Availability of outpatient mental health care by pediatricians and child psychiatrists in five U.S. cities. *Int J Health Serv.* 2017:20731417707492

18. Van Cleave J, Le TT, Perrin JM. Point-of-care child psychiatry expertise: the Massachusetts Child Psychiatry Access Project. *Pediatrics.* 2015;135(5):834–841

19. Zhou C, Crawford A, Serhal E, Kurdyak P, Sockalingam S. The impact of Project ECHO on participant and patient outcomes: a systematic review. *Acad Med.* 2016;91(10):1439–1461

20. Hodgkinson S, Godoy L, Beers LS, Lewin A. Improving mental health access for low-income children and families in the primary care setting. *Pediatrics.* 2017;139(1):e20151175

21. Ader J, Stille CJ, Keller D, Miller BF, Barr MS, Perrin JM. The medical home and integrated behavioral health: advancing the policy agenda. *Pediatrics.* 2015;135(5):909–917

22. Briggs RD, ed. *Integrated Early Childhood Behavioral Health in Primary Care: A Guide to Implementation and Evaluation.* New York, NY: Springer Publications; 2017

23. Tyler ET, Hulkower RL, Kaminski JW. *Behavioral Health Integration in Pediatric Primary Care: Considerations and Opportunities for Policymakers, Planners, and Providers.* New York, NY: Milbank Memorial Fund; 2017. https://www.milbank. org/publications/behavioral-health-integration-in-pediatric-primary-care-considerations-and-opportunities-for-policymakers-planners-and-providers. Accessed January 4, 2018

24. Burns BJ, Costello EJ, Angold A, et al. Children's mental health service use across service sections. *Health Aff (Millwood).* 1995;14(3):147–159

25. Foy JF, Earls MF. A process for developing community consensus on the diagnosis and management of attention-deficit/hyperactivity disorder. *Pediatrics.* 2005;115(1):e97–e104

26. Child abuse and neglect fatalities 2015: statistics and interventions. Child Welfare Information Gateway Web site. https://www.childwelfare.gov/pubs/factsheets/ fatality. Published 2017. Accessed January 4, 2018

27. Ten leading causes of death and injury. Centers for Disease Control and Prevention Web site. https://www.cdc.gov/injury/wisqars/LeadingCauses.html. Updated May 2, 2017. Accessed January 4, 2018

28. American Academy of Pediatrics Disaster Preparedness Advisory Council. Medical countermeasures for children in public health emergencies, disasters, or terrorism. *Pediatrics.* 2016;137(2):e20154273

29. American Academy of Pediatrics Committee on Pediatric Emergency Medicine, American College of Emergency Physicians Pediatric Emergency Medicine Committee. Pediatric mental health emergencies in the emergency medical services system. *Pediatrics.* 2006;118(4):1764–1767

30. Institute of Medicine. *Emergency Care for Children: Growing Pains.* Washington, DC: National Academies Press; 2007

31. Allen MH, Carpenter D, Sheets JL, Miccio S, Ross R. What do consumers say they want and need during a psychiatric emergency? *J Psychiatr Pract.* 2003;9(1):39–58

32. Zeanah CH, Lieberman A. Defining relational pathology in early childhood: the *Diagnostic Classification of Mental Health and Developmental Disorders of Infancy and Early Childhood DC:0–5* approach. *Infant Ment Health J.* 2016;37(5):509–520

33. American Psychiatric Association. *Diagnostic and Statistical Manual of Mental Disorders*. 5th ed. Washington, DC: American Psychiatric Association; 2013

34. Implementation of the Mental Health Parity and Addiction Equity Act (MHPAEA). Substance Abuse and Mental Health Services Administration Web site. https://www.samhsa.gov/health-financing/implementation-mental-health-parity-addiction-equity-act. Updated January 24, 2017. Accessed April 17, 2018

35. American Academy of Pediatrics Task Force on Mental Health, American Academy of Child and Adolescent Psychiatry Committee on Health Care Access and Economics. Improving mental health services in primary care: reducing administrative and financial barriers to access and collaboration [published correction appears in *Pediatrics*. 2009;123(6):1611]. *Pediatrics*. 2009;123(4): 1248–1251

Effective Communication Methods: Common Factors Skills

Lawrence S. Wissow, MD, MPH

"In this approach, the clinician provides a setting in which patient concerns can be expressed, patients take the lead in developing goals and the strategies to attain them, and information is offered when patients say they are ready to hear it."

Approximately 15% of school-aged children and adolescents in the United States are thought to have an emotional or behavioral disorder.[1,2] Nearly two-thirds of those who have disorders receive no formal mental health care, and only one-half receive counseling or some other form of assistance at school.[3] Providing adequate care for this group of young people requires several strategies, including reducing stigma and financial barriers, educating young people and their families about the benefits of seeking care, and increasing the availability of effective services in accessible settings.[4]

One way of broadening access and reducing both financial barriers and psychological barriers involves promoting the detection, and in some cases treatment, of mental health problems by primary care clinicians (PCCs) (ie, pediatricians, family physicians, internists, nurse practitioners, and physician assistants at the front lines of pediatric practice). Primary care visits offer many potential advantages for helping families with mental health problems. Primary care's philosophy of promoting and tracking healthy development fits well with the task of preventing and monitoring for emerging mental health issues. Longitudinal relationships have the potential to build trust and willingness to share sensitive information. Long-term relationships also mean that mental health care can be delivered episodically as needed, in a familiar setting, and in the context of care for medical issues.

However, many young people (and their parents) do not disclose their emotional problems to their primary care physicians.[5] Parent and clinician assessments of child and adolescent mental health often do not agree,[6] and estimates suggest that families follow through with only approximately

40% of the mental health referrals made by PCCs.[7] These challenges are not surprising when considering how pediatric primary care is structured. Visits are relatively short, and many competing concerns need to be addressed. If problems are found, referral sources may be limited, and PCCs report low levels of confidence in managing mental health problems themselves.[8]

The skills presented in this chapter were chosen to help PCCs efficiently uncover and clarify mental health needs, have therapeutic encounters with people who feel demoralized or angry, and give advice about mental health problems, including making referrals, that will be accepted and followed. The skills offer an approach to clinical interaction that contrasts with the style of most routine encounters. The traditional pediatric style is energetic and directive. It assumes that patients and their families come with questions and needs and that clinicians should respond with a straightforward diagnosis and plan for treatment. This approach works much of the time, especially for situations in which few emotional over-lays exist. However, it can fail when people feel ambivalent, ashamed, or anxious, or if they believe that their freedom is being challenged. In these situations, patients do not always admit what really concerns them, they may react to offers of care in unexpected ways, and they may resist advice that is offered. Ambivalence, shame, and anxiety accompany many common concerns, especially those linked to traumatic experiences. Individuals experiencing trauma are often on alert for interactions in which they could feel unsupported or experience further vulnerability. Similar feeling can occur when the trauma people experience stems from the myriad hassles and indignities associated with poverty and racism.

An alternative to a directive style is what has been called either *patient centered* or *quiet and curious*.[9,10] In this approach, the clinician provides a setting in which patient concerns can be expressed, patients take the lead in developing goals and the strategies to attain them, and information is offered when patients say they are ready to hear it. This approach can be an efficient method for helping people institute change in their lives, and it helps clinicians and patients work together during times when change is not yet possible.

The techniques described in this chapter are framed in the context of emotional and behavioral concerns, but their respective uses are not limited to visits with an explicit mental health agenda. They have wide applications to situations in which families and clinicians are trying to understand each other's attitudes and develop mutually acceptable plans of action. Many of the skills will seem intuitive or already part of common practice, such as motivational interviewing[11]; others may seem new. The results of many studies suggest that these sorts of skills can be learned fairly quickly; however, not surprisingly, opportunities for practice, feedback, and self-assessment lead to greater clinical effectiveness.[12]

The patient-centered style discussed in this chapter draws heavily from the "common factors" literature in mental health care.[13] *Common* refers to aspects of patients, clinicians, and their interactions that are shared across successful treatments for a wide variety of mental health problems, including the use of medication. Though there are many formulations of these factors, they can be summarized as attitudes and interactions that promote both the patient's engagement and the provider's engagement in care (individually and as a team), their optimism that care will lead to mutually desired outcomes, and their agreement on how to attain those outcomes. Clinician behaviors that promote common factors seem to have a dual influence on outcomes; that is, they seem to be directly therapeutic and they potentiate the effect of specific treatments.[14] Recognizing the potential of common factors skills to assist pediatric PCCs in addressing a broad array of mental health concerns at many points throughout pediatric visits, the American Academy of Pediatrics (AAP) Task Force on Mental Health (TFMH) incorporated them into their conceptualization of pediatricians' mental health competencies and clinical process algorithms.[1,15] Box 5-1 describes the HELP mnemonic, which was introduced by the AAP TFMH to summarize the common factors approach.

Box 5-1. Common Factors Mnemonic: HELP Build a Therapeutic Alliance

H = Hope

E = Empathy

L^2 = Language, Loyalty

P^3 = Permission, Partnership, Plan

Adapted with permission from American Academy of Pediatrics. *Addressing Mental Health Concerns in Primary Care: A Clinician's Toolkit.* Elk Grove Village, IL: American Academy of Pediatrics; 2010. For the fully annotated mnemonic, please refer to Appendix 5.

Some clinicians may not be able to imagine themselves using the exact phrases described in the following sections or taking this approach in every visit. Approaches can be tailored to each clinician's own style, selectively used by different clinicians sharing a practice, and, of course, applied to the needs and desires of particular patients and their families. Effective practices structure their approach to care around the talents and interests of their staff members.[16] Helping patients with difficult emotional and behavioral problems is rarely a solo effort and can include front desk staff, medical assistants, nursing staff, and colocated mental health professionals. The techniques described in this chapter can be used effectively by anyone with patient contact, and, in fact, as tools to help the clinical workplace be more secure and supportive for staff as well.[17,18]

Efficiently Eliciting an Agenda and Settling on a Topic for the Visit

Many, if not most, patients never tell their clinician their full list of concerns.[5,19] Clinicians, especially when pressed for time, may cut short disclosures by prematurely taking over discussions, and, consciously or not, disregarding patients' comments that seem off topic but that might in fact be hints that there is something else to bring up.[20] Why might patients be so hesitant to speak up? People can be ambivalent about disclosing distressing situations. One aspect they may fear in particular is losing control of the situation; that is, if they admit they have a problem, then someone will tell them what to do about it or do something themselves before the patient can object. Evidence suggests, for example, that some patients do not tell clinicians about depression because they are afraid that the clinician will pressure them or their child into taking medication.[21] Families who have experienced trauma may fear that disclosure will have unwanted consequences or put them at further risk.

Many methods can be used to elicit a full range of concerns. Despite being busy, the clinician can show interest and attention through closing the door, sitting down before speaking, and making good eye contact. These actions show not only interest but a demonstration of respect. If there is a need to consult a paper chart or fill in an electronic record during the visit, the clinician can ask the parent and patient for their permission to take a minute to do so, rather than trying to listen and simultaneously look. These efforts suggest that the clinician has time to listen (even if the clinician believes time is limited). Initial greetings can be open-ended: "How have things been since the last time?" "How can I be of help?" or "What is most important for you today?" rather than "So I see we are here for shots today." Introductions, when needed, or comments suggesting that the clinician remembers the patient and is glad to see the patient again, help establish a commitment to a personal relationship. Children may appreciate a brief period of informal talk that gives them a chance to relax in what may still be frightening surroundings.

Once patients have begun to speak, the clinician can show interest by nodding, allowing a brief pause that encourages them to continue, or summing up what has been said and asking for more detail. Perhaps the most important techniques include not jumping in prematurely with a focused question and not ignoring hints about bigger problems. Patients can interpret focused questions asked too early as a sign of what they *should* be discussing, decreasing the chance they will spontaneously disclose key concerns or information. Similarly, hints often represent patients' desire to go beyond what they believe is the PCC's agenda for the visit. If the practice is using previsit screening for mental health, development, or somatic concerns, this can be a good time to scan the results. One can note that the parent or patient has indicated some concerns and ask if they should be discussed at this visit; if no concerns have been raised, this understanding can be briefly confirmed with the door left open for any future related issues.

Of course, the main reason PCCs do not always ask open-ended questions to elicit concerns or follow up on hints is the fear that they will lose control of time. Families may disclose far more concerns than can be discussed in a short visit, or they may appear to ramble about things that, to the PCC, seem only tangentially related. Sometimes it seems obvious that the multiple concerns all relate to a single underlying issue. The clinician can speculate on this possibility, check for the patient's agreement, and then ask about which aspect is the most troubling or ask which the patient would like to start with.

> You've raised several things related to how he is doing in school, that is, paying attention in class, sitting still, doing his homework. Do you see one of these things as most important at this point? Perhaps we should start by thinking about that.

If several concerns are elicited and their relationship is not clear, the clinician can play back the list and the impression of what seems to be the most important.

> You've mentioned several things, but it seems that your worry about his staying out late is what concerns you the most: Is that right? Maybe that worry is what we should focus on today. [Conversely, if a priority is not clear...] You've mentioned several concerns: Which ones did you want to make sure we talked about today?

When patients seem to be having trouble organizing their thoughts, of if the clinician genuinely needs to move the visit along more quickly, it is possible to gently interrupt, summarize what has been heard so far, and ask for additional concerns.

> I'm sorry to interrupt, but so we don't run out of time, let me see if I understand your concerns. [The clinician can recite the list and get confirmation.] OK, good. Now, was there anything else that concerned you?

Visits often involve both adults and children (or adolescents, collectively called *children* in this chapter unless otherwise specified). Children may be reluctant participants; they rarely initiate visits in which emotional or behavioral topics are likely to be brought up.[22] Connecting with them, however, is likely to be crucial to ensuring their collaboration with any treatment that results. It is important to remember that children may have little knowledge of what happens in a medical visit. Children whose predominant experience of health care is limited to child health supervision visits may be distracted by worries about getting "shots" and find themselves puzzled and even anxious when discussion turns to their feelings or behavior.[23] Without a chance to make a connection with the clinician, and without some explanation of the visit's purpose and possible outcomes, they may choose not to participate. Parents are also more satisfied, children learn more, and outcomes may be improved when clinicians give information to both parents and children.[24] In addition, children and parents provide contrasting information about many problems; that is, parents report more overt behavioral problems than children do, but they tend to lack knowledge of children's mood problems and underestimate the extent to which children have been exposed to stresses outside the home.[25,26]

In many cultures, not only parents and children but grandparents, godparents, or "aunties" may come to visits and have strong opinions about the nature of problems and what should be done about them. Thus, the PCC needs to make an effort to engage everyone who is present and make a connection with each person: a specific greeting for each and a handshake, if appropriate. While talking, the clinician should shift eye contact and body position to address everyone; the clinician should also get all parties' names if unclear and use their names when addressing them. The visit agenda should be developed from talking with all parties, not just the parent. Each person (including the child) should be invited to add to the list or validate the priorities. New patients or those who have not had a visit for a long time can benefit from a review of standards for confidentiality and participatory decision-making. Depending on the child's age, the child and parents' desires, and prevailing practices in the community, either the parents or the child may be invited to speak first, or given opportunities to speak with the clinician alone.

Timing and Delivery of Advice

Even when people seem to be clearly stating a concern or directly asking for advice, they may not always accept suggestions given in response. Both patients and clinicians can create problems at this stage in a visit.[27] Patients may not be ready to take action, even when they are quite concerned about something. They may not see the problem as the most important concern that they face, they may see equally strong reasons not to act, or they may have little confidence in their ability to make a change. Even patients who are ready to change may feel cornered, challenged, shamed, or otherwise disempowered by well-intentioned clinicians whose advice seems, to them, formulaic or comes with a label that patients are not ready to assume. People are generally more likely to act when they develop their own motivation to do so, rather than when they believe that they are being pushed or actively persuaded.[11]

Thus, advice has to be tailored to where individuals are in their readiness to make a change, to their confidence that they can do it, and to their particular goals and values. Although providing advice this way is not nearly as complicated as it sounds (and is not necessarily any more time-consuming than straightforward offering of advice), it does require a few steps.

First, time should be taken to understand why something is a problem for the family, what they think is causing it, what they see as the relative importance of addressing it now, and how confident they are that they can make a change.

> I know that this is something that you want to act on, but tell me first a little bit about what has brought you to want to act on it now. How confident do you feel that you can do something about it now? Does anything make you worry that this might not be the time to act (or that you shouldn't do anything about this problem)?

Second, the clinician should find out the issues about which patients have been thinking. Most people come to a PCC for advice after already having tried various things or asking family members or friends for help. Ideally, the PCC should have an opportunity to validate and reinforce something that the patient has already decided to do. In addition, learning about the patient's opinion may help the clinician avoid or be more tactful about suggesting something the patient already thinks is not likely to work or about which the patient has strong feelings.

> I am happy to give you some ideas, but first I wonder what sorts of things you have been thinking about or have heard about? Is there anything that you have already tried or anything that you feel has or hasn't worked for this?

At this point in the visit can be a good point to seek agreement with the family about things they have already tried but that might not have worked: Might they be willing to try it again if the clinician can give them some advice on modifications, or are they willing to move on to a different intervention?

Third, the clinician should try to present ideas as a range of choices. Even if the choices overlap or appear to be variants on the same thing, patients feel more in control if they perceive that room is available to choose. Even if they reply by asking what the clinician thinks is best, patients still have the knowledge that alternatives exist and that the clinician believes in the importance of their preferences.

Fourth, the clinician should ask about potential barriers to carrying out the advice. Often, people agree to things that they know will be difficult or impossible for them to do. The clinician can help families find telephone numbers or plan how they will get to a referral. It can be worthwhile to go back over the rationale for interventions, so family members present at the visit can feel comfortable about explaining them to important people in their lives.[28]

Finally, the clinician should engage children as much as possible in developing and troubleshooting treatment plans. Language that children can understand should be used while filling in more details for the parent as needed. When developing a treatment plan, the clinician can ask children to walk through it to determine what part they want to play. Feedback on specific parts should be elicited, making a note of specific aspects to follow up with the child at subsequent visits.[24] For example,

> So, it seems that you and your mom agree that we should try medicine to see if it can help you do better in school. That's going to mean taking a pill every morning. How are you at taking pills? Are you good at remembering things? Do you have any ideas about how we should do that? Next time, can you tell me how that plan you had for remembering worked out?

When People Seem Ambivalent About Acting on a Problem

In some instances, ambivalence is obvious: people tell the clinician that they cannot make up their minds about how they feel or what they want to do. Sometimes the clinician can read it only in their expressions. These situations present 3 challenges: first, avoiding turning ambivalence into resistance; second, getting permission to provide information that may help resolve the ambivalence; and, ultimately, turning ambivalence into a decision to act. Throughout the process, the clinician communicates empathy with the difficulty of deciding and acting, a willingness to provide information and support, and patience during a decision-making process that may span more than one visit.

One approach at this point is to circle back and ask for a restatement of the parent's or child's initial concerns. "OK, let's make sure we understand things clearly.…" That can give all involved a chance to rethink their priorities and not feel rushed into a decision.

The Elicit-Provide-Elicit model[27] is another way of getting permission to give information that might help people decide, thus avoiding a lecture that could result in further ambivalence or even resistance. First, the clinician elicits a request for information.

> You mentioned that you were worried about his mood but that you were not a real fan of counselors or of medicines. Would you like to hear some thoughts about those things?

Next, the clinician provides information in a neutral way, keeping it simple and slow-paced. Finally, the clinician elicits a response: "What do you make of that? Does any of that make sense to you?" The clinician should be ready to hear the response and initiate another cycle if doing so seems helpful.

Also helpful is to quantify both the patient's feeling that taking action is important and the patient's confidence in his or her ability to act. Patients can be asked to rate, on a scale of 0 to 10, with 0 being the least important and 10 being the most important, the importance of an issue and their confidence in their ability to address it. These exercises have 3 goals: they help elicit self-affirming statements about resolve and confidence, they help people define for themselves factors that would motivate them to act, and they generate numbers that can be used as benchmarks for further discussion. If the number is low but not zero (ie, low importance or confidence), the clinician should ask, "That is not a lot, but what are the things that make it not zero?" "What would have to happen to increase the importance [or confidence] by a couple of points?" If the number is relatively high (ie, high importance or confidence), the clinician should ask, "Why is it so high?" "How could you move it up even higher?" "What stops you from moving up higher?"

Next, the clinician can examine the pros and cons.[27] In this exercise, which may develop information similar to the information generated by quantifying, people are asked to consider the pros and cons (or potential benefits and costs) of leaving a problem as it is and the pros and cons of making an effort to change. The clinician can jot down a 2×2 chart as patients talk. An important point to remember is that this exercise is not meant to induce some simple weighing of the good and bad and coming up with a decision. For example, the goal is not to have someone say that, on the whole, smoking looks good because it makes his or her social interactions go better and therefore he or she will not attempt to quit. Rather, the goal is for the clinician to be able to empathize with the dilemma that the patient faces and at the same time to help the patient focus on what the decision really involves.

> I can see why this is a difficult decision for you. Smoking makes it easier to socialize, and you are afraid that if you stop you will gain weight, but, at the same time, you recognize that it is not good for your health. That's a tough place to be. Does thinking about it leave you with any new ideas or questions?

When People Seem Unaware of a Problem

In some instances, the clinician may think that someone has a problem, but the patient does not agree. An example might be a parent who uses physical punishment to an extent that the clinician thinks is unproductive. The goal is to help the parents identify for themselves the reasons why they might want to recognize the issue as a problem. However, the advice is likely to be heard politely and ignored, or rejected outright, if the clinician approaches it head-on with a *prescription*.

One way to start a discussion is to use the Elicit-Provide-Elicit model described previously.

> You mentioned that sometimes you use spanking to get her to behave. That's an area that people have a lot of thoughts about: Would you like to hear some more about it?

Another way is to ask how the issue has caused a problem for the patient, the parent, or the family.[10] The question is deliberately phrased as *how* rather than *if*, with the tacit assumption that problems exist. If the patient answers, the clinician should amplify it with, "What else have you noticed?"

> So that's probably been a mixed blessing for you. It gets her to behave but everyone feels bad afterward....

Answers to either of these approaches can be an opening into helping people focus on both dilemmas and discrepancies posed by their behavior. How current behaviors contrast with stated goals and values is gently and respectfully pointed out. Notably, this approach is different from warnings and negative predictions. Instead, the clinician's comments are always framed as empathetic speculations.

> I remember your telling me that you would like to be a lawyer when you grow up. I was wondering how that fits with the kind of grades you are getting now? [or] You have talked about how important it is to feel respected; it seems like your friends might not respect you when they see how you behave when you drink. Can you tell me a little more about how respect works among your friends?

Contrast these comments with

> See, even you acknowledge that your drinking isn't consistent with your career plans or how you want your friends to see you.

When Advice Seems to Be Rejected Overtly or Subtly

The clinician's goal is, of course, to avoid resistance by first eliciting patients' concerns and attitudes, giving advice when people are ready, and working to avoid barriers to action. However, none of these approaches works all the time. How does the clinician know that the advice is being rejected? Patients may overtly argue, become defensive, deny or minimize problems, or simply ignore what the clinician is saying.[10] Why might this circumstance happen? A common view of resistance is that it reflects lack of motivation, personality issues, or limited insight or education. Although all these factors may play some role, patients usually have understandable reasons with which the clinician could empathize if they were made explicit. In particular, individuals may become resistant

▶ As a defense against feeling ashamed of their current or past behaviors

▶ If they believe that they are being coerced, cornered, or rushed

▶ If they fear some unstated consequence of what is being suggested

▶ If they do not want to lose face in front of or have to disagree with another family member who is in the room

A variety of ways can be used to *roll with resistance*.[10] One alternative is to reflect the thought back: "So you have heard some bad things about this medication." In many instances, people will then come back to the clinician with a statement that offers some kind of opening. They may go into detail about their concern, providing the clinician an opportunity to show respect for their position, provide information, and understand parameters that might form an alternative plan. They may become more conciliatory, revealing that they, in fact, see both sides of the issue. This action also opens a possible path to a workable solution. As a second alternative, the clinician can also apologize and back up.

I am sorry if I got ahead of where you were thinking. It is perfectly fine to put this issue aside until you feel that you have all the information that you need. Where do you think we should start?

As a third alternative, the clinician can agree but "with a twist."

You are right, medicines certainly can be a problem if they are not used carefully. Those cases you have heard about in which children had problems with medicine, do you know anything about the dose the children were using or how their families were checking for side effects?

When Parents or Children or Teens Believe They Have Been Coerced Into Coming

Children and teens often say that coming to the PCC for a particular problem was not their idea. Parents sometimes have been told by an agency, a school, or a court that they must see the clinician for counseling or medication. The clinician can often empathize with patients and families in this situation but should avoid doing so in a way that puts down the referring source, such as the following clinician statements:

The school people think every kid needs medication.

The social services people seem to refer everyone whether they need it or not.

Although these statements may contain a grain of truth from the clinician's perspective, they can undermine the legitimacy of the whole therapeutic system, including the clinician's part in it. Perhaps worse, they can reinforce the patient's or family's role as a victim, which ultimately is not helpful. An alternative goal is to start a process through which the patient or family can regain a sense of control. This process can be seen as having

3 stages: acknowledging anger, distancing tactfully from the coercive referral, and offering choice.[27]

> I would be angry too if I felt that someone was telling me what to do that way. I know that I can't make anyone do anything she or he doesn't want to do. Teachers know a lot about children and classroom behavior, so I respect their concerns, but I am your clinician, and my first responsibility to you is to figure out what is right for you. Let's first take a good, broad look at the situation and decide what you think is best to do. I will be glad to talk with the school and explain to them whatever we decide.

A variant for a child or teen might be

> I realize that it wasn't your idea to come, but I am really interested in hearing how you feel about this issue. Would you want to talk with me alone now or with your mother here? I guess it is doubly hard getting told you have to talk with someone and then not even having the choice of who that is. Do you think you might feel more comfortable with someone else? I can help you set that up if you would like.

Helping People Who Say They Are Stuck or Hopeless, or Have Tried Everything

Anger, low mood, and anxiety cause tunnel vision that makes seeing a way out of problems difficult; hopelessness and demoralization become vicious cycles.[29] Focusing on goals for the future and how to get there can initially be more productive than a detailed analysis of how problems came about; focusing on goals is sometimes all that is needed. Solution-focused therapy grew out of a need for ways to help people in the course of brief interactions.[30,31]

Asking specifically about just how bad patients are feeling as well as if patients feel in danger of being hurt, hurting themselves, or hurting someone else is always important. These problems need to be addressed immediately. If a patient reports a major fall in mood, energy, self-esteem, or interest in daily affairs, the patient may be depressed, and further treatment may be warranted. For many individuals, however, more transient periods of low mood and discouragement can be helped by identifying and building on strengths and past successes, by reframing events and feelings so negative attributions about the patient can be made positive or at least neutral, and by breaking down distant and diffuse goals into small, concrete steps that are more readily accomplished.

At least 2 key elements exist to solution-focused interactions. First, the patient is considered to be the expert both on desired goals and on ways to get there; the clinician is a facilitator and coach. Following from this point, the patient, often through telling the story of the problem, provides the outlines of the solution. Second, solution-focused interactions look at observable behavior that either leads to or is part of a desired goal. This element is in comparison with focusing on stopping an undesired behavior or focusing on having poorly observable goals such as *attitude*. For example, "I would like him to work on his homework for 15 minutes before he takes a break," is more effective than, "He needs to stop being so distracted when he does his homework."

Solution-focused interactions often start with asking someone to tell the story of the person's problem. In a clinical setting, *story* means the patient's understanding of how he or she came to be in a particular situation. Although many people will initially say that they do not know, the clinician can prompt the parent or patient to simply describe when the problem started and how it has evolved: "I know that we could probably talk about this for hours, but in a few minutes, starting at the beginning, tell me how you got to this point."

The first, and often only, response necessary is your ability to play the story back in a way that provides validation and empathy. To change, people need to feel understood and supported. The clinician need not agree with everything the patient did, but the difficulty of the situation and the strengths that the person has demonstrated can be supported, and how the problems make sense, given the circumstances, can be pointed out.

> So, here you are, a single parent trying to hold down 2 jobs, with a child who you've told me is not the easiest in the world to manage. Then, on top of that, your own mother gets sick and needs you. What a tough situation.

A related technique is to look for situations that seem important to the clinician but glossed over in the family's or patient's account. For example, a parent tells the story of progressive difficulties with a child's behavior and quickly mentions in the middle of the account that his own parent died during that time. In the clinician's playing back of the story, this factor is noted with the thought that it must have had an effect: "So in the middle of all these difficulties with the school, you lose your own mother. That must have made things particularly hard." Patients or parents who offer corrections or provide more information that changes the clinician's interpretation do not present a problem; this correction or addition is part of the conversation. What matters in this exchange is that patients have a chance to clarify the story in their own minds.

A third technique when listening to stories is to observe and comment on "shoulds." "Shoulds" can be stated explicitly, as in "whenever he does X, I have to do Y"; as regrets, as in "I should have done…"; or implicitly, through a pattern of behavior that recurs in a story.[32]

> So you are saying that every time he gets into trouble it is your job to bail him out. That sounds like an important rule that you are following: Where did it come from?

In using this comment, the clinician is not suggesting that the rule is bad or even an alternative point of view. However, by asking the parent or patient whether this procedure really is a rule that is followed and asking the parent or patient to comment on its origin, the clinician presents an opportunity and grants permission to make a modification.

Eliciting stories usually segues into "So where do we go from here?" or "So what do you want to have happen next?" The clinician can help families set concrete, observable goals. In general, useful goals have the following characteristics:

▶ People develop goals for themselves.

▶ Goals are framed with positive behaviors that are observable.

▶ Goals are often framed in very small steps. "What is the first change in that direction that you would like to see?"

▶ Goals can be counted or documented objectively; thus, progress can be assessed.

When people say that they are at a loss for a goal, the clinician can ask them what they believe would be the first, small sign that things were beginning to improve, preferably so small that they feel confident they could achieve it.[31] For example, if a father's lack of participation in a child's bedtime is the focus of disagreement between parents, a first achievable step might be seeing whether the father would be the one to get the child a cup of water while the mother is reading the bedtime story. The clinician can also ask for a highly detailed account of the problem, look at the sequence of events that leads up to it, and identify places where a behavior or response might be changed. People can also be asked to recall exceptions, that is, a time when the desired outcome or state actually occurred, even if only briefly. The discussion can then move on to what might have been happening then and whether these circumstances might be recreated.

When Parents and Children Argue During the Visit

Parent-child arguments during a visit can derail plans for diagnosis and treatment, and they often leave everyone involved feeling impotent and in a bad mood. In some instances, arguments can be prevented by taking steps at the outset of the visit to ensure that everyone gets a chance to speak. Clinicians can provide this opportunity informally by shifting their gaze and body position from parent to child and back, implying that the clinician is listening to and expecting to hear from everyone. If the parent interrupts the child or vice versa, he or she can be asked to wait briefly while the other finishes.

One way to break up arguments is to interrupt them to point out areas of agreement.

> I hear you both saying that relationships in the family are important, but you [the teen] are concerned about being respected by your parents and you [the parent] are concerned about how much time he spends at home. Do you think there is a common thread to those things that we could talk about?

Arguments can also be normalized to take some of the emotion out of them.

> It's pretty common for parents and children to disagree about curfews and calling to say where you are. It's part of the whole process of learning how to be independent and responsible. How has your family been handling that?

If one or both parties seem particularly angry or are saying things that seem hurtful, several methods can be used to appeal for a calmer approach. One technique is to suggest that the argument is happening in the context of a caring relationship.

> This must be hard; it's difficult when 2 people care a lot about each other but really disagree. Is there a way you could tell X how you feel but also let him know how much you care about him?

Another technique is to point out the use of polarizing or black-and-white words and thinking. These terms tend to promote escalating insults; they also obscure concerns that might be the focus of a plan. Examples include, "He is always late; he never picks up after himself." "He is lazy; he doesn't care about anyone else in the family." Responses on your part can be

> *Ever, never, always*—those words have a way of putting people on the defensive. Can you try telling her those concerns again but without using those words?[32] [or] People often get upset if they feel you are labeling them, and it can really stick with kids, even if they tell you they don't care. Can you tell him what he does that upsets you without using that label to explain why he does it?

Conclusion

Building communication skills is an endeavor that spans a career. Endless variations in clinical situations and patient and family personalities offer the opportunity to learn new skills and analyze new experiences. As PCCs mature, they develop new insights and new relational preferences that change the way they interact with their patients and families. They grow older, but the patients and parents in their care stay relatively young, by comparison. The growing gap both enriches the patient-clinician relationship and creates hurdles to be overcome. Continuing to work on communication skills remains an important component of clinical practice.

Many of the communication techniques described in this chapter are described in detail in the books *The Family Is the Patient: Using Family Interviews in Children's Medical Care* and *Health Behavior Change: A Guide for Practitioners*.[32,33] Detailed suggestions about general approaches to mental health issues in primary care and information about assessment and treatment for a range of commonly occurring behavioral and developmental problems may be found throughout this book. Conferences and training courses in effective communication and motivational enhancement techniques are available at www.aachonline.org and www.aap.org/mentalhealth. Opportunities to apply the communication techniques described in this chapter are noted in many chapters of this book and introduced in Chapter 1, Integrating Preventive Mental Health Care Into Pediatric Practice, and Chapter 2, Pediatric Care of Children and Adolescents With Mental Health Problems.

Acknowledgments: Work on this chapter was supported by National Institute of Mental Health grant MH 062469.

References

1. Lahey BB, Flagg EW, Bird HR, et al. The NIMH Methods for the Epidemiology of Child and Adolescent Mental Disorders (MECA) Study: background and methodology. *J Am Acad Child Adolesc Psychiatry.* 1996;35(7):855–864

2. Costello EJ, Edelbrock C, Costello AJ, Dulcan MK, Burns BJ, Brent D. Psychopathology in pediatric primary care: the new hidden morbidity. *Pediatrics.* 1988;82(3, pt 2):415–424

3. Wu P, Hoven CW, Bird HR, et al. Depressive and disruptive disorders and mental health service utilization in children and adolescents. *J Am Acad Child Adolesc Psychiatry.* 1999;38(9):1081–1090

4. National Advisory Mental Health Council Workgroup on Child and Adolescent Mental Health Intervention Development and Deployment. *Blueprint for Change: Research on Child and Adolescent Mental Health.* Rockville, MD: National Institute of Mental Health; 2001

5. Horwitz SM, Leaf PJ, Leventhal JM. Identification of psychosocial problems in pediatric primary care: do family attitudes make a difference? *Arch Pediatr Adolesc Med.* 1998;152(4):367–371

6. Murphy JM, Kelleher K, Pagano ME, et al. The family APGAR and psychosocial problems in children: a report from ASPN and PROS. *J Fam Pract.* 1998;46(1):54–64

7. Rushton J, Bruckman D, Kelleher K. Primary care referral of children with psychosocial problems. *Arch Pediatr Adolesc Med.* 2002;156(6):592–598

8. Olson AL, Kelleher KJ, Kemper KJ, Zuckerman BS, Hammond CS, Dietrich AJ. Primary care pediatricians' roles and perceived responsibilities in the identification and management of depression in children and adolescents. *Ambul Pediatr.* 2001;1:91–98

9. Stewart M. Patient-physician relationships over time. In: Stewart M, Brown JB, Weston WW, MacWhinney YR, McWilliam CL, Freeman TR, eds. *Patient-Centered Medicine: Transforming the Clinical Method.* Thousand Oaks, CA: Sage Publications; 1995

10. Miller WR, Rollnick S. *Motivational Interviewing: Preparing People to Change Addictive Behavior.* New York, NY: Guilford Press; 1991

11. Rollnick S, Mason P, Butler C. *Health Behavior Change: A Guide for Practitioners.* Edinburgh, Scotland: Churchill Livingstone; 1999

12. Gysels M, Richardson A, Higginson IJ. Communication training for health professionals who care for patients with cancer: a systematic review of training methods. *Support Care Cancer.* 2005;13(6):356–366

13. Castonguay LG, Beutler LE. Principles of therapeutic change: a task force on participants, relationships, and techniques factors. *J Clin Psychol.* 2006;62(6): 631–638

14. Krupnick JL, Sotsky SM, Simmens S, et al. The role of the therapeutic alliance in psychotherapy and pharmacotherapy outcome: findings in the National Institute of Mental Health Treatment of Depression Collaborative Research Program. *J Consult Clin Psychol.* 1996;64(3):532–539

15. American Academy of Pediatrics Committee on Psychosocial Aspects of Child and Family Health and Task Force on Mental Health. The future of pediatrics: mental health competencies for pediatric primary care. *Pediatrics.* 2009;124(1):410–421

16. Crabtree BF, Miller WL, Tallia AF, et al. Delivery of clinical preventive services in family medicine offices. *Ann Fam Med.* 2005;3(5):430–435

17. Brown JD, King MA, Wissow LS. The central role of relationships to trauma-informed integrated care for children and youth. *Acad Pediatr.* 2017;17(7S): S94–S101

18. Brown JD, Wissow LS, Cook BL, Longway S, Caffery E, Pefaure C. Mental health communications skills training for medical assistants in pediatric primary care. *J Behav Health Serv Res.* 2013;40(1):20–35

19. Barsky AJ III. Hidden reasons some patients visit doctors. *Ann Intern Med.* 1981;94(4, pt 1):492–498

20. Levinson W, Gorawara-Bhat R, Lamb J. A study of patient clues and physician responses in primary care and surgical settings. *JAMA.* 2000;284(8):1021–1027

21. Rost K, Zhang M, Fortney J, Smith J, Coyne J, Smith GR Jr. Persistently poor outcomes of undetected major depression in primary care. *Gen Hosp Psychiatry.* 1998;20(1):12–20

22. van Dulmen AM. Children's contributions to pediatric outpatient encounters. *Pediatrics.* 1998;102(3, pt 1):563–568

23. Polk S, Horwitz R, Longway S, et al. Surveillance or engagement: children's conflicts during health maintenance visits. *Acad Pediatr.* 2017;17(7):739–746

24. Lewis CC, Pantell RH, Sharp L. Increasing patient knowledge, satisfaction, and involvement: randomized trial of a communication intervention. *Pediatrics.* 1991;88(2):351–358

25. MacLeod RJ, McNamee JE, Boyle MH, Offord DR, Friedrich M. Identification of childhood psychiatric disorder by informant: comparisons of clinic and community samples. *Can J Psychiatry.* 1999;44(2):144–150

26. Richters JE, Martinez P. The NIMH community violence project: I. Children as victims of and witnesses to violence. *Psychiatry.* 1993;56(1):7–21

27. Pill R, Rees ME, Stott NC, Rollnick SR. Can nurses learn to let go? Issues arising from an intervention designed to improve patients' involvement in their own care. *J Adv Nurs.* 1999;29(6):1492–1499

28. McKay MM, McCadam K, Gonzalez JJ. Addressing the barriers to mental health services for inner city children and their caretakers. *Community Ment Health J.* 1996;32(4):353–361

29. Elliott R, Rubinsztein JS, Sahakian BJ, Dolan RJ. The neural basis of mood-congruent processing biases in depression. *Arch Gen Psychiatry.* 2002;59(7): 597–604

30. Walter JL, Peller JE. *Becoming Solution-Focused in Brief Therapy.* New York, NY: Brunner/Mazel; 1992

31. Klar H, Coleman WL. Brief solution-focused strategies for behavioral pediatrics. *Pediatr Clin North Am.* 1995;42(1):131–141

32. Allmond BW Jr, Tanner JL, Gofman HF. *The Family Is the Patient: Using Family Interviews in Children's Medical Care.* 2nd ed. Baltimore, MD: Williams & Wilkins; 1999

33. Rollnick S, Mason P, Butler C. *Health Behavior Change: A Guide for Practitioners.* Edinburgh, Scotland: Churchill Livingstone; 1999

CHAPTER 6

Iterative Mental Health Assessment

Penelope Knapp, MD; Danielle Laraque-Arena, MD;
and Lawrence S. Wissow, MD, MPH

> "*The psychosocial assessment in pediatric primary care is an iterative process with multiple components.... These components can be envisioned as gauges on a dashboard....*"

Introduction: Unique Opportunities for Mental Health Assessment in Primary Care

In the mental health system, the initial diagnostic assessment typically requires 1 to 2 hours. The mental health specialist conducts an interview with the patient and family, reviewing the individual's primary concern and psychosocial history, which includes a mental status examination and may incorporate information from collateral sources (such as teachers), as appropriate. Its purpose is to establish the patient's diagnosis, if any, and to develop an intervention plan collaboratively with the family.

By contrast, pediatricians, family physicians, internists, nurse practitioners, and physician assistants at the front lines of pediatrics (collectively called *primary care clinicians,* abbreviated as PCCs in this chapter) have a longitudinal relationship with *children* (a term used in this chapter to encompass all age-groups from infancy through adolescence, unless otherwise specified) and their families. Assessment of the child's state of mental health is iterative, based on clinical observations, evolving developmental and patient/family psychosocial history, screening results, collateral information from school or child care providers, and responses to primary care interventions. The purpose of the mental health assessment in this context is prevention, not diagnosis: (1) primary prevention, whenever possible—reinforcing strengths, recognizing and ameliorating risks to the child's development—and (2) secondary prevention—recognizing emerging psychosocial problems before they become impairing or reach the threshold for a disorder.[1,2] The mental health assessment in primary care can be assisted by systematically scrutinizing several factors in the child's situation and the child's manifestations, as a driver would observe information on the dashboard of his or her vehicle. "Gauges" on the Mental Health Dashboard include previsit questionnaires, screening tools, interviews, observations, periodic functional assessment, collateral information, and responses to primary care interventions. Together they provide the PCC with an assessment of the child's well-being over time, in the context of his or her family, school, and community.

Elements of Primary Care Assessment

To assess the risks to a child's mental health or determine whether the child needs mental health intervention, the PCC must consider both the child's situational context, that is, the child's family, caregiver, and community, and the child's emotional and behavioral manifestations. The concept of the Mental Health Dashboard is developed because the many factors in the child's situation and the child's clinical manifestations are complex and interrelated. By arraying information from the history and the clinical observations in a systematic way, it may be easier to construct an overview that incorporates strengths and concerns in each domain.

The Child's Situation: Family, Caregiver, and Community Context

Table 6-1 summarizes the environmental forces affecting the child. It indicates strengths and expectable status for each factor. Red flags indicate concerns that require a response; they also bear noting on the child's problem list and in a practice registry to ensure appropriate follow-up. Risk factors (abuse, neglect, witnessing violence in the home, family discord or divorce, parents with poor health habits, unsafe schools, and unsafe neighborhoods) may be counterbalanced with assets (stable relationships with caring adults, anchor in a faith or spiritual belief or community, involvement in school, and available recreational opportunities). Children continually adapt, and their adaptive repertoire increases with age if they have a solid base on which to build. It is usually beyond the power of the PCC to prevent the family's misfortune, but noting

Table 6-1. Mental Health Dashboard: Child's Situation

Dashboard Domain	Strength	Expectable Status	Red Flag for Risk/Problem
Psychosocial environment, supports, and relationships	≥1 strong parental attachment to child; nurturing, stimulating environment; or supportive school and community	Stable and safe home, school, and community	Family disruption, foster care, poor school and peer connectedness, bullying, racism, or homophobia
ACEs and traumatic experiences (eg, abuse/neglect, exposure to domestic violence or other frightening situations)	Never, none, or, if any: resilience, without symptoms	Usual stressors and average resilience, with some symptoms	Low resilience or significant behavioral and emotional symptoms related to past traumas
Primary support (how the child is cared for by parents [eg, parenting style, discipline, household routines; caregivers' health, mental health, substance use, support system])	Unusually good, with healthy parents, effective parenting, solid support system, or predictable routines with flexibility to adapt to special circumstances	Average or good enough	≥1 parent stressed, overworked, or with limited availability; child maltreatment or neglect; sibling with special health care need or mental disorder; ineffective or inconsistent parenting; maternal depression; parental intellectual disability; substance abuse or mental illness; parent incapable of providing for child's emotional needs; or weak or no support system
Caregiving (how the child is cared for by others) (eg, child care, sitters, after-school care)	Unusually loving, consistent, and reliable	Average or good enough	Poor quality child care; self-care; sibling care; or erratic sitters

Table 6-1. Mental Health Dashboard: Child's Situation *(continued)*

Dashboard Domain	Strength	Expectable Status	Red Flag for Risk/Problem
Change in child's living environment (eg, birth of sibling, illness, separation or divorce of parents, loss of significant relationship, no home, foster care)	Healthy adjustment or new relationships and support system well underway	Transient sadness or worry, ≥1 new relationship, or prospects for building new support system	Child or parents or both stressed, distracted, or manifesting symptoms of anxiety or depression
Physical, legal, economic, and virtual environment, and culture (factors outside the family [eg, housing, exposure to toxins, food, income, virtual environment, immigration status, custody, other legal issues])	No stressors or exposures	Some stressors, but family able to manage	Unstable housing or homelessness, or unsafe neighborhood; strained resources or food insecurity; manifestations of environmental or media exposure; or several/many stressors and limited supports
Events (eg, community disaster, violence, immigration, recent move to new community, loss of a parent secondary to deployment or incarceration)	Events in child's life, but ≥1 parent buffers them well and child adjusts without symptoms	Events in child's life, and ≥1 parent does not buffer them well, while child shows some symptoms	Exposure to event such as community disaster or violence, immigration, recent move, or loss of a parent causing distress to ≥1 parent and marked symptoms in child
Health status of the child	No active health concerns	No serious health concerns	Chronic or acute medical conditions

Abbreviation: ACE, adverse childhood experience

potential risk factors is important, and the more important question is how the family and child are coping.

Psychosocial Environment, Supports, and Relationships

This domain of the Mental Health Dashboard spans the range of social supports and relationships available to the child within the family, school, neighborhood, and broader community. Considering the factors listed in this domain, the PCC can assess whether the interpersonal relationships surrounding the child provide emotional security.

Family Relationships

Attachment theory provides an important lens for viewing the basis of the relationships between the developing child and vital adults that surround and nurture the child. See the Sequelae of Trauma Exposure section later in this chapter for discussion of poor attachment and its consequences for the child.

School

School-aged children spend most of their days in an educational environment that may be safe, supportive, and stimulating or that may threaten them, leave them feeling confused or unsure, and fail to engage their minds. The parent and the PCC need to know about the quality and environment of the school and whether the school has academic and social resources to optimize students' learning. It is important for the clinician to be aware of the quality of the child's school as well as to know how the child experiences school. Does the child feel that the teacher and other children like him or her? Does the child feel able to do the work? Has he or she experienced bullying?

School administrators and staff should be aware of bullying if it occurs, because 85% of the time other children witness bullying. Bullying is not a random event; individual child characteristics and family factors may be predictive.[3] Children who are bullied show signs of distress and problems adjusting; these signs may be the cause or effect of being bullied. Bullying persists and can be stable across ages, and the mental health effects of childhood bullying may persist until late adolescence. It is associated with internalizing mental health symptoms,[4] including low self-esteem, self-harm, aggressive behavior, and trauma-associated psychotic symptoms. This association is true for the child who is bullied and, to some extent, the bully, who may also have been abused or bullied. The PCC should inquire about the quality of school and the child's experience, including bullying and, especially for adolescents, cyberbullying. A history of poor quality school, negative school experience, or bullying is a red flag. A good school and positive school experience are strengths.

Neighborhood and Community

The child's neighborhood provides contact with other adults and children, as well as opportunities for play, learning, and community experiences. Impoverished and unsafe neighborhoods limit those experiences. Disorganized neighborhoods with large numbers of youths (children, adolescents, and young adults) in trouble pose actual danger. Children growing up in dangerous neighborhoods may be denied opportunities for exploration because their parents seek to protect them from harm. The same factors that jeopardize children's readiness for school or success in school may pose risk for gang activity in neighborhoods. Disorganized neighborhoods with large numbers of children who have poor relationships with their parents, who have a low attachment to school, and who have associations among peers involved in delinquent activities such as violence and drug use are neighborhoods vulnerable to gang presence.

The PCC should be informed of or inquire about the quality of the neighborhood and how parents cope with potential dangers. Safe neighborhoods with good resources will be highlighted as a strength, while neighborhood violence, gangs, and drug traffic are red flags. Note that some of these stresses may constitute actual trauma as discussed in the next section of this chapter, Adverse Childhood Experiences and Traumatic Experiences.

Bright Futures: Guidelines for Health Supervision of Infants, Children, and Adolescents[5] provides information and resources on promoting community relationships. It also guides PCCs to resources for vulnerable families who are recent immigrants or who have limited English proficiency.

A good psychosocial environment nurtures the family and child through strong community support systems. At minimum, the environment should be safe and provide some resources in the school and community for a family living in adequate housing. Environmental red flags are raised if resources are strained, if there is toxic exposure or violence in the community, if racism or homophobia affects the family, and if the parents are concerned that they cannot keep their child safe.

Adverse Childhood Experiences and Traumatic Experiences

Children may be exposed to many types of traumatic experiences. Refer to the National Child Traumatic Stress Network for a summary of types of traumatic stress in childhood.[6]

Personal or internal trauma includes physical or sexual abuse and neglect. These are traumatic experiences inflicted upon or experienced by the child. Such trauma may be associated with profound damage to the attachment system, discussed in the following paragraphs.

Subtler personal trauma occurs if the child is being reared by a parent with a mental health or substance use disorder or who experienced ACEs himself or herself. The child is intermittently or continuously deprived of a safe and solid relationship with a special adult who puts the child's needs first and is emotionally available to respond in ways that allow the child to build neuronal connections in an organized way within a secure attachment. Such kinds of toxic early experiences present an unfortunate "natural" experiment, seen in children taken into protective custody. Because normal language and cognitive development are contingent on environmental stimulation through earliest relationships, most young children coming into foster care show speech and language delays, and almost half show cognitive delays. However, these risks do not apply exclusively to foster children. Early recognition of parental problems is an important preventive measure.

External trauma may affect the child from his or her community (eg, violence, brutal acts such as rape and shootings), at school, in the home (eg, domestic or intimate partner violence [IPV]), as a result of natural disaster, in the context of war or refugee experience, or in a medical setting.

Many children experience multiple traumas or prolonged trauma, both called *complex trauma*, which may be chronic and may occur within the primary care system, with resulting emotional dysregulation and lasting impact on later development. Traumatic experiences befalling newborns, infants, and children 6 years or younger are referred to as *early childhood trauma*.

It is difficult to estimate the prevalence of IPV between parents and children's witnessing domestic violence among others in the home, but that IPV presents powerful toxicity to the child's emotional environment is well-documented. Families with physical abuse between parents are likelier to be families with child maltreatment, and psychological abuse between parents is also strongly related to maltreatment of children.[7] Even when one partner perpetrates physical abuse toward only the other, the odds of child neglect have been found to be 5.29 times as great as in families with no psychological abuse. A PCC who uncovers a situation involving violence in the home should question whether the child has witnessed it, whether the child's safety is jeopardized, and whether the mother feels safe or has a plan if she does not feel safe.

Childhood exposure to IPV is a toxic stress associated with poor social-emotional child health outcomes and significantly more externalizing, internalizing, and total behavioral problems.[8] Both the age at which a child is first exposed to violence at home and the amount of violence the child witnesses in his or her lifetime have been found to be significantly related to behavioral problems. Cumulative violence exposure has been shown to have a greater effect[9] and to mediate the relationship between early exposure and later externalizing behavioral problems. This culmination may include excessive exposure to violence through media.

Thus, exposure to physical and psychological abuse between parents is an example of environmental stress that is both formative at an early age and cumulative during childhood. Recognizing such exposure presents an opportunity for prevention: identifying and intervening in families with mothers experiencing abuse may prevent the development of problems for their children, as well as ensure the safety and well-being of the child and mother.

It is important that the PCC inquire about exposure to trauma and about the child's resilience. Open-ended questions may elicit this information, for example: "Sometimes when there are disagreements or fights between adults, children are upset; does this ever happen at home?" If there is no exposure, or if the family has shown resilience in the face of exposure, the clinician can highlight this as a family strength. Many families face stressors, and even if the child is resilient and has some symptoms, the clinician should make note of this. A red flag is raised if there has been serious trauma exposure and the child has significant behavioral and emotional symptoms related to this exposure. Younger children are more vulnerable.

Primary Support (Health, Mental Health, and Capacity of Parents)

Parenting Style

The culture within the family will shape the relationship and learning environment for the child. Families have individually distinct beliefs, rituals, and routines related to health and discipline. This fact applies regardless of family composition (eg, single parent, gay parents,[10] intergenerational parenting). Baumrind's classical description of 4 parenting styles is widely used.[11] Authoritative parents are comfortably consistent in providing limits and guidance to shape children's behavior and support their learning; they both demand that children adhere to developmentally appropriate clear standards and respond warmly to children's needs. Authoritarian parents, by contrast, demand but do not respond; they impose noncontingent or punitive discipline that children may experience as arbitrary, unfair, or confusing. Permissive parents are responsive but not demanding; these parents fail to provide their children with consistent rules or discipline, so the children struggle with their own impulses without predictable controls. Uninvolved parents, also termed *rejecting-neglecting parents,* neither demanding nor responsive, do not provide emotional scaffolding to help children understand the effects of their emotions and feelings.

Children depend on their parents' control of the family emotional environment and on their engagement and stimulation for basic learning. This dependence has measurable effects on learning: young children whose parents have low responsiveness to their developmental activities have delayed vocabulary development.[12] Numerous instruments are available for assessing parenting style. In the Suggested Reading section at the end of this chapter, see Johnson et al[13] for a review and Kemper and Kelleher for approaches to family psychosocial screening.[14]

As noted in other chapters, family routines for meals and bedtimes are important, and parents should have strategies for managing children's urges and demands, for example, for too much screen exposure. Each parent will approach these daily events with his or her own style. The PCC should observe parenting style in the office and ask about parenting stresses and challenges and can then reinforce observed strengths, such a warm rapport, awareness of the child's needs, and sensitive efforts, to help the child's communication with the clinician. A red flag is raised if the parents are stressed, have medical or mental illness, are overworked, use substances sometimes to the level of a substance use disorder, or have limited availability (or any combination thereof). Inability to provide for the child's emotional needs, inconsistent parenting, and, as noted previously, neglect or maltreatment also raise red flags. Negative effects on the mental health of children are discussed in the Discipline section and Parental Mental Health: Maternal Depression and Substance Use section. If significant parenting concerns are noted, consider referral to a mental health specialist for fuller assessment.

Discipline

Child-rearing is challenging. Primary care clinicians should inquire about discipline and support positive parenting strategies. Nonetheless, parents must at times set limits and provide consequences to guide their child to safe and prosocial behaviors. In what ways and how often parents set limits and provide discipline for their children depends on characteristics of the parents, the behaviors or predilections of the child, and the social context. Among these, parental characteristics such as warmth, protectiveness, and authoritarianism may be the most influential in determining the type of discipline used.[15,16]

Limit setting and discipline are necessary elements of rearing most children. Each parent, and each family, develops a style for these, with a range from nonverbal demonstration of disapproval, to scolding, to spanking. The American Academy of Pediatrics (AAP) recommends against corporal punishment, yet it is endorsed or used at some point by most parents in the United States. Frequent corporal punishment is associated with other parenting risk factors, including whether parents considered abortion and whether there is neglect, physical and psychological maltreatment, IPV, maternal stress, substance use, and depression.

The style of discipline of children is influenced by culture. In a study of low-income white, black, and Mexican American families of toddlers, both spanking and verbal punishment were found to vary by maternal race and ethnicity.[17] The PCC should ask about parents' views on discipline, specifically for what behaviors, how, and how often they discipline their children. A strength is noted if discipline is age appropriate and logically linked to the concerning behavior. A red flag is raised if discipline is harsh, inconsistent, or inappropriate to the child's developmental level.

Parental Mental Health: Maternal Depression and Substance Use

For infants and young children, the environment is created and embodied by the parents, particularly the mothers. Parental mental illness powerfully affects the emotional environment and possibly the physical environment in the home. The 12-month prevalence of mental illness in adults in the United States is estimated at 32.4%,[18] and Nicholson and colleagues noted in 2004 that two-thirds of these individuals are parents.[19] A child whose parent has a mental illness is more likely to have developmental delay, difficulty regulating emotions, or problems with relationships (or any combination thereof).[19] One-fifth of children in the general population have a psychiatric diagnosis,[20] but 30% to 50% of children with parents with mental illness have a psychiatric diagnosis, so recognition of parental mental disorder is necessary to prevent or minimize childhood psychiatric disorders.

Because babies are wholly dependent on a caregiving adult for survival, they are at greatest risk for abuse, neglect, and inadequate medical care. Babies' earliest reciprocal experiences shape the developing brain. Many mothers with depression work hard to meet their children's needs, but some infants of mothers with depression are at risk for developmental delay, impaired social interaction, attachment problems, behavioral problems, and later problems with cognitive and social-emotional development.

Growing up in the environment created by a mother with depression may also affect children before and beyond infancy.[21] Riley and colleagues[22] in evaluating combined reports (mother, father, and teacher) about children whose mothers were depressed found that their adaptive skills were significantly poorer than those of socio-demographically similar children whose mothers were not depressed. Parents reported more emotional and behavioral problems among these children. Measured family stressors did not mediate the association with children's psychosocial problems, but the quality of mothers' parenting did.

Maternal depression is a cumulative risk factor because it sets in motion multiple risk processes. These processes have been described and explained by the "launch-and-grow" cascade model through which the earlier risk factor, exposure to maternal depression before age 12 years, was demonstrated to predict other adverse processes, that is, stress, altered family relationships, and reduced self-worth, that set the course for children to develop depressive symptoms over time.[22,23]

The prevalence of substance use disorders (SUDs) among adults who are parenting children is difficult to estimate, but the likelihood of child maltreatment leading to out-of-home placement is higher in these families.[24] From the child's perspective, the parent with an SUD inevitably provides a fluctuating interpersonal environment, depending on whether the parent is under the influence or experiencing withdrawal. Children exposed to a mother with SUD experience both nonspecific risk and, in the case of alcohol exposure leading to fetal alcohol spectrum disorder, specific neurodevelopmental harm. Parental SUD is part of a cluster of risks[25]: it is often associated with a chaotic, harsh, and stressed environment; exposure to interpersonal violence; and dysregulating experiences that prevent minimally adequate or consistent care for the child. Also, parental SUDs are related to parental depression or trauma, so even if the situation does not lead to active maltreatment, the home environment poses a threat to the child's adjustment. Early recognition of parental problems is an important preventive measure. The PCC should screen for maternal depression during the newborn period and infancy using a validated tool (see Chapter 23, Maternal Depression) and observe for or ask about parental depression, interpersonal or domestic violence, and substance use at subsequent visits. Additional screening tools may also be useful.

The clinician should ask how things are in the family, how the parents cope with the demands of child-rearing, and if they have emotional problems or use substances. If the parent or parents report that they are coping well and don't have a mental or substance use problem, this is a strength. If the parents report that they are stressed, or overworked; that they can give their child only limited availability; and that their parenting is inconsistent or ineffective, a red flag is raised. If they report child maltreatment or neglect, a sibling with a special health care need or mental disorder, maternal depression, parental intellectual disability or substance abuse or mental illness, any of which may cause them to be incapable of providing for the child's emotional needs, a red flag is also raised.

Caregiving (How the Child Is Cared for by Others)

Parental Employment: The Working Mother

According to the US Department of Labor, mothers are sole or primary earners for 40% of households. Seventy percent of mothers with children younger than 18 years are employed; more than 75%, full-time.[26]

Although, overall, research does not support the concern that family relationships, attachment to children, or children's development is harmed by a mother's work alone, some fatigue and strain inevitably accompany working, and if the quality of child care is inadequate, children's developmental opportunities will be compromised. Primary care clinicians can support working parents by assessing how they balance demands of work and home, determining whether they have adequate child care options, and providing advice about finding quality child care. This discussion may lessen the extent to which parents' work may draw away their available energy and the emotional resources needed for parenting.

The PCC should ask about hours of parental work, strain associated with work, and how the parent and child are dealing with it. A strength is noted if the parent is able to provide for the child's needs for learning and love. If the parent cannot manage this provision, a red flag is raised, particularly if the parent resorts to letting the child have screen exposure to occupy the time required to prepare meals and manage household chores.

Child Care

Most young children receive care from adults outside the family, in child care, with sitters, or in after-school programs. If this care is loving, consistent, and reliable, the PCC can acknowledge and reinforce it as a strength. A red flag is raised if children are left alone at a young age, or in the care of siblings too young for this responsibility; if children are in a child care setting of poor quality; or if sitters are erratic.

Quality of child care is an important factor for preschool-aged children. Studies have shown that high-quality care attenuates negative effects of economic disadvantage on children's early academic trajectory.[27] For children whose mothers had low levels of education, formal child care led to higher receptive vocabulary, reading and math achievement scores, and school readiness than for those cared for by their parents. Although children experiencing higher-quality child care have better language and cognitive development, and are more cooperative than those in low-quality care,[28] long hours in child care, even of high quality, may take a toll. Children with higher combined numbers of hours in nonmaternal care showed relatively more behavioral problems in both child care classrooms and kindergarten classrooms than did those who had spent fewer hours away from their mothers. Cognitive and language development was found to be somewhat better for children who attended child care centers, but, also, these children showed more behavioral problems in child care and kindergarten classrooms than did children who were placed in other nonmaternal child care arrangements.

Child care is an early watershed for children with social-emotional problems, and it may either add to the child's positive experience or exacerbate risks.[29] Young children in preschool have 3 times the expulsion rate of children and adolescents in kindergarten through 12th grade. Expulsion rates of 4-year-olds are 50% higher than for 3-year-olds, and boys are 4 times likelier to be expelled than are girls.[30]

The PCC should ask whether the child care setting is formal or informal, how confident the parent feels in the child care providers, how many hours per week the child spends there, and what happens during the child's day (eg, if much of the time is spent in front of a television [TV] set).

Change in Child's Living Environment

On the dashboard, this domain is a strength if the environment is stable and fosters the child's thriving and is expectable if there are transient changes that require adjustment, yet the child and family are coping with this change. Red flags are raised if environmental changes are disrupting the child's functioning or if the parents are sufficiently stressed and distracted to have difficulty with the demands of parenting. Some of these environmental changes are discussed in this section.

Family Disruption, Dissolution, and Variation: Cohabitation, Divorce, and Blended Families

When a family shatters or scatters, the child is threatened and challenged to adapt. Disputes and tension may precede family disruption, and children, even very young ones, are affected.

The negative effect on the mental health of the child results from the subsequent, sometimes rapid, changes in family status that may occur, pose adjustment challenges, or threaten loss of important relationships for the child. The PCC should ask about the economic effect and time course of family changes and help the parent understand and alleviate their effects on the child, considering the child's developmental level. A strength is noted if the parent or parents are able to sensitively address the stress experienced by the child or children as a result of radical changes in the family composition. A red flag is raised if they are unaware of or unconcerned about the children's reactions and if the children manifest emotional or behavioral symptoms.

Children in Foster or Kinship Care

Removal of a child from his or her home is typically preceded by toxic or troubled attachments, so separation from the parent or parents is a loss for an already stressed child, as described by Szilagyi.[31] The PCC caring for a child in foster or dependent care should expect complex issues. Optimizing the physical, emotional, developmental, and mental health status of children in dependent care requires extra attention to screening and documentation. Guidelines found in the second edition of the AAP publication *Fostering Health: Health Care for Children and Adolescents in Foster Care* provide further detail.

Mental health implications are considerable. Newborns, infants, and younger children in out-of-home placement are most vulnerable. In the United States, maltreatment presents the highest risk of morbidity and mortality for infants and toddlers.[32] These young children have usually had experiences that put the development of robust foundations for relationships at grave risk. Early recognition will enable early intervention (EI), but often the PCC is appealed to for pharmacological intervention to reduce children's troubled and troubling behaviors. However, evidence-based interventions to support foster parents can help avert the socially destructive process of multiple foster home placements for children with troubled attachments.[33,34]

Abuse is a red flag. As a mandated reporter of abuse, the PCC must recognize the threshold for reporting, but, also as a clinician who knows the child in the medical home, he or she can put together the child's story to understand the effect of timing of stress in relation to the child's developmental stage. If the child in out-of-home placement has settled well, formed an attachment to the parents now caring for him or her, and is free of emotional or behavioral symptoms, this progress is a strength.

Juvenile Justice

Children in juvenile justice settings are separated from their families, experience interruption of peer and school relationships, and must cope with an environment that is rarely nurturing or able to provide age-appropriate experiences. Involvement in the juvenile justice system is always a red flag. The prevalence of mental disorders among youths in juvenile justice settings is high: 50% to 75% of children encountering the juvenile justice system met criteria for a mental disorder.[35]

Physical, Legal, Economic, and Virtual Environment and Culture: Factors Outside the Family

Factors outside the family may challenge even mature, capable, and loving parents. The PCC should inquire about stressful physical, economic, legal, and cultural factors. The absence of these stresses, or the family's resilience in the face of these stresses, is a family strength. If there are many or severe stresses, and the family has limited supports to deal with them, such that their parenting functions are strained, a red flag is raised. Supporting parents' coping will directly benefit the child, and helping parents build children's resilience will counter the effect of environmental stress on the child.

Physical and Legal Environments

Environmental threats to the developing child may begin in utero. Exposure to toxic environmental agents such as lead, allergens, poor air quality, and pesticides is ubiquitous but disproportionately affects minority, vulnerable, and underserved populations. Almost all parents strive to do their best for their children, but many work against daunting odds.

Unemployment, Underemployment, and Poverty

As noted previously, inquiring about whether the family's current financial situation affects parenting, parents' hours of work or work strain, and neighborhood quality will identify risk factors. Children and single mothers are increasingly overrepresented among the poor. Direct effects of material impoverishment, such as inadequate nutrition leading to developmental delay, are compounded by the increased likelihood that children in poverty will be exposed to other hazards, such as substandard housing, lead poisoning, parental psychological distress, inadequate child care arrangements, or neglect and abuse.[36]

Furthermore, it is more difficult for low-income parents without social supports to meet the basic needs of very young children and those with special health care needs. Parents of any economic level who have experienced ACEs in their own early years may be at risk for poor or maladaptive parenting, may have diminished capacity to respond to stress in a healthy way, and have a higher risk of health, mental health, or substance use problems. In addition, if a parent is working multiple jobs or is too depressed, tired, or detached to engage with children in challenging settings, the parent may resort to allowing excessive screen time or substituting media for parent-child interaction.

Job loss, with associated financial strain and hardship, affects families greatly and is more common during economic recession.[37] Stressors in the aftermath of job loss include depression and decline in the quality of the parents' relationship. For 2-parent families, both the parent seeking employment and his or her partner may experience depression and reduced relationship satisfaction.[38] The economic environment may affect the child, even if parents are capable and affectionate.

Compromised parental mental health, particularly maternal distress and depression, is more common in low-income families. Parental mental health problems may disrupt the parent-child relationship on which a child's social, emotional, and cognitive development is founded. Not surprisingly, children in low-income neighborhoods, with poor housing conditions, high unemployment, and high crime rates, have higher rates of behavioral problems that affect their school readiness and performance.

Although a strength may be noted if the child has no symptoms, and a red flag raised if symptoms are severe or out of proportion to the stresses the child is experiencing, it is important to recognize that a child's developmental or mental health "symptoms" may be reasonable adaptations to the stresses of his environment and that such adaptations should be understood and addressed before a psychiatric problem is considered.

The Virtual Environment

Regardless of the home environment and the school and neighborhood environments, children may be exposed to the virtual environment of media by exposure to TV, video games, and the Internet. The positive or negative effects on the child depend on the timing, quantity, and quality of this exposure.

For very young children whose language development is progressing most rapidly, exposure to baby DVDs and videos cannot substitute for reciprocal language interaction with adults and other children.[39] For older children, screen media exposure (TV and video games) has been found to be significantly associated with teacher-reported attention problems,[40,41] controlling for gender and earlier attention problems.

For children and adolescents with good adjustment, online activity may be an asset. Thus, consistent with developmental theory, there is cross-situational continuity in the social behaviors of children and adolescents, and this continuity extends to the online domain. However, they may be pursued as potential targets by pedophiles via online contact, and risk for this may be higher for youths whose family support and adjustment are compromised.[42] The online environment also enables cyberbullying. In a large, diverse sample of urban middle- and high-school students,[43] half (49.5%) indicated they had been bullied online, and 33.7% reported that they had bullied others online. Most bullying was by and toward friends, and generally students did not tell anyone about the bullying. After being bullied online, they reported feeling sad, angry, and depressed. Those who bullied others online reported that they did so to feel popular, powerful, or funny, but many reported feeling guilty afterward.

The PCC should discuss with the family and the child what type of media exposure the child has and how it influences her or him. Specific questions about media use should explore whether the media diet is healthy; if it is, this is noted as a strength. However, if the child or adolescent turns to media because of loneliness, lack of interaction in the home, or difficulties with peer relationships, a red flag is raised.

Events

Events that affect the family will affect the child. These include disaster, exposure to violence, disruption of the family, and medical illness, topics already covered. Two other events are common and important for children: immigration and military deployment.

Immigration

Cultural and economic adaptation of families new to the United States, along with immigration uncertainty, may cause significant psychological stress. In caring for newborns and infants, the PCC should inquire about the parent's support system, as families may be separated from their support networks. In addition, it is well to be aware of family customs and beliefs about diet, discipline, and stimulation of young children. A strength is noted if the family is adapting well and connecting to a social network. However, a red flag is raised if the family is struggling with problems that directly stress the child or create strain on the parents that may interfere with their parenting.

Military Deployment

Primary care clinicians who care for patients in military families, whether active duty, veteran, or reserve, or who practice in groups that contract with programs serving veterans or reserve families, will need to recognize and respond to child and family stress that may be associated with the military environment or National Guard service.

Frequent moves, multiple deployments, and injury or loss of a parent are facts of military life that inflict psychological stress on children and their parents.[44] Stress related to deployment is associated with increased incidence of marital problems (44% among active duty and 39% among reserve), and military families' rates of mental disorders and trauma are higher than national rates. In families of enlisted Army soldiers, child maltreatment was found to be 42% higher during deployment than during non-deployment.

In particular, the wartime deployment of a parent is highly stressful for a child. One-fourth of children with deployed parents experience depression and one-fifth exhibit academic problems. Parents remaining behind experience stress, of which even young children are aware. Children's difficulties are proportional to the mental health difficulties and coping problems of the parent; their mental health symptoms include externalizing and internalizing problems. For veteran partners returning with post-traumatic stress disorder (PTSD), interpersonal violence rates are higher, and their partners experience higher caregiver burden.

A strength is noted if the family adjusts smoothly to the mobility and strain of military life and if its children adapt well. However, mental health resources available to military families, including reserve and National Guard families, are often insufficient to meet families' needs. If the parents are stressed and cannot identify mental health resources, and if this lack of treatment is associated with behavioral or emotional symptoms in the child, a red flag is raised.

Health Status of the Child

Health concerns are the domain of pediatric care. Psychological effects of health concerns and the stresses on children with chronic illness and special health care needs have been well studied.[45,46] The pediatric medical home mediates the needs of children with special health care needs among specialists. This mediation includes recognizing and seeking support for children's mental health symptoms and their parents' caregiving burdens.[47]

The Child's Manifestations: The Mental Status Examination

The mental status examination organizes clinical observations.[48] Its components are the domains of developmental level, cognition and language, attention and executive function, control of impulses, anxiety and sequalae of trauma exposure, mood, capacity for relationships, self-regulation, and adolescent addiction: substance use and the Internet. These domains are summarized in Table 6-2.

Children's behavioral and emotional manifestations evolve as they develop. For example, separation anxiety is a sign of healthy attachment in an 8-month-old and tantrums are not uncommon in 2-year-olds as they navigate development of autonomy. Both behaviors are uncommon in school-aged children and adolescents and would be cause for concern. For each of the categories in Table 6-2, the PCC will adjust expectations for the child's capacities to that child's developmental level.

The use of standardized mental health screening tools in pediatric practice has been widely advocated[9] and is logistically feasible,[24] but these

Table 6-2. Mental Health Dashboard: Child's Manifestations			
Dashboard Domain	Strength	Expectable Status	Red Flag for Risk/ Problem
Developmental level	Gifted child Precocious	Average range or age appropriate	Area of delay Lagging, inconsistent, or immature
Cognition and language	Strong verbal and cognitive ability	Average range Able to perform and express self at age level	Area of delay or disability Psychotic thought process
Attention and executive function	Above-age abilities to concentrate and learn	Focuses on tasks at age level and eager to learn	Distractible; not persistent; forgetful; or inconsistent
Control of impulses	Child mature for age in managing his or her strong urges or feelings	Redirectable, able to wait, able to name feelings, and knows "good" from "bad"	Impulsive, reckless, frequent unintentional injuries, or aggressive
Anxiety and sequelae of trauma exposure	Resilient and able to maintain equilibrium under stress	Untroubled by anxiety or trauma exposure, or has recovered promptly when stressed	Subject to fears and worries, difficult to reassure, and trauma-related symptoms (may additionally or alternatively appear in other domains)
Mood	Well modulated with good range Ability to control, express, and understand feelings	Reacts as expected to positive or negative events Good range and modulation of moods	Mood swings, irritability or persistent sadness, thoughts of self-harm, or overreaction to events
Capacity for relationships	Deep and diverse relationships Strong, intense, and well-modulated interactions	Age-expected range of relationships Expressive, reciprocal, and capacity for empathy	Isolated, avoidant, or confrontational; lack of empathy; cruel; or chronic or significant peer problems

Table 6-2. Mental Health Dashboard: Child's Manifestations (*continued*)			
Dashboard Domain	**Strength**	**Expectable Status**	**Red Flag for Risk/Problem**
Self-regulation	Able to maintain adequate sleep and appetite, even when under stress	Age-expected self-control Recovers from stress-related disruptions Maintains regular sleep and eating routines	Sleep or appetite easily and persistently disrupted by emotions or events
Adolescent addiction: substance use and the Internet	None	Some experimentation	Frequent or solitary use of drugs or interfering with function
Gender and sexual development	Confident, clear gender identity Age-appropriate sexual interests	Age-appropriate embarrassment	Gender dysphoria, anxiety, confusion, or conflict with parents

tools are infrequently used.[49] Screening results may suggest or confirm the observations of the child's strengths and risk factors and contribute to the assessment of the child in one or multiple domains. A number of validated tools are available; some are general screeners (eg, Pediatric Symptom Checklist [PSC], Strengths and Difficulties Questionnaires [SDQ]), while others focus on specific symptom clusters such as inattention and impulsivity, depression, or anxiety (eg, NICHQ Vanderbilt attention-deficit/hyperactivity disorder [ADHD] assessment scales, PHQ-9 [Patient Health Questionnaire-9] Modified for Teens, SCARED [Screen for Child Anxiety Related Disorders]). Tools that assist in screening and assessment are listed in Appendix 2, Mental Health Tools for Pediatrics. Boxes 1-8 and 1-9 in Chapter 1, Integrating Mental Health Care Into Pediatric Practice, offer guidance in their use. Whichever tools are used to screen for symptoms, functional assessment is also important. Examples are given in Appendix 2.

As part of the mental status examination, the PCC may pose questions to pursue specific elements, such as brief orientation and memory items, or follow-up questions about anxiety (eg, "What scares you?") or mood (eg, "Do you ever feel sad or hopeless or think about harming yourself?").

Office routines for collecting collateral data as needed are discussed in Chapter 3, Office and Network Systems to Support Mental Health Care. The PCC should ask the parent to sign a release for exchange of information with other agencies that may be serving the child, for example, EI, social services (particularly for children in foster care or with a history of abuse or neglect), and the school (eg, Individualized Education Programs [IEPs], 504 plans, report cards, teacher questionnaires such as the NICHQ Vanderbilt ADHD assessment scales and SDQ). Any of these reports can serve as a gauge of the child's mental health status, and several incorporate functional assessment. Brief descriptions of the domains of child manifestations follow. Part 4 of this book, Chapters 13 through 32, includes a full discussion of presenting symptoms in each of these domains. The American Academy of Child and Adolescent Psychiatry (commonly known as AACAP) has developed a series of Facts for Families for PCCs and families, with summaries of specific problem areas.[50] Whenever a child manifests impairing symptoms or findings that suggest a disorder, this manifestation raises a red flag. The concern should be addressed and noted in the child's problem list and the practice registry to assure appropriate follow-up. All children manifesting mental health problems should be triaged for a psychiatric or social emergency.

Developmental Level

Social development has both a biological basis and neurobiological consequences. Normative theories of child development describe the progression from the newborn's complete dependence on parents through the acquisition of strengths, knowledge, and skills to pursuit of independence and relationships outside the family during childhood and adolescence. This progression, propelled by physical and neurological maturation, is well-known to the pediatrician, and the pediatrician's role in helping the parent understand and facilitate the child's development has been well established.[24] To optimize biologically driven maturation, a fuller understanding of the critical influence of the child's interpersonal and social environment is also necessary, because psychological and social development is necessarily interpersonal and mediated by experience.[51] The PCC should routinely and systematically assess the parents' and caregivers' understanding of the child's developmental capacity.

The fifth edition of the *Diagnostic and Statistical Manual of Mental Disorders* (*DSM-5*)[52] separately classifies neurodevelopmental disorders to include intellectual disability (formerly called *mental retardation*), communication disorders, autism spectrum disorder (ASD), specific learning disorders, ADHD, developmental coordination disorder, stereotypic movement disorder, and tic disorders. Early recognition of neurodevelopmental disorders that negatively affect the developmental trajectory is vital for EI. Intellectual disability may include deficits in either intellectual functioning or adaptive functioning (or both). Deficits in intellectual functions include difficulty with reasoning, problem-solving, planning, abstract thinking, judgment, academic learning, and learning from experience. If a deficit is suspected, the child should be referred for individual standardized intelligence testing. Deficits in adaptive functioning are marked by the child's failure to meet developmental and sociocultural standards for developing independence and social responsibility.

Assessment and screening of child development is familiar to the PCC, and the AAP has provided tools to assist.[53] A strength is noted if the child is on track or ahead developmentally; a red flag, if there are areas of delay.

Cognition and Language

Children with strengths in this domain think and communicate clearly at their age levels. A red flag is raised if difficulties as listed herein are noted.

Knowledge and language skills are routinely assessed in preschool and school settings. Milestones are widely familiar to PCCs and early childhood educators. Difficulties in these areas are commonly brought to the PCC's attention, and they may be encountered, for example, as language delays, communication or reading problems, troubles with generalization of learning or frustration, and excessive problems with change in daily routine.

In interacting with the child and through history from the parents, the PCC can consider the child's language development, ability to learn, problem-solving ability, and cognitive flexibility. As part of the mental status examination, the PCC should evaluate whether the child's vocabulary and fund of knowledge are developmentally appropriate, noting her speech spontaneity, her articulation, and the content and connectedness of her thought processes. Typically, problems in this domain are recognized in preschool and school settings. Still, the PCC may need to advocate for parents to pursue testing by the school.

Communication disorders include language disorder, speech sound disorder, and fluency disorder (eg, stuttering). Social, or pragmatic, communication disorders functionally limit effective communication with peers and in the classroom. For example, the child may have difficulty using communication socially, in a way that fits the social context; may have difficulties following rules for conversation and storytelling; and may have trouble understanding what is not explicitly stated.

The *DSM-5* regards autism as a spectrum, no longer distinguishing Asperger syndrome or pervasive developmental disorders. Replacing "mild," "moderate," and "severe," the clinician now uses specifiers to indicate the child's strengths, weaknesses, and co-occurring conditions, for example, the severity of symptoms, accompanying intellectual or language impairment. Other chapters in this book provide guidance for the assessment and care of children presenting with learning difficulties (see Chapter 21, Learning Difficulty) and speech and language concerns (see Chapter 29, Speech and Language Concerns).

Psychosis typically emerges in late adolescence, young adulthood, or early adulthood (ages 15–30). Prodromal symptoms include unusual thinking (eg, paranoia, delusions), perceptual disturbances (eg, hearing or seeing things others don't see or hear), negative symptoms (eg, withdrawal, loss of motivation), disorganized symptoms (eg, vague, racing, or slow speech; difficulty staying on track; neglect of personal hygiene), mood or anxiety symptoms, and decline in functioning. These may occur for short periods with varying intensity, sometimes generating the need for emergency intervention.

Attention and Executive Function

The saying "a mother's attention span is as long as that of her youngest child," while humorous, reflects both the challenge of parenting and the fact that good-enough parents accommodate to their child's needs. Parents can readily report on their child's attention capacities and, while these vary with fatigue, illness, and stress, this variability is expected development. Likewise, the constellation of cognitive capacities (eg, memory, persistence, problem-solving, flexibly adaptive approaches to new challenges) that are broadly called *executive function* manifest themselves daily in the child's behavior.

Responsive parents accommodate to their children's limitations or proudly report their children's accomplishments, so an important part of the PCC's assessment is asking about how the parent manages a typical day with the child. This inquiry may reveal habitual adaptations, which the parent may regard as routine, even though they are necessary scaffolding to prevent problems. For example, the mother of a school-aged child with ADHD might say she would never leave him alone at another child's birthday party because she knows her son will become too rambunctious or impulsive.

Although a cardinal feature of the ADHD diagnosis is that symptoms occur in 2 or more settings, the child may or may not be overtly hyperactive, impulsive, or inattentive in the examining room. Diagnosis of ADHD relies on history to learn if these behaviors occur in multiple settings. Many PCCs use parent and teacher questionnaires to confirm suspected ADHD. In the *DSM-5* classification, ADHD is now positioned as a neurodevelopmental disorder. The older subtypes (eg, "predominantly hyperactive") are now specifiers of the child's current presentation.

Capacities for attention and executive function are also set awry by the hypervigilance or avoidance and numbing brought about by PTSD. The PCC may not initially know the cause of attention or executive function problems, but recognition that they are present and that they are age inappropriate is an important first step toward a differential diagnosis. Children with strengths in this domain deploy their attention as flexibly and persistently as expected for their ages. A red flag is raised if the child shows symptoms of inattention, impulsivity, impersistence, or hyperactivity more than children of the same age do, and it behooves further assessment.

Chapter 20, Inattention and Impulsivity, provides guidance in the assessment and care of children presenting with inattention and impulsivity.

Control of Impulses

Control of impulses is a recognized requirement of bringing a child to adulthood. Children with strengths in this domain can control their impulses and are generally cooperative and considerate. A red flag is raised if they show symptoms as described herein.

Normally, a frustrated preschooler who swats a peer reaching for his toy becomes a school-aged child who protests, "It's not fair,'" and then a preadolescent who is more strategic in achieving his goals. These behaviors are expected for these stages. If a preschool-aged child can never "use his words" to deal with frustration; a school-aged child steals, defies adults, and initiates physical fights; or an adolescent destroys property, harms others, steals, and seriously violates rules, in spite of a family and neighborhood context that doesn't teach him to do these things, impulse control problems are significant. The PCC can get information about control of urges, anger, and impatience from the child and, often more readily, from the parent.

Oppositional defiant disorder (ODD) is a pattern of uncooperative, hostile, and defiant behavior toward parents and authority figures that seriously interferes with daily functioning. The child may frequently argue, defy, annoy, and spite or blame others, even when he has nothing to gain by this behavior. Parents may have noticed from an early age that the child was more rigid and demanding. Behaviors are frequently worse at home, but young children may be kicked out of child care or preschool, and school-aged children incur disciplinary action. The problem is not transient, and referral for parent management, individual or family therapy, or cognitive problem-solving skills training may be indicated. Parents need support and guidance to raise children with these difficult behaviors.

Intermittent explosive disorder (commonly known as IED), with onset in later childhood or adolescence, is characterized by disproportionate, uncontrolled, sudden anger and aggression with little if any apparent provocation. The child or adolescent has low frustration tolerance and describes himself as being overcome with anger and feeling out of control. Previous trauma is a risk factor.

Conduct disorder is particularly challenging. The callous disregard for and aggression toward others may begin with biting, pushing, and hitting in early childhood and progress to cruelty, bullying, and violence in adolescence. Risk factors are childhood abuse, neglect or inconsistent or coercive parenting, and neighborhood violence, peer delinquency, or rejection by peers. Children with parents who have ADHD, substance use disorder, or other serious mental disorders are at greater risk. For guidance in the assessment and care of children presenting with impulsivity, see Chapter 20, Inattention and Impulsivity; for the assessment and care of children presenting with disruptive behavior and aggression, see Chapter 15, Disruptive Behavior and Aggression.

Anxiety and Sequelae of Trauma Exposure

Anxiety

Anxiety is an expectable neurobiological reaction to stress and is therefore a universal experience that likely mobilizes the individual in adaptive ways. How a child develops the capacity to contain, explain, and rebound from anxiety-provoking experiences depends greatly on the buffering and support of the adults who care for him. Neglect, particularly emotional neglect, leaves the child to struggle alone with this frightening state. Trauma, particularly recurrent trauma, brings about a re-set of anxiety thresholds that may be enduring. Some children have anxiety that ignites too easily and is too hard to assuage, and this tendency is a greater dilemma for them if their parents are also anxious and cannot help them modulate this feeling.

On mental status examination, the child may report worries and fears, feeling keyed up or on edge, inability to concentrate, susceptibility to fatigue, or muscle tension. Outward signs of anxiety are varied: the child may have stomachaches, trouble sleeping, fidgetiness, or trouble focusing in class. Regardless of the etiologic origin, the PCC can inquire of the child and family about the child's fears and worries and determine whether they are appropriate reactions or inappropriately severe or persistent.

Most infants and young children between 6 and 18 months of age may show distress on separation from a major attachment figure; this distress is a hallmark of attachment. However, a young child who is extremely unwilling to separate, becoming highly anxious, afraid of harm to himself or parents, perhaps with nightmares and somatic symptoms such as trembling, sweating, headaches, or stomachaches, may have separation anxiety disorder.

Other childhood anxiety disorders are generalized anxiety disorder (GAD), panic disorder, selective mutism, social phobia, and obsessive-compulsive disorder. The child with GAD worries excessively and cannot control his worrying about a wide variety of issues. The symptoms are present most days, lasting at least 6 months.

Panic disorder is diagnosed if intense episodes of fear and unease occur with physical symptoms such as increased heart rate, chest pain, sweating, trembling, or trouble breathing. Panic attacks are sudden and recurring and lead to avoidance of situations that the child thinks might trigger them. Cognitive behavioral treatments are effective.

Specific phobias are intense irrational fears of certain things or certain situations, with anxiety expressed by crying, clinging, freezing, or tantrums.

Persistent failure to speak in specific social situations, such as at school or with peers, despite the child's ability to speak in other situations, is called *selective mutism*.

Beyond shyness, social phobia is intense fear of being embarrassed or humiliated in social situations. It typically begins in childhood or early adolescence and disrupts age-appropriate school or social relationships.

Obsessive-compulsive disorder is marked by recurrent intrusive thoughts (obsessions) and repeated behaviors (compulsions) that are distressing, are time-consuming, and impair daily functioning. Common obsessions are fears of contamination, self-doubt, and aggression and needing to have things in a particular order. Repetitive behaviors, such as handwashing, checking, counting, praying, or ordering things, have the goal of reducing or preventing the anxiety, but they do not provide pleasure.

Children with strengths in this domain do not have the symptoms just described. A red flag is raised if they do. For guidance in the assessment and care of children presenting with symptoms of anxiety, see Chapter 14, Anxiety and Trauma-Related Distress.

Sequelae of Trauma Exposure

Reactive attachment disorder may result from extremes of insufficient care, such as neglect or deprivation, rearing in unusual settings, or repeated change in caregivers. It manifests as either emotionally with-drawn and inhibited behavior (eg, reduced responsiveness, limited affect, irritability, fearfulness, sadness) or indiscriminately socially disinhibited behavior (eg, lack of reticence with unfamiliar adults). This second type is now a distinctive separate disorder in the *DSM-5* called *disinhibited social engagement disorder.* PCCs who care for very young children who have experienced disruptive or disrupted parenting should be aware of this disorder.

Children of any age actively adapt to their relationship environment, and within the constellation of that interpersonal environment, they develop self-regulation and automatic expectations about others. Original studies of attachment indicate that most infants and toddlers have secure attachments with their primary caregiver. Children with insecure attachment styles fall into 3 groups, termed *insecure and avoidant, resistant and ambivalent,* and *disorganized and disoriented.* Attachment types are specific between an infant and a particular caregiver, are predictable from normal caregiving behavior in the first year after birth, and remain stable to at least 6 years of age. Sensitive, responsive care leads to secure attachment. Rejecting caregiving leads to insecure and avoidant attachment. Inconsistent caregiving leads to resistant and ambivalent attachment.

If the constellation of intimate parent-child interactions is troubled, or disturbed enough to be characterized as attachment disorder, the child is at high risk for developing self-perpetuating troubled patterns of interactions with other children and adults. The PCC must recognize disordered attachment, not only because the child's development is contingent on reciprocal interactions in an attached relationship[54] but also because without EI, disordered attachment may jeopardize or distort later close relationships. The *DSM-5*[52] recognizes 2 types of attachment disorders: reactive attachment disorder and disinhibited social engagement disorder; these have previously been described as nonattachment and indiscriminate sociability.[55] This pattern of shallow, friendly, engaging behavior may result from cycling through multiple caregivers before removal from the parent and multiple foster placements thereafter. Reactive attachment disorder may resemble internalizing disorders, with a lack of or incompletely formed preferred attachments to caregiving adults and a dampened expression of joy or happiness. Disinhibited social engagement disorder more closely resembles ADHD and may occur in children who do not lack attachments or who have established or even secure attachments. Children with disordered attachment may exhibit symptoms ranging from withdrawn behavior to angry, aggressive behavior.

Children with both patterns of attachment disorder are very challenging to parent, as they have difficulties with self-regulation along with disruptive or disturbing behavior, and they cannot return the love and trust that their parents try to give them, leaving the parents feeling ineffective and distressed.

Measures of attachment are available for both adults[56] and children.[57] If the PCC is concerned about the quality of the child-parent attachment, a fuller history or use of a screening tool is indicated, followed by referral to a mental health professional for further assessment. Ideally, the PCC would identify problems of attachment early in the child's life. For guidance in assessing young children manifesting emotional or behavioral disturbances, see Chapter 17, Emotional or Behavioral Disturbance in Children Younger Than 5 Years.

Post-traumatic stress disorder is an intense and disabling response to a catastrophic traumatizing event, one in which the individual has been injured or feels overwhelmingly threatened. Symptoms fall into 3 clusters: reexperiencing (intense memories, nightmares, and flashbacks); avoidance of reexposure, perhaps with psychological numbing; and a constant hyperalert state, with increased startle, sleep difficulties, irritability, or anger. Children experiencing repeated trauma may develop emotional numbing or dissociation. Depersonalization and derealization may also be features of PTSD. The *DSM-5* has lowered the threshold for diagnosing PTSD in preschool-aged children to improve recognition.

Acute stress disorder has similar features to PTSD and lasts at least 3 days or up to a month. Adjustment disorder is diagnosed if a child develops clinically significant behavioral or emotional symptoms in response to an identifiable stress, not of traumatic degree, that has occurred within 3 months, and if these symptoms cause impairment in functioning. In the *DSM-5,* the symptoms are specified as being depressive, being anxious, or occurring with conduct disturbance (or any combination thereof). For guidance in the assessment and care of children experiencing trauma-related distress, see Chapter 14, Anxiety and Trauma-Related Distress.

Mood

The PCC will see many sad children in practice. Some have mood disorders. The prevalence of mood disorders is 14% among 13- to 18-year-old adolescents, and, of these, 4.7% have severe disorders. Girls are likelier

(18.1%) than boys (10.1%) to be affected, and there are no statistically significant differences by race.[58] The Bright Futures/AAP *Recommendations for Preventive Pediatric Health Care* (periodicity schedule) recommends routine screening for depression at all adolescent health supervision visits. This screening is important because there is an established link between depression and suicide, and suicide among adolescents is on the rise, with 14.5% of the 9th to 12th grade students in the United States in 2007 reporting suicidal ideation and 6.9% reporting at least one suicide attempt during the previous year.[58]

Major depressive disorder (MDD) is marked by sad, empty, irritable mood, persisting at least 2 weeks. A child with symptoms that include crying, low self-esteem, lack of energy, or loss of interest in formerly pleasurable activities (or any combination thereof) that significantly interfere with functioning might have MDD. Accompanying cognitive changes may include problems with concentration, guilt, and belief that he or she is worthless. Accompanying somatic changes may include change in sleeping or eating habits. If these symptoms are mild and chronic, with a low mood almost daily over a span of at least 2 years, the child may have persistent depressed mood (formerly called *dysthymia*). Adjustment disorder with depressed mood may have similar symptoms, and it appears after an identifiable event or stressor. If depressed periods alternate with at least weeklong periods of mania (euphoria, abnormally happy states, agitation, excessive energy or irritability, impulsive decisions, reduced need to sleep, racing thoughts, rapid uninterruptable speech, and high-risk behaviors, including hypersexuality), a bipolar disorder may be present. Hypomania, a milder form, is defined as at least 4 days of manic symptoms.

In evaluating mood, the PCC should note the dominant type of mood (sadness, elation, or irritability) and the range and modulation of moods. For example, a child who is sad may show intervals of brightness and demonstrate capacity to move to other feeling states. Poorly modulated mood does not adjust or align to events, including the interview. Observation of depression is always an indication for inquiring about suicidal ideation. Mood swings from depression to manic energy and irritability may require evaluation by a mental health professional.

For guidance in the primary care assessment and treatment of children presenting with low mood, see Chapter 22, Low Mood.

Depression can occur in children as young as 3 years of age. A small child who is sad, grouchy, and unable to enjoy activities and play, or who has low energy, changed sleep or appetite, and talk or play of themes about death or killing himself, should be evaluated for depression.[59] See Chapter 17, Emotional or Behavioral Disturbance in Children Younger Than 5 Years, for discussion of the assessment and care of young children presenting with symptoms of emotional or behavioral disturbance.

Irritability is a troubling and troublesome symptom. When irritability is severe (eg, tantrums), frequent (eg, ≥3 times a week), persistent (most of every day), chronic (eg, lasting weeks), and out of proportion in duration and intensity to the situation, disruptive mood dysregulation disorder (DMDD) may be present.[52] Disruptive mood dysregulation disorder is diagnosed if a child is at least 6 years of age, and symptoms must appear before age 10 and be present at least a year. The DMDD diagnosis has been developed because bipolar disorders were frequently diagnosed in school-aged children, but children with DMDD experience a different course, and they are not specifically benefitted by treatments of bipolar disorders. Again, consultation with a mental health specialist is indicated.

Capacity for Relationships

Capacity for relationships begins with the earliest attachment. A lens through which to view the infant's earliest relationships is the transactional model,[60,61] which provides a comprehensive view of the interaction between nature and nurture, focusing on relations between the genotype (ie, the individual's biological organization), the phenotype (ie, the individual's personal organization), and the environtype (ie, the organization of experience).

The child's behavior is seen as a product of transactions among the genotype, phenotype, and environtype. The transactional model provides a framework for EI that can emphasize, depending on the nature of the relationship problem, remediation of the child's behavior, redefinition of the parents' interpretation of the child's behavior, or reeducation of the parents to change their behavior to the child.

The PCC will observe the child's manner of relating during the interview, but, importantly, history from the parents will inform him or her about whether the child's relationships are deep and diverse, whether the child has empathy for others, or whether the child is isolated, avoidant, confrontational, or cruel.

Children with a variety of mental health conditions often have impairment in their ability to form and maintain relationships. For children with ASD or conduct disorder, the capacity for relationships is severely limited. Children with reactive attachment disorder, as described previously, and those with disorders of impulse control, and mood disorders, experience disruption of their relationships as well.

Self-regulation

Anticipatory guidance about sleep, eating patterns, toileting, and discipline is familiar to PCCs. Progression from the newborn or young infant's requirement that all these be managed by the parent to the older child's ability to manage them independently is expected. However, the child must also learn to self-regulate his or her attention, urges, fears, anger, exuberance, and aggression. This process takes place through the innumerable interactions with parents in daily exchanges around learning patience, perseverance, self-calming, and self-restraint. Thus, it depends on the interaction of a more or less intact child nervous system with generally consistent and nurturing parenting. A neglected infant who cries exhausted to sleep, hungry and wet, does not learn how to self-soothe; a toddler who may be unpredictably either ignored or punished for age-appropriate behavior does not learn self-restraint; a frantic or distressed young child who receives no comfort or explanation cannot easily learn to modulate his or her feelings. The PCC, by inquiring about how typical challenges are managed at home, can gain information about the child's self-regulation and how parents may assist or impair its development.

Eating disorders are a serious disruption of self-regulation. The lifetime prevalence of eating disorders among 13- to 18-year-olds is 2.7%, with a 2.5 times predominance of girls.[62] They include anorexia nervosa, bulimia nervosa, and binge-eating disorder. The PCC will begin by asking, "How do you feel about your weight?" taking note of the child or adolescent's response, both verbal and nonverbal. This question may be followed by simple screening questionnaires, such as the SCOFF (sick, control, one, fat, food).[63]

Anorexia nervosa is marked by weight loss of at least 15% below minimal normal level; intense fear of weight gain, even if the child or adolescent has underweight; disturbance in perception of body weight or shape and inability to recognize the seriousness of low body weight; and, in adolescent girls, absence of at least 3 consecutive menstrual periods. Bulimia nervosa is marked by recurring food binging and purging, occurring at least twice a week for 3 months.

For guidance in the assessment and care of children with eating abnormalities, see Chapter 16, Eating Abnormalities. Inpatient treatment should be considered if there is bradycardia (pulse <50 beats/min at daytime, <45 beats/min at night), hypotension (blood pressure <90/45 mm Hg), hypothermia, orthostasis, electrocardiographic (commonly known as ECG) abnormalities (eg, prolonged corrected QT interval >460 msec), electrolyte abnormalities, or other acute medical events such as syncope, GI (gastrointestinal) bleeding, or dehydration.

Sleep is important to a child's mental health, as well as the health of the child's caregivers, and poor sleep may be a manifestation of mental health problems. For these reasons, a sleep history is an important piece of the mental health assessment. For an extensive discussion of sleep abnormalities and their association with mental health, see Chapter 28, Sleep Disturbances.

Adolescent Addiction: Substance Use and the Internet

Addiction may seriously affect adolescent functioning. Formal screening for use of substances should be a routine part of health supervision for all adolescents and for those presenting with psychosocial symptoms or impairment in psychosocial functioning. (See Appendix 2.) For further discussion, see the 3 chapters on substance use: Chapter 30, Substance Use 1: Use of Tobacco and Nicotine; Chapter 31, Substance Use 2: Use of Other Substances; and Chapter 32, Substance Use 3: Specialty Referral and Comanagement.

Internet use is described previously in this chapter, in discussion of the virtual environment. Increasing concern about pathological Internet use has received considerable press. Signs for concern are excessive (eg, >40 hours a week) Internet use that interferes with sleep, family relationships, homework, and outside activities; irritability when deprived of Internet access; or lying about time spent online.

Gender and Sexual Development

Brief mention is made in this section of mental health aspects of gender and sexual development. Developmentally, by about age 2 years, children are aware of physical differences between boys and girls, and at about age 3 they easily label themselves as a boy or girl and differentiate toys preferred by boys or girls. For some young children, articulating the wish to be another gender may be a temporary phenomenon. This phenomenon most commonly resolves by around age 9 or 10. If children are gender nonconforming and persistently, consistently, and insistently say they wish they were the other gender, they are more likely to become a transgender adult. If an adolescent wishes to pursue medical transition to the other gender, the PCC should assist in referring to a counselor or therapist experienced in supporting transgender youths, and a pediatric endocrinologist, ideally just before puberty.[64] Chapter 19, Gender Expression and Identity, provides guidance on care of children with gender expression and identity issues.

Sexual orientation refers to the pattern of the child's or adolescent's romantic or sexual attractions, whether the same sex, the opposite sex, or both sexes. Both nonconforming gender identity and same-sex orientation may render a child vulnerable to bullying and discrimination, which typically leads to anxiety and depression.

A strength is noted if the parents are accepting and supportive of their child's wishes and choices. A red flag is raised if children or adolescents are distressed about themselves because of their gender identities or if there is family conflict around the issue.

Gauges

Gauges can include the full array of data-gathering tools available to PCCs, in addition to clinical observations during the visit. Chapter 1, Integrating Preventive Mental Health Care Into Pediatric Practice, describes how these can be integrated into the flow of primary care visits. Following are examples of gauges the PCC can use.

Previsit Questionnaires

Previsit questionnaires are essential aids to organizing what the parent knows and what the PCC wants to know about the child. They engage parents in reflecting on their child's development and well-being and identifying concerns. This engagement, in turn, facilitates joint focus with the PCC during the office visit. To make effective use of questionnaires, PCCs will need to review responses with children, adolescents, and parents to clarify and reflect any concerns in the their own words and those of their family. Appendix 2 lists questionnaires in common use. The Tools for Practice section at the end of this chapter includes examples of questionnaires tailored to the dashboard concept (Tables 6-4 and 6-5).

Screening Tools

Early recognition and screening for emerging mental health problems has been facilitated by the work of the AAP Task Force on Mental Health, including a summary of mental health screening and assessment tools for primary care. See Appendix 2 for a list of those readily applied to the primary care setting. Screening results may confirm the PCC's observations of the child's strengths and risk factors or call attention to unrecognized strengths, risk factors, or symptoms.

Interview

Screening provides a springboard to further assessment. Primary care clinicians need to clarify and reflect any positive findings. When a problem is identified, whether through screening or an expressed concern of the youth or family, the PCC can ask for more detail to understand its impact and the risk factors that underlie it. If a symptom is reported, she or he can ask about its frequency, duration, intensity, context, and progression, and whether previous treatment has been sought. The PCC can also ask about the impact of the symptom on the family, school performance, and peer relationships.

With input from the family, the PCC can construct an understanding of predisposing, precipitating, and perpetuating risk factors. For example, for the symptom of anxiety, predisposing factors might be gender (female), temperament (inhibited), and the attachment pattern (anxious). Precipitating factors might be a traumatic event, peer abuse, neighborhood violence, anxious parents, and a pattern of avoidance than interferes with mastery.

It is important to make note of strengths; for example, a child with high verbal skills can be better reassured or helped to understand his symptoms. Finally, for each symptom, the PCC can inquire about the parents' explanatory model for the symptom. For example, the father of an anxious child might say, "Her mother coddles her too much," and the mother might say, "Her dad yells at her when he thinks she is being a coward." In this way, the clinician builds a common understanding with the family and creates a foundation for further assessment and treatment planning.

Observations

The alert and sensitive PCC takes in a great deal of information by observing parent-child interactions, the child's behavior in the examining room, and the child and family's responses to the provider and other office staff. Bright Futures visit documentation forms provide an approach for each age-group.

The PCC will note the child's developmental level. The conversation in the interview will allow the PCC to estimate the child's cognition and language development. The child's attention and executive function are also observed, and information about how the child is doing in school is an important corollary. How the child controls his or her impulses can be directly observed, and, again, history is an important factor, as children's behavior may be relatively subdued in an office setting. The PCC will observe the child's anxiety level and general mood. Through the relationship the child develops with the PCC, his or her capacity for relationships can be observed, as well as the relationship with the parents. The child's self-regulation is primarily estimated by asking the child about sleep, appetite, loss of temper, and ability to feel calm or contained, and history from the parents is vital to assess whether the child is generally stable and self-regulating or the parents must devote considerable energy to keeping the child "on an even keel."

Response to Primary Care Interventions

Experienced PCCs who have acquired "common factors" skills, described in Chapter 5, Effective Communication Methods: Common Factors Skills, and summarized by the HELP mnemonic (Appendix 5), can be effective in reducing parental distress and improving child functioning across a range of undifferentiated mental health problems.[65] This information can empower the PCC who wants to assist a family that may be resistant to mental health specialty care, or to provide help while they await specialty care. The common factors approach can be applied to commonly presenting symptoms, such as anxiety, disruptive behavior and aggression, inattention and impulsivity, and low mood, as described in Part 4 of this book, the common signs and symptoms part (Chapters 14, 15, 20, and 22, respectively). Note that these are domains of child manifestations in the dashboard. If the child and family fail to respond to this type of primary care intervention, this is another gauge of the difficulties faced by the child.

Periodic Functional Assessment

Symptoms are important to note, but the PCC must pay attention to how the child is functioning as well and whether he or she is tackling age-appropriate challenges. Much of this information comes out in the interview, but rating scales and screening tools that assess functioning assist in anchoring the child's functional adaptation in relation to age-expected levels. See Appendix 2.

Collateral Information

Office routines for collecting collateral data, as needed, are discussed in Chapter 3, Office and Network Systems to Support Mental Health Care. The PCC can ask the parent to sign a release for exchange of information with other agencies that may be serving the child, for example, EI, social services (particularly for children in foster care or with a history of abuse or neglect), and the school (eg, IEPs; 504 plans; report cards; teacher questionnaires such as the NICHQ Vanderbilt ADHD assessment scales, PSC, and SDQ, all of which have teacher versions).

Integrating the Assessment

Red Flags in a Single Domain

Chapter 2, Pediatric Care of Children and Adolescents With Mental Health Problems, of this book describes general principals and processes for providing care to children with mental health problems, and the chapters following it provide guidance for the content of that care when faced with common signs and symptoms. This guidance includes triaging for a psychiatric or social emergency in any child identified with a mental health problem. In addition to addressing flagged concerns, PCCs should add them to the child's problem list in the medical record and to the practice registry, which will trigger office protocols and alert the PCC to address the concern at future visits.

Red Flags in Multiple Domains
Comorbidity and Complexity

In contrast to categorical diagnostic schemes such as the fourth revised edition of the *Diagnostic and Statistical Manual of Mental Disorders* (commonly known as *DSM-IV-TR*), or the fourth edition of the primary care version of the *Diagnostic and Statistical Manual of Mental Disorders* (commonly known as *DSM-PC*), dimensional approaches have been invoked to extend diagnostic capacity to children, as the boundaries between types of behaviors and emotions and behaviors may be less definable, especially for preschool-aged children. This approach has been termed "breaking apart the phenotype"[66] to more flexibly consider development, adaptation, social context, and emerging scientific findings. A dimensional approach allows recognition of subclinical conditions, and if protective factors are included in the dimensions, the assessment will point to directions for selective prevention and early intervention. The *DSM-5* provides a dimensional approach to some extent. Problems in multiple domains create a situation commonly classified as comorbidity (defined as co-occurrence of $\geq$2 psychological disorders[67]) but more recently better conceptualized as *homotypic* and *heterotypic* disorder patterns. Homotypic disorders are those that co-occur in the externalizing spectrum (eg, ADHD plus ODD) or the internalizing spectrum (eg, both anxiety disorders and depressive disorders); heterotypic disorders co-occur from both internalizing and externalizing groups, such as conduct disorder and MDD. New knowledge about neurodevelopmental mechanisms points to common neural and genetic effects that influence homotypic and heterotypic disorders, and it accounts for overlapping symptoms in these disorders. (See Knapp and Mastergeorge[68] for a summary.)

The dashboard concept lends itself to observing clusters of problems without counting symptoms and imposing cutoffs to meet criteria for *DSM* diagnostic specification. This model is consistent with latent class analysis or latent profiles analysis.[69]

That said, when a child has multiple red flags, some prioritization will be necessary. The PCC should begin by considering potential emergency issues, those affecting the child's safety, and then consider issues jeopardizing family stability or the child's placement in the family. The PCC should prioritize issues that would require referral to a mental health specialist. The PCC should be mindful of areas of strength that might enable resolution of the difficulties; for example, a child with strong attachment and good verbal skills would be a good candidate for psychotherapeutic treatment.

The Clinical Wild Card

The traumatized child may not seem to fit into any clear category. Symptoms following neglect, abuse, and trauma are pleomorphic. These experiences mold plastic neural connections in the developing brain in lasting ways, with important implications for social-emotional function, psychopathology, and resilience.[70,71] The higher prevalence of psychiatric disorders among foster children and other child risk groups is associated with their higher exposure to such events, often associated with insufficient parental buffering. The dashboard captures elements of the child's life experience and relationships and places them in relationship to symptom clusters that may have emerged because of early dysregulation.

Indications for Full Diagnostic Assessment

The PCC must treat the whole child, provide preventive anticipatory guidance, and know when to pursue more rigorous diagnostic clarity and when to intervene. Carrying out these functions is a tall order, and to carry them out while deploying a large number of screening or diagnostic tools, and articulating with fragmented or insufficient mental health services, requires navigating unmarked and occasionally treacherous territory. By recording findings in a format such as Table 6-3, incorporated into the medical record, the PCC can rapidly focus on the child's overall functioning ("engine"), the progress she or he is making ("fuel level, odometer, and speed"), and the direction of intervention ("GPS"). Just as dashboard readings in a vehicle do not provide all the information about the workings of the engine or the behavior of other drivers, the Mental Health Dashboard does not substitute for full diagnostic evaluation or evidence-based treatment. However, as an indicator it can be a helpful device for sharing information from and with the child and parent.

Table 6-3. Primary Care Provider's Mental Health Dashboard Summary				
Psychosocial Assessment	Dashboard Domain	Strength	Expectable Status	Red Flag for Risk/Problem
Child's situation	Psychosocial environment, supports, and relationships			
	ACEs and traumatic experiences			
	Primary support			
	Caregiving			
	Change in child's living environment			
	Physical and legal environments			
	Events			
	Health status of the child			
Child's manifestations	Developmental level			
	Cognition and language			
	Attention and executive function			
	Control of impulses			
	Anxiety and sequelae of trauma exposure			
	Mood			
	Capacity for relationships			
	Self-regulation			
	Adolescent addiction: substance use and the Internet			
	Gender and sexual development			

Abbreviation: ACE, adverse childhood experience.

Red flags may point to indications for full diagnostic evaluation by a mental health specialist, or, in the case of delayed development, a full developmental evaluation if the situation is urgent—for example, suspected abuse or neglect, risk of homicide—in addition to specialty referral; additional immediate action mandated by state law is necessary (eg, reporting to social services or legal authorities).

Conclusion

The busy clinician must be diagnostically nimble and efficient. She or he cannot conduct extensive multidisciplinary diagnostic assessments in thick clinical traffic. The psychosocial assessment in pediatric primary care is an iterative process with multiple components: previsit questionnaires, screening tools, interview, observations, response to primary care interventions, periodic functional assessment, and collateral information. These components can be envisioned as gauges on a dashboard: collectively, over time, they provide the PCC with an overview of the child's situation and mental status. Individually, each gauge prompts the clinician to acknowledge and reinforce strengths and to identify red flags that warrant immediate attention or monitoring or both.

Tools for Practice

Table 6-4. Questionnaire: Parent Form

My Child	About My Child	Circle the best response.			Parent Comment
My child's experiences	Trauma	Never	Mild	Severe	
	Separations from parent	Never long	>1 mo	Out-of-home placement	
	Parent stresses: (Specify.)	No	Mild	Serious	
	Parent with depression: Mother___ Father___ Other parenting figure___	No	Mild	Significant	
	Parent with mental health or substance abuse concerns	No	Mild	Significant	
	Divorce or separation	No	Yes	Currently	
	Someone harmed my child.	Never	A little bit	Seriously	
My child's health		Circle the best answer.			
		0	1	2	
		No	Yes, not a problem now	Yes, and still is a problem	
	Illness or health problem	None	Mild or occasional	Severe or ongoing	
	Asthma or respiratory condition	No	Mild or occasional	Severe or ongoing	
	Other medical problem	No	Mild or occasional	Severe or ongoing	

My child's development	I have concerns about how my child is developing.	No	Possibly	Yes
	I am concerned whether my child has autism spectrum disorder.	No	Possibly	Yes
	I know where to get support for my child's development.	Yes	Possibly	No
My child's feelings and behavior	**Compared with other children, my child**			
	Has trouble learning or communicating	No	Somewhat	Yes
	Is overactive	No	Somewhat	Yes
	Has trouble paying attention	No	Somewhat	Yes
	Is impulsive or has risky behaviors	No	Somewhat	Yes
	Has negative or aggressive behaviors	No	Somewhat	Yes
	Is anxious/has fears	No	Somewhat	Yes
	Is sometimes too sad or too happy	No	Somewhat	Yes
	Has trouble getting along with others	No	Somewhat	Yes
	Is shy or withdrawn	No	Somewhat	Yes
	Has had traumatic experiences	No	Somewhat	Yes
	Has trouble with sleep, eating, or caring for himself/herself	No	Somewhat	Yes
My family and neighbors	I have someone to rely on in an emergency.	Yes	Maybe	No

Table 6-5. Questionnaire: Provider Form

Child/Patient	History/Observations	0	1	2	Scoring/Comment
Child's life experiences	Trauma	No	At risk	Confirmed	**Total experience:** *For each of the 7 items, score 0, 1, or 2. Compute total.*
	Separations from parent	Never for long	>1 mo	Out-of-home placement	
	Parent stresses: (Specify.)	No	Mild	Serious	
	Parent with depression: Mother ____ Father ____ Other parenting figure ____	No	Suspected	Significant/confirmed	
	Parent with mental health concerns	No	Suspected	Significant/confirmed	
	If 2-parent household, involvement of both parents in child's care	Yes	Somewhat	No	
	Abuse or neglect	No	Suspected	Confirmed	
Child's health	Child's overall health status	OK	Significant problems in past	Ongoing problems	**Total health:** *For each of the 4 items, score 0, 1, or 2. Compute total.*
	Child's use of health care services	Up-to-date	Episodic	Usual care is urgent care/ED.	
	Medical vulnerability (eg, asthma)	No	Mild or intermittent	Severe or ongoing	
	Child with special health care needs	No	Yes, with medical home	Yes, but no medical home	

		On track	Some delays	Global delay	Total development: *For each of the 4 items, score 0, 1, or 2. Compute total.*
Child's development	Developmental status				
	Assessment	No	Checklist	Standardized measure	
	ASD or PDD	No	Possible	Yes	
	Developmental support or resources	Not needed	Receives services (eg, EI, MH, ECE)	Needs but does not receive services	
		0 Strengths/ no problem	**1** Child has symptoms or other concerns requiring time for advice.	**2** Active problem receiving treatment	Total social-emotional-behavioral: *For each of the 13 items, score 0, 1, or 2. Compute total.*
Social-emotional-behavioral	Communication or learning problem	No	Needs some extra support	Diagnosis of LD	
	Hyperactivity	No	Somewhat	ADHD diagnosis	
	Inattention	No	Somewhat	ADHD diagnosis	
	Impulsive or risky behaviors	No	Upper bounds of reference range	Active problem	
	Negativity or aggression	No	Somewhat	ODD, CD, or DBD	
	Anxiety	No	Appropriate to age or experience	Significant, with functional impairment	

Table 6-5. Questionnaire: Provider Form (continued)

Child/Patient	History/Observations	0	1	2	Scoring/Comment
	Mood: sad, depressed, labile, or manic	No	Appropriate to age or experience	Significant, with functional impairment	
	Shy or withdrawn	No	Occasional or in some situations	Limits age-appropriate experiences	
	Relationship difficulties	No	Occasional or in some situations	Limits age-appropriate experiences	
	Traumatic exposure	No	Yes, but no trauma-specific symptoms	Yes, with ongoing symptoms	
	Regulatory problems: sleep, eating, or self-care	No	Appropriate to age or experience	Significant, with functional impairment	
	Referral for mental health services	Not needed	Referred and receiving prescription	Needs, but not receiving prescription	
	Psychotropic medication	Not needed	Receives and is responding	Needs, but not receiving or not responding	
Family resources and support	Adequate social support network	Yes	Maybe	No	

Abbreviations: ADHD, attention-deficit/hyperactivity disorder; ASD, autism spectrum disorder; CD, conduct disorder; DBD, disruptive behavior disorder; ECE, early childhood education; ED, emergency department; EI, early intervention; LD, learning disability; MH, mental health; ODD, oppositional defiant disorder; PDD, pervasive developmental disorder.

AAP Policy

American Academy of Pediatrics Council on Children With Disabilities, Section on Developmental Behavioral Pediatrics, Bright Futures Steering Committee, and Medical Home Initiatives for Children With Special Needs Project Advisory Committee. Identifying infants and young children with developmental disorders in the medical home: an algorithm for developmental surveillance and screening. *Pediatrics.* 2006;118(1):405–420. Reaffirmed August 2014 (pediatrics.aappublications.org/content/118/1/405)

Chun TH, Mace SE, Katz ER; American Academy of Pediatrics Committee on Pediatrics Emergency Medicine, American College of Emergency Physicians Pediatric Emergency Medicine Committee. Evaluation and management of children and adolescents with acute mental health or behavioral problems. Part I: common clinical challenges of patients with mental health and/or behavioral emergencies. *Pediatrics.* 2016;138(3):e20161570 (pediatrics.aappublications.org/content/138/3/e20161570)

Chun TH, Mace SE, Katz ER; American Academy of Pediatrics Committee on Pediatrics Emergency Medicine, American College of Emergency Physicians Pediatric Emergency Medicine Committee. Evaluation and management of children with acute mental health or behavioral problems. Part II: recognition of clinically challenging mental health related conditions presenting with medical or uncertain symptoms. *Pediatrics.* 2016;138(3):e20161573 (pediatrics.aappublications.org/content/138/3/e20161573)

Garner AS, Shonkoff JP; American Academy of Pediatrics Committee on Psychosocial Aspects of Child and Family Health; Committee on Early Childhood, Adoption, and Dependent Care; and Section on Developmental Behavioral Pediatrics. Early childhood adversity, toxic stress, and the role of the pediatrician: translating developmental science into lifelong health. *Pediatrics.* 2012;129(1):e224–e231 (pediatrics.aappublications.org/content/129/1/e224)

Shonkoff JP, Garner AS; American Academy of Pediatrics Committee on Psychosocial Aspects of Child and Family Health; Committee on Early Childhood, Adoption, and Dependent Care; and Section on Developmental Behavioral Pediatrics. The lifelong effects of early childhood adversity and toxic stress. *Pediatrics.* 2012;129(1):e232–e246. Reaffirmed July 2016 (pediatrics.aappublications.org/content/129/1/e232)

Weitzman C, Wegner L; American Academy of Pediatrics Section on Developmental Behavioral Pediatrics, Committee on Psychosocial Aspects of Child and Family Health, and Council on Early Childhood; Society for Developmental Behavioral Pediatrics. Promoting optimal development: screening for behavioral and emotional problems. *Pediatrics.* 2015;135(2):384–395 (pediatrics.aappublications.org/content/135/2/384)

References

1. Tolan PH, Dodge KA. Children's mental health as a primary care and concern: a system for comprehensive support and service. *Am Psychol.* 2005;60(6):1–14
2. Williams J, Klinepeter K, Palmes G, Pulley A, Foy JM. Diagnosis and treatment of behavioral health disorders in pediatric practice. *Pediatrics.* 2004;114(3):601–606

3. Arseneault L, Bowes L, Shakoor S. Bullying victimization in youths and mental health problems: "much ado about nothing"? *Psychol Med.* 2010;40(5):717–729

4. Arseneault L, Milne BJ, Taylor A, et al. Being bullied as an environmentally mediated contributing factor to children's internalizing problems: a study of twins discordant for victimization. *Arch Pediatr Adolesc Med.* 2008;162(2):145–150

5. Hagan JF Jr, Shaw JS, Duncan PM, eds. *Bright Futures: Guidelines for Health Supervision of Infants, Children, and Adolescents.* 4th ed. Elk Grove Village, IL: American Academy of Pediatrics; 2017

6. Types of traumatic stress. National Child Traumatic Stress Network Web site. http://www.nctsn.org/trauma-types. Accessed January 16, 2018

7. Chang JJ, Theodore AD, Martin SL, Runyan DK. Psychological abuse between parents: associations with child maltreatment from a population-based sample. *Child Abuse Negl.* 2008;32(8):819–829

8. Bair-Merritt MH, Jennings JM, Chen R, et al. Reducing maternal intimate partner violence after the birth of a child: a randomized controlled trial of the Hawaii Healthy Start Home Visitation Program. *Arch Pediatr Adolesc Med.* 2010;164(1):16–23

9. Lannon CM, Flower K, Duncan P, Moore KS, Stuart J, Bassewitz J. The Bright Futures Training Intervention Project: implementing systems to support preventive and developmental services in practice. *Pediatrics.* 2008;122(1): e163–e171

10. American Academy of Pediatrics Committee on Psychosocial Aspects of Child and Family Health. Promoting the well-being of children whose parents are gay or lesbian. *Pediatrics.* 2013;131(4):827–830

11. Baumrind D. Rearing competent children. In: Damon W, ed. *Child Development Today and Tomorrow.* San Francisco, CA: Jossey-Bass Publishers; 1989:349–378

12. Camp BW, Cunningham M, Berman S. Relationship between the cognitive environment and vocabulary development during the second year of life. *Arch Pediatr Adolesc Med.* 2010;164(10):950–956

13. Johnson M, Stone S, Lou C, et al. Family assessment in child welfare services: instrument comparisons. *J Evid Based Soc Work.* 2008;5(1–2):57–90

14. Kemper KJ, Kelleher KJ. Family psychosocial screening: instruments and techniques. *Ambul Child Health.* 1996;1(4):325–339

15. Wade TD, Kendler KS. Parent, child, and social correlates of parental discipline style: a retrospective, multi-informant investigation with female twins. *Soc Psychiatry Psychiatr Epidemiol.* 2001;36(4):177–185

16. Kendler KS, Sham PC, MacLean CJ. The determinants of parenting: an epidemiological, multi-informant, retrospective study. *Psychol Med.* 1997;27(3):549–563

17. Berlin LJ, Ispa JM, Fine MA, et al. Correlates and consequences of spanking and verbal punishment for low-income white, African American, and Mexican American toddlers. *Child Dev.* 2009;80(5):1403–1420

18. NCS-R twelve-month prevalence estimates. National Comorbidity Survey Web site. https://www.hcp.med.harvard.edu/ncs/index.php. Accessed January 16, 2018

19. Nicholson J, Biebel K, Katz-Levy J, Williams VF. The prevalence of parenthood in adults with mental illness: implications for state and federal policymakers, programs and providers. In: Manderscheid R, Henderson M, eds. *Mental Health,*

United States, 2002. Rockville, MD: Substance Abuse and Mental Health Services Administration; 2004

20. Hammen C. Risk and protective factors for children of depressed parents. In: Luthar SS, ed. *Resilience and Vulnerability: Adaptation in the Context of Childhood Adversities.* New York, NY: Cambridge University Press; 2003

21. Kaplan LA, Evans L, Monk C. Effects of mothers' prenatal psychiatric status and postnatal caregiving on infant biobehavioral regulation: can prenatal programming be modified? *Early Hum Dev.* 2008;84(4):249–256

22. Riley AW, Coiro MJ, Broitman M, et al. Mental health of children of low-income depressed mothers: influences of parenting, family environment, and raters. *Psychiatr Serv.* 2009;60(3):329–336

23. Garber J, Cole DA. Intergenerational transmission of depression: a launch and grow model of change across adolescence. *Dev Psychopathol.* 2010;22(4):819–830

24. Schonwald A, Huntington N, Chan E, Risko W, Bridgemohan C. Routine developmental screening implemented in urban primary care settings: more evidence of feasibility and effectiveness. *Pediatrics.* 2009;123(2):660–668

25. Smith DK, Johnson AB, Pears KC, Fisher PA, Degarmo DS. Child maltreatment and foster care: unpacking the effects of prenatal and postnatal parental substance use. *Child Maltreat.* 2007;12(12):150–160

26. DeWolf M. 12 stats about working women. US Department of Labor Blog Web site. Published March 1, 2017. https://blog.dol.gov/2017/03/01/12-stats-about-working-women. Accessed January 16, 2018

27. Magnuson KA, Waldfogel J. Early childhood care and education: effects on ethnic and racial gaps in school readiness. *Future Child.* 2005;15(1):169–196

28. NICHD Study of Early Child Care and Youth Development (SECCYD) sunsetted/ for reference only. Eunice Kennedy Shriver National Institute of Child Health and Human Development Web site. https://www.nichd.nih.gov/research/supported/Pages/seccyd.aspx. Accessed January 16, 2018

29. National Institute of Child and Health and Human Development. *The NICHD Study of Early Child Care and Youth Development. Findings for Children Up to Age 4½ Years.* Rockville, MD: National Institute of Child Health and Human Development; 2006. NIH publication 05-4318. https://www.nichd.nih.gov/publications/pubs/documents/seccyd_06.pdf. Accessed January 16, 2018

30. Gilliam WS. *Prekindergarteners Left Behind: Expulsion Rates in State Prekindergarten Systems.* New York, NY: Foundation for Child Development; 2005. https://www.fcd-us.org/prekindergartners-left-behind-expulsion-rates-in-state-prekindergarten-programs. Accessed January 16, 2018

31. Szilagyi M. The pediatrician and the child in foster care. *Pediatr Rev.* 1998;19(2):39–50

32. Statistics on child abuse and neglect fatalities. Child Welfare Information Gateway Web site. https://www.childwelfare.gov/topics/systemwide/statistics/can/stat-fatalities. Accessed January 16, 2018

33. Dozier M, Lindheim O, Akerman JP. Attachment and biobehavioral catch-up: an intervention targeting empirically identified needs of foster infants. In: Berlin LJ, Ziv Y, Amaya-Jackson L, Greenberg MT, eds. *Enhancing Early Attachments: Theory, Research, Intervention, and Policy.* New York, NY: Guilford Press; 2005:178–194

34. Fisher PA, Chamberlain P. Multidimensional treatment foster care: a program for intensive parenting, family support, and skill building. *J Emot Behav Disord.* 2000;8(3):155–164

35. Underwood LA, Washington A. Mental illness and juvenile offenders. *Int J Environ Res Public Health.* 2016;13(2):228

36. *Poverty and Hunger Fact Sheet.* Chicago, IL: Feeding America; 2017. http://www.feedingamerica.org/hunger-in-america/hunger-facts/hunger-and-poverty-statistics.aspx. Accessed January 16, 2018

37. Sell K, Zlotnik S, Noonan K, Rubin D. *The Recession and Child Health.* Philadelphia, PA: Foundation for Child Development; 2010

38. Howe GW, Levy ML, Caplan RD. Job loss and depressive symptoms in couples: common stressors, stress transmission, or relationship disruption? *J Fam Psychol.* 2004;18(4):639–650

39. Zimmerman FJ, Christakis DA, Meltzoff AN. Associations between media viewing and language development in children under age 2 years. *J Pediatr.* 2007;151(4):364–368

40. Swing EL, Gentile DA, Anderson CA, Walsh DA. Television and video game exposure and the development of attention problems. *Pediatrics.* 2010;126(2):214–221

41. Pagani LS, Fitzpatrick C, Barnett TA, Dubow E. Prospective associations between early childhood television exposure and academic, psychosocial, and physical well-being by middle childhood. *Arch Pediatr Adolesc Med.* 2010;164(5):425–431

42. Finkelhor D, Mitchell KJ, Wolak J. *Online Victimization: A Report on the Nation's Youth.* Durham, NH: Crimes Against Children Research Center; 2000

43. Mishna F, Cook C, Gadalla T, Daciuk J, Solomon S. Cyber bullying behaviors among middle and high school students. *Am J Orthopsychiatry.* 2010;80(3):362–374

44. Sogomonyan F, Cooper JL. *Trauma Faced by Children of Military Families: What Every Policymaker Should Know.* New York, NY: National Center for Children in Poverty; 2010

45. Chandra A, Lurie N. Falling short: continued challenges in meeting the mental health needs of children with special health care needs. *Health Serv Res.* 2008;43(3):803–809

46. Ghandour RM, Perry DF, Kogan MD, Strickland BB. The medical home as a mediator of the relation between mental health symptoms and family burden among children with special health care needs. *Acad Pediatr.* 2011;11(2):161–169

47. Ring A, Dowrick CF, Humphris GM, Davies J, Salmon P. The somatising effect of clinical consultation: what patients and doctors say and do not say when patients present medically unexplained physical symptoms. *Soc Sci Med.* 2005;61(7):1505–1515

48. Lempp T, de Lange D, Radeloff D, Bachmann C. The clinical examination of children, adolescents and their families. In: Rey JM, ed. *IACAPAP Textbook of Child and Adolescent Mental Health.* Geneva, Switzerland: International Association for Child and Adolescent Psychiatry and Allied Professions; 2015. http://iacapap.org/iacapap-textbook-of-child-and-adolescent-mental-health. Accessed January 16, 2018

49. Habis A, Tall L, Smith J, Guenther E. Pediatric emergency medicine physicians' current practice and beliefs regarding mental health screening. *Pediatr Emerg Care.* 2007;23(6):387–393

50. Facts for Families Guide. American Academy of Child and Adolescent Psychiatry Web site. http://www.aacap.org/aacap/families_and_youth/facts_for_families/FFF-Guide/FFF-Guide-Home.aspx. Accessed January 16, 2018

51. Weitzman C, Wegner L. American Academy of Pediatrics Section on Developmental and Behavioral Pediatrics, Committee on Psychosocial Aspects of Child and Family Health, and Council on Early Childhood; Society for Developmental and Behavioral Pediatrics. Promoting optimal development: screening for behavioral and emotional problems. *Pediatrics.* 2015;135(2)384–395

52. American Psychiatric Association. *Diagnostic and Statistical Manual of Mental Disorders.* 5th ed. Arlington, VA: American Psychiatric Association; 2013:31–87

53. American Academy of Pediatrics Council on Children With Disabilities, Section on Developmental Behavioral Pediatrics, Bright Futures Steering Committee, and Medical Home Initiatives for Children With Special Needs Project Advisory Committee. Identifying infants and young children with developmental disorders in the medical home: an algorithm for developmental surveillance and screening. *Pediatrics.* 2006;118(1):405–420

54. Denham SA. Emotional competence in preschoolers: implications for social functioning. In: Luby JL, ed. *Handbook of Preschool Mental Health: Development, Disorders, and Treatment.* New York, NY: Guilford Press; 2006:23–44

55. American Psychiatric Association. *Diagnostic and Statistical Manual of Mental Disorders.* 4th rev ed. Arlington, VA: American Psychiatric Association; 2000

56. Adult Attachment Scale (AAS). Statistic Solutions Web site. http://www.statisticssolutions.com/adult-attachment-scale-aas. Accessed January 16, 2018

57. O'Connor TG, Zeanah CH. Attachment disorders: assessment strategies and treatment approaches. *Attach Hum Dev.* 2003;5(3):223–244

58. Any mood disorder in children. National Institute of Mental Health Web site. https://www.nimh.nih.gov/health/statistics/prevalence/any-mood-disorder-in-children.shtml. Accessed January 16, 2018

59. Luby JL, Belden AC. Mood disorders: phenomenology and a developmental emotion reactivity model. In: Luby JL, ed. *Handbook of Preschool Mental Health: Development, Disorders, and Treatment.* New York, NY: Guilford Press; 2006: 209–230

60. Sameroff AJ. Developmental systems: contexts and evolution. In: Kessen W, ed. *Handbook of Child Psychology.* 4th ed. New York, NY: John Wiley & Sons; 1983:238–294. *History, Theories, and Methods;* vol 1

61. Sameroff AJ, Fiese BH. Models of development and developmental risk. In: Zeanah CH Jr, ed. *Handbook of Infant Mental Health.* 2nd ed. New York, NY: Guilford Press; 2000:3–20

62. Eating disorders. National Institute of Mental Health Web site. https://www.nimh.nih.gov/health/topics/eating-disorders/index.shtml. Accessed January 16, 2018

63. Morgan JF, Reid F, Lacey JH. The SCOFF questionnaire: a new screening tool for eating disorders. *West J Med.* 2000;172(3):164–165

64. Gender non-conforming and transgender children. HealthyChildren.org Web site. https://www.healthychildren.org/English/ages-stages/gradeschool/Pages/Gender-Non-Conforming-Transgender-Children.aspx. Updated June 4, 2015. Accessed January 16, 2018

65. Wissow L, Anthony B, Brown J, et al. A common factors approach to improving the mental health capacity of pediatric primary care. *Adm Policy Ment Health.* 2008;35(4):305–318

66. Knapp P, Jensen PJ. Recommendations for *DSM-V.* In: Jensen PJ, Knapp P, Mrazek DA, eds. *Toward a New Diagnostic System for Child Psychopathology: Moving Beyond the* DSM. New York, NY: Guilford Press; 2006:162–182

67. Angold A, Costello J, Erkanli A. Comorbidity. *J Child Psychol Psychiatry.* 1999; 40(1):57–87

68. Knapp PK, Mastergeorge AM. Clinical implications of current findings in neurodevelopment. *Psychiatr Clin North Am.* 2009;32(1):177–197

69. Acosta MT, Castellanos FX, Bolton KL, et al. Latent class subtyping of attention-deficit/hyperactivity disorder and comorbid conditions. *J Am Acad Child Adolesc Psychiatry.* 2008;47(7):797–780

70. Heim C, Nemeroff CB. The role of childhood trauma in the neurobiology of mood and anxiety disorders: preclinical and clinical studies. *Biol Psychiatry.* 2001;49(12):1023–1039

71. Perry DB, Pollard RA, Blakley TL, Maker WL, Vigilante D. Childhood trauma: the neurobiology of adaptation and "use-dependent" development of the brain: how "states" become "traits." *Infant Ment Health J.* 1995;16(4):271–291

CHAPTER 7

Psychosocial Therapies

W. Douglas Tynan, PhD, and Meghan McAuliffe Lines, PhD

"Properly carried out, effective psychosocial therapies have excellent long-term benefits that extend years beyond the termination of therapy and can positively influence a child's overall developmental course."

This chapter first provides an overview of the evidence-based nonpharmacological treatments available for the common mental disorders of childhood. In the parlance of the mental health community, they may be called *psychotherapy* or simply *therapy;* in this chapter they will be called *psychosocial therapies.* These treatments may be delivered by a variety of mental health professionals (eg, licensed clinical psychologists, social workers, professional counselors, marriage and family therapists, child psychiatrists) trained in the specific techniques of that therapy. Interactive Web-based programs show promise as additional or alternative sources of these therapies.

Second, the chapter draws from these evidence-based psychosocial therapies common elements that are effective across a number of disorders and potentially applicable to the treatment of children and adolescents (collectively referred to as *children* in this chapter unless otherwise specified) with emerging or undifferentiated symptoms, as they might present in the primary care setting. Practical resources are offered to support pediatric clinicians in applying these common elements to the care of these children, to children referred for and awaiting care in the mental health specialty system, and to children for whom the appropriate mental health specialty resources are inaccessible.

Separate chapters in this book describe other nonpharmacological mental health interventions: Chapter 8, Self-regulation Therapies and Biofeedback, and Chapter 9, Complementary and Integrative Medical Therapies.

History

The origin of modern psychosocial therapies for children and adolescents (collectively called *children* in this chapter unless otherwise specified) is usually attributed to the pioneering work of Sigmund Freud at the turn of the 20th century. Freud's ideas about the importance of early childhood experiences and his publication of case studies with both adults and children framed the field, and the influence of his psychoanalytic and psychodynamic concepts is still evident. Behavioral therapy concepts arose early in the 20th century in Mary Cover Jones and J.B. Watson's work on conditioning and learning. They based this work on Pavlovian conditioning models of learned fears and maladaptive emotional responses. Both psychodynamic theory approaches and learning theory approaches focused on early traumatic experiences as causal to later behavioral problems. In the mid-20th century, work arose on behavioral interventions, based both on early Pavlovian theories of learned emotional responses and on B.F. Skinner's writings on positive operant conditioning and voluntary responses to improve behaviors. This launched a variety of behavioral approaches, ranging from using early reward systems to providing parents and teachers with strategies for positively oriented behavior modification.[1] During the same era, various play therapies, dramatic therapies, and relationship therapies emerged as additional strategies to help ameliorate children's emotional and behavioral problems.

Current approaches to etiologic theory are more complex. It is generally accepted that variations in behavior may have origins in temperamental differences, early patterns of attachment, parent-child interaction difficulties, and social factors, along with early traumatic experience.[2] As more was learned about multiple etiologic factors of childhood disorders, multiple therapy approaches were developed to address those factors. By the start of the 21st century, Alan Kazdin[3] identified 551 differently named psychosocial therapy approaches that are used with children. This is a vast number that does not even include eclectic approaches to treatment, in which elements of several therapies are combined—the approach most commonly used by clinicians.

Clearly, the practice of psychosocial therapies grew much more quickly than did research into their effectiveness. However, in the past decade, research has emphasized documenting the critical elements of therapeutic approaches in treatment manuals and then testing these treatment modalities in representative patients. This research of manualized therapy using written reminders of specific approaches has revealed common elements of effective therapy. More important, these therapies specify what behavior changes need to occur for true treatment progress to be achieved. The American Academy of Pediatrics (AAP) Task Force on Mental Health used the common elements of effective treatment as the basis for the guidance it provided to primary care clinicians (ie, pediatricians, family physicians, internists, nurse practitioners, and physician assistants at the front lines of pediatrics) for the initial management of mental health problems.[4] This guidance has now been incorporated into several chapters in this book (Chapters 14, 15, 17, 20, 22, and 31). Within the mental health professions, the concept of combining components of evidence-based therapies that have been proven effective in treating specific disorders, to address the needs of individual patients, has been advanced as a modular approach. Thus, for a child demonstrating both anxiety and oppositional behavior, elements of evidence-based cognitive behavioral therapy (CBT), to manage the anxiety, and parent training, to address the oppositional behavior, would be implemented. Chorpita and Daleiden[5] have developed a model that includes training and treatment monitoring using this modular approach.

Internalizing and Externalizing Behavioral Disorders in Children

Because all psychosocial disorders are not the same, it is critically important to identify the key symptoms for which children typically present for treatment, in order to systematically research effective therapeutic strategies. The most commonly diagnosed emotional and behavioral disorders of childhood can be largely divided into 2 broad categories: externalizing behavioral disorders and internalizing behavioral disorders.[6] *Externalizing behavioral disorders* refers to the group of disorders that are manifested in children's display of negative outward behavior, including aggression, oppositional behavior, defiance, delinquency, and hyperactivity. Children with externalizing disorders are frequently nonadherent, have difficulty following rules, are restless, and are overly active. The most common referrals for psychosocial therapies, making up 50% to 75% of all children referred,[7] are for disruptive behavioral problems. The diagnoses that typically fall into this category are attention-deficit/hyperactivity disorder (ADHD), oppositional defiant disorder (ODD), conduct disorder, bipolar disorders, and other specified disruptive, impulse-control, and conduct disorders.

In contrast, *internalizing behavioral disorders* in children represent the group of emotional disorders of which the symptoms primarily affect a child's internal psychological environment. Rather than acting out, children with internalizing disorders often display anxious, depressed, withdrawn, or inhibited behavior. Anxiety disorders are among the most common forms of psychopathology in children and adolescents.[1,8] Specific internalizing disorders that may emerge in childhood include anxiety disorders (eg, separation anxiety disorder, generalized anxiety disorder, specific phobia, obsessive-compulsive disorder, selective mutism, other specified anxiety disorders) and depressive disorders (eg, major depressive disorder, disruptive mood dysregulation disorder, persistent depressive disorder, other specified depressive disorders).

Although the distinction between the categories of internalizing and externalizing disorders is important for case conceptualization, treatment decisions, and research, these disorders are not necessarily mutually exclusive. In fact, there is often significant comorbidity between externalizing and internalizing disorders in children.[9] However, research on evidence-based treatments for childhood disorders has demonstrated that the most effective types of treatment differ according to the type of problem. A helpful summary is the table "Evidence-Based Child and Adolescent Psychosocial Interventions," originally developed by the Hawaii Department of Health. A snapshot is included as Appendix 6 of this book, updated twice yearly by PracticeWise, LLC, and posted by the AAP at www.aap.org/en-us/Documents/CRPsychosocialInterventions. pdf. This resource demonstrates the psychosocial interventions that are most and least helpful for the various categories of child emotional and behavioral difficulties according to a summary of the research in the field. In the case of children who seem to be exhibiting symptoms of both internalizing difficulties and externalizing difficulties, a best practice recommendation is to treat the primary symptoms first (ie, symptoms that are causing the most significant impairment).

Psychosocial Therapy of Externalizing Disorders in Children

Parent Management Training

An evidence-based treatment for a school-aged child diagnosed as having both ADHD and ODD may include guidance for parents on behavior management and medication, in order to address the impulsivity and lack of focus.

Of the therapies used, parent management training (PMT), a therapeutic technique centered around teaching parents to modify their child's behavior using evidence-based strategies, has been proven effective for disruptive behavior in a variety of settings and methods of implementation. *Parent management training*[7] is a term that encompasses a number of evidence-based programs. All PMT programs that have been proven effective include all 6 of the following components:

▶ **Increasing positive interaction between parent and child using special playtime strategies.** This approach is found in all evidence-based PMT programs and is also common to many other therapies designed to encourage positive parent-child interaction, including Greenspan's Developmental, Individual Differences, and Relationship-based Floortime model[10] and Brazelton's Touchpoints.[11] For parents who are frustrated with constant arguments and battles with their children, establishing a positive relationship is an essential first step.

▶ **Teaching parents how to record and monitor behavior accurately.** Change comes with learning, which can be enhanced and accelerated by teaching parents reinforcement and reward skills, but it still requires some time to change patterns of behavior. Parents often respond emotionally in the heat of the moment. It is only when they document and track gradual change that they can maintain their own efforts to bring about change.

▶ **The use of reinforcement and rewards to increase the rate of desirable behaviors.** Although parents often present with their list of problem behaviors, they usually have lost sight of what they want their children to do instead. Identifying the desired positive behaviors and using social rewards such as praise, hugs, and more time with parents helps reinforce positive behaviors quickly and can change the overall tone of the parent-child relationship.

▶ **Teaching parents how to give directions and commands that are effective.** One of the difficulties noted in observational studies of parents and children in conflict is the difficulty some parents have recognizing what children can comprehend and simply giving clear, direct, understandable commands. This component, although brief in most programs, is essential.

▶ **Coaching and training in the use of mild, nonphysical punishments such as time-out to reduce undesirable behaviors.** Research shows that parents use physical punishment inconsistently and that their use of time-out, loss of privileges, or contingent work chores is more effective and less emotionally damaging to the parent-child relationship. This component is also aligned with current AAP[12] policy on disciplining children.

▶ **All the skills are taught within a context of typical child development for age.** Parents often overestimate their child's abilities, skills, and motivation and require psychoeducation on typical child development. Thus, effective PMT programs either include specific information about developmental skills or are designed for specific age ranges. Although various effective programs may place a different emphasis on specific skills, all effective programs implement the complete set of all 6 elements in discussion, role-playing, and the use of video or active coaching to teach parents new behavior patterns. Programs use a variety of strategies, including intensive individual coaching (eg, Parent-Child Interaction Therapy, Helping the Noncompliant Child), group format with video (eg, Incredible Years), and variations of group and individual family formats (eg, PMT – Oregon Model, Triple P – Positive Parenting Program), as well as these strategies in combination with other therapeutic interventions (problem-solving skills + PMT).[7,13–17]

Psychosocial Therapy of Internalizing Disorders in Children

Cognitive Behavioral Therapy

Internalizing disorders in children, encompassing the anxiety and depressive disorders, comprise the second core group of psychosocial difficulties that often lead to referrals for mental health treatment. Across diagnostic categories, CBT has consistently received the best support for reducing internalizing symptoms in children.[18] Although the primary approach for addressing externalizing behavior in children is to provide parents with skills to shape the child's behavior through modifying the environment, research has demonstrated that, for internalizing symptoms, it is critical to address the child's thoughts, feelings, and behaviors directly.

The specific treatment strategies vary by treatment program, but a number of common components are present across CBT programs. According to Kendall,[19,20] the primary components of all CBT programs are strategies designed to address changes in thinking, feeling, and behavior, as well as an enactive component. Cognitive behavioral therapy programs for children with internalizing difficulties typically address

▶ **Cognitions.** Children with anxiety and depression often have faulty cognitions, including distorted thinking about themselves and the world around them and negative, automatic thoughts that cause them to feel fearful or distressed. One aspect of CBT is to help children learn to identify these cognitions and cope with or even change them.

▶ **Feelings.** Another important aspect of CBT is to help children learn affective recognition and coping strategies for unpleasant emotions.

▶ **Behavior.** Behavioral strategies typically used in CBT include coping skills to help children manage some of their distressing emotional experiences. Behavioral strategies might include relaxation techniques, scheduling of pleasurable activities, and problem-solving strategies.

▶ **Practice.** A key element of CBT is opportunities to practice new strategies and evaluate them. Although internalizing disorders are, by definition, manifested in symptoms that are within the child, it is important to consider the social context and provide opportunities for social practice with new strategies. Research has demonstrated that these components can be effectively delivered in individual or group settings.[18,19]

An example of a well-supported CBT program for anxiety in children is the Coping Cat program.[19] In Coping Cat, children learn to recognize the physiologic and cognitive symptoms of anxiety, learn cognitive and behavioral strategies for coping with the anxiety, and practice the skills taught.

Cognitive behavioral therapy programs have been developed for the treatment of depression in children and adolescents as well.[21] One example includes the Taking Action program, through which children learn to identify emotions, learn coping skills for unpleasant emotions, learn problem-solving strategies, and learn to restructure negative cognitions.[22] This treatment is performed in a group setting, providing opportunities to practice.

For CBT to be an effective treatment strategy, the child must have the cognitive capacity to engage in the treatment. Studies indicate that school-aged children (typically developing children aged ≥7 years) are able to benefit, provided that they have adequate language skills. The therapy requires being able to label emotions, use language to develop an action plan, and use language to evaluate success.

Psychosocial Therapy of Post-traumatic Conditions

Post-traumatic emotional responses are now better recognized as underlying a number of symptoms of both internalizing disorders and externalizing disorders. Fortunately, the National Child Traumatic Stress Network (NCTSN) has developed a directory of appropriate screening and assessment measures and has documented psychosocial interventions (http://nctsnet.org). Of the many effective therapies cited on the NCTSN Web site, trauma-focused CBT has the longest history of clinical research to support its use.[23]

Common Elements of Evidence-Based Psychosocial Therapies

A criticism of evidenced-based approaches is that they have been developed in randomized controlled trials (RCTs) for single disorders and often come with a lengthy, detailed manual that leads the therapist and patient through a stepwise series of goals in a specific course of treatment, often for a fixed number of sessions. Clinical practice, however, is marked by comorbidity of more than one diagnosis and requires some flexibility in implementation to match the needs of the family. In practice, often the approach is to have the family successfully complete one goal before moving on to the next, and the goal is often determined by immediate need. Thus, a therapist working from an evidence-based perspective needs the elements of each approach available in a modular format that can be presented in the order needed by the patient.[24,25] The common elements approach is best captured in the PracticeWise[26] program, which incorporates evidence-based approaches to treating anxiety, depression, trauma, and conduct problems in a single set of treatment modules. Included in this program are descriptions of the disorders and detailed guidelines for therapists to guide sessions, as well as handouts for patients and their parents on identifying emotions, problem-solving and cognitive strategies for managing depression and anxiety, and the common elements of PMT (described previously). This program is a comprehensive approach to using modules shown to be effective so that a therapist can construct a treatment approach individualized for each child's particular set of symptoms.[27]

Chapter 10, Adapting Psychosocial Interventions to Primary Care, discusses the adaptation of this common elements approach to primary care settings, in which it can be used to address clinical and subclinical presentations of internalizing and externalizing disorders, as well as the effects of trauma.

Treatments Lacking a Research Evidence Base

One of the hallmarks of the therapies cited as evidence-based is manualized therapies. This kind of systematic approach, which lends itself to standardization across patients, is more easily studied in an RCT than are more individualized treatments such as play therapy, various creative arts therapies, and individualized psychosocial therapies. These latter kinds of approaches lend themselves to analysis on a case-by-case, N-of-1, or anecdotal basis. In some circumstances, the RCT is not an appropriate research method, and highly individualized therapy (eg, treatment individualized to a patient rather than following a manual) is among those circumstances. As a result, a number of therapies show promise with some patients but have no specific evidence regarding their effectiveness. In some situations, therapy can result in harm or worsening of the condition.[28] As with any other type of treatment, there can be iatrogenic effects.

Along with providing information about the treatment methods with the greatest support, recent outcomes research has a second benefit: to provide guidance about which forms of treatment do not work well, or may even potentially cause harm. Across disorders, at this time, there is little to no research support for the use of play therapy or psychodynamic therapy with children, and there is no support for eye movement desensitization and reprocessing.

Mode of treatment delivery can also influence outcomes. Cognitive behavioral therapy and some other treatment modalities addressing anxiety and depression are effective in a group setting. However, research has demonstrated that for children with disruptive behavior disorders, including ODD, some types of group therapy are potentially harmful. A review and study showed that unstructured groups for adolescents with conduct disorder tended to increase deviant and oppositional behavior.[29] For children with disruptive behavior, more structured groups that have specific goals for self-control strategies can result in positive therapeutic effects.[30]

Primary care clinicians can help promote the optimal health and well-being of their patients by providing research-informed guidance to parents when selecting mental health professionals and by developing a list of established professionals who practice evidence-based approaches to treatment of child psychosocial problems.[4]

In general, although one-to-one, individual unstructured psychosocial therapies or counseling with children is the preferred modality of treatment by many mental health specialists, review of research does not support this form of treatment; statistically, there is no improvement when compared with receiving no treatment.[31] Active structured therapies, with clear goals and procedures that involve working with parents (and other involved adults), are most effective in shaping behavior.[7] For children aged 7 years and older who have typical cognitive and language skills, teaching coping skills and strategies with targeted goals is also effective.[19] Indeed, these approaches have a more extensive body of supportive research than other treatments do, including many medication treatments. Properly carried out, effective psychosocial therapies have excellent long-term benefits that extend years[14,27] beyond the termination of therapy and can positively influence a child's overall developmental course.

References

1. Lazarus AA. *Behavior Therapy and Beyond.* New York, NY: McGraw-Hill; 1971
2. Mash EJ, Barkley RA, eds. *Child Psychopathology.* 3rd ed. New York, NY: Guilford Press; 2014
3. Kazdin AE. The state of child and adolescent psychotherapy research. *Child Adolesc Ment Health.* 2002;7(2):53–59
4. American Academy of Pediatrics Task Force on Mental Health. *Addressing Mental Health Concerns in Primary Care: A Clinician's Toolkit.* Elk Grove Village, IL: American Academy of Pediatrics; 2010
5. Chorpita BF, Daleiden EL. Building evidence-based systems in children's mental health. In: Weisz JR, Kazdin AE, eds. *Evidence-Based Psychotherapies for Children and Adolescents.* 2nd ed. New York, NY: Guilford Press; 2010:482–499
6. Rescorla L, Achenbach T, Ivanova MY, et al. Behavioral and emotional problems reported by parents of children ages 6 to 16 in 31 societies. *J Emot Behav Disord.* 2007;15(3):130–142
7. Kazdin AE. *Parent Management Training: Treatment for Oppositional, Aggressive and Antisocial Behavior in Children and Adolescents.* New York, NY: Oxford University Press Inc; 2005
8. Kendall PC, Aschenbrand SG, Hudson JL. Child-focused treatment of anxiety. In: Kazdin AE, Weisz JR, eds. *Evidence-Based Psychotherapies for Children and Adolescents.* New York, NY: Guilford Press; 2003:81–100
9. Lilienfeld SO. Comorbidity between and within childhood externalizing and internalizing disorders: reflections and directions. *J Abnorm Child Psychol.* 2003;31(3):285–291
10. Greenspan SI. *Great Kids: Helping Your Baby and Child Develop the Ten Essential Qualities for a Healthy, Happy Life.* Philadelphia, PA: Da Capo Press, Perseus Books Group; 2007
11. Brazelton TB. *Touchpoints: Birth to Three.* 2nd ed. Philadelphia, PA: Da Capo Press, Perseus Books Group; 2006
12. American Academy of Pediatrics. Committee on Psychosocial Aspects of Child and Family Health. Guidance for effective discipline. *Pediatrics.* 1998;101(4, pt 1):723–728
13. Pelham WE Jr, Fabiano GA. Evidence-based psychosocial treatments for attention-deficit/hyperactivity disorder. *J Clin Child Adolesc Psychol.* 2008;37(1):184–214
14. Eyberg SM, Nelson MM, Boggs SR. Evidence-based psychosocial treatments for children and adolescents with disruptive behavior. *J Clin Child Adolesc Psychol.* 2008;37(1):215–237
15. Thomas R, Zimmer-Gembeck MJ. Behavioral outcomes of Parent-Child Interaction Therapy and Triple P—Positive Parenting Program: a review and meta-analysis. *J Abnorm Child Psychol.* 2007;35(3):475–495
16. Menting AT, Orobio de Castro B, Matthys W. Effectiveness of the Incredible Years parent training to modify disruptive and prosocial child behavior: a meta-analytic review. *Clin Psychol Rev.* 2013;33(8):901–913
17. Higa-McMillan CK, Francis SE, Rith-Najarian L, Chorpita BF. Evidence base update: 50 years of research on treatment for child and adolescent anxiety. *J Clin Child Adolesc Psychol.* 2016;45(2):91–113

18. Silverman WK, Pina AA, Viswesvaran C. Evidence-based psychosocial treatments for phobic and anxiety disorders in children and adolescents. *J Clin Child Adolesc Psychol.* 2008;37(1):105–130

19. Kendall PC. *Cognitive-Behavioral Therapy for Anxious Children: Therapist Manual.* 2nd ed. Ardmore, PA: Workbook Publishing; 2000

20. Kendall PC. Guiding theory for therapy with children and adolescents. In: Kendall PC, ed. *Child and Adolescent Therapy: Cognitive Behavioral Procedures.* 3rd ed. New York, NY: Guilford Press; 2006:3–32

21. David-Ferdon C, Kaslow NJ. Evidence-based psychosocial treatments for child and adolescent depression. *J Clin Child Adolesc Psychol.* 2008;37(1):62–104

22. Stark KD, Schnoebelen S, Simpson J, Hargrave J, Molnar J, Glenn R. *Treating Depressed Children: Therapist Manual for ACTION.* Ardmore, PA: Workbook Publishing Inc; 2005

23. Cohen JA, Mannarino AP, Deblinger E. *Treating Trauma and Traumatic Grief in Children and Adolescents.* New York, NY: Guilford Press; 2006

24. Barth RP, Lee BR, Lindsey MA, et al. Evidence-based practice at a crossroads: the timely emergence of common elements and common factors. *Res Soc Work Pract.* 2012;22(1):108–119

25. Weisz JR, Gray JS. Evidence-based psychotherapy for children and adolescents: data from the present and a model for the future. *Child Adolesc Ment Health.* 2008;13(2):54–56

26. Chorpita BJ, Weisz JR. Modular approach to therapy for children with anxiety, depression, trauma, or conduct problems. PracticeWise Web site. http://www.practicewise.com/portals/0/MATCH_public/index.html. Accessed February 7, 2018

27. Chorpita BF, Weisz JR, Daleiden EL, et al; Research Network on Youth Mental Health. Long-term outcomes for the Child STEPs randomized effectiveness trial: a comparison of modular and standard treatment designs with usual care. *J Consult Clin Psychol.* 2013;81(6):999–1009

28. Lilienfeld SO. Psychological treatments that cause harm. *Perspect Psychol Sci.* 2007;2(1):53–70

29. Dishion TJ, McCord J, Poulin F. When interventions harm. Peer groups and problem behaviors. *Am Psychol.* 1999;54(9):755–764

30. Nelson WM, Finch AJ, Ghee AC. Anger management in child and adolescent cognitive behavior therapy. In: Kendall PC, ed. *Child and Adolescent Therapy: Cognitive Behavioral Procedures.* 3rd ed. New York, NY: Guilford Press; 2006

31. Weisz JR, Weiss B, Donenberg GR. The lab vs the clinic: effects of child and adolescent psychotherapy. *Am Psychol.* 1992;47(12):1578–1585

CHAPTER 8

Self-regulation Therapies and Biofeedback

Denise Bothe, MD, and Karen N. Olness, MD

"The mind-body skills learned with hypnosis can give a child the capacity to change attitudes, emotions, behavior, habits, autonomic reactivity, and biological functions."

Children and adolescents learn self-regulation therapies easily. They can apply them to managing everyday life stressors and to solving problems such as acute and chronic pain, undesirable habits, anxiety associated with chronic illnesses such as hemophilia or cancer, performance anxiety, and enuresis. Many self-regulation techniques involve hypnosis (Box 8-1). Training in hypnosis has been used for many years by athletes and other performers and by pediatricians since 1976. Child and adolescent self-hypnosis is applicable to a wide range of clinical conditions (Box 8-2), discussed in greater detail in the Clinical Applications section of this chapter. The teaching and application of self-hypnosis is enhanced by the

---

Box 8-1. Terms Used to Describe Self-regulation Techniques Involving Hypnosis

- Self-hypnosis
- Mind-body skills training
- Self-regulation
- Biofeedback
- Relaxation
- Progressive relaxation
- Meditation
- Visual imagery
- Guided imagery
- Cyberphysiology
- Mindfulness

Box 8-2. Clinical Applications of Child Hypnosis

- Pain
  - Acute (eg, injury, illness, procedural)
  - Chronic or recurrent (eg, chronic illness, disability, trauma, recurrent procedures)

- Habit problems and disorders (eg, thumb-sucking, nail-biting, hairpulling [trichotillomania], habitual coughs, tics)

- Behavioral problems (eg, attention problems, anger management)

- Medical-biobehavioral disorders (eg, asthma, migraine, Tourette syndrome, inflammatory bowel disease, warts, pruritus)

- Anxiety (eg, performance anxiety [eg, examinations, stage fright, sports], anxiety disorders, PTSD, phobias)

- Psychophysiological problems (eg, enuresis, encopresis, conditioned nausea and vomiting, IBS, sleep disorders)

- Chronic disease, multisystem disease, terminal illness (eg, cancer, hemophilia, AIDS, cystic fibrosis, diabetes, chronic renal disease)

Abbreviations: IBS, irritable bowel syndrome; PTSD, post-traumatic stress disorder.

Derived from Kohen DP, Olness KN. Self-regulation therapy: helping children help themselves. *Ambul Child Health.* 1996;2(1):43–58; and Sugarman LI, Wester WC II, eds. *Therapeutic Hypnosis With Children and Adolescents.* 2nd ed. Carmarthen, UK: Crown House Publishing Ltd; 2013.

addition of biofeedback, which provides proof to the patient that changes in thinking result in changes in body responses. Children, adolescents, and their families can gain an increased sense of control and participation in their respective treatments by learning effective coping strategies such as those available through self-hypnosis, with or without biofeedback.

History

Hypnosis techniques have been used since the late 18th century. The Franklin Commission, which investigated the claims of Franz Mesmer, included experiments involving children and adolescents (collectively called *children* in this chapter unless otherwise specified). In the 1840s, 2 British surgeons, John Elliotson and James Braid, both reported surgical procedures on children during which hypnosis was the sole anesthesia method.[1,2] In the late 19th century, European physicians reported successfully treating negative habits and pain in children with hypnosis.[3] The first research studies of children using hypnosis were in the 1960s and assessed hypnotizability.[4] Since then, researchers have recognized that children generally learn hypnosis more quickly and easily than do adults. The first use of biofeedback with children was reported in the 1970s, and since the 1970s, increasing research has documented the ability of children to use hypnosis, with or without biofeedback, to treat many clinical conditions.[5]

Three-day workshops training child health professionals to teach hypnosis to children were first offered in 1976 by what is now the National Pediatric Hypnosis Training Institute (NPHTI) (www.nphti.org) and have been available annually since. Training emphasizes the necessity of selecting an approach that relates to the child's developmental level. Small group practice focuses on specific exercises such as slow abdominal breathing, imagining a special place, or adding metaphors such as a focus on the positive characteristics of superheroes. After completion of the NPHTI workshops, participants have access to an active and useful e-mail list (Listserv) to assist them with their patients. A recent paper has reviewed the history of pediatric hypnosis education and recent improvements in educational methods.[6]

Definitions

Hypnosis is defined as a focused state of awareness, sometimes involving relaxation, during which the individual has enhanced ability to facilitate specific physiologic and behavioral outcomes. *Hypnotherapy* is defined as a treatment modality that uses hypnosis by integrating that focused state of awareness into treatment.

Many terms have been used to describe the process of hypnosis (see Box 8-1). *Mesmerism* was the original term used to describe the clinical work of Franz Mesmer. James Braid, an English surgeon, first coined the term *hypnosis. Hypnos* came from the Latin root for "sleep," implying that the person in hypnosis is asleep. However, this implication is not the case, as one is fully awake and aware when in a state of hypnosis. Still, often hypnosis remains misunderstood. Since then, many other terms (see Box 8-1) such as *self-regulation* and *mind-body skills training* have been used. *Cyberphysiology* is another term coined in the 1980s to describe these same techniques. The prefix *cyber* is derived from the Greek *kybernan,* which means "to steer or take the helm"; thus, cyberphysiology refers to a person's ability to steer or regulate a physiologic or behavioral response.[7]

Some of the more common misconceptions about hypnosis include

▶ Hypnotists exert mind control over passive participants.

▶ Hypnosis is magic.

▶ When under hypnosis, the participant is sleeping.

▶ Only a few people are able to be hypnotized.

None of these statements is true. The participant is fully awake during hypnosis and aware of the environment. The mind and mental imagery of the person using these mind-body skills causes the physiologic changes. Although some people find these skills easier to acquire than other people, anyone can learn self-hypnosis.

Biofeedback is a term coined in 1969 to describe the procedure of using a physiologic response measure, or signal from the body, to give feedback to the person. This feedback increases the awareness of the body and how it is functioning. Biofeedback is a useful tool in training individuals to strengthen their mind-body connection and learn self-regulation skills. Although biofeedback is a useful adjunct, training in biofeedback requires self-hypnosis instructions, which lead to the desired physiologic changes.

Measures of physiologic response include skin temperature, galvanic skin response (GSR) or electrodermal activity, electroencephalographic (EEG) data, breathing, heart rate, and heart-rate variability (HRV). Simple skin-temperature monitors make an inexpensive and effective biofeedback tool. Nocturnal enuresis alarms are essentially biofeedback tools. Heart-rate variability is the measure of time interval between heartbeats and has become a very popular biofeedback tool.

A popular biofeedback computer program that was originally designed for adults and has also been successful with children is the emWave (formerly Freeze Framer) program (www.heartmath.com). A finger sensor connected to the computer measures the HRV. As the person relaxes, the image on the computer screen gives positive feedback. For example, a rainbow comes down and fills a pot with coins, and in another a hot-air balloon floats up and across a field as the player relaxes. The program has a graphical representation that shows the details of the session with HRV over time and percentage of time during which the participant was at low, medium, and high levels of relaxation. Feedback can then be compared with the data from other sessions from the same subject to determine progress. HeartMath also makes a portable emWave personal stress reliever biofeedback device.

Common Ground

Pediatric clinicians (in this chapter a term encompassing pediatric subspecialists, as well as primary care pediatricians, family physicians, internists, nurse practitioners, and physician assistants who provide health care to children and adolescents) use many terms such as *imagery, relaxation imagery, progressive relaxation, meditation,* and *mindfulness* among others, all of which refer to the same process by which hypnosis is induced, which often includes deep breathing, relaxing the body, and asking the child to imagine something. Although great confusion and disagreement exists in the definitions of the variety of terms used, common ground can be found among terms. For example, hypnosis often uses relaxation and imagery techniques, and biofeedback can be used to augment a person's body-physiologic awareness during hypnosis. In addition, imagery and relaxation techniques, which are hypnosis methods, are used in biofeedback to help increase the person's focus and awareness. Culbert and colleagues describe the biofeedback-hypnosis interface and the rationale for integrating these self-regulation or cyberphysiologic techniques with children and adolescents.[8] These skills all foster empowerment, mastery, and self-control. Many athletes use these skills to improve performance, and many patients use them to improve their health and body functions.

Guidelines for Learning and Teaching Self-hypnosis

Before training a patient in self-regulation skills, the pediatric clinician should prepare the patient and family (Box 8-3). The choice of strategies for teaching self-hypnosis to children and adolescents (all encompassed in the terms *child* or *children* in this chapter unless otherwise specified) varies, depending on the child's age and developmental stage, the preferred type of mental imagery (ie, visual, auditory, kinesthetic, olfactory), learning

---

Box 8-3. When Teaching a Child Self-regulation Techniques

1. Conduct a thorough diagnostic evaluation to understand the effects of the problem on the child and the significance of symptoms for the family.

2. Understand the child by learning about the child's personality, interests, likes, dislikes, and developmental stage, as well as any learning disabilities.

3. Emphasize the need for practice by explaining that becoming proficient in self-hypnosis requires practice, similar to learning (eg, a sport or music skill).

4. Emphasize that the child, not the parent, is the client; thus, parents should be supportive but should not remind their child to practice.

5. Throughout the process, emphasize the child's control because the child being in control is the principal key to success.

Derived from Kohen DP, Olness KN. Self-regulation therapy: helping children help themselves. *Ambul Child Health.* 1996;2(1):43–58.

---

style, preferred activities, dislikes, and personality. The clinician who provides coaching or teaching of hypnosis should emphasize that the child is in control and can choose when and where to use self-hypnosis. The clinician should be knowledgeable about the basic problem of the child before embarking on a hypnotherapeutic intervention. For example, a primary care clinician (PCC) (ie, pediatrician, family physician, internist, nurse practitioner, or physician assistant at the front lines of pediatrics) should be able to assess whether all necessary diagnostic tests have been completed for the patient presenting with problems of abdominal pain, headache, or enuresis before offering training in self-hypnosis. A PCC would not teach self-hypnosis to a child with post-traumatic stress disorder (PTSD) unless working closely with a child psychiatrist or psychologist who was experienced in assessment and treatment of PTSD.

Training in self-hypnosis is helpful to a pediatric clinician interested in using these skills to help children. Much can be learned about the language used to promote mind-body control and self-confidence in a child. The language used should be permissive, allowing the child to feel a sense of control. However, many techniques that use mind-body or hypnosis methods can be used in a primary care setting without formal training. Understanding a child's needs, increasing the child's understanding of mind-body control, and helping the child feel comfortable will promote a sense of control and increase the child's ability to regulate her or his body and behavior. Techniques that help a child focus and relax may be taught as part of hypnosis (Box 8-4). Slow deep breathing, sometimes called *diaphragmatic breathing* or *belly breathing*, is a powerful way to focus the child's attention and start the relaxation process. Progressive muscle relaxation is useful for older children who understand the instructions. Young children may respond better to *becoming floppy* as they relax. Kuttner[9] has described strategies for working with preschool children in pediatric practice.

Imagery techniques work best when the clinician has an understanding of the child's developmental stage, likes, dislikes, and fears. The clinician should help each child choose relaxation and imagery methods that suit him or her. It is recommended that a child practice 10 to 20 minutes twice daily for 1 month and then once daily for the second month. Because biofeedback and hypnosis are designed to promote self-control, the parents should not remind their child to practice; children should develop their own reminder system (eg, a ribbon around the neck of a favorite stuffed animal). Adding a biofeedback measure (eg, to monitor pulse and HRV, peripheral temperature, or GSR) may help the child improve. An audio recording may also be an effective reinforcer.

Clinical Applications

Mind-body interventions constitute a major portion of the overall use of complementary and integrative medicine by the public. National survey data published in 2004 showed that 5 relaxation techniques along with imagery, biofeedback, and hypnosis, taken together, were used by more than 30% of the adult US population.[10]

Box 8-4. Techniques to Help a Child Focus and Relax

- Deep breathing
- Relaxation (eg, progressive muscle relaxation)
- Mental imagery
- Guided imagery
- Therapeutic suggestions
- Adjunct biofeedback

Hypnosis and biofeedback are generally categorized in the mind-body aspects of complementary and integrative medicine; however, increasingly, medical institutions are considering hypnosis and biofeedback as part of mainstream medicine. Pediatric clinicians see many children who exhibit symptoms of high stress levels, including such symptoms as anxiety, depression, headaches, abdominal pain, and school avoidance. Children and parents often feel out of control, with busy lives, worries, or chronic health problems. Children and adolescents may attempt to cope in self-injurious ways, such as with the use of alcohol, nicotine, and drugs.

A thorough medical evaluation should precede hypnosis, with or without biofeedback treatment. Children referred for integrative treatment may not have had adequate diagnostic evaluations. In a study that reviewed 200 cases of children referred specifically for treatment with hypnosis, biofeedback, or both, 25% of the children had unrecognized biological bases for symptoms such as enuresis, headache, anxiety, and recurrent abdominal pain.[11] Some of the children referred for hypnosis to control headaches proved to have sinusitis, food allergies, brain tumor, or carbon monoxide poisoning.

Children have been taught self-hypnosis for a wide range of problems (see Box 8-2). The mind-body skills learned with hypnosis can give a child the capacity to change attitudes, emotions, behavior, habits, autonomic reactivity, and biological functions. This self-regulation offers techniques that facilitate their ability to

▶ Direct their behavior.

▶ Modulate physiologic changes in desired directions.

▶ Control their thoughts for the purpose of symptom control.

▶ Attain and maintain health and wellness.

▶ Improve function or enhance performance.

Pain Management

Pain is a subjective experience, and children exhibit different tolerance levels. Hypnosis techniques can be used for pain control, for example, in emergency departments[12] or for children with cancer who are undergoing procedures.[13]

When in acute pain, children are in a more focused state of awareness and are highly motivated to feel better. Because of this motivation, they may be more likely to respond to suggestions that increase their sense of control, which they can then use to decrease their sensation of pain. Helping children *dissociate* by imagining that they are in a favorite place can have a calming effect. In some situations, such as a first-time migraine, it can be difficult to work with a child who is acutely miserable. While not always possible, it is preferable overall to teach children these techniques when they are well, allowing them to prepare themselves for the possible acute episode. Some of these effective self-regulatory techniques are described in the literature.[14] A resource by Kuttner (*Child in Pain: What Health Professionals Can Do to Help*) offers guidance for child health care professionals to help children in pain using self-regulation techniques.

Chronic pain and recurrent pain are more difficult to manage than acute pain. A child who experiences pain over a long period or learns to expect the pain to return again and again may become increasingly anxious and develop feelings of hopelessness. Teaching self-regulation is more complicated in these situations because of the need to address both the severity and the negative expectancy that accompany chronic pain. If the self-regulatory techniques seem ineffective for the child with chronic or recurrent pain, the clinician should reevaluate the situation. The pain may be serving a protective psychological purpose. Significant mental health issues, such as PTSD, depression, or abuse, may exist, and psychotherapeutic evaluation and intervention may be needed (Box 8-5).

The efficacy of 3 promising psychological neuromodulatory treatments, that is, neurofeedback, meditation, and hypnosis, when provided to young people with chronic pain were studied and showed that hypnotic treatments are effective in reducing pain intensity for a variety of pediatric chronic pain problems, but more clinical trials are needed to evaluate the effects of neurofeedback and meditation training.[15] It has been shown[16] that children will benefit more and require less training if they are offered training very early, ideally within a few days, after diagnosis of a chronic or life-threatening disease. *No Fears, No Tears* and *No Fears, No Tears: 13 Years Later* are 2 video productions produced by the Canadian Cancer Society in 1986 and 1999, respectively, that illustrate

---

Box 8-5. Case Report: Abdominal Pain

Sarah, a 6-year-old girl, was brought to the PCC by her mother because of severe abdominal pain of 2 months' duration. The pains started suddenly one day in the morning after breakfast and before school. They occurred many mornings of the week and lasted for 1–2 h. Sarah would clutch her abdomen and bend over with pain. She did not have vomiting or diarrhea or fever. After the pain resolved, each day she appeared healthy. She had no history of constipation. Medical workup was negative for any medical causes of her pain.

A complete history revealed that Sarah did not want to go to school. She was afraid because a classmate on her school bus was saying things to scare her. The abdominal pain kept her home and protected her from the child who was scaring her.

Sarah's PCC spoke with her mother about addressing this issue with school officials and then asked Sarah if she wanted to learn a way to help herself prevent the pain from arising and decrease the intensity when it occurred. Sarah was interested. She liked dolls and stuffed animals; thus, she was asked if she had one that was very soft and squishy, and she did. Sarah was taught to take slow, deep breaths "into her belly" and then advised to "make her belly very soft" like her squishy stuffed animal. This exercise would help her belly work better and prevent the pain from coming. Sarah demonstrated in the office that she was able to perform this task. She was then advised to practice this deep breathing and making her belly soft at home. (This teaching took approximately 5 min of the office visit.)

One month later, Sarah's mother brought her back for a child health supervision visit. Sarah had had only one more episode of abdominal pain after learning how to relax herself and her abdomen. She has not had similar recurrent abdominal pains since. Sarah's mother also addressed the issue of the child who was scaring Sarah by talking with the principal, teacher, and bus driver. Sarah now enjoys going to school and does well with her friends and schoolwork.

Abbreviation: PCC, primary care clinician.

---

the use of self-regulation strategies with children who have cancer. Children and adolescents with cancer undergo many repeated and invasive medical procedures that are often painful and highly distressing. Techniques such as distraction, cognitive-behavioral strategies, and hypnosis have been identified as effective for reducing pain and increasing coping in children.[17]

Habit Problems

Habit problems are common in children. Habit problems such as thumb-sucking, nail-biting, hairpulling (trichotillomania), or habitual cough are potentially responsive to hypnotherapy. In a retrospective study, a significant number of children with habitual cough responded well to hypnosis, with resolution of their symptoms of cough.[18]

Some types of habits, such as tics or hairpulling, often begin during a stressful experience and initially carry with them emotional significance. In most instances, the emotional significance disappears, yet the habit remains. Habits such as habitual cough may begin with an upper respiratory tract infection but persist long after the infection is gone. Others, such as thumb-sucking, may have begun as a comfort measure in young childhood and have become habitual. Unless a motivation exists behind the habit (eg, if the habit helps the child avoid school) and provided that the child is motivated to change (not just the parent), hypnosis techniques are effective in extinguishing the habit. Emphasizing the child's control in mastering the problem is crucial to success in eliminating the problem.

Enuresis

Before considering hypnotherapy for enuresis, the clinician should distinguish whether the enuresis is primary or secondary and whether the enuresis occurs during both day and night or only at night only. Organic causes such as urinary tract infection, diabetes, and constipation must be ruled out. Primary enuresis may be considered a maturational issue, whereas secondary enuresis, after a period of dryness, may be associated with a significant stressor in the child's life. Enuresis that has no organic cause is expected to resolve spontaneously over time. Depending on the age of the child, enuresis can be quite frustrating and interfere with activities such as sleepovers. Children with nocturnal enuresis often feel shame or guilt. Various methods have been used for children and parents who wish to stop enuresis; these include motivational behavior management (including reward systems, the child helping in cleanup of the wet bed, and bed-wetting alarms) and medications such as desmopressin.[19] Hypnotherapy is helpful for many children with enuresis. In a study that compared 2 groups of children treated with hypnotherapy vs imipramine, comparable results were seen with each group. At long-term follow-up, the group treated with hypnotherapy had a significantly larger positive response.[20] Drugs such as imipramine can have significant adverse effects and can be life-threatening. Desmopressin has negligible known adverse effects, but some parents are reluctant to give their child medication. The bed-wetting alarm is a type of conditioning device and is quite effective, although some children find the alarm to be aversive. Hypnosis as a treatment is at least as effective, has longer duration, and is not life-threatening. As a treatment option for enuresis, self-regulation therapy or hypnosis is the least invasive, and many children respond favorably.

Behavioral and Attention Disorders

Self-regulation has value as an adjunct in management of behavioral problems. In addition to therapeutic interventions, such as counseling and behavior modification, teaching self-regulation techniques to a child can be a constructive way to build self-esteem and more effectively control the maladaptive behaviors. Attention-deficit/hyperactivity disorder (ADHD) is one of the most common behavioral problems encountered in children. Recommended management usually involves behavior modification and primarily stimulant medication. A review of research studies that use of neurofeedback for ADHD shows potential for short- and long-term improvement from ADHD symptoms.[21] One study using biofeedback and hypnosis techniques has demonstrated beneficial effects of EEG biofeedback on measures of intelligence, behavioral rating scales assessing the frequency of core symptoms of ADHD, computerized tests of attention (eg, the Test of Variables of Attention [commonly known as TOVA]), and quantitative EEG measures of cortical arousal.[22] Evidence is promising for neurofeedback as a treatment alternative for ADHD, but more research needs to be done to be certain about efficacy of neurofeedback.[23]

Stress Management and Anxiety

Self-regulation skills are an excellent way to manage stress. Relaxation and hypnosis are useful for helping children and adolescents with symptoms of anxiety. Many parents bring children to their PCCs for symptoms related to high stress levels. Stress and anxiety can manifest in a variety of ways, including somatic concerns, behavioral issues, and poor sleep. Helping children learn self-hypnosis can give them a coping skill they can use anywhere and anytime. When learned at a young age, these stress-management skills can be used for a lifetime to help with daily or extraordinary stressors.

Culbert and Kajander have created kits to help children manage stress, sleep problems, and pain (*Be the Boss of Your Pain: Self-care for Kids,* 2007; *Be the Boss of Your Stress: Self-care for Kids,* 2007; and *Be the Boss of Your Sleep: Self-care for Kids,* 2007). The contents of the kit include helpful stress-relieving tools such as finger puppets, small acupressure devices, squeeze balls, paper, crayons, small dolls, and blowing devices. Contents vary somewhat, depending on the purpose and the country.

A study looking at the effects of a stress management intervention on elementary school children found significantly improved HRV and lower scores on an anxiety questionnaire. During the intervention, the class of students in third grade learned the stress management technique with their teacher and practiced daily as a group for 10 minutes for about 4 months. The measures were obtained before the intervention, immediately after the 4 months, and again the following year in fourth grade when they were no longer getting the intervention. These positive findings persisted into the next year of school, showing an even better HRV, indicating that these children mastered a skill that they were then using in their daily lives to help cope with stressors. The children had many positive comments about how using this technique helped them at school during recess and test times, and at home. The control group did not have any improvements in HRV or the anxiety questionnaire; in fact, they had a worsening of their HRV after 1 year.[24] (See Box 8-6.)

With children who have an anxiety disorder, such as generalized anxiety disorder, separation anxiety disorder, or selective mutism, hypnosis techniques can be a useful adjunct along with therapeutic counseling.

Box 8-6. Case Report: Anxiety

Dan, a 16-year-old boy, was referred to learn self-hypnosis for control of test anxiety. He had been an excellent student during all his school years until a year earlier, when he began to perform poorly on examinations. No changes occurred in his studying habits. He did very well on homework. No family changes had occurred. He got along well with 2 older siblings, both of whom are now in college. Dan had a girlfriend, a classmate, who was also a good student and was looking forward to college.

Dan's mother described him as having always been "perfectionistic." She said that he began expressing worry about examinations when his older brother was taking student aptitude tests. Dan said that he studied and felt that he knew the material but that he froze during the examinations and was unable to think clearly. He also said that he slept poorly on nights before examinations.

Dan said that he enjoyed reading, drawing, playing computer games, swimming, and soccer. He said that his dream was to become an architect. He said that he had been afraid of dogs as a young child, but this was no longer so. Dan also said he got approximately 6 h of sleep on school nights and slept 10–12 h a night on weekends.

The PCC explained to Dan that she was able to teach him self-hypnosis to reduce test anxiety and that his daily practice would be required. She described the use of self-hypnosis by Olympic athletes and the type of practice that was required. The PCC emphasized that Dan's parents were not allowed to remind him to practice. Dan said that he wished to learn and was willing to practice.

The PCC taught Dan a self-hypnosis method involving progressive relaxation and focus on a winning soccer game. She asked that he practice this method twice daily and return in a week. When Dan returned, he said he had been practicing regularly. At this visit, Dan was hooked to a temperature sensor and was able to watch a screen that demonstrated the increase in his peripheral temperature as he relaxed and achieved self-hypnosis. The PCC then taught him specific suggestions to use before his examinations, including suggestions related to sleeping well, and to include future programming of pleasant events associated with successful examinations.

Dan continued to practice daily and was followed up by telephone every 2 wk for 2 mo. At that time, Dan had no further test anxiety, was achieving high scores on tests, and had good grades.

Abbreviation: PCC, primary care clinician.

Self-regulation and ADHD

Attention-deficit/hyperactivity disorder is a common child and adolescent diagnosis. Finding methods to help children improve attention is of great interest. Some studies are showing neurofeedback as a promising attention-training treatment intervention for children with ADHD. A recent study used a smart tablet–based neurofeedback training program and found long-term improvements on scores on several neuropsychological tests and parent behavioral rating scales in the training group but not in the control group, indicating that this type of technique might improve cognitive function in children with attention problems.[25]

A randomized controlled study that looked at the short- and long-term effects of computer attention training on symptoms of ADHD compared neurofeedback and cognitive training with a control group. They found that children who received neurofeedback showed significant improvement of their ADHD symptoms compared with control groups, whereas children who received cognitive training showed no improvement compared with control groups. A long-term follow-up of this study showed that neurofeedback participants had more prompt and greater improvements in ADHD symptoms, sustained at the 6-month follow-up, than did cognitive training participants or those in the control group. These 2 studies also monitored stimulant medication use and found that children who received neurofeedback had minimal to no increase in their medication dosage, whereas children with cognitive training or the control group had significant increases in dosages. More research needs to be done using neurofeedback as an intervention for ADHD, but these results are promising.[26,27]

Mindfulness

Mindfulness is a technique described by Kabat-Zinn as a way of paying attention and being in "present moment" and has been used by adults for many years. There is some interest in applying these techniques to children and adolescents, but research is still limited regarding the effectiveness with small sample sizes and lack of control groups. Mindfulness programs have be used in the school setting. There is interest in mindfulness techniques to help children with ADHD in gaining better self-control.[28–30]

Medical Problems

Some diseases respond well to self-regulation techniques. One group of diseases can be classified as *biobehavioral disorders* because they have clear pathophysiologic origins, as well as significant psycho-emotional components. Examples of these conditions include asthma, migraine, and irritable bowel syndrome (IBS). Relaxation and self-hypnosis help promote a sense of self-control and a reduction of symptoms in children with biobehavioral disorders.

Children and adolescents with asthma can learn self-hypnosis to reduce wheezing in acute episodes. Research using hypnosis, with and without biofeedback, has demonstrated decreased functional morbidity, with fewer emergency department visits, fewer missed school days, and a better sense of control in children who were taught to use these techniques.[31] Hypnosis has been reported to be useful within the field of pediatric respiratory medicine as a primary and an adjunctive therapy.[32]

Functional abdominal pain (FAP) and IBS are quite common in children. Studies have shown that hypnotherapy is an effective treatment for reducing symptoms of FAP and IBS.[33,34] A long-term study found that children who were treated using gut-directed hypnotherapy had significantly sustained improvements in their symptoms, with 68% still in remission after almost 5 years, compared with standard medical treatment, with only 20% still in remission.[35]

Chronic headaches in adolescents respond well to hypnosis treatment after little to no benefit from pharmacological and other nonpharmacological therapies.[36] Children with migraines have been shown to respond well, with a significant decrease in frequency of their headaches after self-regulation training when compared with propranolol and placebo.[37] (See Box 8-7.)

Warts are another common condition seen in primary care pediatrics. Warts are reported to respond to many interventions and often resolve by themselves. In many instances, children will undergo numerous topical treatments without success or with recurrences. A study comparing self-hypnosis and topical treatment found no difference in immediate resolution of the warts. However, after 6 months the topical treatment group had a much higher rate of recurrence than did the self-hypnosis group.[38] (See Box 8-8.)

Box 8-7. Case Report: Migraine

Anne, an 11-year-old girl, had a history of migraines for 3 y. Her mother also had migraines since childhood. Anne was evaluated by a child neurologist who, at various times, had prescribed propranolol, cyproheptadine (Periactin), and amitriptyline (Elavil). He also suggested regular sleep and avoidance of certain foods.

Anne did well in school and had many friends. She enjoyed music and played the piano. She had 2 younger siblings, aged 8 and 6. She said that she was afraid of thunder.

At the initial visit, Anne was having a migraine episode at least once a week. Most episodes were preceded by a visual aura, and they lasted approximately 12 h. They were accompanied by nausea and sometimes vomiting. Anne said that she would sleep as soon as possible after a migraine began and would usually awaken without the pain but with a shaky feeling that lasted for several hours thereafter.

Anne was interested in learning self-hypnosis for control of her migraines. Anne chose to focus on music for her hypnotic induction. She imagined her favorite music as she gradually relaxed all her muscles. She did well during the first practice.

At her second visit, Anne's finger temperature was monitored during her examination. Her peripheral temperature increased 2.2°C (4°F) during this practice, proof that she was relaxing. She learned about pain signals and was offered options for turning the signals off, if she should develop a migraine episode.

The third visit took place 3 wk later. Anne had had 1 migraine during the period between visits, a significant decrease. Subsequently, she was followed up by telephone. In the 6-mo follow-up period, she had 2 migraine episodes, both associated with sleep deprivation.

Diabetes

A child with diabetes must cope with frequent blood tests, a special diet, and daily injections. When a child with diabetes feels out of control, adherence with diet and medicines can prove inadequate. Hypnotherapy can provide a child with a way to learn to cope and gain a sense of mastery, both of which may help reduce anxiety and improve adherence.

Box 8-8. Case Report: Warts

David, a 7-year-old boy, had had warts on his hands and legs for 2 y. He had been treated by a dermatologist with topical treatments and freezing the warts. Each time, the warts recurred. David had 3 warts on his left leg, 3 on his right leg, 2 on his left hand, and 5 on his right hand.

David was in second grade. He enjoyed school and had friends in both school and the neighborhood. He liked bicycle riding, playing soccer, and ice-skating. David had an older sister and a younger brother. He said he wanted to get rid of the warts because he did not like the way they looked and because the previous treatments hurt.

David was told that many children had eliminated warts by doing a relaxation exercise and giving a message to themselves to stop feeding the warts. He was told about practice at home and about the need for a good reminder system for the practice; his mother was told not to remind him to practice.

David imagined himself playing soccer as a hypnotic induction and was asked to imagine playing until the game was won and then to tell himself to stop feeding each of the 13 warts.

David returned in 2 wk. At this point, David had 7 warts and was very pleased. He continued practice for another month, and 12 of the warts were gone. No new warts appeared. After 3 mo, all the warts were gone.

Medical Procedures

Medical procedures are usually a source of anxiety for children and are often painful. These procedures include routine immunization injections, venipuncture, and pelvic examinations. Reductions in anxiety and pain have been noted in children who were taught skills using hypnosis techniques.[39,40] A randomized controlled study assessing the effects of hypnosis on distress of children undergoing a voiding cystourethrogram procedure found significant reductions in distress for the group of children who received hypnosis.[41] Distraction and hypnosis are also efficacious in reducing needle-related pain and distress in children.[42]

Hypnosis as an adjunctive treatment for pediatric patients undergoing anesthesia is also useful for reducing anxiety, shortening hospital stays, and lessening long-term pain and discomfort in children.[43]

Hypnosis in the Primary Care Pediatric Office Visit

Integrating self-regulation techniques into primary care practice[44] offers the opportunity for PCCs to facilitate a sense of mastery and competency in the children under their care. Although many PCCs may not realize it, they have long been applying some of the hypnotic principles and using some of the sensitive language in their clinical work with children. In an introductory course on hypnosis, clinicians become aware of the importance of carefully selecting their language and monitoring the timing and pacing with which to introduce new words in their encounters with children. Clinicians often realize that integrating these techniques will be easier and faster than they may have originally believed.[45]

Brief self-regulation interventions can be integrated into primary care practice. Following are some examples of simple techniques that can be used to make a child more comfortable during routine office procedures, such as receiving shots or undergoing throat cultures or just being examined by a stranger.

▶ Having a child *blow away* pain by using a pinwheel, bubbles, or a pretend candle is an effective tool for decreasing a child's experience of pain during injections or venipuncture.

▶ Bubbles can also be used to get the attention of the young child who starts screaming as soon as the PCC walks into the room and to help the child feel more comfortable.

▶ A stuffed animal or doll can be used as an example before examining a child. By pointing out how the doll or stuffed animal is comfortable being examined, the PCC can often help the child become more comfortable when being examined.

▶ A child who needs a throat culture may be able to use slow, deep breaths while focusing on a pleasant thought to keep still while keeping his or her mouth open.

▶ Allowing the child to select and listen to a favorite piece of music during procedures may help the child focus and relax.

How can the PCC learn to use hypnosis in the practice?

1. *Take a basic 3-day hypnosis-training workshop.* See Box 8-9.

2. *Identify and stay in touch with a mentor after the first workshop.* Most of the workshops will offer mentoring assistance to encourage the new learner and provide advice regarding clinical situations. Workshops also have an active Listserv resource for child health care professionals who share knowledge about using hypnosis in a pediatric setting.

3. *Take follow-up workshops, read textbooks and hypnosis journals, and attend annual hypnosis scientific meetings.*

4. *Take a board-certified examination in hypnosis.* Examinations are available from the American Board of Medical Hypnosis, American Board of Psychological Hypnosis, American Board of Dental Hypnosis, and American Hypnosis Board for Clinical Social Work. Information can be obtained from the American Society of Clinical Hypnosis or the Society for Clinical and Experimental Hypnosis.

Research in Child Hypnosis

Active research in child hypnosis has taken place over the past 40 years. Initial research examined measures of child hypnotic susceptibility, such as the Stanford Children's Hypnotic Susceptibility Scale. Most subsequent research has been clinical research documenting the efficacy of hypnosis with children in areas such as pain management, habit problems, wart reduction, and performance anxiety. The variability in preferences, learning styles, and developmental stages complicates the design of research protocols for the study of hypnosis with children. These protocols are often written to describe identical hypnotic inductions, often recorded, to

---

Box 8-9. Hypnosis-Training Organizations

- National Pediatric Hypnosis Training Institute (www.nphti.org)
- Society for Clinical and Experimental Hypnosis (www.sceh.us)
- American Society of Clinical Hypnosis (training workshops bimonthly) (www.asch.net)

be used at prescribed times. Measured variables do not address whether a child likes the induction or listens to the tape or whether the child focuses on entirely different mental imagery of the child's own choosing. Furthermore, learning disabilities are often subtle and may not be recognized without detailed testing that is not usually done before research studies involving child hypnosis. Learning disabilities, such as auditory processing disorder, may interfere with the ability of children to learn and remember self-hypnosis training. Each of these variables complicates efforts to perform meta-analyses on hypnosis and related interventions. Interventions called *relaxation imagery, imagery, visual imagery,* or *progressive relaxation* each lead to a hypnotic state. The proper analysis of studies on the efficacy of hypnosis in children should combine all studies that describe strategies for inducing hypnosis in children.

Some research studies are defined as controlled but mix therapeutic interventions. For example, Scharff et al[46] reported on "[a] controlled study of minimal-contact thermal biofeedback treatment in children with migraine." Children were randomly assigned to thermal biofeedback, attention, or wait-list control groups. The hand-warming biofeedback group received 4 sessions of cognitive behavioral stress management training, thermal biofeedback, progressive muscle relaxation, imagery training on warm places, and deep-breathing techniques. Thus, children were also being taught self-hypnosis.

Several controlled laboratory studies have demonstrated that an association exists between learning self-hypnosis and changes in humoral immunity or in cellular immunity (or in both) in children. In one study, Olness and colleagues[47] examined the self-regulation of salivary immunoglobulin A by children, demonstrating that self-hypnosis can facilitate some immunomodulation in children. This work was the basis for a clinical trial by Hewson-Bower, who demonstrated that training in self-hypnosis for children with frequent upper respiratory tract infections resulted in a reduction of infectious episodes and fewer illness days when upper respiratory tract infections occurred.[48]

Landry and Raz reviewed 38 neuroimaging studies (positron emission tomography and functional magnetic resonance imaging) to evaluate current opinions concerning the neurobiological underpinnings of hypnosis. They concluded that neuroimaging studies of hypnosis revealed a top-down modulation indexed by Prefrontal cortex and anterior cingulate cortex (ACC) activity. These studies indicate that hypnotic induction without task-specific or indirect suggestions mainly engages the frontal and thalamic areas. When suggestions are given, specific brain regions relevant to hypnotic responses are engaged. For example, suggestions to alter pain perception are manifested in somatosensory areas and the ACC, both areas involved in pain perception. Authors point out that most studies did not differentiate whether subjects scored high or low on hypnotic susceptibility tests. Future studies should follow more tightly controlled experimental designs, including individual differences.[49]

References

1. Elliotson J. *Numerous Cases of Surgical Operations Without Pain in the Mesmeric State.* Philadelphia, PA: Lea and Blanchard; 1843
2. Braid J. *Neurypnology, or the Rationale of Nervous Sleep.* New York, NY: Julian Press; 1960 (original publication 1843)
3. Bramwell JM. *Hypnotism: Its History, Practice, and Theory.* New York, NY: Julian Press; 1903 (reissued with new introduction 1956)
4. London P. *Children's Hypnotic Susceptibility Scale.* Palo Alto, CA: Consulting Psychologists Press; 1963
5. Dikel W, Olness K. Self-hypnosis, biofeedback, and voluntary peripheral temperature control in children. *Pediatrics.* 1980;66(3):335–340
6. Kohen DP, Kaiser P, Olness K. State-of-the-art pediatric hypnosis training: remodeling curriculum and refining faculty development. *Am J Clin Hypn.* 2017;59(3):292–310
7. Culbert T, Olness K, eds. *Integrative Pediatrics.* Oxford University Press: New York, NY; 2010
8. Culbert TP, Reaney JB, Kohen DP. "Cyberphysiologic" strategies for children: the clinical hypnosis/biofeedback interface. *Int J Clin Exp Hypn.* 1994;42(4):97–117
9. Kuttner L. Helpful strategies in working with preschool children in pediatric practice. *Pediatr Ann.* 1991;20(3):120–122, 124–127
10. Wolsko PM, Eisenberg DM, Davis RB, Phillips RS. Use of mind-body medical therapies. *J Gen Intern Med.* 2004;19(1):43–50
11. Olness K, Libbey P. Unrecognized biologic bases of behavioral symptoms in patients referred for hypnotherapy. *Am J Clin Hypn.* 1987;30(1):1–8
12. Kohen DP. Applications of relaxation/mental imagery (self-hypnosis) in pediatric emergencies. *Int J Clin Exp Hypn.* 1986;34(4):283–294
13. LeBaron S, Hilgard JR. *Hypnotherapy of Pain in Children With Cancer.* Los Altos, CA: William Kaufman; 1984
14. Kuttner L. *A Child in Pain: How to Help, What to Do.* Point Roberts, WA: Hartley and Marks; 1996
15. Miró J, Castarlenas E, de la Vega R, et al. Psychological neuromodulatory treatments for young people with chronic pain. *Children (Basel).* 2016;3(4):E41

16. Olness K, Singer L. Five-year follow-up of 61 children taught cyberphysiologic strategies as adjunct management in cancer. *Top Pediatr*. 1989;7:2–6

17. Flowers SR, Birnie KA. Procedural preparation and support as a standard of care in pediatric oncology. *Pediatr Blood Cancer*. 2015;62(suppl 5):S694–S723

18. Anbar RD, Hall HR. Childhood habit cough treated with self-hypnosis. *J Pediatr*. 2004;144(2):213–217

19. Wootton J, Norfolk S. Nocturnal enuresis: assessing and treating children and young people. *Community Pract*. 2010;83(12):37–39

20. Banjeree S, Srivastav A, Palan BM. Hypnosis and self-hypnosis in the management of nocturnal enuresis: a comparative study with imipramine therapy. *Am J Clin Hypn*. 1993;36(2):113–119

21. Fox DJ, Tharp DF, Fox LC. Neurofeedback: an alternative and efficacious treatment for attention deficit hyperactivity disorder. *Appl Psychophysiol Biofeedback*. 2005;30(4):365–373

22. Monastra VJ, Lynn S, Linden M, Lubar JF, Gruzelier J, LaVaque TJ. Electro-encephalographic biofeedback in the treatment of attention-deficit/hyperactivity disorder. *Appl Psychophysiol Biofeedback*. 2005;30(2):95–114

23. Nash J. Commentary on neurofeedback. *Biofeedback Self Regul*. 2008;36:15

24. Bothe DA, Grignon JB, Olness KN. The effects of a stress management intervention in elementary school children. *J Dev Behav Pediatr*. 2014;35(1):62–67

25. Shin MS, Jeon H, Kim M, et al. Effects of smart-tablet-based neurofeedback training on cognitive function in children with attention problems. *J Child Neurol*. 2016;31(6):750–760

26. Steiner NJ, Frenette EC, Rene KM, Brennan RT, Perrin EC. Neurofeedback and cognitive attention training for children with attention-deficit hyperactivity disorder in schools. *J Dev Behav Pediatr*. 2014;35(1):18–27

27. Steiner NJ, Frenette EC, Rene KM, Brennan RT, Perrin EC. In-school neurofeedback training for ADHD: sustained improvements from a randomized control trial. *Pediatrics*. 2014;133(3):483–492

28. Perry-Parrish C, Copeland-Linder N, Webb L, Sibinga EM. Mindfulness-based approaches for children and youth. *Curr Probl Pediatr Adolesc Health Care*. 2016;46(6):172–178

29. Burke CA. Mindfulness based approaches with children and adolescents: a preliminary review of current research in an emergent field. *J Child Fam Stud*. 2010;19(2):133–144

30. Perry-Parrish C, Copeland-Linder N, Webb L, Shields AH, Sibinga EM. Improving self-regulation in adolescents: current evidence for the role of mindfulness-based cognitive therapy. *Adolesc Health Med Ther*. 2016;7:101–108

31. Kohen DP. Relaxation/mental imagery (self-hypnosis) for childhood asthma: behavioral outcomes in a prospective controlled study. HYPNOS. *Swed J Hypn Psychother Psychosom Med*. 1995;22:133–144

32. McBride JJ, Vlieger AM, Anbar RD. Hypnosis in paediatric respiratory medicine. *Paediatr Respir Rev*. 2014;15(1):82–85

33. Rutten JM, Reitsma JB, Vlieger AM, Benninga MA. Gut-directed hypnotherapy for functional abdominal pain or irritable bowel syndrome in children: a systematic review. *Arch Dis Child*. 2013;98(4):252–257

34. Gulewitsch MD, Müller J, Hautzinger M, Schlarb AA. Brief hypnotherapeutic-behavioral intervention for functional abdominal pain and irritable bowel syndrome in childhood: a randomized controlled trial. *Eur J Pediatr.* 2013;172(8):1043–1051

35. Vlieger AM, Rutten JM, Govers AM, Frankenhuis C, Benninga MA. Long-term follow-up of gut-directed hypnotherapy vs. standard care in children with functional abdominal pain or irritable bowel syndrome. *Am J Gastroenterol.* 2012;107(4):627–631

36. Kohen DP. Chronic daily headache: helping adolescents help themselves with self-hypnosis. *Am J Clin Hypn.* 2011;54(1):32–46

37. Olness KN, MacDonald JT, Uden DL. Comparison of self-hypnosis and propranolol in the treatment of juvenile classic migraine. *Pediatrics.* 1987; 79(4):593–597

38. Felt B, Hall H, Schmidt W, Olness K, et al. Warts in children. Self-hypnosis compared to other approaches. *Am J Clin Hypn.* 1998;40:88–96

39. Schechter NL, Bernstein BA, Zempsky WT, Bright NS, Willard AK. Educational outreach to reduce immunization pain in office settings. *Pediatrics.* 2010;126(6):e1514–e1521

40. Kohen D, Olness K. *Hypnosis and Hypnotherapy With Children.* 4th ed. New York, NY: Routledge; 2011

41. Butler LD, Symons BK, Henderson SL, et al. Hypnosis reduces distress and duration of an invasive medical procedure for children. *Pediatrics.* 2005;115(1): e77–e85

42. Birnie KA, Noel M, Parker JA, et al. Systematic review and meta-analysis of distraction and hypnosis for needle-related pain and distress in children and adolescents. *J Pediatr Psychol.* 2014;39(8):783–808

43. Kuttner L. Pediatric hypnosis: pre-, peri-, and post-anesthesia. *Paediatr Anaesth.* 2012;22(6):573–577

44. Sugarman LI. Hypnosis in a primary care practice: developing skills for the "new morbidities." *J Dev Behav Pediatr.* 1996;17(5):300–305

45. Kohen DP, Olness KN. Self-regulation therapy: helping children help themselves. *Ambul Child Health.* 1996;2(1):43–58

46. Scharff L, Marcus DA, Masek BJ. A controlled study of minimal-contact thermal biofeedback treatment in children with migraine. *J Pediatr Psychol.* 2002;27(2):109–119

47. Olness KN, Culbert T, Uden D. Self-regulation of salivary immunoglobulin A by children. *Pediatrics.* 1989;83(1):66–71

48. Hewson-Bower B. *Psychological Treatment Decreases Colds and Flu in Children by Increasing Salivary IgA* [thesis]. Perth, Western Australia: Murdoch University; 1995

49. Landry M, Raz A. Hypnosis and imaging of the living human brain. *Am J Clin Hypn.* 2015;57(3):285–313

Complementary and Integrative Medical Therapies

Jane R. Hull, MD

> *"Integrative medicine seeks to use the best of scientifically based medical therapies along with compassion and attention to the patient's spiritual and emotional needs, as well as appropriate complementary approaches when they enhance conventional medicine."*

Despite opposition from some skeptics in the scientific community, interest in complementary and integrative medicine (CIM) continues to grow, particularly among people affected by mental health symptoms and the clinicians who care for them. Formerly unconventional therapies such as acupuncture and acupressure, biofeedback, guided imagery, and hypnotherapy have been integrated into pediatric care in many clinics and hospitals (see Chapter 8, Self-regulation Therapies and Biofeedback). Other therapies such as herbs, essential oils, dietary supplements, massage, and chiropractic care are widely used by the public and are increasingly available at conventional hospitals. Health care quality measures now acknowledge the importance of respecting spirituality and culturally based healing traditions in daily practice. The growing practice of providing care in a medical home emphasizes the importance of patient- and family-centered care that is at the heart of both pediatrics and integrative medicine. Pediatrics, more than most other specialties, embraces integrative medicine's emphasis on prevention and health promotion.

Ninety-six percent of pediatricians surveyed in July 2004 reported having patients who use CIM therapies, but only 37% of pediatricians routinely ask about the use of CIM therapies. Most (84%) wanted to learn more about CIM therapies so that they might appropriately counsel families interested in them.[1] Specialists as well as generalists need to know about integrative care because the use of CIM therapies is particularly high among children with multiple chronic conditions who seek specialist care.[2]

Most parents desire to discuss CIM with their respective *pediatric clinicians* (a term used in this chapter to encompass pediatric subspecialists, pediatricians, family physicians, internists, nurse practitioners, and physician assistants who provide health care to children and adolescents). The group of parents desiring discussion of CIM includes more than 80% of those who use CIM for their children. However, fewer than one-half of these parents report having done so.[3] Lack of communication may compromise the quality of care.

Pediatric integrative medicine (commonly known as PIM) represents one of the newest subspecialties in the care of children and adolescents (collectively called *children* in this chapter unless otherwise specified). In North America alone, there are more than 16 academic pediatric programs in which clinical care, resident teaching, and research in CIM are conducted.[4] However, pediatric clinicians do not need to be content experts on every CIM therapy and product or seek specialized training. Nor do they need to reject their training in biopsychosocial medicine or critical thinking. The tremendous growth in demand for CIM plus use of the Internet and mass media for health information suggests the need for new competencies in pediatric care. The 21st-century pediatric clinician should have the capacity to

▶ Focus on patient and family health goals in addition to diagnostic labels.

▶ Inquire regarding CIM use.

▶ Counsel on CIM from an evidence-based perspective using proven behavioral techniques to foster healthy lifestyles.

▶ Partner with and refer appropriately to CIM practitioners.

▶ Monitor for potential adverse effects.

This chapter defines CIM and describes how to inquire, counsel, partner, and refer. For pediatric clinicians who seek further skills development, Box 9-4 at the end of the chapter cites additional training opportunities.

Complementary and Integrative Medicine

Complementary and integrative medicine includes all health care systems, therapies, and products that are not considered part of conventional medicine as practiced in the United States. These therapies can be used to supplement conventional care, thus the term *complementary*. When prescribed by clinicians as part of a comprehensive treatment plan, they are considered integrative. Because the term *alternative* meant in place of conventional medical care, the term has been dropped by most physicians and the National Institutes of Health (NIH). The term *integrative medicine* has been adopted by the American Academy of Pediatrics (AAP) and is represented by the Section on Integrative Medicine.

Integrative medicine represents the ideal of a higher-order system of care rather than simply the addition of complementary therapies to conventional care.[5] The Academic Consortium for Integrative Medicine & Health, which consists of 71 academic medical centers and affiliate institutions in North America, defines integrative medicine as follows:

> Integrative medicine reaffirms the importance of the relationship between practitioner and patient, focuses on the whole person, is informed by evidence, and makes use of all appropriate therapeutic and lifestyle approaches, healthcare professionals and disciplines to achieve optimal health and healing.[6]

Integrative medicine emphasizes the centrality of the therapeutic relationship, the importance of prevention, and the healing power of nature. Integrative medicine seeks to use the best of scientifically based medical therapies along with compassion and attention to the patient's spiritual and emotional needs, as well as appropriate complementary approaches when they enhance conventional medicine.[7] Some argue that integrative medicine is simply good pediatric care.[8]

The NIH 2001 survey of 31,044 adults assessed and ranked the use of 5 categories of CIM: mind-body medicine, biologically based therapies, manipulative and body-based methods, alternative medical systems, and energy therapies. However, since 1996, pediatric clinicians have embraced a more synergistic model of 4 categories of integrative and complementary medicine and conventional therapies[9]: lifestyle (healthy habits in a healthy habitat), biochemical (medications and supplements), biomechanical (surgery, massage, and manipulative therapies), and bio-field (acupuncture, prayer, and homeopathy).

Lifestyle Strategies

Healthy lifestyle habits are the keys to good health throughout the life span. Healthy habits include

▶ Healthy nutrition

▶ Healthy physical activity

▶ Healthy sleep

▶ Healthy emotional and mental self-regulation

▶ Healthy social relationships

▶ Healthy environment (including avoiding toxins)

A healthy habitat refers to the physical, psychological, social, educational, and political environment. For example, music and spending time in nature offer therapeutic benefits to children of all ages.

This chapter will focus on healthy emotional and mental self-regulation. Although conventional care typically refers to mental and behavioral health, psychotherapy, and support groups, integrative care also includes mind-body strategies such as biofeedback, meditation, hypnosis, guided imagery, and yoga. The purpose of using these strategies is to achieve optimal mental and emotional health and enhance resilience.

Mind-body medicine includes all therapies that activate emotional, mental, spiritual, and behavioral factors to modulate positively physiologic mechanisms, including immune and endocrine function.[10] More than 35 years ago, Green et al stated that

> …every change in the physiologic state is accompanied by an appropriate change in the mental-emotional state, conscious or unconscious, and every change in the mental-emotional state is accompanied by an appropriate change in the physiologic state.[11]

The bidirectional influences of mind on body and body on mind can have significant mediating effects, both positive and negative, on health outcomes for children. In the past 20 years, mind-body therapies have become recognized as safe and effective for many pediatric conditions, including headaches, asthma, enuresis, sleep problems, pain, and stress-related symptoms.[12–18] These therapies may reduce autonomic hyperarousal, which may be of benefit in children with attention-deficit/hyperactivity disorder (ADHD).[19]

According to the NIH, spiritual and religious practices such as prayer represent the most prevalent complementary therapies in the United States. Nearly 80% of US adults believe religion helps patients and families cope with illness.[20] Nearly 75% of the public think that praying for someone else can help cure that person's illness, and 56% of adults state that faith has helped them recover from illness, injury, or disease.[20] Spirituality may or may not involve formal religion. Spiritual concerns arise in clinical settings when important connections with self, others, nature, or a higher power, or any combination of those connections, are threatened or disrupted. Spiritual beliefs are frequently important in medical decisions.[21] Spiritual well-being is closely linked to successful coping,[22] faster recovery,[23] and higher quality of life.[24] Many patients desire help with meaning, hope, or overcoming fears,[25] and unmet spiritual needs are associated with despair[26] and increased mortality.[27] Parents often have significant spiritual needs around the life-threatening illness or death of a child.[28]

A growing body of research has demonstrated the benefits of various kinds of meditative practices to train the mind and regulate the emotions, resulting in less pain and fewer symptoms in children and adults.[29] For example, training in mindfulness-based stress reduction and mindfulness-based cognitive behavioral therapy decreased psychological distress among adolescents with psychiatric disorders and decreased hostility and stress among adolescents and young adults living in urban communities.[30,31] Moving meditation practices such as tai chi and yoga can also improve behavior, mental health, physical symptoms, and physical fitness.[32]

Relaxation responses can be elicited by having patients repeat a word, phrase, sound, prayer, or muscular activity that has meaning for them. The patient should passively disregard intrusive thoughts that come to mind and return to the repetitive focus. Physiologic effects of the relaxation response include decreased metabolism, decreased rate of breathing, decreased blood pressure, decreased muscle tension, decreased heart rate, and increased slow brain waves.[33]

Creative arts or expressive therapies such as music, art, dance, drama, and poetry have been used in psychotherapy and counseling for more than 70 years. Art therapy is using visual arts materials and media in counseling and rehabilitation. Drama therapy is using drama and theater processes to achieve symptom relief, personal growth, or emotional and physical integration. Poetry and other literary forms can be used for healing and personal growth. Dance therapy has been shown to cause changes in feelings, cognition, physical functioning, and behavior. Nia, a sensory-based movement practice, initially stood for nonimpact aerobics, but it has evolved to include neurological integrative practices and teachings. Nia combines martial arts, modern dance arts, and yoga.[34] Child life and play therapists can be used to help children cope with illness or psychosocial difficulties.

Music and music therapy, that is, the intentional use of melody, rhythm, harmony, timbre, form, and style for healing, are important contributors to well-being. In preterm newborns and infants, music therapy can lower heart and respiratory rates, increase oxygen saturation, improve sleep patterns, improve sucking behaviors, improve caloric intake and weight gain, and decrease salivary cortisol and distress behaviors. Music can also significantly reduce the stress parents associate with preterm newborn and infant care.[35-39] In patients, intraoperatively and postoperatively, music reduces both pain and pharmaceutical requirements, including use of both sedatives and analgesics.[40,41] This outcome seems to be true for procedures as well.[42] In pediatric oncology patients, music therapy can reduce pain and suffering and improve both mood and attitude.[43-47] In intensive care units, music reduces patient anxiety and depression,[48-51] and for patients who are dying, music therapy has been shown to improve the quality of life.[52-54]

Many government agencies and national organizations have started to focus on the need for Americans to increase their physical activity levels. The American College of Sports Medicine has developed a global health initiative called Exercise is Medicine. Resources for participating in this initiative can be found at www.exerciseismedicine.org. The focus is encouraging all health care professionals to include physical activity in their treatment plans. The national physical activity guidelines for children and adolescents 6 to 17 years of age recommends 60 minutes of moderate to vigorous physical activity per day. Muscle strengthening activities should be included in the 60 minutes about 3 times per week. The AAP recommends no screen time for newborns, infants, and children younger than 2 years and no more than 2 hours per day for children older than 2 and adolescents. Bright Futures guidelines for physical activity of children can be found in Table 9-1.

Every patient should be assessed using the following physical activity vital sign:

1. On average, how many days per week do you engage in moderate to vigorous physical activity? _____ days per week

2. On average, how many minutes do you engage in physical activity at this level? _____ minutes per day

3. Total activity = days per week · minutes per day = _____ minutes per week

Table 9-1. Age-Appropriate Physical Activities		
Age	Motor Skills Being Developed	Appropriate Physical Activities
5–6 y	Fundamental: running, galloping, jumping, hopping, catching, skipping, throwing, catching, striking, kicking	Activities that focus on having fun and developing motor skills rather than competition Simple activities requiring little instruction Repetitive activities that do not require complex motor and cognitive skills
7–9 y	Fundamental transitional: throwing for distance or accuracy	Activities that focus on having fun and developing motor skills rather than competition Activities with flexible rules Activities that require little instruction Activities that do not require complex motor and cognitive skills
10–11 y	Transitional complex: playing basketball, soccer	Activities that continue to focus on having fun and developing motor skills Activities that require entry-level complex motor and cognitive skills Activities that continue to emphasize motor skill development but begin to incorporate instruction on strategy and teamwork

Reprinted with permission from Promoting physical activity. In: Hagan JF Jr, Shaw JS, Duncan PM, eds. *Bright Futures: Guidelines for Health Supervision of Infants, Children, and Adolescents*. 4th ed. Elk Grove Village, IL: American Academy of Pediatrics; 2017: 201.

Physical exercise has been found to decrease depressive symptoms; however, a study of children with untreated ADHD showed a blunted catecholamine response to exercise.[55,56]

Mind-body therapists may include physicians, psychologists, meditation instructors, nurses, social workers, chaplains, music therapists, and registered yoga teachers. Frequently, master's level and higher levels of education in these fields include training in one or more mind-body therapies. Formal graduate-level training is required for both chaplaincy and music therapy certification.

Biochemical Therapies

Biochemical therapies include both medications and natural products such as herbs, vitamins, and other supplements. Vitamin K is recommended for all newborns to prevent hemorrhagic disease of the newborn, and supplemental vitamin D is recommended for all exclusively breastfed newborns and infants.[57] The most recent data show that 46.2% of 1,280 interviewed adolescents had used dietary supplements in their lives, with 29.1% having used a supplement in the previous month. Nearly 10% of adolescents report using supplements with prescription medications in the previous month.[58] Teens are more likely to use supplements that claim to aid in weight loss, increase energy, and improve sports performance. About 10% of infants are given teas or botanical supplements and about 40% of children aged 2 to 8 are given dietary supplements.[59] Children with mental health concerns or chronic or recurrent illnesses often turn to herbs and other dietary supplements.[60–68]

The most frequently used supplements in children (aside from vitamins D and K) are multivitamins, single vitamins, and minerals (eg, vitamin C, iron, and calcium). The most frequently used herbal products in children include chamomile (most commonly *Matricaria chamomilla* or German chamomile and *Chamaemelum nobile* or Roman chamomile), peppermint (*Mentha x piperita*), echinacea (*Echinacea purpurea*, *Echinacea angustifolia*, and *Echinacea pallida*), and aromatherapies such as lavender (*Lavendula officinalis*). Commonly used dietary supplements are found in Table 9-2. Timothy Culbert, MD, former chair of Integrative Medicine at Children's Minnesota, collected data from 2005–2006 that showed the use of weight-loss supplements and creatine in adolescents is closely linked to attempts to change body shape. Vitamin and mineral

Table 9-2. Commonly Used Dietary Supplements (Nutraceuticals)		
Supplement	**Proposed Use**	**Comments**
5-HTP	Possibly: depression Insufficient evidence: anxiety, headaches, insomnia, ADHD, PMS	Risk of eosinophilia-myalgia syndrome
DHEA	Possibly: bipolar depression, depression in those with comorbid physical disease, aging skin Possibly ineffective: physical performance Likely ineffective: mental function	Hormone May cause mania in patients with mood disorder May lower HDL levels May worsen PCOS symptoms
EPA derived from krill oil	Possibly: unipolar and bipolar depression, borderline personality disorder, to decrease healing time Possibly ineffective: eclampsia, asthma, hypertension	Fatty acid found in cold-water fish
Fish oil (Ω-3 fatty acids)	Effective: to lower triglyceride levels, to raise HDL levels Likely: heart disease, autoimmune disease Possibly: ADHD, bipolar and unipolar depression, developmental coordination disorder, dysmenorrhea, dyspraxia, hypertension, psychosis Insufficient evidence: asthma, allergies	Some preparations are available by prescription.[a–c] High doses may decrease immune function.
Inositol	Possibly: panic disorder; OCD; psoriasis induced by lithium therapy; elevated cholesterol levels; PCOS Likely ineffective: diabetic neuropathy Insufficient evidence: ADHD	Vitamin-like substance thought to balance chemicals in the brain; high doses may worsen bipolar disorders.

272

Mental Health Care of Children and Adolescents: A Guide for Primary Care Clinicians

Table 9-2. Commonly Used Dietary Supplements (Nutraceuticals) (*continued*)		
Supplement	Proposed Use	Comments
Lithium orotate (low dose)	Possibly: reduces impulsive and aggressive behaviors	—
Methyl folate/folate	Likely: to reduce homocysteine levels Possibly: macular degeneration, depression, hypertension, gum disease As an adjunct, improved symptoms associated with depression and schizophrenia	High doses may increase risk of myocardial infarction, seizures, and cancer.[d]
Melatonin (*N*-acetyl-5-methoxytryptamine)	Likely: sleep disorder in patients with blindness; delayed sleep phase syndrome; sleep-wake cycle disturbance Possibly: endometriosis, hypertension, jet lag, anxiety Likely ineffective: depression	Fluvoxamine, sertraline, and OCPs can potentiate drowsiness; melatonin should be avoided, or dose decreased.
N-acetylcysteine	Acetaminophen OD, atelectasis Possibly: depression; to reduce homocysteine levels; flu symptoms; hair pulling	May slow blood clotting, may cause bronchospasm in people with asthma
SAMe	Depression, other mood disorders, arthritis	Naturally occurring in the body, acts similarly to noradrenergic antidepressants[d] Can induce mania in patients with bipolar disorders
Spirulina/phycocyanin	To reduce inflammation	Decreased LPS induced release of LDH and expression of TNF-α and IL-6[e]
Zinc	Likely: diarrhea, Wilson disease Possibly: insomnia, acne, ADHD, depression, URTI (to decrease duration of symptoms, not risk of), macular degeneration	High doses may cause fever, cough, stomach pain, fatigue. May increase risk of prostate cancer.

Table 9-2. Commonly Used Dietary Supplements (Nutraceuticals) (*continued*)

Abbreviations: 5-HTP, 5-hydroxytryptophan; ADHD, attention-deficit/hyperactivity disorder; DHEA, dehydroepiandrosterone; EPA, eicosapentaenoic acid; HDL, high-density lipoprotein; OCP, oral contraceptive pill; OCD, obsessive-compulsive disorder; OD, overdose; PCOS, polycystic ovary syndrome; PMS, premenstrual syndrome; LDH, lactate dehydrogenase; LPS, lipopolysaccharide; SAMe, *S*-adenosyl methionine; TNF-α, tumor necrosis factor-α; IL-6, interleukin-6; URTI, upper respiratory tract infection.

[a] Manor I, Magen A, Keidar D, et al. The effect of phosphatidylserine containing Omega3 fatty-acids on attention-deficit hyperactivity disorder symptoms in children: a double-blind placebo-controlled trial, followed by an open-label extension. *Eur Psychiatry*. 2012;27(5):335–342.

[b] Koski RR. Omega-3-acid ethyl esters (Lovaza) for severe hypertriglyceridemia. *P T*. 2008;33(5):271–303.

[c] Hirayama S, Terasawa K, Rabeler R, et al. The effect of phosphatidylserine administration on memory and symptoms of attention-deficit hyperactivity disorder: a randomised, double-blind, placebo-controlled clinical trial. *J Hum Nutr Diet*. 2014;27(suppl 2):284–291.

[d] Qureshi NA, Al-Bedah AM. Mood disorders and complementary and alternative medicine: a literature review. *Neuropsychiatr Dis Treat*. 2013;9:639–658.

[e] Chen JC, Liu KS, Yang TJ, Hwang JH, Chan YC, Lee IT. Spirulina and C-phycocyanin reduce cytotoxicity and inflammation-related genes expression of microglial cells. *Nutr Neurosci*. 2012;15(6):252–256.

Data from WebMD. Vitamins and supplements center. https://www.webmd.com/vitamins-supplements/default.aspx. Accessed February 7, 2018.

deficiencies can cause significant symptoms, but some holistic providers are recommending high doses even with normal levels. Vitamin D regulates calcium metabolism and may play a role in chronic inflammatory conditions such as autoimmune disorders.[69] Vitamin D deficiencies have been associated with fatigue and depression.[70,71] Vitamin B_{12} deficiency can lead to megaloblastic anemia, and it can have serious neurological consequences.[72] Low levels of vitamin B_{12}, vitamin B_6, iron, zinc, and folate have been linked to depression.[73,74] Low vitamin B_{12}, vitamin D, and folate levels are also associated with poor memory and cognitive dysfunction.[74] Low total serum cholesterol levels have been associated with a higher risk of depression, suicidality, impulsivity, and aggression.[75,76]

Since the passage of the Dietary Supplement Health and Education Act (DSHEA) of 1994, supplements have been regulated by the US Food and Drug Administration (FDA) with requirements more akin to foods than drugs. Good Manufacturing Practice regulations are identical to those for food. Unlike food and drugs, dietary supplements can be sold without premarket approval and do not require a specific post-marketing study. Companies do not have to prove that a supplement will do what is claimed, or even that it contains what it is supposed to contain. Supplements can be sold on the basis of evidence of safety in the possession of the manufacturer. Supplements can be removed from the market only if the FDA can prove them to be unsafe under ordinary conditions of use. This removal occurred in April 2004 when the FDA banned the sympathomimetic herb ephedra (*Ephedra sinica* and related plants), which had been widely marketed for weight reduction. A Utah judge overturned the ban in April 2005, but in August 2006 the US Court of Appeals upheld the ban. The FDA issued a recommendation in October 2010, and then again in September 2016, warning consumers on the use of homeopathic teething tablets and gels. The concern revolves around the use of belladonna (*Atropa belladonna*) in these products and the possibility of varied amounts of this ingredient. Hyland's is no longer distributing their teething tablets in the United States. CVS has voluntarily withdrawn all brands of teething tablets sold in their stores and online.

Under DSHEA, herbal medicines can be sold for *stimulating, maintaining, supporting, regulating,* and *promoting health* rather than for treating disease. As dietary supplements rather than drugs, herbal medicines may not claim to restore normal function or to correct abnormal function. Additionally, herbs may not claim to *diagnose, treat, prevent, cure,* or *mitigate.* For example, an herbal medicine company can assert that its product supports cardiovascular health but not that it lowers cholesterol levels. To do so would suggest that the product is for treating a disease (hypercholesterolemia) and is therefore subject to FDA pharmaceutical regulations. However, most herbs are used by the public for the treatment of a disease or symptoms of a disease (Table 9-3). Only functional foods (eg, oat bran, soy, cranberries, certain processed butter-like spreads) can claim specific health benefits. Such approvals require significant supporting clinical data and FDA approval.

Licensed practitioners who promote herbal medicine use include naturopaths and chiropractors for whom advanced training often exists as part of their degree programs or continuing education programs. Not all naturopaths, however, are graduates of accredited naturopathic medical schools. Reliable resources (Box 9-1) describing herbal medicine and supplements are useful.

Biomechanical Therapies

Manipulative and body-based methods include all therapies that focus on manipulation and movement of one or more parts of the body. The

Table 9-3. Claimed Benefits of Commonly Used Herbal Therapies

Common Name (Latin Name)	Common Uses	Comments
Aloe (*Aloe vera*)	Burns, minor wounds, skin irritations, aphthous stomatitis, constipation, gastric and duodenal ulcers	—
Astragalus (*Astragalus* species)	Immune booster	—
Bergamot oil (*Citrus bergamia*)	Anxiolytic, promoted to boost mood	Comparative study with diazepam.[a] Effects of blend with lavender oil.[b]
Calendula (*Calendula officinalis*)	Skin soother	—
Cascara (*Rhamnus purshiana*)	Constipation	Cramps, diarrhea; long-term use can cause dehydration and electrolyte disturbances.
Cayenne (*Capsicum frutescens*)	Topical treatment for pain and postherpetic neuralgia, as nasal spray for headaches	Ingestion can cause vomiting and diarrhea; topically, can cause swelling.
Chamomile (*Matricaria recutita*)	Sedative, anti-inflammatory, antispasmodic, may soothe mouth ulcers; colic	Drowsiness; vomiting in large doses
Clove oil (*Syzygium aromaticum*)	Teething pain	—
Coffee (*Coffea* species)	Stimulant, ADHD, bronchodilator	—

Table 9-3. Claimed Benefits of Commonly Used Herbal Therapies (*continued*)

Common Name (Latin Name)	Common Uses	Comments
Curcumin (the family Zingiberaceae)	Anti-inflammatory, antioxidant	From turmeric
Dandelion (*Taraxacum officinale*)	Mild diuretic, liver tonic	—
Dill (*Anethum graveolens*)	Antispasmodic, promoted to provide colic relief and decrease flatulence	—
Echinacea (*Echinacea* species)	Immune stimulation, anti-inflammatory	—
Ephedra (ma huang) (*Ephedra* species)	Vasoconstriction; allergy; URTI; asthma; appetite suppressant	Banned by FDA, NCAA, NFL, and IOC
Eucalyptus (*Eucalyptus* species)	Oil can be used on scalp for lice but must be diluted.	*Eucalyptus smithii* is least toxic; high concentrations can cause vomiting, lethargy, and seizures.[c]
Evening primrose oil (*Oenothera biennis*)	Eczema, PMS	—
Fennel (*Foeniculum vulgare*)	Colic, promoted to decrease flatulence	—
Fenugreek (*Trigonella foenum-graecum*)	Promoted to increase milk supply for breastfeeding mothers	—
Feverfew (*Tanacetum parthenium*)	Migraines, rheumatoid arthritis	—

Garlic (*Allium sativum*)	Antimicrobial, cholesterol level lowering	—
Geranium oil (*Pelargonium graveolens*)	Promoted to balance hormones, elevates mood, skin care	—
Ginger (*Zingiber officinale*)	Antiemetic, anti-nauseant	—
Ginkgo (*Ginkgo biloba*)	Promoted to enhance blood flow past clogged arteries, prevent memory loss, and treat ADHD and depression	—
Ginseng (*Panax* species)	Stimulant, adaptogen; promoted to enhance endurance and performance	—
Hawthorn (*Crataegus oxyacantha*)	Cardiac stimulant, promoted to enhance cardiac contractility	—
Hops (*Humulus lupulus*)	Sedative	—
Jasmine oil (*Jasminium* species)	Relaxation, balances mood, abdominal pain	—
Kava kava (*Piper methysticum*)	Anxiolytic	—
Lavender (*Lavendula* species)	Sedative, antimicrobial; promoted to alleviate anxiety, balance gut microflora, and alleviate headaches	Effects of blend with bergamot oil.[b] Study comparing inhaled oil vs placebo in patients with migraines.[d]

Table 9-3. Claimed Benefits of Commonly Used Herbal Therapies (*continued*)		
Common Name (Latin Name)	Common Uses	Comments
Lemon balm (*Melissa officinalis*)	Sedative, colic, menstrual cramps, nausea, anxiety	—
Licorice (*Glycyrrhiza* species)	Anti-inflammatory, antiviral, demulcent	—
Milk thistle (*Silybum marianum*)	Hepatic protection against cirrhosis and hepatitis	—
Neroli oil (*Citrus aurantium*)	Improves mood, anxiety, stress headaches, sleep, skin care	—
Oats (*Avena sativa*)	Antipruritic; eczema, varicella	—
Peppermint (*Mentha* × *piperita*)	Headaches, promoted to improve IBS symptoms	Shown to have cooling effect, increase blood flow, and inhibit 5-HTP.[c] No significant difference found in comparison to peppermint oil vs acetaminophen in tension headaches.[e] Extensively studied for use in patients with IBS.[f]
Pine bark extract (*Pinus* species)	Antioxidant, promoted to improve focus	—
Rhubarb root (*Rheum officinale*)	Constipation, chronic renal failure	—
Siberian golden root (*Rhodiola rosea*)	May improve menopausal symptoms, elevate mood; mild stimulant	Evidence for use in the treatment of mood disorders.[g]

Saffron (*Crocus sativus*)	Depression, PMS, cough	—
St John's wort (*Hypericum perforatum*)	Depression, antiviral, anxiety, fatigue, insomnia, somatization disorder, wound healing	May make OCPs less effective. Use in patients with mood disorders.[9]
Skullcap (*Scutellaria species*)	Sedative	—
Slippery elm bark (*Ulmus fulva*)	Demulcent; pharyngitis	—
Stinging nettle (*Urtica dioica, Urtica urens*)	Hay fever	—
Sweet basil (*Ocimum basilicum*, linalool chemotype)	Antimicrobial, anti-inflammatory, antioxidant	Estragole chemotype (exotic basil) is carcinogenic.
Tea tree oil (*Melaleuca alternifolia*)	Topical antimicrobial; promoted to treat acne, minor skin infections (including fungal and yeast infections), and lice	—
Thyme (*Thymus vulgaris*)	Antimicrobial, expectorant; promoted to treat colds, sore throats, and cough	—
Valerian (*Valeriana officinalis*)	Sedative, sleep disorders and insomnia	—

Table 9-3. Claimed Benefits of Commonly Used Herbal Therapies (*continued*)

Common Name (Latin Name)	Common Uses	Comments
Witch hazel (*Hamamelis virginiana*)	Antiseptic (topical), anti-inflammatory	—
Ylang ylang oil (*Cananga odorata*)	Promoted to help with anger, fear, mood, insomnia, and stress	—

Abbreviations: 5-HTP, 5-hydroxytryptophan; ADHD, attention-deficit/hyperactivity disorder; FDA, US Food and Drug Administration; IBS, irritable bowel syndrome; IOC, International Olympic Committee; NCAA, National Collegiate Athletic Association; NFL, National Football League; OCP, oral contraceptive pill; PMS, premenstrual syndrome; URTI, upper respiratory tract infection.

[a] Saiyudthong S, Marsden CA. Acute effects of bergamot oil on anxiety-related behaviour and corticosterone level in rats. *Phytother Res*. 2011;25(6):858–862.

[b] Hongratanaworakit T. Aroma-therapeutic effects of massage blended essential oils on humans. *Nat Prod Commun*. 2011;6(8):1199–1204.

[c] Göbel H, Schmidt G, Dworschak M, Stolze H, Heuss D. Essential plant oils and headache mechanisms. *Phytomedicine*. 1995;2(2):93–102.

[d] Sasannejad P, Saeedi M, Shoeibi A, Gorji A, Abbasi M, Foroughipour M. Lavender essential oil in the treatment of migraine headache: a placebo-controlled clinical trial. *Eur Neurol*. 2012;67(5):288–291.

[e] Göbel H, Fresenius J, Heinze A, Dworschak M, Soyka D. [Effectiveness of oleum menthae piperitae and paracetamol in therapy of headache of the tension type]. *Nervenarzt*. 1996;67(8):672–681.

[f] National Center for Complementary and Integrative Health. Peppermint oil. National Center for Complementary and Integrative Health Web site. https://nccih.nih.gov/health/peppermintoil. Updated December 1, 2016. Accessed February 7, 2018.

[g] Qureshi NA, Al-Bedah AM. Mood disorders and complementary and alternative medicine: a literature review. *Neuropsychiatr Dis Treat*. 2013;9:639–658.

Data from WebMD. Vitamins and supplements center. https://www.webmd.com/vitamins-supplements/default.aspx. Accessed February 7, 2018.

Box 9-1. Web Resources for Herbal Medicines and Dietary Supplements

- American Botanical Council (www.herbalgram.org)
- Consumer Lab (www.consumerlab.com)
- Memorial Sloan Kettering Cancer Center "About Herbs" (www.mskcc.org/cancer-care/integrative-medicine/about-herbs)
- Natural Medicines Comprehensive Database (www.naturaldatabase.com)
- Natural Medicines (https://naturalmedicines.therapeuticresearch.com)
- National Library of Medicine MedlinePlus (www.nlm.nih.gov/medlineplus)
- NIH Office of Dietary Supplements (www.ods.od.nih.gov)
- US Pharmacopeia (www.usp.org)
- Cochrane Complementary Medicine (http://cam.cochrane.org)
- Vintage Remedies Learning Center (https://vintageremedies.com)
- Franklin Institute of Wellness (https://franklininstituteofwellness.com)
- Herbs and Dietary Supplements Across the Lifespan (https://herbs-supplements.osu.edu)
- Vitamins and Supplements Center (http://www.webmd.com/vitamins-supplements/default.aspx)
- Herbs2000 (www.herbs2000.com)

Abbreviation: NIH, National Institutes of Health.

---

best-known examples are chiropractic, osteopathic, and massage. All examples incorporate touch, an essential human need with therapeutic, interpersonal, and cultural dimensions. Massage is one of the oldest health care practices and was used in ancient times in India, China, Arabia, Egypt, and Greece. Experience at one of the largest pediatric CIM programs at a children's hospital in the Midwest suggests that massage and other forms of bodywork are among the most popular options, either inpatient or outpatient, selected by children and teens.[77-81] Similar observations have been documented in pediatric oncology patients[82] and adolescents.[83] Massage may be provided most often by parents or other family members. The appropriate amount of massage has not yet been measured, but family members frequently appreciate the chance to learn a skill that can contribute to the comfort and well-being of the patient.

Massage can also include many different techniques and forms that require more significant training, including structural integration (Rolfing), movement integration (eg, Feldenkrais method and Alexander technique), pressure point techniques (shiatsu and acupressure), cranial sacral therapy, reflexology, myofascial release (commonly known as MFR) and others.

The manipulation, compression, and stretching of the skin, muscles, and joints activates a variety of mechanisms that support and promote health, including

▶ Mechanical: Enhances blood flow to the muscles and soft tissues and enhances lymphatic flow.[84]

▶ Immunologic: Enhances specific immune cell functions such as natural killer cell activity.[85]

▶ Neurological: Triggers relaxation response and lowers sympathetic nervous system arousal, reduces serum cortisol levels, enhances endogenous serotonin and dopamine levels,[86] and modulates pain perception.[87]

▶ Energetic: According to traditional thought, certain massage practices can provide balance and improve the flow of life force energy, or chi.

Massage can be enhanced with a biochemical therapy, that is, aromatherapy, the therapeutic application of essential oils distilled from plants. Specific scents are targeted to specific symptoms, such as lavender or chamomile for relaxation, ginger (*Zingiber officinale*) or spearmint (*Mentha spicata*) for nausea, and peppermint or lemon for fatigue.

Chiropractors are licensed in all 50 states, and their services are widely covered by insurance, including Medicaid. Most chiropractic schools offer courses in pediatric care. Chiropractors can receive extra training and certification in pediatrics. Chiropractors can use special pediatric tables and gentle techniques, or they can treat the children in their parents' laps. Massage therapists are also licensed in all 50 states, but training and licensure requirements are quite variable. The largest professional national organization of bodyworkers is the American Massage Therapy Association. Membership requires training in an accredited school and completion of 500 hours of training.

Bio-field Therapies

Bio-field therapies include practices that invoke, stimulate, or alter an invisible energy, spirit, or information to achieve a health goal. In conventional medicine, radiation therapy is used to treat cancer and invisible rays are used to diagnose illnesses with radiographs and ultrasound. In Asian cultures, an invisible energy or life force is known as chi, which can be affected by acupuncture and related practices. In some religious and secular traditions, healing energy can be sent by prayer, good wishes, the laying on of hands, therapeutic touch, healing touch, or reiki. In homeopathy, an original compound that causes a symptom is diluted so much that what remains has energy or information to combat that symptom.

Among major teaching hospitals that have a pediatric pain service, 33% offer acupuncture therapy to treat pain.[88] Additional indications may include constipation[89] and traumatic brain injury.[90] Acupuncture is quite safe,[91] even with cancer-associated thrombocytopenia,[92] and can be an effective and well-accepted intervention with children and teens. Use of the term *acu-point stimulation* may prevent eliciting fear of needles. Acu-point stimulation can be achieved by massage, comfortable electrical stimulation, stickers with beads, or very thin (>30 gauge) non-hollow acupuncture needles. In many instances, after the acupuncturist gradually establishes comfort and trust with a noninvasive approach, children and teens will agree to needle insertion. Acupuncture, when done correctly, is virtually painless and well tolerated for older children.[93]

Acupuncturists are licensed in more than 40 states. In most states, licensed health care professionals such as physicians can practice acupuncture. Insurance plans increasingly offer acupuncture for chronic pain and chemotherapy-induced nausea and vomiting.

Therapeutic Touch

Therapeutic touch, healing touch, and reiki are all secular forms of laying-on-of-hands healing. Actual touching of the patient does not always take place because the human energy field, like the electromagnetic field, extends beyond the skin into the space surrounding the body. Therapeutic touch was invented in the 1970s by a New York University nursing professor, Dolores Krieger, and a lay healer, Dora Kunz. On the basis of their observations of numerous religious healers, they distilled the process into

5 steps that practitioners might bring to healing outside of a specific religious faith or belief. These steps are

1. Having a clear and conscious intent to be helpful and heal

2. Being centered in a peaceful state of mind

3. Using hands to assess the patient's energy (typically moving the hands 3 to 8 cm [1–3 in] away from the body in a slow downward sweep from the head to the toes)

4. Using hands to help restore the patient's energy to a balanced, harmonious, peaceful state

5. Releasing the patient to complete the healing process while the healer returns to the healer's own centered, peaceful state of mind

Nurses and other health care professionals in more than 80 countries have received training in therapeutic touch from its founders. It is currently taught in nursing schools across the United States. Nursing practice in many hospitals, including children's hospitals, includes policies and procedures for performing therapeutic touch.

Additional techniques have been added to therapeutic touch in a group of treatments called healing touch, which is largely practiced by holistic nurses. Small studies have suggested that healing touch can help decrease stress and improve autonomic balance in pediatric oncology patients.[94]

Reiki is a similar practice that comes from a Japanese tradition. Practitioners are trained by a reiki master through apprenticeship and spiritual and energetic initiation. Neither therapeutic touch nor reiki has national certifying examinations or state licensure. Therapeutic touch and healing touch are typically provided by nurses in both inpatient settings and outpatient settings. Reiki is typically provided by lay practitioners outside of medical settings. No reports of adverse effects have been documented from such treatments. The primary clinical benefits of therapeutic touch are increased relaxation, diminished anxiety, diminished pain, and enhanced sense of well-being.[95–98]

In addition to therapeutic touch and reiki, some practitioners use electromagnetic or static magnet fields to reduce pain or speed healing. For example, pulsed electromagnetic fields are used to promote union of long-bone fractures.[99] There is growing research on the use of pulsed electromagnetic fields for fracture and wound healing in pediatrics.[100,101] Growing research also supports the use of static magnetic fields to reduce pain and inflammation.[102–104]

Homeopathy

Homeopathy is a system of medical treatment invented in the early 1800s by the German physician Samuel Hahnemann. Homeopathy was frequently taught and practiced in US medical schools until criticized in the 1910 Flexner Report. Currently, homeopathy is popular in Europe, Russia, India, and South America.

Homeopathy is based on 2 principles: the *Law of Similars* or *like cures like* and the *Law of Dilutions.* The Law of Similars means that a remedy that would cause a symptom in a healthy person is used to treat the same symptom in a sick person. For example, a treatment or *remedy,* made from the poison ivy plant (*Rhus toxicodendron*) might be used to treat a child with eczema. Although pediatric clinicians might be concerned about dangerous-sounding homeopathic medications such as belladonna, serious adverse effects from homeopathic treatment are exceedingly rare, far less common than adverse effects from standard over-the-counter and prescription medications.

Homeopathy's safety is attributable to homeopathy's second principle, the Law of Dilutions, which states that the more a remedy is diluted, the more powerful it becomes. Dilutions of 1 to 10 are designated by the roman numeral X ($1X = 1/10$, $3X = 1/1,000$, $6X = 1/1,000,000$). Similarly, dilutions of 1 to 100 are designated by the roman numeral C ($1C = 1/100$, $3C = 1/1,000,000$, and so on). Most remedies today range from 6X to 30X, but some products are as dilute as 200C. Dilutions beyond 12X or 24C contain none of the original molecules. Common over-the-counter remedies include combination products for teething, colic, allergies, and bed-wetting.

Homeopaths think that these highly dilute solutions contain an energy, or information, that the patient uses to heal symptoms. Many clinicians think that the remedies are placebos that trigger the patient's psychoneuroimmunologic healing systems. Randomized controlled trials suggest some support for homeopathic remedies for diarrhea[105] and otitis media[106] but not for ADHD.[107]

The private, nonprofit Council for Homeopathy Certification reviews homeopathic programs. Certification in homeopathy is given after testing by the council. The American Institute of Homeopathy and American Board of Homeotherapeutics certifies physicians. Nonphysicians are registered with the North American Society of Homeopaths.

Talking With Patients About Complementary and Integrative Medicine

Although many pediatric clinicians are concerned that families who use CIM may be dissatisfied with mainstream medical care and fear they may abandon effective therapies in favor of unproved alternatives, data do not support these concerns. Fifty-five percent of all surveyed adults think that CIM therapies would support health when used with conventional medical treatments.[108] For the most part, families seek therapies that are consistent with their respective values, worldviews, and cultures, and they seek care from therapists who respect them as individuals and who offer them time and attention.[109,110] Families continue to highly value the care they receive from compassionate, comprehensive primary care clinicians (PCCs) (ie, pediatricians, family physicians, internists, nurse practitioners, and physician assistants at the front lines of pediatric health care), and they seek additional information on healthy lifestyles, dietary supplements, and environmental therapies over which they may exert some control.[111] They also seek care from therapists who offer personal attention, hope, time, and therapies that are consistent with their cultures and values. Families who seek out CIM therapies rarely abandon their PCCs, but they may not feel comfortable discussing these therapies if they perceive the PCC to be antagonistic or judgmental toward them.

To provide the best care, pediatric clinicians should ask all patients about all therapies they use to promote health. This task is best accomplished in a seamless, structured, and nonjudgmental manner during the medical interview. To set a positive tone, the clinician can begin new patient interviews with questions about the number of meals eaten together as a family, fun things the family does together, hopes and dreams for the child, and aspects of the child of which they are most proud. At each return visit, a helpful question would be, "Since the last visit, which other health care professionals has your child visited?" As with all good interviewing, listening for understanding rather than agreement or disagreement enhances the therapeutic alliance.

Social History

During the social history, the clinician should inquire about

- ▶ Diet, exercise, and environment (including use of music to manage stress) to provide insight about risks and actions taken to promote health
- ▶ Illness care at home
- ▶ Any special foods, teas, rubs, prayers, or rituals that are helpful for the patient's family
- ▶ Any mind-body therapies to manage stress, reduce chronic symptoms, or promote well-being, such as deep breathing, yoga, meditation, or prayer

One such question might be, "When you are stressed, what is most helpful for you? Which of your activities do you find is best for your health?" To assess psychological wellness, stress and time management, self-esteem, and self-concept, a thorough academic history and questions about learning style, friends, hobbies, and extracurricular activities should be included.

Questions regarding spirituality can be inserted at this point in the inquiry, as appropriate. Several mnemonics exist to guide clinicians in their interviews to understand the patient's or family's source of meaning, purpose, richness, and direction (an example is given in Box 9-2). Conscious choices expressed in the social history represent strengths that can be used for achieving health goals. Clearly, ethical boundaries exist around faith and spirituality. The clinician's role is not to provide answers but to support the search for answers.

This point of the inquiry is also the time for assessing all potential environmental factors contributing to health and illness in children.[112] A useful mnemonic for an environmental history is ACHHOO, with each letter representing a potential exposure site to known toxins, such as lead, mercury, secondhand tobacco smoke, pesticides, and other contaminants.

Box 9-2. Spiritual Assessment Tool

HOPE

H: Hope—What are your sources of hope, meaning, strength, peace, love, and connection? What do you hold onto during difficult times?

O: Organization—Do you consider yourself part of an organized religion? How important is this to you?

P: Personal spirituality and practices—What aspects of your spirituality or spiritual practices do you find most helpful?

E: Effects—How do your beliefs affect the kind of medical care you would like me to provide?

Adapted with permission from Anandarajah G, Hight E. Spirituality and medical practice: using the HOPE questions as a practical tool for spiritual assessment. *Am Fam Physician.* 2001;63(1):81–89.

► Activities

► Community

► Household

► Hobbies

► Occupation

► Oral behaviors

Allergies and Current and Past Medications

When documenting current and past medication use, additional questions to ask in routine practice include

1. Do you use multivitamins, for example, Poly-Vi-Sol or Flintstones chewable vitamins?

2. Do you use over-the-counter medications, for example, any medications for colds, pain, or constipation?

3. Do you use herbal medicines, for example, any herbs such as echinacea or chamomile?

4. Do you take specific vitamins and minerals, for example, vitamin C, D, or E? Do you take any mineral supplements, such as calcium, iron, magnesium, or selenium?

5. Do you take dietary supplements, for example, any supplements such as fish oils, melatonin, or probiotics?

Follow-up questions include

▶ What brand?

▶ What dose?

▶ How often?

▶ What directions are you following?

▶ What goals are you hoping to achieve by taking it?

▶ Are you using any other remedies now?

Understanding the supplements used and the patient's or family's source of information for making treatment decisions can be quite helpful for comprehending what is important to the family.

Interviewing for supplement use is crucial for identifying patients who are at risk for interactions with prescription medications or for excessive bleeding in surgery. Too frequently, professionals and patients follow a *don't ask, don't tell* policy. *Ask, provide an example, and then ask again* is a practice policy that is foundational to safe and effective patient care. Patients should be asked to bring all remedies with them to every visit so the chart can be updated and use monitored. Patients with special risks of drug interactions include those who take anticoagulants, hypoglycemics, antidepressants, sedative-hypnotics, antihypertensives, and medications with narrow therapeutic windows, such as digoxin and theophylline.

Medical History

In addition to immunizations, surgeries, and hospitalizations, the interview for the medical history is a good time to ask about other therapies that often require multiple visits, such as chiropractic, massage, and acupuncture. Understanding what worked or did not work for the patient provides further insights into what is important for the patient and family. Additionally, questioning during this portion of the inquiry can help identify health issues that may be important to address in the context of a holistic approach to health.

Counseling Families About Complementary and Integrative Medicine

The goal of counseling is to strengthen the clinician-patient relationship through honest dialogue that is clinically responsible, ethically appropriate, and legally defensible. Parental inclusion of CIM therapies for their children, in and of itself, does not constitute child neglect.[113] Similarly, clinician provision of complementary and integrative therapies does not, in itself, represent professional misconduct.

Increasingly, pediatric clinicians will find themselves sharing patients with massage therapists, chiropractors, acupuncturists, and others. Pediatric patient advocacy requires assessing for safety and efficacy and respecting the autonomy of the parent-child relationship. When patients or families report seeing other health care professionals and describe current CIM use, clinicians should follow 3 steps in response to the answers provided.

Step 1. Determine whether the therapy represents a rejection of standard care for a serious or life-threatening disease for which a reasonable chance exists of cure or if use of the therapy will delay proven treatment. In such cases, the first step is to protect the child while understanding the parents' goals. Reporting requirements for abuse and neglect may apply.

Step 2. Determine whether the therapies used are known to be unsafe, ineffective, or both. Excellent Web-based resources include "Are You Considering a Complementary Health Approach?" (https://nccih.nih.gov/health/decisions/consideringcam.htm) and "Integrative Therapies" (http://ccw.columbia.edu).

In the event of use of a known toxic agent or an ineffective agent with possible harm, the clinician's responsibility is to counsel from the documented evidence that the therapy should be stopped. Resistance to such advice may place the parents at risk for charges of negligence or abuse.

In the absence of data on toxicity or efficacy, the clinician's role is to monitor as clinically appropriate. This role can include scheduling telephone follow-up or office visits. In both cases, document the following information in the medical record:

▶ Therapy used and the goal of the therapy.

▶ Patient or family preferences and expectations regarding the therapy.

▶ Provider of the therapy, location, and treatment plan (as known by the family). This information should include names, telephone numbers, any other contact information, and specialties.

▶ Review of the safety and efficacy issues of the therapy from the medical literature.

▶ Results of counseling, including the pediatric clinician's treatment plan for monitoring the treatment and its results.

▶ Advice provided or resources recommended for further information.

Step 3. Ensure that the patient's or family's decision to use a therapy is based on a fully informed judgment and that their verbal consent was obtained and documented. This documentation includes what options have been discussed, offered, tried, or refused. (General guidelines for counseling are found in Box 9-3.) Counseling on spiritual concerns requires special consideration for clinical and ethical reasons. Although clinicians talking with patients about spirituality is not classically part of medical training, adults in the United States consistently report that it is appropriate.[114,115] Eighty-three percent of 921 primary care patients surveyed in Ohio reported that they wanted physicians to ask about spiritual beliefs in certain circumstances, such as with serious illness or the loss of loved ones.[116]

Spirituality may be understood as connection with a higher power. Spirituality may or may not include formal religion. Spiritual concerns arise with threatened losses or disruptions of such connections. These issues can include key relationships with parents, other family members, and friends or can include what the child thinks God to be. For efficient and effective clinical care when spiritual issues are present, the following guidelines should be kept in mind:

1. Anticipate the presence of spiritual concerns with every illness. These concerns can include those of the patient, the family, and the care team members, as well as one's own concerns.

> **Box 9-3. How to Talk With Patients About Complementary and Integrative Therapies**
>
> ❶ *Do* talk about the different kinds of therapies families may have tried to help their children.
>
> ❷ *Do not* wait for families to bring it up.
>
> ❸ Ask in an open-minded, nonjudgmental fashion. Avoid using potentially pejorative terms such as *unproved, unconventional,* or *alternative.*
>
> ❹ Elicit further information with questions about specific therapies. For example, "Have you tried any *herbal* therapies, such as echinacea or ginkgo?" "Have you tried any *dietary* therapies, such as avoiding wheat or milk?" "Have you sought care from any *other health care professionals,* such as acupuncturists or chiropractors?"
>
> ❺ Elicit the values, beliefs, and influences that led parents to these therapies. For example, were these suggested by family members? Were they consistent with the parents' religious, spiritual, or cultural beliefs? What is the value of natural or organic approaches? Do they have a fear of adverse effects of mainstream treatments?
>
> ❻ Whenever possible, join with the parents and support their decision to pursue avenues that may help their child. Be an ally rather than a tyrant.
>
> ❼ Ask how well the family thinks the therapies worked or did not work *before* offering your opinion.
>
> ❽ Offer to talk with other therapists involved in the child's care to maintain coordinated, comprehensive care.
>
> ❾ Offer to learn more to help answer the family's questions.
>
> ❿ Offer families additional information and resources to address their questions about complementary and integrative therapies.

2. Comprehend how the patient's or family's faith or spirituality can be a resource during illness.

3. Seek to understand how the patient's or family's cultural and spiritual worldview influence understanding of the disease, the appropriate treatment, and the recovery process.

4. Determine what effect, positive or negative, the patient's or family's spiritual orientation or interpretation has on perceived needs.

5. Partner with, and refer to, chaplains or the patient's or family's preferred spiritual care provider for assistance with significant spiritual concerns.

To achieve these goals, open-ended questions are always helpful. The clinician should create a safe environment in which patients and families can articulate their questions. For spiritual concerns, solving problems and providing answers are rarely helpful. The best answers are found rather than given. The clinician's role is to support the search for answers.

How to Partner With Other Practitioners

Because of increasing interest and evidence of safety and efficacy, pediatric clinicians will want to partner with and refer to a growing number of diverse practitioners. This task is quite easy when credentialed practitioners exist in conventional settings such as hospital-based integrative pediatric clinics or consultation services. Some communities will have networking opportunities for providers interested in more holistic or integrative care. When a pediatric clinician provides the therapy, or refers to practitioners in the community, the State Medical Board Guidelines apply.[113] Key points include documenting the following information in the medical record:

1. Parity of evaluation (medical history and physical examination as thorough as for conventional care).

2. Informed consent (review of diagnosis and all medical options for that diagnosis; discussion of risks and benefits of the recommended treatment, including potential interference with ongoing conventional care; and disclosure and discussion of any applicable financial interests).

3. Treatment plan objectives and goals (expected favorable outcomes and monitoring plan for duration of treatment). Pediatric clinicians should refer only to licensed or otherwise state-regulated health care practitioners with the requisite training and skills to use the therapy being recommended. Clinicians are expected to not sell, rent, or lease health-related products or engage in personal branding. Clinicians must also be able to demonstrate a basic understanding of the medical scientific knowledge connected with any recommended therapy.

Clinicians are not liable for any negligence on the part of another provider unless the clinician's referral to the other provider delayed necessary conventional treatment, the referring clinician knew the provider was not competent to provide the therapy, or the clinician employed the provider or provided joint treatment with the provider.[113]

When referring children with complex chronic illness, chronic pain, or mental health conditions, pediatric clinicians must carefully prioritize and schedule necessary conventional therapies. They must also coordinate care with all subspecialists. It is equally important for pediatric clinicians to consider the effect on time and expenses of families who are vulnerable as they seek any available therapies for their children. The clinician should set appropriate expectations, support appropriate hope, and avoid over-scheduling and overtreating children.

Clinician Self-care

An important part of caring for patients is caring for self. Contrary to what clinicians may have been told most of their careers, caring for self is not selfish. It is difficult to give to others if we do not take care of ourselves. According to Lisa Chu, MD, there are 5 principles of self-care.

1. Establish boundaries. Take responsibility only for your role in your own reality.

2. Move from reactive to creative mode. Affirm your sense of self before reacting to others.

3. Listen to your body, your intuition, and your experience. Listen to your whole being, not just your knowledge.

4. Find out what restores you. Restorative activities engage the body and mind and can result in freedom and joy. Listening to your inner voice will lead you to new experiences.

5. Give yourself permission to feel good and to want what you want. It may take time and practice to allow yourself to feel good. Health care professionals have long been trained to put everyone else's needs before their own.[117]

Pamela Wible, MD, is a physician who speaks and writes about physician self-care. She speaks out about the tragedy of physician suicide and how it can be prevented. There are many resources on her Web site: www.idealmedicalcare.org.

Conclusion

Increasingly, the public expects pediatric clinicians to provide wise counsel on all reasonable available therapies and to appropriately refer based on scientific evidence and families' values and goals. There are many opportunities for pediatric clinicians to seek additional training to enhance their clinical practice (Box 9-4). The AAP, the NIH, and many other organizations provide additional resources to support pediatric service excellence.

Box 9-4. Educational Opportunities in Complementary and Integrative Medicine

Hypnosis and Biofeedback

- American Society of Clinical Hypnosis (www.asch.net)
- Association for Applied Psychophysiology and Biofeedback (www.aapb.org)
- Biofeedback Certification International Alliance (formerly Biofeedback Certification Institute of America) (www.bcia.org)
- National Pediatric Hypnosis Training Institute (www.nphti.net)
- Society for Developmental and Behavioral Pediatrics (www.sdbp.org)

Meditation

- The Center for Mind-Body Medicine (www.cmbm.org)
- Center for Mindfulness in Medicine, Health Care, and Society (www.umassmed.edu/cfm)
- Mind-Body Medical Institute (www.mbmi.org)
- "Prevention and Treatment of Stress-Related Disorders Through the Transcendental Meditation Technique" (http://scientiacme.org/cmecoursecontent.php?ID=164)
- American Meditation Institute (http://americanmeditation.org)

Spirituality

- The George Washington Institute for Spirituality and Health (www.gwish.org)

Acupuncture

- American Academy of Medical Acupuncture (www.medicalacupuncture.org)
- Helms Medical Institute (www.hmieducation.com)

> **Box 9-4. Educational Opportunities in Complementary and Integrative Medicine (*continued*)**
>
> Integrative and Functional Medicine
>
> - Academic Consortium for Integrative Medicine & Health (http://imconsortium.org)
> - National Center for Integrative Primary Healthcare (http://nciph.org)
> - Office of Cancer Complementary and Alternative Medicine (https://cam.cancer.gov)
> - National Center for Complementary and Integrative Health (https://nccih.nih.gov)
> - The Institute for Functional Medicine (www.functionalmedicine.org)
> - Integrative Medicine for Mental Health (www.immh.org)
> - The Wahls Protocol (http://terrywahls.com)
> - Integrative Healthcare Symposium (www.ihsymposium.com/annual-conference)
> - American Board of Integrative Medicine (www.abpsus.org/integrative-medicine)

AAP Policy

American Academy of Pediatrics Committee on Children With Disabilities. Counseling families who choose complementary and alternative medicine for their child with chronic illness or disability. *Pediatrics*. 2001;107(3):598–601. Reaffirmed May 2010 (pediatrics.aappublications.org/content/107/3/598)

American Academy of Pediatrics Committee on Pediatric Workforce. Scope of practice issues in the delivery of pediatric health care. *Pediatrics*. 2013;131(6):1211–1216. Reaffirmed October 2015 (pediatrics.aappublications.org/content/131/6/1211)

American Academy of Pediatrics Section on Complementary and Integrative Medicine and Council on Children With Disabilities. Sensory integration therapies for children with developmental and behavioral disorders. *Pediatrics*. 2012;129(6):1186–1189 (pediatrics.aappublications.org/content/129/6/1186)

American Academy of Pediatrics Section on Integrative Medicine. Mind body therapies in children and youth. *Pediatrics*. 2016;138(3):e20161896 (pediatrics.aappublications.org/content/138/3/e20161896)

Kemper KJ, Vohra S, Walls R; American Academy of Pediatrics Task Force on Complementary and Alternative Medicine and Provisional Section on Complementary, Holistic, and Integrative Medicine. The use of complementary and alternative medicine in pediatrics. *Pediatrics*. 2008;122(6):1374–1386. Reaffirmed January 2013 (pediatrics.aappublications.org/content/122/6/1374)

References

1. Sawni A, Thomas R. Pediatricians' attitudes, experience and referral patterns regarding complementary/alternative medicine: a national survey. *BMC Complement Altern Med.* 2007;7:18

2. Adams D, Dagenais S, Clifford T, et al. Complementary and alternative medicine use by pediatric specialty outpatients. *Pediatrics.* 2013;131(2):225–232

3. Sibinga EM, Ottolini MC, Duggan AK, Wilson MH. Parent-pediatrician communication about complementary and alternative medicine use for children. *Clin Pediatr (Phila).* 2004;43(4):367–373

4. Vohra S, Surette S, Mittra D, Rosen LD, Gardiner P, Kemper KJ. Pediatric integrative medicine: pediatrics' newest subspecialty? *BMC Pediatr.* 2012;12:123

5. Bell IR, Caspi O, Schwartz GE, et al. Integrative medicine and systemic outcomes research: issues in the emergence of a new model for primary health care. *Arch Intern Med.* 2002;162(2):133–140

6. Academic Consortium for Integrative Medicine and Health Web site. https://www.imconsortium.org. Accessed February 7, 2018

7. Snyderman R, Weil AT. Integrative medicine: bringing medicine back to its roots. *Arch Intern Med.* 2002;162(4):395–397

8. Kemper KJ. Holistic pediatrics = good medicine. *Pediatrics.* 2000;105(1, pt 3): 214–218

9. Kemper KJ. Separation or synthesis: a holistic approach to therapeutics. *Pediatr Rev.* 1996;17(8):279–283

10. Astin JA, Forys K. Psychosocial determinants of health and illness: integrating mind, body, and spirit. *Adv Mind Body Med.* 2004;20(4):14–21

11. Green E, Green A, Walters E. Voluntary control of internal states: psychological and physiologic. *J Transpersonal Psych.* 1970;2:1–26

12. Sussman D, Culbert T. Pediatric self-regulation. In: Levine MD, Carey WB, Crocker AC, eds. *Developmental-Behavioral Pediatrics.* 3rd ed. Philadelphia, PA: WB Saunders; 1999

13. Astin JA, Shapiro SL, Eisenberg DM, Forys KL. Mind-body medicine: state of the science, implications for practice. *J Am Board Fam Pract.* 2003;16(2):131–147

14. Morgenthaler T, Kramer M, Alessi C, et al; American Academy of Sleep Medicine. Practice parameters for the psychological and behavioral treatment of insomnia: an update. An American Academy of Sleep Medicine report. *Sleep.* 2006;29(11):1415–1419

15. Andrasik F, Schwartz MS. Behavioral assessment and treatment of pediatric headache. *Behav Modif.* 2006;30(1):93–113

16. Tsao JC, Zeltzer LK. Complementary and alternative medicine approaches for pediatric pain: a review of the state-of-the-science. *Evid Based Complement Alternat Med.* 2005;2(2):149–159

17. Mellon M, McGrath M. Empirically supported treatments in pediatric psychology: nocturnal enuresis. *J Pediatr Psychol.* 2000;25(4):219–224

18. Lehrer PM, Vaschillo E, Vaschillo B, et al. Biofeedback treatment for asthma. *Chest.* 2004;126(2):352–361

19. Sawni A. Attention-deficit/hyperactivity disorder and complementary/alternative medicine. *Adolesc Med State Art Rev.* 2008;19(2):313–326

20. Rakel D. *Integrative Medicine.* 4th ed. Philadelphia, PA: Elsevier; 2017

21. Silvestri GA, Knittig S, Zoller JS, Nietert PJ. Importance of faith on medical decisions regarding cancer care. *J Clin Oncol.* 2003;21(7):1379–1382

22. Koenig HG, Cohen HJ, Blazer DG, et al. Religious coping and depression among elderly, hospitalized medically ill men. *Am J Psychiatry.* 1992;149(12):1693–1700

23. Koenig HG, George LK, Peterson BL. Religiosity and remission of depression in medically ill older patients. *Am J Psychiatry.* 1998;155(4):536–542

24. Fisch MJ, Titzer ML, Kristeller JL, et al. Assessment of quality of life in outpatients with advanced cancer: the accuracy of clinician estimations and the relevance of spiritual well-being—a Hoosier Oncology Group Study. *J Clin Oncol.* 2003;21(14):2754–2759

25. Moadel A, Morgan C, Fatone A, et al. Seeking meaning and hope: self-reported spiritual and existential needs among an ethnically-diverse cancer patient population. *Psychooncology.* 1999;8(5):378–385

26. McClain CS, Rosenfeld B, Breitbart W. Effect of spiritual well-being on end-of-life despair in terminally-ill cancer patients. *Lancet.* 2003;361(9369):1603–1607

27. Pargament KI, Koenig HG, Tarakeshwar N, Hahn J. Religious struggle as a predictor of mortality among medically ill elderly patients: a 2-year longitudinal study. *Arch Intern Med.* 2001;161(15):1881–1885

28. Meert KL, Thurston CS, Briller SH. The spiritual needs of parents at the time of their child's death in the pediatric intensive care unit and during bereavement: a qualitative study. *Pediatr Crit Care Med.* 2005;6(4):420–427

29. Sibinga EM, Kemper KJ. Complementary, holistic, and integrative medicine: meditation practices for pediatric health. *Pediatr Rev.* 2010;31(12):e91–e103

30. Tan L, Martin G. Taming the adolescent mind: preliminary report of a mindfulness-based psychological intervention for adolescents with clinical heterogeneous mental health diagnoses. *Clin Child Psychol Psychiatry.* 2013;18(2):300–312

31. Sibinga EM, Kerrigan D, Stewart M, Johnson K, Magyari T, Ellen JM. Mindfulness-based stress reduction for urban youth. *J Altern Complement Med.* 2011;17(3):213–218

32. Birdee GS, Yeh GY, Wayne PM, Phillips RS, Davis RB, Gardiner P. Clinical applications of yoga for the pediatric population: a systematic review. *Acad Pediatr.* 2009;9(4):212–220.e1–9

33. Anandarajah G, Hight E. Spirituality and medical practice: using the HOPE questions as a practical tool for spiritual assessment. *Am Fam Physician.* 2001;63(1):81–89

34. The Center for Nia and Yoga. The Center for Nia and Yoga Web site. http://nia-yoga.com. Accessed February 7, 2018

35. Standley JM. A meta-analysis of the efficacy of music therapy for premature infants. *J Pediatr Nurs.* 2002;17(2):107–113

36. Standley JM, Moore RS. Therapeutic effects of music and mother's voice on premature infants. *Pediatr Nurs.* 1995;21(6):509–512, 574

37. Block S, Jennings D, David L. Live harp music decreases salivary cortisol levels in convalescent preterm infants. *Pediatr Res.* 2003;53(4, pt 2):469a

38. Kemper KJ, Hamilton C. Live harp music reduces activity and increases weight gain in stable premature infants. *J Altern Complement Med.* 2008;14(10):1185–1186

39. Loewy J, Stewart K, Dassler AM, Telsey A, Homel P. The effects of music therapy on vital signs, feeding, and sleep in premature infants. *Pediatrics.* 2013;131(5): 902–918

40. Koch ME, Kain ZN, Ayoub C, Rosenbaum SH. The sedative and analgesic sparing effect of music. *Anesthesiology.* 1998;89(2):300–306

41. Nilsson U, Rawal N, Unosson M. A comparison of intraoperative or postoperative exposure to music—a controlled trial of the effects on postoperative pain. *Anesthesia.* 2003;58(7):699–703

42. Nguyen TN, Nilsson S, Hellström AL, Bengtson A. Music therapy to reduce pain and anxiety in children with cancer undergoing lumbar puncture: a randomized clinical trial. *J Pediatr Oncol Nurs.* 2010;27(3):146–155

43. Barrerra ME, Rykov MH, Doyle SL. The effects of interactive music therapy on hospitalized children with cancer: a pilot study. *Psychooncology.* 2002;11(5): 379–388

44. Magill L. The use of music therapy to address the suffering in advanced cancer pain. *J Palliat Care.* 2002;17(3):167–172

45. Beck SL. The therapeutic use of music for cancer-related pain. *Oncol Nurs Forum.* 1991;18(8):1327–1337

46. Standley JM, Hanser SB. Music therapy research and applications in pediatric oncology treatment. *J Pediatr Oncol Nurs.* 1995;12(1):3–8

47. Kemper KJ, Hamilton CA, McLean TW, Lovato J. Impact of music on pediatric oncology outpatients. *Pediatr Res.* 2008;64(1):105–109

48. Guzzetta CE. Effects of relaxation and music therapy on patients in a coronary care unit with presumptive acute myocardial infarction. *Heart Lung.* 1989;18(6): 609–616

49. Evans D. The effectiveness of music as an intervention for hospital patients: a systematic review. *J Adv Nurs.* 2002;37(1):8–18

50. Vickers AJ, Cassileth BR. Unconventional therapies for cancer and cancer-related symptoms. *Lancet Oncol.* 2001;2(4):226–232

51. Chlan L. Effectiveness of a music therapy intervention on relaxation and anxiety for patients receiving ventilatory assistance. *Heart Lung.* 1998;27(3):169–176

52. Halstead MT, Roscoe ST. Restoring the spirit at the end of life: music as an intervention for oncology nurses. *Clin J Oncol Nurs.* 2002;6(6):332–336

53. Hilliard RE. The effects of music therapy on the quality and length of life of people diagnosed with terminal cancer. *J Music Ther.* 2003;40(2):113–137

54. Lindenfelser KJ, Hense C, McFerran K. Music therapy in pediatric palliative care: family-centered care to enhance quality of life. *Am J Hosp Palliat Care.* 2012;29(3):219–226

55. Korczak DJ, Madigan S, Colasanto M. Children's physical activity and depression: a meta-analysis. *Pediatrics.* 2017;139(4):e20162266

56. Wigal SB, Nemet D, Swanson JM, et al. Catecholamine response to exercise in children with attention deficit hyperactivity disorder. *Pediatr Res.* 2003;53(5): 756–761

57. Wagner CL, Greer FR; American Academy of Pediatrics Section on Breastfeeding and Committee on Nutrition. Prevention of rickets and vitamin D deficiency in infants, children, and adolescents. *Pediatrics.* 2008;122(5):1142–1152

58. Wilson KM, Klein JD, Sesselberg TS, et al. Use of complementary medicine and dietary supplements among U.S. adolescents. *J Adolesc Health.* 2006;38(4):385–394

59. National Center for Complementary and Integrative Health. Children and the use of complementary health approaches. National Center for Complementary and Integrative Health Web site. https://nccih.nih.gov/health/children. Updated March 2017. Accessed February 7, 2018

60. Pitetti R, Singh S, Hornyak D, Garcia SE, Herr S. Complementary and alternative medicine use in children. *Pediatr Emerg Care.* 2001;17(3):165–169

61. Breuner CC, Barry PJ, Kemper KJ. Alternative medicine use by homeless youth. *Arch Pediatr Adolesc Med.* 1998;152(11):1071–1075

62. Lanski SL, Greenwald M, Perkins A, Simon HK. Herbal therapy use in a pediatric emergency department population: expect the unexpected. *Pediatrics.* 2003; 111(5, pt 1):981–985

63. Sawni-Sikand A, Schubiner H, Thomas RL. Use of complementary/alternative therapies among children in primary care pediatrics. *Ambul Pediatr.* 2002;2(2): 99–103

64. Sanders H, Davis MF, Duncan B, et al. Use of complementary and alternative medical therapies among children with special health care needs in southern Arizona. *Pediatrics.* 2003;111(3):584–587

65. Hagen LE, Schneider R, Stephens D, Modrusan D, Feldman BM. Use of complementary and alternative medicine by pediatric rheumatology patients. *Arthritis Rheum.* 2003;49(1):3–6

66. Heuschkel R, Afzal N, Wuerth A, et al. Complementary medicine use in children and young adults with inflammatory bowel disease. *Am J Gastroenterol.* 2002;97(2):382–388

67. Kelly KM, Jacobson JS, Kennedy DD, Braudt SM, Mallick M, Weiner MA. Use of unconventional therapies by children with cancer at an urban medical center. *J Pediatr Hematol Oncol.* 2000;22(5):412–416

68. Reznik M, Ozuah PO, Franco K, Cohen R, Motlow F. Use of complementary therapy by adolescents with asthma. *Arch Pediatr Adolesc Med.* 2002;156(10): 1042–1044

69. Agmon-Levin N, Theodor E, Segal RM, Shoenfeld Y. Vitamin D in systemic and organ-specific autoimmune diseases. *Clin Rev Allergy Immunol.* 2013;45(2): 256–266

70. Sawni A, Breuner CC. Complementary, holistic, and integrative medicine: depression, sleep disorders, and substance abuse. *Pediatr Rev.* 2012;33(9):422–425

71. Nowak A, Boesch L, Andres E, et al. Effect of vitamin D_3 on self-perceived fatigue: a double-blind randomized placebo-controlled trial. *Medicine (Baltimore).* 2016;95(52):e5353

72. Green R. Vitamin B_{12} deficiency from the perspective of a practicing hematologist. *Blood.* 2017;129(19):2603–2611

73. Hall-Flavin DK. What's the relationship between vitamin B-12 and depression? Mayo Clinic Web site. http://www.mayoclinic.org/diseases-conditions/depression/ expert-answers/vitamin-b12-and-depression/FAQ-20058077. Published November 23, 2016. Accessed February 7, 2018

74. Qureshi NA, Al-Bedah AM. Mood disorders and complementary and alternative medicine: a literature review. *Neuropsychiatr Dis Treat.* 2013;9:639–658

75. Partonen T, Haukka J, Virtamo J, Taylor PR, Lönnqvist J. Association of low serum total cholesterol with major depression and suicide. *Br J Psychiatry.* 1999;175: 259–262

76. Troisi A. Low cholesterol is a risk factor for attentional impulsivity in patients with mood symptoms. *Psychiatry Res.* 2011;188(1):83–87

77. Field T. Massage therapy for skin conditions in young children. *Dermatol Clin.* 2005;23(4):717–721

78. Khilnani S, Field T, Hernandez-Reif M, Schanberg S. Massage therapy improves mood and behavior of students with attention-deficit/hyperactivity disorder. *Adolescence.* 2003;38(152):623–638

79. Diego MA, Field T, Hernandez-Reif M, et al. Aggressive adolescents benefit from massage therapy. *Adolescence.* 2002;37(147):597–607

80. Field T. Preterm infant massage therapy studies: an American approach. *Semin Neonatol.* 2002;7(6):487–494

81. Field T. Massage therapy. *Med Clin North Am.* 2002;86(1):163–171

82. McCurdy EA, Spangler JG, Wofford MM, Chauvenet AR, McLean TW. Religiosity is associated with the use of complementary medical therapies by pediatric oncology patients. *J Pediatr Hematol Oncol.* 2003;25(2):125–129

83. Wilson KM, Klein JD. Adolescents' use of complementary and alternative medicine. *Ambul Pediatr.* 2002;2(22):104–110

84. Hansen TI, Kristensen JH. Effect of massage, shortwave diathermy and ultrasound upon 133Xe disappearance rate from muscle and subcutaneous tissue in the human calf. *Scand J Rehabil Med.* 1973;5(4):179–182

85. Ironson G, Field T, Scafidi F, et al. Massage therapy is associated with enhancement of the immune system's cytotoxic capacity. *Int J Neurosci.* 1996;84(1–4):205–217

86. Field T, Hernandez-Reif M, Diego M, Schanberg S, Kuhn C. Cortisol decreases and serotonin and dopamine increase following massage therapy. *Int J Neurosci.* 2005;115(10):1397–1413

87. Jain S, Kumar P, McMillan DD. Prior leg massage decreases pain responses to heel stick in preterm babies. *J Paediatr Child Health.* 2006;42(9):505–508

88. Lin YC, Lee AC, Kemper KJ, Berde CB. Use of complementary and alternative medicine in pediatric pain management service: a survey. *Pain Med.* 2005;6(6): 452–458

89. Anders EF, Findeisen A, Nowak A, Rüdiger M, Usichenko TI. Acupuncture for treatment of hospital-induced constipation in children: a retrospective case series study. *Acupunct Med.* 2012;30(4):258–260

90. Wong V, Cheuk DK, Lee S, Chu V. Acupuncture for acute management and rehabilitation of traumatic brain injury. *Cochrane Database Syst Rev.* 2013;(3):CD007700

91. Adams D, Cheng F, Jou H, Aung S, Yasui Y, Vohra S. The safety of pediatric acupuncture: a systematic review. *Pediatrics.* 2011;128(6):e1575–e1587

92. Ladas EJ, Rooney D, Taromina K, Ndao DH, Kelly KM. The safety of acupuncture in children and adolescents with cancer therapy-related thrombocytopenia. *Support Care Cancer.* 2010;18(11):1487–1490

93. Kemper KJ, Sarah R, Silver-Highfield E, Xiarhos E, Barnes L, Berde C. On pins and needles? Pediatric pain patients' experience with acupuncture. *Pediatrics.* 2000;105(4, pt 2):941–947

94. Kemper KJ, Fletcher NB, Hamilton CA, McLean TW. Impact of healing touch on pediatric oncology outpatients: pilot study. *J Soc Integr Oncol.* 2009;7(1):12–18

95. Kemper KJ, Kelly EA. Treating children with therapeutic and healing touch. *Pediatr Ann.* 2004;33(4):248–252

96. Giasson M, Bouchard L. Effect of therapeutic touch on the well-being of persons with terminal cancer. *J Holist Nurs.* 1998;16(3):383–398

97. Wilkinson DS, Knox PL, Chatman JE, et al. The clinical effectiveness of healing touch. *J Altern Complement Med.* 2002;8(1):33–47

98. Lafreniere KD, Mutus B, Cameron S, et al. Effects of therapeutic touch on biochemical and mood indicators in women. *J Altern Complement Med.* 1999;5(4):367–370

99. Assiotis A, Sachinis NP, Chalidis BE. Pulsed electromagnetic fields for the treatment of tibial delayed unions and nonunions. A prospective clinical study and review of the literature. *J Orthop Surg Res.* 2012;7:24

100. Boyette MY, Herrera-Soto JA. Treatment of delayed and nonunited fractures and osteotomies with pulsed electromagnetic field in children and adolescents. *Orthopedics.* 2012;35(7):e1051–e1055

101. Vásquez CE, Tomita T, Bedin A, Castro RA. [Subdural anesthesia after epidural puncture: two case reports.] *Rev Bras Anestesiol.* 2003;53(2):209–213

102. László JF, Farkas P, Reiczigel J, Vágó P. Effect of local exposure to inhomogeneous static magnetic field on stomatological pain sensation—a double-blind, randomized, placebo-controlled study. *Int J Radiat Biol.* 2012;88(5):430–438

103. Kovács-Bálint Z, Csathó A, László JF, Juhász P, Hernádi I. Exposure to an inhomogeneous static magnetic field increases thermal pain threshold in healthy human volunteers. *Bioelectromagnetics.* 2011;32(2):131–139

104. Ross CL, Harrison BS. The use of magnetic field for the reduction of inflammation: a review of the history and therapeutic results. *Altern Ther Health Med.* 2013;19(2):47–54

105. Jacobs J, Jonas WB, Jiménez-Pérez M, Crothers D. Homeopathy for childhood diarrhea: combined results and metaanalysis from three randomized, controlled clinical trials. *Pediatr Infect Dis J.* 2003;22(3):229–234

106. Jacobs J, Springer DA, Crothers D. Homeopathic treatment of acute otitis media in children: a preliminary randomized placebo-controlled trial. *Pediatr Infect Dis J.* 2001;20(2):177–183

107. Jacobs J, Williams AL, Girard C, Njike VY, Katz D. Homeopathy for attention-deficit/hyperactivity disorder: a pilot randomized-controlled trial. *J Altern Complement Med.* 2005;11(5):799–806

108. Barnes PM, Powell-Griner E, McFann K, Nahin RL. Complementary and alternative medicine use among adults: United States, 2002. *Adv Data.* 2004;(343):1–19

109. Astin JA. Why patients use alternative medicine: results of a national study. *JAMA.* 1998;279(19):1548–1553

110. Neuberger J. Primary care: core values. Patients' priorities. *BMJ.* 1998;317(7153):260–262

111. Kaptchuk TJ, Eisenberg DM. The persuasive appeal of alternative medicine. *Ann Intern Med.* 1998;129(12):1061–1065

112. American Academy of Pediatrics Council on Environmental Health. *Pediatric Environmental Health.* 3rd ed. Etzel RA, ed. Elk Grove Village, IL: American Academy of Pediatrics; 2012

113. Cohen MH, Kemper KJ. Complementary therapies in pediatrics: a legal perspective. *Pediatrics.* 2005;115(3):774–780

114. King DE, Bushwick B. Beliefs and attitudes of hospital inpatients about faith healing and prayer. *J Fam Pract.* 1994;39(4):349–352

115. Ehman JW, Ott BB, Short TH, Ciampa RC, Hansen-Flaschen J. Do patients want physicians to inquire about their spiritual or religious beliefs if they become gravely ill? *Arch Intern Med.* 1999;159(15):1803–1806

116. McCord G, Gilchrist VJ, Grossman SD, et al. Discussing spirituality with patients: a rational and ethical approach. *Ann Fam Med.* 2004;2(4):356–361

117. Chu L. 5 principles of self-care for health professionals. KevinMD.com Web site. http://www.kevinmd.com/blog/2010/07/5-principles-selfcare-health-professionals. html. Published July 20, 2010. Accessed February 7, 2018

CHAPTER 10

Adapting Psychosocial Interventions to Primary Care

W. Douglas Tynan, PhD, and Rebecca Baum, MD

> *"...strategies from evidence-based practices..., proven to be effective in the treatment of mental disorders and related subclinical symptoms, can be easily adapted to the pediatric primary care setting, and a growing body of literature documents their effectiveness."*

Of the top 6 health problems resulting in childhood disability, 3 are mental health conditions: attention-deficit/hyperactivity disorder (ADHD), behavioral and conduct problems, and mood problems.[1] Among children with diagnosable conditions, between 13% and 20% experience mental health problems that lead to distress and impairment in daily activities each year,[2] and an equal or greater number of children have subclinical problems that impair functioning and cause distress for them and their families. While referral to mental health services may seem the obvious path, it may not always be feasible or appropriate. Access to mental health services is often limited because of provider shortages, and for children and adolescents (collectively called *children* in this chapter unless otherwise specified) who have emerging or subclinical symptoms, specialty mental health services may not be appropriate. The persistent stigma regarding mental disorders prevents many families from accessing treatment. Treatment in the pediatric medical home, either through integrated mental health services or first-line interventions delivered by primary care clinicians (PCCs) (ie, pediatricians, family physicians, internists, nurse practitioners, and physician assistants at the front lines of pediatrics) can help reduce these barriers to care.

For many PCCs, the treatment of mental health problems seems daunting, in part because of limited training and perceived complexity and comorbidity. However, strategies from evidence-based practices (EBPs), proven to be effective in the treatment of mental disorders and related subclinical symptoms, can be easily adapted to the pediatric primary care setting,[3] and a growing body of literature documents their effectiveness.[4–8] Common elements of EBPs are specific treatment strategies that can be applied across a number of mental health problems frequently encountered in pediatrics, such as anxiety, depression, disruptive behavior, inattention, substance use, and emotional and behavioral disturbances in young children. These approaches can improve provider comfort and deliver elements of effective interventions in a timely manner within a pediatric setting. They also address treatment challenges related to the presence of comorbid symptoms, as more than one symptom can be addressed simultaneously.

Developing a Plan of Care

First-line Strategies

Several first-line strategies can be considered general or universal approaches to children and adolescents with social-emotional and mental health problems (ie, they are effective regardless of the disorder or presenting symptom). These strategies include the following strategies.

Engaging the Child and Family in Care

Studies show that engagement is essential to promote adherence and improve treatment outcomes. Engagement is an especially important consideration for mental health treatment: families may feel shame or embarrassment when discussing mental health concerns, parents may worry that "it's their fault," and older children may be concerned about being different from their peers. The HELP mnemonic (Box 10-1)

Box 10-1. Common Factors Mnemonic: HELP Build a Therapeutic Alliance

H = Hope

E = Empathy

L^2 = Language, Loyalty

P^3 = Permission, Partnership, Plan

Adapted with permission from American Academy of Pediatrics. *Addressing Mental Health Concerns in Primary Care: A Clinician's Toolkit.* Elk Grove Village, IL: American Academy of Pediatrics; 2010. For the fully annotated mnemonic, please refer to Appendix 5.

summarizes the "common factors" that are important for building a therapeutic alliance and facilitating behavior change: hope, empathy, language, loyalty, permission, partnership, and plan. These have been drawn from EBPs of family therapy, cognitive therapy, motivational interviewing, family engagement, family-focused pediatrics, and solution-focused therapy.

It is important to note that the evaluation process can inadvertently lead to an undue focus on deficits and symptoms. Purposefully and regularly highlighting the child and family's strengths can serve as an engagement strategy, contributing to their hopefulness and confidence in taking action. With the child and family's help, the PCC can identify goals for treatment that are achievable and precise, so progress can be monitored. Framing goals as both short- and long-term plans can help difficult problems seem more surmountable.

Offering Psychoeducation

Myths regarding mental health problems persist. Children and families are reassured by the knowledge that mental health problems are common, treatable, and not caused by character flaws or "bad parenting." Although some mental health conditions have a heritable component, families should be reassured that family history serves as a risk factor rather than a predetermined condition, and protective factors should also be elicited. Understanding family concerns and perceptions can be helpful in addressing underlying worries that may not be shared initially. Many families are unaware that mental health concerns can be addressed in the primary care setting. If referral to mental health services is warranted, families also appreciate ongoing support and partnership that can be provided by primary care.

Encouraging Healthy Habits

Encouraging healthy habits is important in promoting overall well-being but also because sleep, nutrition, and other aspects of wellness can affect and be affected by mental health problems. Maintaining routines is particularly helpful for children with anxiety and for children who have trouble following directions, as it helps them understand what to expect. Similarly, habits such as limiting screen time, engaging in social interaction with family members and peers, and being physically active should be promoted for all children and should also be part of the care plan for children with mental health concerns.

Reducing Overall Stress

Taking care of children can be stressful, and growing up can be stressful too. By acknowledging these facts, practitioners provide empathy and normalcy to the family's experience. Stress can amplify existing symptoms, so addressing stress can be an important first step in treatment. Taking with families about what would "lighten the load" can elicit the family's input regarding stressors that are important to them, thereby increasing engagement and follow-through.

Offering Initial Intervention

Regardless of whether mental health referral is planned or treatment will occur in the pediatric setting, PCCs can initiate care. This care might include one or more problem-solving sessions with the family around difficult behaviors or conflicts (eg, fighting among siblings, bedtime, media use, homework, adolescent boundaries), measures to relieve stress in either the child or any family members, or interventions targeting specific symptoms, using common elements from EBPs. All can be implemented in the pediatric practice as part of the care plan.

Providing Resources

The PCC can offer the child and parents educational resources to assist them with self-management. Providers should also provide contact numbers and resources in case of an emergency, if appropriate.

Monitoring Progress

It is important for the PCC to check in with the child and family about progress they're making toward goals identified at the start of treatment. For some conditions, screening instruments or functional assessment scales, completed by the child or adolescent, family members, or any teachers (or any combination thereof), can be used to monitor symptoms over time. (See Appendix 2, Mental Health Tools for Pediatrics.) The PCC can reassure the family by reminding them that each day can have ups and downs, but a trend toward progress is most important.

Involving Specialists When Needed

Appendix 4, Sources of Key Mental Health Services, describes the types of mental health and social service providers that may be useful to the patient and family. Several factors may weigh into the decision to involve mental health specialty care, including severity, chronicity, and degree of comorbidity of the condition; the PCC's training and confidence in managing it; and the family's preferences. The presence of significant family stressors or limited supports may necessitate a higher level of care. When a referral is made, PCCs can increase the likelihood of a completed referral by explaining the process and reason for the referral. Written material describing the credentials and roles of various mental health specialists may also be helpful. Forwarding appropriate records (after consent has been obtained) can also facilitate the exchange of information between the primary care staff and the mental health office staff.

Practical Guidance in Using Common Elements of Evidence-Based Practices

Chapter 7, Psychosocial Therapies, provides an overview of EBPs in the psychosocial therapy of children and adolescents with common mental health problems, and Appendix 6, PracticeWise Table of Evidence for Psychosocial Therapies, summarizes the strength of evidence supporting each EBP. Common elements of these EBPs amenable to use in pediatric practice are summarized in Appendix 7, Common Elements of Evidence-Based Practice Amenable to Primary Care: Indications and Sources. This table also notes the chapters in this book that describe the elements more fully and provide guidance for incorporating them into a plan of care. The following discussion highlights practical considerations in using a few of the most pediatric-friendly common elements within pediatric practice and offers suggestions for educating parents about them.

Anxiety, Depression, and Trauma-Related Distress

Children with anxiety demonstrate low self-esteem and cognitive distortion of everyday events, they perceive life to be very stressful, and they may withdraw socially. Children with depression demonstrate many of the psychosocial deficits associated with depression in adults, such as low self-esteem, negative and irrational thoughts, high levels of stressful life events, social withdrawal, impaired social abilities, and low activity level. Both depression and anxiety in children can be marked by irritability, which is often the presenting concern by the parents. In many situations involving trauma, there may be ongoing threats to safety and security. The actual traumatic threat may still be present, or there may have been disruptions to safety and routines because of trauma.

Common elements helpful in managing anxiety, depression, and trauma-related distress are drawn from cognitive behavioral therapy (commonly known as CBT) and mind-body therapies. These elements require that parents model coping skills and children learn specific coping strategies, such as relaxation or self-calming. Problem-solving strategies in which the child learns to identify components of a fearful situation and then determines which coping skills to use are important for long-term maintenance of progress. In addition, parents should identify situations difficult for their child and praise and reward effort by the child to over-come those situations. Improved communication skills, including identi-fying and accurately labeling emotions, are also helpful. One of the key points in managing anxiety is not to give in readily to the fears, which will reinforce avoidance and make the problem worse. Instead, parents should work on helping their child confront and face these fears, starting with the easier ones. Box 10-2 summarizes guidance to offer parents in the use of these approaches.

When caring for children exposed to trauma, the PCC can make a plan with the family to help restore or maintain security and normalcy to the extent possible. It is important to acknowledge that trauma to one family member may be felt by others who were not directly affected: in particu-lar, the PCC should ask about siblings and include them in plans for support.

Disruptive Behavior and Inattention

Research has consistently shown that the most effective therapeutic approach to help children with disruptive behaviors, including ADHD, oppositional behavior, and conduct problems, is to teach parents more effective, consistent child behavior management skills. A wealth of infor-mation on a number of parenting interventions has been proven effective

> **Box 10-2. Common Elements of Evidence-Based Practices for Depression and Anxiety Suggestions for Parents**
>
> - Provide consistency and routines.
> - Model "brave" behavior, and have other adults and siblings do the same.
> - Teach your child coping skills, relaxation, problem-solving, and self-talk, and practice these skills with your child regularly.
> - Accurately label emotions and improve communication with your child.
> - Increase pleasant events and activities in your child's daily living schedule.
> - Always praise verbally and reward efforts by your child to cope with difficult situations.
> - Help your child deal with fears in steps, starting with the easier ones to cope with.
> - Discourage avoidance of fear-producing situations.
> - Be empathic and validate and label the emotions, but don't endorse the behavior of avoiding or escaping.
> - Prepare your child for fearful or stressful situations with a plan.

in more than a 40-year history of research and intervention.[9] These programs include the Strengthening Families Program, The Incredible Years, Parent Corps, the Triple P – Positive Parenting Program, and Parent-Child Interaction Therapy. Essential components of these programs include increasing positive parent-child interactions, teaching emotional communication skills to parents, and requiring parents to practice new skills with their children during parent training sessions. For parents of children who have disruptive behaviors, the following additional components are also essential: teaching parents to use time-out correctly, teaching parents the importance of parenting consistency, and practicing these skills. Description of these skills and a video library demonstrating them are publicly available at www.cdc.gov/parents/essentials/videos/video_timeout_vig.html. These approaches are consistent with current American Academy of Pediatrics policies on parenting and with the treatment guidelines of the American Academy of Child and Adolescent Psychiatry.

Emotional or Behavioral Disturbance in Young Children

Given the high frequency of visits during early childhood, PCCs play an important role in preventing, identifying, and addressing emotional and behavioral problems in young children. These problems may include difficulties with self-regulation, extreme tantrums or aggression, activity and impulsivity levels that are excessive for developmental age, irritability or low mood, or anxiety out of proportion for age, including difficulties with separation, excessive shyness, and fears. Primary care clinicians can provide education regarding general parenting practices and should be comfortable addressing mild clinical problems and supporting families who encounter more severe symptoms. A number of EBPs have been developed for young children and their families, including Child-Parent Psychotherapy and Trauma-Focused Psychotherapy, as well as the parent intervention programs mentioned previously. Common elements used in these programs include

▶ *Apply positive parenting principles.* These principles include giving positive attention for positive behaviors, removing attention for low-level behaviors, and providing safe, consistent, and calm consequences for unacceptable or unsafe behaviors.

▶ *Reframe the child's behaviors.* Parents may feel that the child's challenging behavior is purposeful and directed at them. Parents with depression or those who are experiencing significant amounts of stress may be especially sensitive to difficult behavior and more inclined to misinterpret it. Helping the parent understand reasons behind the child's behavior can allow the parent to focus on positive parenting principles instead.

▶ *Use relaxation and anxiety management techniques.* Playing quiet music, introducing a soothing toy, or blowing bubbles to practice deep breathing can help calm a child who is anxious or agitated.

See Chapter 17, Emotional or Behavioral Disturbance in Children Younger Than 5 Years, for further discussion of these parenting interventions.

Summary

Evidence-based interventions for common childhood mental health morbidities can be adapted to brief interventions in pediatric practice and delivered effectively by trained PCCs.[4] These interventions can be augmented with print and video resources that can facilitate parents' practicing skills at home. These brief interventions, delivered quickly and efficiently in primary care, are all that many parents need to reach their goals. For families who require further professional help, referrals to skilled child mental health providers are the next step in care.

AAP Policy

American Academy of Pediatrics Committee on Substance Use and Prevention. Substance use screening, brief intervention, and referral to treatment. *Pediatrics.* 2016;138(1):e20161210 (pediatrics.aappublications.org/content/138/1/e20161210)

American Academy of Pediatrics Section on Integrative Medicine. Mind-body therapies in children and youth. *Pediatrics.* 2016;138(3):e20161896 (pediatrics. aappublications.org/content/138/3/e20161896)

Gleason MM, Goldson E, Yogman MW; American Academy of Pediatrics Council on Early Childhood, Committee on Psychosocial Aspects of Child and Family Health, and Section on Developmental Behavioral Pediatrics. Addressing early childhood emotional and behavioral problems. *Pediatrics.* 2016;138(6):e20163023 (pediatrics. aappublications.org/content/138/6/e20163025)

Harstad E, Levy S; American Academy of Pediatrics Committee on Substance Abuse. Attention-deficit/hyperactivity disorder and substance abuse. *Pediatrics.* 2014;134(1): e293–e301 (pediatrics.aappublications.org/content/134/1/e293)

Levy SJ, Williams JF; American Academy of Pediatrics Committee on Substance Use and Prevention. Substance use screening, brief intervention, and referral to treatment. *Pediatrics.* 2016;138(1):e20161211 (pediatrics.aappublications.org/content/138/1/e20161211)

References

1. Halfon N, Houtrow A, Larson K, Newacheck PW. The changing landscape of disability in childhood. *Future Child.* 2012;22(1):13–42
2. Merikangas KR, He JP, Brody D, Fisher PW, Bourdon K, Koretz DS. Prevalence and treatment of mental disorders among US children in the 2001-2004 NHANES. *Pediatrics.* 2009;125(1):75–81
3. Kazdin AE. Evidence-based psychosocial treatment: advances, surprises, and needed shifts in foci. *Cogn Behav Pract.* 2016;23(4):426–430

4. Leslie LK, Mehus CJ, Hawkins JD, et al. Primary health care: potential home for family focused preventive interventions. *Am J Prev Med.* 2016;51(4)(suppl 2): S106–S118

5. Turner KM, Sanders MR. Help when it's needed first: a controlled evaluation of brief, preventive behavioral family intervention in a primary care setting. *Behav Ther.* 2006;37(2):131–142

6. Tully LA, Hunt C. Brief parenting interventions for children at risk of externalizing behavior problems: a systematic review. *J Child Fam Stud.* 2015;25(3):705–719

7. Perrin EC, Sheldrick RC, Mcmenamy JM, Henson BS, Carter AS. Improving parenting skills for families of young children in pediatric settings. *JAMA Pediatr.* 2014;168(1):16

8. Lavigne JV, Lebailly SA, Gouze KR, et al. Treating oppositional defiant disorder in primary care: a comparison of three models. *J Pediatr Psychol.* 2007;33(5):449–461

9. Haslam D, Mejia A, Sanders MR, de Vries PJ. Parenting programs. In: Rey JM, ed. *IACAPAP e-Textbook of Child and Adolescent Mental Health.* Geneva, Switzerland: International Association for Child and Adolescent Psychiatry and Allied Professions; 2016:1–29

CHAPTER 11

Psychotropic Medications in Primary Care

Mark A. Riddle, MD; Susan dosReis, PhD; Gloria Reeves, MD;
Lawrence S. Wissow, MD, MPH; David Pruitt, MD; and
Jane Meschan Foy, MD

> "...the pediatric primary care clinician must judge whether
> each of the 4 components of diagnosis, that is,
> symptoms, duration, impairment, and non-normality,
> crosses a diagnostic threshold that warrants
> a recommendation for medication."

Introduction

In a policy statement published in July 2009, the American Academy of Pediatrics (AAP) recommended that primary care pediatricians achieve competence in initiating care not only for children and adolescents with attention-deficit/hyperactivity disorder (ADHD) but also for those with anxiety, depression, and substance use or use disorder.[1] In addition, the statement recommended that pediatricians achieve competence in providing a medical home for children and adolescents with the full range of pediatric mental health conditions. Implicit in these recommendations is the necessity for pediatric primary care clinicians (PCCs) (ie, pediatricians, family physicians, internists, nurse practitioners, and physician assistants who provide frontline care to children and adolescents) to be knowledgeable about pediatric psychopharmacology in general and to use psychotropic medications safely and effectively in certain clinical situations.

The goal of this chapter is to offer a clear, rational, and evidenced-based framework for using psychotropic agents in children and adolescents (collectively called *children* in this chapter unless otherwise specified) with psychiatric diagnoses. Although many pediatric PCCs are already using these medications, there remains a wide variance of comfort with, confidence in, and knowledge about how drugs are initiated, titrated, and monitored across care settings. This chapter, although not a how-to manual, provides a unifying approach grounded in the most up-to-date research, filling in the who, what, and why aspects of psychopharmacological management. The intention is not to dictate practice specifics but rather to offer a methodological approach that can best serve a wide range of pediatric PCCs who, after completing a thorough diagnostic assessment in which medication-responsive illness is identified, must then make decisions regarding medication treatment options for children, adolescents, and their families.

Getting Started: Prerequisites for Prescribing Medication

The safe and effective use of psychiatric medications in the primary care setting requires several conditions, outlined in Box 11-1.

Determining Whether to Prescribe Medication: The Diagnostic Threshold

An accurate diagnosis of medication-responsive disorders (ie, disorders for which, at a minimum, there is sufficient evidence of a clinically meaningful reduction of symptom severity in response to medication) is important in pediatric psychopharmacology. This diagnostic accuracy ensures that children who may benefit from medication are offered a trial, and it prevents needless use of medication in children who will not benefit from such treatment. Even with an accurate diagnosis and evidence-based treatments, there is no completely sensitive and specific way to determine which child will respond to medication or any other evidence-based therapy for psychiatric disorders; nor is there a way to predict who will experience adverse events or what type of adverse event may emerge.

The uncertainty underlying these issues presents clinical challenges for the prescribing PCC. A relatively simple approach to assessing whether to recommend medication is outlined in Box 11-2. This approach approximates the fifth edition of the American Psychiatric Association *Diagnostic and Statistical Manual of Mental Disorders* (DSM-5)[2] in terms of essential components or criteria and of practice guidelines for therapies.

> **Box 11-1. Optimal Conditions for Safe and Effective Prescribing of Psychotropic Medications by Pediatric Primary Care Clinicians**
>
> The *disorder* for which medication is prescribed needs to be
> - Sufficiently common for the patient to be seen regularly by a PCC
> - Efficiently and accurately diagnosable by a PCC
>
> The *medication* needs to
> - Have demonstrated efficacy
> - Be relatively safe, as assessed by several parameters
> - Have side effects (adverse events) that are reasonably predictable, readily detected, and readily managed
>
> The *dosing and monitoring* of the medication needs to
> - Follow guidelines that are reasonably established and easily followed
> - Include somatic monitoring that is limited to vital signs, height, and weight
>
> The *prescribing PCC* needs to have
> - Expertise in diagnosing the relevant disorders
> - Knowledge of available psychosocial therapies (eg, parent behavior management training, CBT)
> - Knowledge of the medications prescribed
> - Procedures for monitoring medication clinical response, adverse effects, drug interactions, and adherence
>
> The *system of care* needs to provide
> - Access to pediatric psychopharmacological expertise for consultation on issues beyond the expertise of the pediatrician
> - Access to appropriate, evidence-based psychosocial therapies
> - Adequate payment for services rendered
> - Minimal administrative and regulatory barriers
>
> ---
> Abbreviations: CBT, cognitive behavioral therapy; PCC, primary care clinician.

The term *sufficient* (or *sufficiently*) appears in the first 4 components in Box 11-2. Thus, the PCC must judge whether each of the 4 components of diagnosis, that is, symptoms, duration, impairment, and non-normality, crosses a diagnostic threshold that warrants a recommendation for medication.

Box 11-2. Assessing Whether to Prescribe Psychotropic Medication

1. Does the child have *sufficient* symptoms to support a syndrome or disorder?

2. Have the symptoms been present for a *sufficient* period?

3. Is the child experiencing *sufficient* impairment or distress from the symptoms in ways that negatively affect academic development, family life, interactions with peers, participation in activities, or emotional well-being?

4. Is this disorder *sufficiently* different from normal levels of activity and impulsivity (in contrast with ADHD), worry and concern (in contrast with an anxiety disorder), or demoralization or grief (in contrast with an episode of depression)?

5. Have evidence-based therapies (eg, behavior management training with parents for ADHD, CBT for anxiety or depression) been tried, if available?

Abbreviations: ADHD, attention-deficit/hyperactivity disorder; CBT, cognitive behavioral therapy.

All PCCs struggle with threshold when deciding on a diagnosis and determining whether to initiate a specific treatment. A familiar example in pediatrics is ADHD: all 18 symptoms of ADHD in the *DSM-5* include the term *often,* but there is no specific definition of *often.* Comparable examples in general medicine of the struggle with threshold include diagnosis and treatment of pain and insomnia.

Parent reports and self-reports can provide useful information about a child's symptoms and their severity and are often useful in determining threshold. Among the many available reporting tools, the following ones generally incorporate current *Diagnostic and Statistical Manual of Mental Disorders* criteria and are available as open-access tools: the NICHQ Vanderbilt ADHD assessment scales for parents and teachers; the SCARED (Screen for Child Anxiety Related Disorders), parent and child versions, for symptoms of anxiety; and the Patient Health Questionnaire-9 (commonly known as PHQ-9 Modified for Teens) for symptoms of depression. See Appendix 2, Mental Health Tools for Pediatrics, for more information about these tools.

Also critical to threshold is assessment of the child's functioning: determination of whether the child's symptoms are causing impairment of school performance, relationships with peers and family members, and progress toward developmental goals. Several PCC-friendly tools are available to assist with this assessment, including the impact scale (second page) of the Strengths and Difficulties Questionnaires and the Columbia Impairment Scale, also described in Appendix 2. Use of a tool can break ground for a fuller assessment of functioning and serve as a baseline for monitoring the child's functioning over time.[3]

Assessing Common Disorders

It is important to recognize that there is a hierarchy of difficulty in making accurate diagnoses of specific psychiatric disorders. Among the disorders addressed in this chapter, ADHD is generally the easiest and most straightforward to diagnose because the symptoms of ADHD are observable by multiple informants (eg, parents, teachers) in multiple settings (eg, school, home). Yet, even ADHD can often be confused with comorbid intellectual, language, and learning difficulties and with anxiety or the effects of trauma.

Anxiety disorders may be more difficult to diagnose than ADHD. Although anxiety and depression are both considered internalizing conditions, most symptoms of anxiety can be observed or easily elicited. Physical symptoms (eg, abdominal pain, muscle tension) are common in children with anxiety[4] and are familiar to PCCs. Other symptoms, such as avoiding social situations or phobic stimuli or entering the parents' bedroom or bed at night in response to separation concerns, either are reported by the children to their parents or are readily observed by parents. Asking children what they worry about may reveal anxiety more easily than asking, "Do you worry?"

Depression may be difficult to diagnose because demoralization, grief, and adjustment disorder, which are common in children and adolescents, can mimic the symptoms of depression. Parsing depression from these other conditions requires time and patience. When the differential diagnosis is complex, consultation with a child and adolescent psychiatrist may be needed to confirm the diagnosis of the child or adolescent who is suspected of being depressed.

Information about assessment can be found in other chapters in this book (Chapter 6, Iterative Mental Health Assessment, and symptom-specific chapters of Part 4, Chapters 13–32).

Screening for Adverse Childhood Experiences and Substance Use

Because symptoms of ADHD, anxiety, and depression can result from or be exacerbated by adverse childhood experiences (ACEs), including trauma, it is important to conduct universal screening for ACEs. Adverse childhood experiences may include single incidents (eg, car crash), ongoing traumas (eg, exposure to domestic violence), or a combination of stresses. Screening for ACEs may identify environmental factors that are contributing to a child's mood and behavior and urgent concerns that require safety planning (eg, child abuse reporting). See The Resilience Project "Clinical Assessment Tools" (American Academy of Pediatrics; www.aap.org/en-us/advocacy-and-policy/aap-health-initiatives/resilience/Pages/Clinical-Assessment-Tools.aspx).

A simple screening question that can be incorporated into a standard visit is "Since the last time I saw you, has anything really scary or upsetting happened to you or your family?" For children younger than 8 years, screening optimally relies on parent report, so the analogous question should be asked to parents: "Since the last time I saw your child, has anything really scary or upsetting happened to your child or anyone in your family?" Ultimately, the clinical relevance of a reported ACE depends on the PCC's judgment.[5]

Substance use and experimentation are very common among adolescents. The CDC reports that approximately 25% of high school–aged adolescents report they have bought, sold, or been given drugs on school grounds in the past 6 months (www.cdc.gov/features/YRBS). Preteens and adolescents should be screened for substance use. See Appendix 2 for a description of screening and brief assessment tools.

Substance use and post-traumatic stress disorder (PTSD) may co-occur with other mood or behavioral disorders (eg, ADHD and marijuana use, depression and PTSD). Complex psychopathology may require further mental health consultation for diagnostic evaluation or incorporation of specific psychosocial therapies. It is important to note that there are no US Food and Drug Administration (FDA)–approved pediatric medication treatments for either substance use or PTSD, but there are evidence-based psychosocial interventions.

Early Determinants of Need for Referral

Children with undiagnosed learning disabilities may also present with significant mood or behavioral problems. These problems may be related to school maladjustment (eg, symptoms occur primarily in a school setting, not at home). Parents may benefit from referral to family advocacy programs or support programs available in the school system that can provide information on obtaining learning disabilities evaluations and advocating for disability services.

Finally, children living in families with complex psychosocial situations (eg, parents have mental health or substance use issues, have cognitive impairment, have significantly impaired parenting skills, or have been maltreated or exposed to significant childhood adversities) may need a more thorough evaluation by a mental health specialist. Parents with mental health concerns that have not been addressed may benefit from counseling by the PCC on the positive impact of seeking help for their children as well as themselves. If a parent's mental illness is affecting the child's mental health, referral of the parent for his or her own care and screening for basic child safety and supervision concerns is warranted.

Psychosocial Therapies

Effective evidence-based psychosocial therapies, often described simply as *therapy*, are available for many pediatric psychiatric disorders. See reviews by Ginsburg[6] and Weisz et al[7] for a summary of these therapies and the evidence supporting them and see Chapter 7, Psychosocial Therapies. Psychosocial therapies are often tried before considering medication and are also used in combination with medication. For very young children, guidelines by the American Academy of Child and Adolescent Psychiatry (AACAP) recommend at least 2 trials of psychosocial therapy before starting medication.[8] Evidence from large studies sponsored by the National Institute of Mental Health (NIMH) demonstrate the advantage of combining psychosocial and medication treatments over medication or therapy alone for ADHD (ages 7–9 years),[9] common anxiety disorders (separation anxiety disorder, social phobia, and generalized anxiety disorder [GAD]; ages 7–17 years),[10] and depression (ages 12–17 years).[11]

It is important to consider when psychosocial interventions are preferred over medication. Many children and adolescents present to PCCs with mild depression or anxiety (ie, they meet diagnostic criteria, but symptoms and impairment are minimal) or subthreshold depression or anxiety (ie, they do not meet the diagnostic criteria for the disorder). In general, such a child is likely to benefit from a psychosocial intervention and may not need medication.

Despite the clear effectiveness of psychosocial therapies and the pressing need for them, there are still far too few mental health physicians and therapists with adequate training and experience to provide high-quality evidence-based therapy, and families face many administrative and financial barriers to access. For many PCCs, these factors add pressure to prescribe psychopharmacological therapy as a single first-line treatment. Primary care clinicians can join with families and mental health specialists in their communities to advocate for evidence-based psychosocial services in both public systems and private systems of care. Ideally, psychosocial interventions always accompany pharmacological interventions.[12]

Off-label Prescribing

Before the mid-1990s, very few psychiatric medications had been approved by the FDA for pediatric indications (ie, approved for use in children and adolescents <18 years). Those approved included stimulants for ADHD, tricyclic antidepressants for enuresis, a few antipsychotics for psychosis, and lithium for mania associated with bipolar I disorder. Thus, to treat psychiatric disorders in children and adolescents, it was often necessary to prescribe off-label. Although many medications still lack FDA-approved pediatric indications across the age span, the number of pediatric indications has increased markedly over the past 20 years. This increase has occurred in response to federal legislation, including the Best Pharmaceuticals for Children Act and the Pediatric Research Equity Act. Also, the NIMH began funding large multisite treatment studies in the mid-1990s.

A number of medications are now available with indications for psychiatric disorders in children, including ADHD, depression, obsessive-compulsive disorder (OCD), mania associated with bipolar I disorder, psychosis associated with schizophrenia, and irritability in children with autism spectrum disorder (ASD). Thus, prescribing off-label, especially for a medication that has no indication for any psychiatric disorder in children and adolescents, should be carefully justified and documented in the medical record.

Conceptual Framework for Prescribing Psychiatric Medications

Overview

According to an expert task force comprising representatives from major international and regional (American, Asian, and European) organizations, led by the European College of Neuropsychopharmacology (commonly known as ECNP), 108 psychotropic drugs are available for prescribing. Most of these drugs are approved by the FDA for adults in the United States. This large number of medications can be overwhelming, even for experienced mental health specialists.

The goal of the proposed conceptual framework for prescribing psychotropic medications by pediatric PCCs is to simplify and organize these medications into manageable and targeted groups in accordance with the AAP mental health competencies policy statement.

The first and most important group of psychotropic medications for PCCs (group 1) includes medications for the common psychiatric disorders: ADHD, major depressive disorder (MDD), and anxiety disorders. The best epidemiological data indicate that more than 80% of psychotropic medications prescribed to children are for ADHD, anxiety, and depressive disorders.[13]

Group 1 includes all FDA-approved medications for ADHD in children: 2 stimulants (methylphenidate and amphetamine), 2 α_2-adrenergic agonists (guanfacine and clonidine), and 1 selective norepinephrine reuptake inhibitor (NRI) (atomoxetine). It includes the serotonin-norepinephrine reuptake inhibitor (SNRI) duloxetine, recently FDA approved for GAD. It also includes all FDA-approved medications for depression in children: the 2 selective serotonin reuptake inhibitors (SSRIs) fluoxetine and escitalopram. Also, for anxiety in children, 3 SSRIs are included, that is, fluoxetine, fluvoxamine, and sertraline, that all have at least one high-quality, positive efficacy study for anxiety disorders commonly occurring in children and have FDA approval for OCD, an anxiety-related condition.

Thus, only 10 medications are in group 1 (Table 11-1). It is important to emphasize that these 10 group 1 medications are not a formulary or restricted list of possible medications. However, as will be described in greater detail later, they are the only medications with high-quality scientific evidence supporting their efficacy. Also, these medications are relatively safe.

The second group of medications (group 2) includes all FDA-approved medications for children with other *DSM-5* disorders (ie, not ADHD, anxiety, or depression). Group 2 includes 7 antipsychotics (aripiprazole, olanzapine, quetiapine, risperidone, paliperidone, asenapine, and lurasidone) and the mood stabilizer lithium. These medications are approved for treatment of psychosis in children with schizophrenia, mania associated with bipolar disorder, and, for aripiprazole and risperidone, irritability associated with ASD. However, they are most commonly used in children to treat behavioral problems, especially aggression. Group 2 medications have a higher-risk profile and are associated with more concerning acute and chronic adverse effects than group 1 medications. Primary care clinicians are ideally positioned to monitor the adverse effects of group 2 medications, and some PCCs, for various reasons, will be involved in prescribing them.

The third group of medications includes medications not approved by the FDA for children and thus not included in groups 1 or 2. For group 3 medications, there are about 10 that PCCs are most likely to see in their practices. These 10 medications will be discussed in terms of available efficacy data and adverse-event profile. Other group 3 medications, which are not commonly prescribed, will not be discussed, but their adverse-event profiles can be accessed through electronic media (eg, Drugs@FDA, Epocrates, Micromedex).

Evidence Supporting Efficacy

The evidence base for the treatment of ADHD, common anxiety disorders (GAD, social phobia, and separation anxiety disorder), and depression has been demonstrated in several multisite randomized clinical trials

Table 11-1. Group 1 Psychotropic Medications[a]

Drug (Mode of Action)	Indication[b]	US Food and Drug Administration Approval and Approved Age (y)
Attention-deficit/Hyperactivity Disorder		
Methylphenidate (stimulant)	ADHD	Yes; ≥6[c]
Amphetamine (stimulant)[d]	ADHD	Yes; ≥6[c]
Guanfacine (α_2-adrenergic agonist)	ADHD	Yes; ≥6
Clonidine (α_2-adrenergic agonist)	ADHD	Yes; ≥6
Atomoxetine (selective NRI)	ADHD	Yes; ≥6
Anxiety Disorders		
Duloxetine (SNRI)	GAD	Yes; >7
Fluoxetine (SSRI)	Anxiety[d]	No
	OCD	Yes; >7
Sertraline (SSRI)	Anxiety[d]	No
	OCD	Yes; ≥6
Fluvoxamine (SSRI)	Anxiety[d]	No
	OCD	Yes; ≥10
Major Depressive Disorder		
Fluoxetine	MDD	Yes; ≥8
Escitalopram	MDD	Yes; ≥12

Abbreviations: ADHD, attention-deficit/hyperactivity disorder; GAD, generalized anxiety disorder; MDD, major depressive disorder; NRI, norepinephrine reuptake inhibitor; OCD, obsessive-compulsive disorder; SNRI, serotonin-norepinephrine reuptake inhibitor; SSRI, selective serotonin reuptake inhibitor.

[a] Evidence of efficacy and favorable side-effect (adverse-events) profile and expectation of management of disorder within primary care competencies; for a detailed discussion on pediatric mental health competencies for primary care, see *Pediatrics* (2009;124[1]:410–421).

[b] For each of these disorders, there are also evidence-based psychosocial interventions.

[c] Approved down to age 3 y for some preparations.

[d] GAD, social phobia, separation anxiety disorder.

conducted since the mid-1990s (eg, the Multimodal Treatment Study of ADHD [MTA] Cooperative Group,[9] Walkup et al,[10] March et al[11]).

The research procedure used to demonstrate efficacy (or not) of a medication is the random-assignment, masked ("blinded"), placebo-controlled, properly implemented treatment study (RCT). Additional design features that improve the quality of RCTs include a predetermined primary outcome variable; a sufficiently large number of participants, usually estimated by a power analysis, to accurately test the efficacy hypothesis; multiple performance sites that use comparable methodology; to minimize bias, independent funding (eg, in the United States, the National Institutes of Health [NIH] or another government agency); and use of independent evaluators (IEs) who do not receive any information about medication side effects.

There is no single criterion standard for determining that a medication is efficacious. In adults, 2 well-designed and conducted RCTs that demonstrate superiority of the active medication over placebo is the generally accepted standard and is used by the FDA as a prerequisite for drug approval. For children and adolescents, because there are fewer funding resources and fewer studies, the FDA sometimes relaxes this standard and approves a medication with just 1 large, high-quality, multicenter RCT along with other supportive data. That approach is also used by the GRADE (Grading of Recommendations Assessment, Development and Evaluation) Working Group to evaluate treatments of children and adolescents (www.gradeworkinggroup.org).

One of the widely recognized limitations with this approach to determining efficacy is that, for ethical and practical reasons, RCTs are short-term, although most psychotropic medications are used to treat children and adolescents with chronic disorders that often require long-term treatment. Despite this limitation, the well-designed and conducted RCT is the best method available for demonstrating efficacy.

Table 11-2 summarizes the efficacy data supporting the use of the group 1 medications. As a proxy for the magnitude of effect, the rate of responders on active drug and placebo is listed. It is important to note that a responder is not the same as a remitter. A patient who remits no longer meets diagnostic criteria and has no or very mild residual symptoms, whereas a responder generally meets a severity criterion of "much better"

Table 11-2. Evidence Supporting Short-term Safety and Efficacy of Group 1 Psychotropic Medications in Children and Adolescents

Drug	Indication	Support	Age (y)	Rate of Responders	Independent Evaluator[a]
Methylphenidate: standard formulation	ADHD	Spencer et al (1996): review[b]	6–12	A: ≈70%, P: ≈25%	NA
		MTA Cooperative Group (1999)[c]	7–9	Not specified	No
		Greenhill et al; PATS Team (2006)[d]	3–5	A: 21%, P: 13%	No
Methylphenidate: extended-release formulation	ADHD	Greenhill et al; ADHD Study Group (2002)[e]	6–16	A: 64%, P: 27%	No
		McGough et al (2006): patch[f]	6–12	A: 71%, P: 16%	No
		Findling et al (2010): patch[g]	13–17	A: 66%, P: 21%	No
Amphetamine: standard formulation	ADHD	Spencer et al (1996): review[b]	NA	NA	NA
Amphetamine: extended-release formulation	ADHD	McGough et al (2005)[h]	6–12	Not specified	No
		Domnitei, Madaan (2010)[i]	6–12	A: 70%, P: 18%	No
Guanfacine: standard formulation	ADHD	Scahill et al (2001)[j]	7–15	A: 53%, P: 0%	No
		Arnsten et al (2007): review[k]	NA	NA	NA
Guanfacine: extended-release formulation	ADHD	Biederman et al; SPD503 Study Group (2008)[l]	6–17	A: 50%, P: 26%	No
		Sallee et al; SPD503 Study Group (2009)[m]	6–17	A: 56%, P: 30%	No

Table 11-2. Evidence Supporting Short-term Safety and Efficacy of Group 1 Psychotropic Medications in Children and Adolescents (continued)

Drug	Indication	Support	Age (y)	Rate of Responders	Independent Evaluator[a]
Clonidine: extended-release formulation	ADHD	Jain et al (2011)[n]	6–17	NA	No
		Kollins et al (2011)[o]	6–17	NA	No
Atomoxetine	ADHD	Michaelson et al; Atomoxetine ADHD Study Group (2001)[p]	8–18	Not specified	No
Fluoxetine	Anxiety	Birmaher et al (2003)[q]	7–17	A: 61%, P: 35%	No
	MDD	Emslie et al (1997)[r]	7–17	A: 56%, P: 33%	No
		Emslie et al (2002)[s]	8–18	A: 65%, P: 53%	No
		March et al; TADS Team (2004)[t]	12–17	A: 61%, P: 35%	Yes
	OCD	Riddle et al (1992)[u]	8–15	A: 33%, P: 12%	No
		Geller et al; Fluoxetine Pediatric OCD Study Team (2001)[v]	7–17	A: 49%, P: 25%	No
Sertraline	Anxiety	Liebowitz et al (2002)[w]	6–18	A: 57%, P: 27%	Yes
	MDD	Walkup et al (2008)[x]	7–17	A: 55%, P: 24%	Yes
		Wagner et al; Sertraline Pediatric Depression Study Group (2003)[y]	6–17	A: 36%, P: 24%	No
	OCD	March et al (1998)[z]	13–17	A: 42%, P: 26%	No
		POTS Team (2004)[aa]	7–17	A: 21%, P: 4%	Yes

Escitalopram	MDD	Wagner et al (2006)[bb]	6–17	A: 63%, P: 52%	No
		Emslie et al (2009)[cc]	12–17	A: 62%, P: 52%	No
Fluvoxamine	Anxiety	RUPP Anxiety Study Group (2001)[dd]	6–17	A: 76%, P: 29%	No
	OCD	Riddle et al (2001)[ee]	8–17	A: 42%, P: 26%	No
Duloxetine	GAD	Strawn et al (2015)[ff]	7–17	A: 59%, P: 42%	No

Abbreviations: A, active drug recipients; ADHD, attention-deficit/hyperactivity disorder; GAD, generalized anxiety disorder; IE, independent evaluator; MDD, major depressive disorder; MTA, Multimodal Treatment Study of ADHD; NA, not applicable; OCD, obsessive-compulsive disorder; P, placebo recipients; PATS, Preschool ADHD Treatment Study; POTS, Pediatric OCD Treatment Study; RUPP, Research Unit on Pediatric Psychopharmacology; TADS, Treatment for Adolescents With Depression Study.

[a] Use of IEs to rate symptom severity may help reduce bias because these individuals are blinded to patient side effects (adverse events) that could reveal their treatment assignment.

[b] Spencer T, Biederman J, Wilens T, Harding M, O'Donnell D, Griffin S. Pharmacotherapy of attention-deficit hyperactivity disorder across the life cycle. *J Am Acad Child Adolesc Psychiatry.* 1996;35(4):409–432.

[c] A 14-month randomized clinical trial of treatment strategies for attention-deficit/hyperactivity disorder. The MTA Cooperative Group. Multimodal Treatment Study of Children with ADHD. *Arch Gen Psychiatry.* 1999;56(12):1073–1086.

[d] Greenhill L, Kollins S, Abikoff H, et al; PATS Team. Efficacy and safety of immediate-release methylphenidate treatment for preschoolers with ADHD. *J Am Acad Child Adolesc Psychiatry.* 2006;45(11):1284–1293.

[e] Greenhill LL, Findling RL, Swanson JM; ADHD Study Group. A double-blind, placebo-controlled study of modified-release methylphenidate in children with attention-deficit/hyperactivity disorder. *Pediatrics.* 2002;109(3):E39.

[f] McGough JJ, Wigal SB, Abikoff H, Turnbow JM, Posner K, Moon E. A randomized, double-blind, placebo-controlled, laboratory classroom assessment of methylphenidate transdermal system in children with ADHD. *J Atten Disord.* 2006;9(3):476–485.

[g] Findling RL, Turnbow J, Burnside J, Melmed R, Civil R, Li Y. A randomized, double-blind, multicenter, parallel-group, placebo-controlled, dose-optimization study of the methylphenidate transdermal system for the treatment of ADHD in adolescents. *CNS Spectr.* 2010;15(7):419–430.

[h] McGough JJ, Biederman J, Wigal SB, et al. Long-term tolerability and effectiveness of once-daily mixed amphetamine salts (Adderall XR) in children with ADHD. *J Am Acad Child Adolesc Psychiatry.* 2005;44(6):530–538.

[i] Domnitei D, Madaan V. New and extended-action treatments in the management of ADHD: a critical appraisal of lisdexamfetamine in adults and children. *Neuropsychiatr Dis Treat.* 2010;6:273–279.

[j] Scahill L, Chappell PB, Kim YS, et al. A placebo-controlled study of guanfacine in the treatment of children with tic disorders and attention deficit hyperactivity disorder. *Am J Psychiatry.* 2001;158(7):1067–1074.

Table 11-2. Evidence Supporting Short-term Safety and Efficacy of Group 1 Psychotropic Medications in Children and Adolescents (*continued*)

k   Arnsten AF, Scahill L, Findling RL. alpha2-Adrenergic receptor agonists for the treatment of attention-deficit/hyperactivity disorder: emerging concepts from new data. *J Child Adolesc Psychopharmacol.* 2007;17(4):393–406.

l   Biederman J, Melmed RD, Patel A, et al; SPD503 Study Group. A randomized, double-blind, placebo-controlled study of guanfacine extended release in children and adolescents with attention-deficit/hyperactivity disorder. *Pediatrics.* 2008;121(1):e73–e84.

m   Sallee FR, McGough J, Wigal T, Donahue J, Lyne A, Biederman J; SPD503 Study Group. Guanfacine extended release in children and adolescents with attention-deficit/hyperactivity disorder: a placebo-controlled trial. *J Am Acad Child Adolesc Psychiatry.* 2009;48(2):155–165.

n   Jain R, Segal S, Kollins SH, Khayrallah M. Clonidine extended-release tablets for pediatric patients with attention-deficit/hyperactivity disorder. *J Am Acad Child Adolesc Psychiatry.* 2011;50(2):171–179.

o   Kollins SH, Jain R, Brams M, et al. Clonidine extended-release tablets as add-on therapy to psychostimulants in children and adolescents with ADHD. *Pediatrics.* 2011;127(6):e1406–e1413.

p   Michelson D, Faries D, Wernicke J, et al; Atomoxetine ADHD Study Group. Atomoxetine in the treatment of children and adolescents with attention-deficit/hyperactivity disorder: a randomized, placebo-controlled, dose-response study. *Pediatrics.* 2001;108(5):E83.

q   Birmaher B, Axelson DA, Monk K, et al. Fluoxetine for the treatment of childhood anxiety disorders. *J Am Acad Child Adolesc Psychiatry.* 2003;42(4):415–423.

r   Emslie GJ, Rush AJ, Weinberg WA, et al. A double-blind, randomized, placebo-controlled trial of fluoxetine in children and adolescents with depression. *Arch Gen Psychiatry.* 1997;54(11):1031–1037.

s   Emslie GJ, Heiligenstein JH, Wagner KD, et al. Fluoxetine for acute treatment of depression in children and adolescents: a placebo-controlled, randomized clinical trial. *J Am Acad Child Adolesc Psychiatry.* 2002;41(10):1205–1215.

t   March J, Silva S, Petrycki S, et al; Treatment for Adolescents With Depression Study (TADS) Team. Fluoxetine, cognitive-behavioral therapy, and their combination for adolescents with depression: Treatment for Adolescents With Depression Study (TADS) randomized controlled trial. *JAMA.* 2004;292(7):807–820.

u   Riddle MA, Scahill L, King RA, et al. Double-blind, crossover trial of fluoxetine and placebo in children and adolescents with obsessive-compulsive disorder. *J Am Acad Child Adolesc Psychiatry.* 1992;31(6):1062–1069.

v   Geller DA, Hoog SL, Heiligenstein JH, et al; Fluoxetine Pediatric OCD Study Team. Fluoxetine treatment for obsessive-compulsive disorder in children and adolescents: a placebo-controlled clinical trial. *J Am Acad Child Adolesc Psychiatry.* 2001;40(7):773–779.

w   Liebowitz MR, Turner SM, Piacentini J, et al. Fluoxetine in children and adolescents with OCD: a placebo-controlled trial. *J Am Acad Child Adolesc Psychiatry.* 2002;41(12):1431–1438.

x   Walkup JT, Albano AM, Piacentini J, et al. Cognitive behavioral therapy, sertraline, or a combination in childhood anxiety. *N Engl J Med.* 2008;359(26):2753–2766.

y   Wagner KD, Ambrosini P, Rynn M, et al; Sertraline Pediatric Depression Study Group. Efficacy of sertraline in the treatment of children and adolescents with major depressive disorder: two randomized controlled trials. *JAMA*. 2003;290(8):1033–1041.

z   March JS, Biederman J, Wolkow R, et al. Sertraline in children and adolescents with obsessive-compulsive disorder: a multicenter randomized controlled trial. *JAMA*. 1998;280(20):1752–1756.

aa Pediatric OCD Treatment Study (POTS) Team. Cognitive-behavior therapy, sertraline, and their combination for children and adolescents with obsessive-compulsive disorder: the Pediatric OCD Treatment Study (POTS) randomized controlled trial. *JAMA*. 2004;292(16):1969–1976.

bb Wagner KD, Jonas J, Findling RL, Ventura D, Saikali K. A double-blind, randomized, placebo-controlled trial of escitalopram in the treatment of pediatric depression. *J Am Acad Child Adolesc Psychiatry*. 2006;45(3):280–288.

cc Emslie GJ, Ventura D, Korotzer A, Tourkodimitris S. Escitalopram in the treatment of adolescent depression: a randomized placebo-controlled multisite trial. *J Am Acad Child Adolesc Psychiatry*. 2009;48(7):721–729.

dd Fluvoxamine for the treatment of anxiety disorders in children and adolescents. The Research Unit on Pediatric Psychopharmacology Anxiety Study Group. *N Engl J Med*. 2001;344(17):1279–1285.

ee Riddle MA, Reeve EA, Yaryura-Tobias JA, et al. Fluvoxamine for children and adolescents with obsessive-compulsive disorder: a randomized, controlled, multicenter trial. *J Am Acad Child Adolesc Psychiatry*. 2001;40(2):222–229.

ff Strawn JR, Prakash A, Zhang Q, et al. A randomized, placebo-controlled study of duloxetine for the treatment of children and adolescents with generalized anxiety disorder. *J Am Acad Child Adolesc Psychiatry*. 2015;54(4):283–293.

or "very much better" but may still have mild to moderate symptoms. Thus, a remitter is generally more improved than a responder. The last column notes whether ratings were done by IEs. An IE is a rater who is not involved in data collection other than to conduct blinded symptom severity ratings at specified times during a study. The use of IEs is thought to reduce bias because the presence or absence of medication side effects (which are not known to the IEs) can help investigators guess the participant's medication status: active or placebo. Finally, all relevant and published NIH-sponsored studies are included in Table 11-2. However, there may be unpublished industry-sponsored studies that are not listed.

Evidence Supporting Safety

There is no criterion standard for assessing safety of medications in children and adolescents. For the purposes of this discussion, 5 parameters will be used for assessing safety.

1. An FDA-approved pediatric indication (a proxy for a minimal standard of research data supporting short-term safety [and efficacy] of a medication for a specified indication)

2. At least 10 years on the market (a proxy for sufficient time to discover rare adverse long-term consequences and rare complications with long-term exposure [ie, greater exposure over time increases the chance to detect rare and harmful events that would not otherwise be detected in brief clinical trials])

3. Minimal overdose harm, determined by a review of the available literature

4. Lack of clinically significant boxed warnings (a formal FDA proxy for rare, major adverse events)

5. Lack of other known or potentially harmful long-term effects, determined by a review of available literature and review of warnings and precautions in the FDA package inserts

Table 11-3 applies these safety parameters to the 4 categories of group 1 medications.

Table 11-3. Safety Profile of Group 1 Psychotropic Medication Classes in Children and Adolescents

Safety Criteria	Stimulants	Adrenergics	SSRIs	Selective NRIs	SNRIs
FDA approval	≥6 y	≥6 y	≥8 y	≥6 y	≥7 y
Years on market[a]	>50 y	>30 y	>25 y	≥10 y	≥10 y
Overdose harm	Low	Low	Very low	Very low	Very low
Boxed warning (major AEs)[b]	Drug abuse potential	None	Suicidality	Suicidality	Suicidality
Long-term risk to health[c,d]	Possible growth deceleration	None known	None known	None known	None known

Abbreviations: AEs, adverse events; FDA, US Food and Drug Administration; NRI, norepinephrine reuptake inhibitor; SNRI, serotonin-norepinephrine reuptake inhibitor; SSRI, selective serotonin reuptake inhibitor.

[a] Measure of exposure in large populations; time to observe potentially harmful events.

[b] Original FDA meta-analysis; 2% for placebo and 4% active in forced dose titration studies (*Arch Gen Psychiatry*. 2006;63[3]:332–339). More recent analysis shows difference of 0.67%, down from 2% difference (*JAMA*. 2007;297[15]:1683–1696).

[c] Lack of studies to assess long-term risk to health, except for stimulants.

[d] Stimulants and growth deceleration: data are not convincing.

Group 1 Medications: Specific Rationale

The group 1 medications for use in the primary care setting belong to 4 different classes of medications. The rationale for using specific medications is presented here.

Stimulants

Despite the numerous products available on the market, there are just 2 distinct stimulant chemical entities: *methylphenidate* and *amphetamine*. The available literature has not shown advantages in efficacy of methylphenidate vs amphetamine. Thus, different preparations (brands) are considered interchangeable except for dose and duration of action. Methylphenidate and amphetamine are available in numerous release preparations that provide a treatment effect ranging from 3 to 12 hours. Preparations with longer time on the market and lower cost may be preferred, but that is a general comment, not a preparation-specific recommendation.

α_2-Adrenergic Agonists

Guanfacine is approved by the FDA for ADHD in children and adolescents. It is relatively specific to the α_{2A} receptor subtype, which mediates attention and other executive functions. *Clonidine* is approved by the FDA for ADHD in children and adolescents. It nonspecifically interacts with α_{2A}, α_{2B}, and α_{2C} receptor subtypes. The B and C receptors mediate the sedation and hypotension or bradycardia adverse effects. Thus, clonidine may have a less favorable adverse-event profile than guanfacine. There are no direct comparative data regarding this issue. Also, regular (not sustained-release) clonidine is associated with acute drops in blood pressure (BP), syncope, and even death following unintentional or intentional ingestions of more than therapeutic quantities.

Selective Norepinephrine Reuptake Inhibitor

Atomoxetine, a selective NRI, has an FDA indication for ADHD. It has more concerning FDA warnings and precautions than the other medications for ADHD included in group 1.

Selective Serotonin Reuptake Inhibitors

Six SSRIs are marketed in the United States: fluoxetine, sertraline, escitalopram, paroxetine, citalopram, and fluvoxamine. Comments regarding the 4 SSRIs included in group 1 follow.

▶ *Fluoxetine:* Has FDA indications in children and adolescents for depression and OCD; high-quality, NIH-sponsored study demonstrating efficacy for the 3 common anxiety disorders in children[14]; the first SSRI marketed in the United States; and longest half-life, so abrupt discontinuation results in slow, safe fall in plasma and brain levels

▶ *Sertraline:* Has FDA indication in children and adolescents for OCD, is second SSRI in the United States, has best data for the 3 common anxiety disorders in children,[10] and offers alternative to fluoxetine when shorter half-life may be indicated (eg, for a child taking multiple medications with further changes likely) or when fluoxetine cannot be used because of interactions with metabolic isoenzymes (eg, inhibition of cytochrome P450 2D6 isozyme [CYP2D6])

▶ *Escitalopram:* Has FDA indication in adolescents for depression and no clinically relevant interactions with hepatic cytochrome P450 isoenzymes

▶ *Fluvoxamine:* Has FDA indication for OCD in children and a high-quality, NIH-sponsored study demonstrating efficacy for the 3 common anxiety disorders in children[15]

Serotonin-Norepinephrine Reuptake Inhibitor

Duloxetine, an SNRI, has an FDA indication for GAD. The main clinical difference between duloxetine and SSRIs is the adverse-event profile.

Prescribing Group 1 Medications in Pediatric Primary Care

The general rationale regarding efficacy and safety of psychotropic medications, especially those in group 1, was described in previous sections. Provided here is a brief introduction to clinical issues associated with prescribing and monitoring of group 1 psychotropic medications in primary care pediatrics.

Informed Consent

Obtaining informed consent from the parent or guardian and assent from the patient can be more complicated and difficult for psychotropic medications than for other medications. This difficulty is caused by parental concerns about the potential effect of medications on the child's developing brain and controversy in the media regarding psychiatric medications. The basic steps involved in obtaining informed consent and assent are the same, no matter what psychotropic medication is recommended. A description of essential and optional areas to cover in the consent process is provided in Box 11-3. In addition to the initial consent process,

---

Box 11-3. A Clinical Approach to Informed Consent for Psychotropic Medication

Essential

- Preamble
  - Conceptualization of signs and symptoms as *illness*.
  - What are the *risks of not treating* with medication?
  - Think *job performance* (eg, home, school, friends).
  - Think *development* (eg, emotional, behavioral, social, cognitive).

- Evidence supporting short-term efficacy and effectiveness
  - A level: 2 RCTs or, in some cases for children and adolescents, 1 well-designed RCT[a]
  - B level: 1 RCT
  - C level: information from open-label studies, case reports, other observations

- Alternative and additional treatments
  - Evidence-based psychosocial therapies
  - Community, family, school system support
  - Other medications

- Adverse effects

Severity	Change Needed	Examples
Mild	Requires no change	Dry mouth, transient nausea
Moderate	Requires dose change	Sedation
Severe	Requires stopping drug	Real suicidal ideation or attempt

- Potential long-term adverse effects
  - Examples: suppression of growth (stimulants), diabetes mellitus, tardive dyskinesia (antipsychotics)
  - Unknown

> ### Box 11-3. A Clinical Approach to Informed Consent for Psychotropic Medication (*continued*)
>
> ◾ Pharmacokinetic issues
> - Convenience: once-daily dosing preferred, no laboratory monitoring preferred
> - Drug-drug interactions: especially involving hepatic cytochrome P450 enzymes
>
> ◾ Adherence
> - The importance of establishing a convenient daily routine for taking the medication
>
> ◾ Your opinion about benefit to risk ratio for this patient
> - Taking into consideration all the above, what options do you recommend?
> - Why?
> - *Think: If this were your child, what would you do?*
>
> <u>Optional</u>
> ◾ Cost
> - Generic vs brand
> - This drug vs others in class
>
> ◾ Evidence supporting long-term efficacy and effectiveness
> - For ethical and practical reasons, no randomized, parallel-group, clinical trial data are available.
>
> ---
>
> Abbreviations: ADHD, attention-deficit/hyperactivity disorder; RCT, placebo-controlled, random-assignment, properly implemented treatment study.
>
> [a] This level applies to all group 1 medications for ADHD, anxiety, and depression.

informed consent is usually an ongoing process that unfolds over time as the patient and caregiver develop new questions and concerns about medications. The initial consent process offers an ideal opportunity to consider a timeline for reevaluating both medication efficacy and side effects and to note that consent will be revisited in light of the patient's initial and ongoing responses to and experiences with the medication, both positive and negative. Thus, consent is an ongoing component of an evolving clinical process.

Dosing

Dosing for all group 1 medications generally follows the same pattern: start with a relatively low dose, increase in relatively small increments about every week, and continue to increase the dose until an optimal benefit to risk ratio is reached. The dosing guidance presented in this chapter for all group 1 medications is derived from the FDA package inserts, with the authors adding detail on points about which the FDA is silent, such as how often or by how much to increase the dose. Dosing recommendations from the FDA can be found in package inserts or at the Drugs@FDA: FDA Approved Drug Products Web site (www.accessdata. fda.gov).

▶ *Methylphenidate preparations* (Table 11-4): For standard-release preparations, starting doses range from 2.5 mg per dose for preschoolers (aged 4–5 years), to 5 mg per dose for school-aged children, to 10 mg per dose for adolescents. Recommended doses for Focalin preparations are half of those for other methylphenidate preparations. Dose increments for increases are generally equivalent to the starting dose. Because response to stimulants may be idiosyncratic, individualized dose titration with interval reports from multiple independent observers is indicated. Optimal benefit to risk ratio is common at a total daily dosage of 0.5 to 1.5 mg/kg/d, although some children respond to lower doses and some adolescents may require higher doses. Some adverse events, such as decreased appetite and insomnia, may be dose sensitive, so higher total daily dosages need to be carefully monitored. Most children and families prefer long-acting preparations, which can usually be given once per day. The smallest daily dosage of the most popular extended-release methylphenidate preparation (osmotic pump) is 18 mg/d; lower dose increments are available with other formulations.

▶ *Amphetamine preparations* (Table 11-4): One milligram of amphetamine is approximately equivalent to 2 mg of methylphenidate. Thus, the dosages given previously for methylphenidate can be used for amphetamine preparations, but they need to be divided by 2. Long-acting preparations of amphetamine are available in a wide range of doses.

▶ *Guanfacine:* For the once-daily preparation, which is preferred by children and families, the starting dosage is usually 1 mg/d. Doses can be increased by 1 mg every few days to a maximum recommended daily dosage of 4 mg for children and 7 mg for adolescents.

▶ *Clonidine:* One-tenth milligram of clonidine is approximately equivalent to 1 mg of guanfacine. Thus, the dosages given previously for

Table 11-4. Stimulant Preparations

Preparation	Duration (h)	Methylphenidate	Amphetamine
Pills			
Standard (immediate) release	3–4 (MPD) 4–6 (AMP)	Ritalin Focal *d*	Adderall Evekeo[a] Zenzedi *d*[a]
Pulse (beads) extended release	7–8	Metadate ER Aptensio XR[a]	Dexedrine Spansule *d*
Pearls (matrix) extended release	8–12	Metadate CD Ritalin LA Focalin XR *d*	Adderall XR
Pump (osmotic) extended release	≤12	Concerta	No preparation available
Modified standard release	≤12	No preparation available	Vyvanse *d*[a,b]
Liquid, Chewable, Disintegrate, and Patch Preparations			
Liquid immediate release	3–5	Methylin	Procentra[a]
Chewable immediate release	3–5	Methylphenidate Chewable[a]	No preparation available
Liquid extended release	8–12	Quillivant XR[a]	Dynavel XR[a]
Chewable extended release	8–12	Quillichew ER[a]	No preparation available
Oral disintegrating extended release	8–12	No preparation available	Adzens XR-ODT[a]
Patch	≤12	Daytrana[a]	No preparation available

Abbreviation: *d*, dextroamphetamine.
[a] Only branded form is available (ie, no generic).
[b] Vyvanse is converted to standard-release dextroamphetamine after the prodrug passes through the gut without being metabolized. Thus, it is a "modified" standard-release preparation.
From *FDA Listing of Authorized Generics*. Silver Spring, MD: US Food and Drug Administration; 2017. https://www.fda.gov/downloads/AboutFDA/CentersOffices/OfficeofMedicalProductsandTobacco/CDER/UCM183605.pdf. Accessed February 7, 2018.

guanfacine can be used for clonidine preparations, but they need to be divided by 10. Recommended dosing for the long-acting preparation of clonidine is twice daily using 0.1- and 0.2-mg preparations, with a maximum daily dosage of 0.4 mg.

▶ *Atomoxetine:* Atomoxetine is dosed once daily. For children and adolescents up to 70 kg, the FDA-recommended initial daily dosage is 0.5 mg/kg; target daily dosage is 1.2 mg/kg, and maximum daily dosage is 1.2 mg/kg. For those more than 70 kg, initial daily dosage is 40 mg; target daily dosage is 80 mg, and maximum daily dosage is 100 mg. Dosage should be adjusted (lowered) for patients known to be CYP2D6 poor metabolizers.

▶ *Fluoxetine:* Fluoxetine is dosed once daily. Starting dose ranges from 2.5 to 10 mg, depending on age and weight. Doses are generally increased every week or so by an amount equivalent to the starting dose until a favorable benefit to risk ratio is achieved. Best effective dose is generally 5 to 20 mg, although higher doses are sometimes required.

▶ *Sertraline:* Sertraline is dosed once daily. Starting dose ranges from 12.5 to 25 mg. Dose increments range from 12.5 to 50 mg. Effective total daily dosage is generally 25 to 200 mg.

▶ *Escitalopram:* Escitalopram is dosed once daily. Starting dose ranges from 2.5 to 5 mg. Dose increments range from 2.5 to 10 mg. Effective total daily dosage is generally 5 to 20 mg.

▶ *Fluvoxamine:* The starting dose is 25 mg at bedtime, with increases of 25 mg every 4 to 7 days as tolerated to maximum effect, not to exceed 200 mg/d (8–11 years) or 300 mg/d (12–17 years). Daily dosages more than 50 mg should be divided. Although an extended-release preparation is available, the FDA package insert states that for "pediatric patients naïve to fluvoxamine maleate—the lowest available dose of Luvox CR capsules may not be appropriate."

▶ *Duloxetine:* Duloxetine is dosed once daily. Recommended starting dose is 30 mg. The target and maximum doses for 7- to 17-year-olds is 60 mg. The capsule must be swallowed whole.

Side Effects or Adverse Events

Adverse events can be evaluated on the basis of either severity or frequency. In package inserts required by the FDA, potential severity of adverse events is emphasized; that is, boxed warnings are more severe than warnings and precautions, which are more severe than adverse reactions. In addition, package inserts describe contraindications and drug interactions.

The most comprehensive and least potentially biased prescribing information about adverse events can be found in FDA-required labels or package inserts. These labels are available in various formats and locations, including in medication packaging and the *Physicians' Desk Reference*. They are available online at the Drugs@FDA: FDA Approved Drug Products Web site (www.accessdata.fda.gov). Since the FDA modified the format for labels a few years ago, each label or insert has a 1-page Highlights of Prescribing Information section that includes relatively complete and essential information about boxed warnings, warnings and precautions, adverse reactions, contraindications, and drug interactions. These highlights can be accessed and reviewed quickly and conveniently and are useful resources.

Rather than reiterate all the details regarding all the adverse events associated with all the medications in group 1, the following 3 sections provide general guidance regarding boxed warnings, warnings and precautions, and adverse reactions. Because contraindications are essentially prohibitions to prescribing, they are not amenable to summarization and should be specifically and carefully considered before prescribing any medication. Likewise, drug interactions, although not prohibitive, are drug specific and generally not amenable to summarization; they should be carefully considered before prescribing any medication.

US Food and Drug Administration Boxed Warnings

The most concerning adverse events are given boxed warnings by the FDA. There is 1 boxed warning for antidepressants (specifically SSRIs and duloxetine), 1 for atomoxetine, 1 for stimulants, and none for α_2-adrenergic agonists. It is important to keep in mind that all the adverse events described in the boxed warnings listed here occur infrequently and may never be seen by an individual PCC. The information in the following sections was taken from the most recent labels available at Drugs@FDA as of March 15, 2017.

Antidepressants (Selective Serotonin Reuptake Inhibitors and Duloxetine) and Atomoxetine and Suicidal Thoughts and Behavior

The FDA boxed warning about increased risk of suicidal thoughts and behavior is an obstacle for many PCCs who consider prescribing SSRIs or duloxetine for anxiety and depression. The boxed warning issued in October 2004 stated that all antidepressants pose significant risk for suicidality (suicidal ideation or behavior, not completed suicides) in children and adolescents and recommended a specific protocol for close monitoring for suicidal thoughts and behaviors. Revised and less specific recommendations for monitoring were described in a revised FDA medication guide in 2007 (www.fda.gov/downloads/Drugs/Drug-Safety/InformationbyDrugClass/ucm100211.pdf). This updated guide focuses on information parents need to know regarding suicidal thoughts and behaviors and antidepressants rather than on specific mandates for monitoring frequency.

Antidepressant-induced suicidality is rare. The original FDA estimate, based solely on data from more than 4,300 research participants in 23 studies, was that 2% of children and adolescents receiving placebo and 4% receiving an antidepressant developed suicidal thoughts or attempted suicide.[16] Thus, the risk difference was 2%. A subsequent analysis based on data from 27 RCTs involving more than 5,300 participants showed a risk difference of just 0.7% (95% confidence interval [CI]: 0.1%–1.3%).[17] The most recent estimate, which was based on data from 35 RCTs involving more than 6,000 participants, showed a risk difference of 0.9% (95% CI: 20.000–0.018), just reaching statistical significance.[18]

Clinical prudence indicates the need to educate patients and parents about suicidal thoughts and behaviors, because they are both target symptoms and potential adverse effects for depressed children and adolescents treated with antidepressants, and to provide careful monitoring during the initial phase of treatment (when the risk for suicidal thoughts and behaviors is generally greatest from both the depression and the medication) and throughout treatment.

Stimulants and Concerns About Abuse and Dependence

The boxed warning for both amphetamines and methylphenidate states that they have a high potential for abuse and that prolonged administration may lead to dependence. Fortunately, there are no reports of children who were treated with therapeutic doses of stimulants developing dependence. Available data suggest that children with ADHD who are treated with stimulants are not more likely than those who did not receive stimulant treatment to develop substance abuse later in life.[19–21] A related problem is diversion, that is, patients selling their prescription stimulants to be used as drugs of abuse.[22]

US Food and Drug Administration Warnings and Precautions
Stimulants

Most warnings and precautions concern events that rarely occur in children and adolescents treated with stimulants. Those most relevant to children taking either methylphenidate or amphetamine preparations include

▶ Serious cardiovascular events (generally only in patients with known structural cardiac abnormalities, cardiomyopathy, serious heart rhythm abnormalities, coronary artery disease, or other serious heart problems)

▶ Increase in BP (This warning and precaution is more common than other warnings and precautions.)

▶ Psychiatric adverse events (primarily emergence of psychotic, manic, or aggressive symptoms)

▶ Exacerbation of tics

▶ Seizures

▶ Priapism (methylphenidate preparations only)

▶ Long-term suppression of growth

CNS stimulants have been associated with weight loss and slowing of growth rate in pediatric patients. Closely monitor growth (weight and height) in pediatric patients treated with CNS stimulants, including Aptensio XR.

Careful follow-up of weight and height in pediatric patients aged 7 to 10 years who were randomized to either methylphenidate or non-medication treatment groups over 14 months, as well as in naturalistic subgroups of newly methylphenidate-treated and non-medication treated pediatric patients over 36 months (to the ages of 10 to 13 years), suggests that consistently medicated pediatric patients (i.e., treatment for 7 days per week throughout the year) have a temporary slowing in growth rate (on average, a total of about 2 cm less growth in height and 2.7 kg less growth in weight over 3 years), without evidence of growth rebound during this period of development.

Published data are inadequate to determine whether chronic use of amphetamines may cause a similar suppression of growth; however, it is anticipated that they likely have this effect as well. Therefore, growth should be monitored during treatment with stimulants, and patients who are not growing or gaining height or weight as expected may need to have their treatment interrupted.[23]

α_2-Adrenergic Agonists

Both guanfacine preparations and clonidine preparations have the following relevant warnings and precautions:

► Hypotension, bradycardia, and syncope

► Sedation and somnolence

► Worsening of some preexisting cardiac conduction abnormalities

In addition, abrupt discontinuation should be avoided with clonidine preparations.

Atomoxetine

Atomoxetine has the following relevant warnings and precautions:

► Severe liver injury

► Serious cardiovascular events

► Effects on BP and heart rate

► Emergent psychotic or manic symptoms

► Bipolar disorder

► Aggressive behavior or hostility

► Possible allergic reactions (in addition to the standard contraindication for hypersensitivity)

► Effects on urine outflow

► Priapism

► Growth

► Concomitant use with potent CYP2D6 inhibitors

Selective Serotonin Reuptake Inhibitors

The SSRIs fluoxetine, sertraline, escitalopram, and fluvoxamine all have the following relevant warnings and precautions:

► Serotonin syndrome

► Activation of mania or hypomania

► Seizures

► Abnormal bleeding

► Hyponatremia

▶ Potential cognitive and motor impairment

▶ Angle-closure glaucoma

Fluoxetine has some additional relevant warnings and precautions: altered appetite and weight, anxiety and insomnia, QT prolongation, and long half-life (thus, changes in dose may not be reflected in plasma for several weeks).

Sertraline, escitalopram, and fluvoxamine all have a warning and precaution regarding discontinuation of treatment, specifically concerns about various withdrawal symptoms with abrupt discontinuation.

Fluvoxamine has a warning and precaution regarding potentially important drug interactions, beyond those described in the Drug Interactions section of the label. These interactions are generally related to inhibiting effect of fluvoxamine on several cytochrome P450 isoenzymes, including 1A2, 2C9, 3A4, and 2C19.

Adverse Reactions

The FDA label uses frequency, rather than severity, to delineate adverse reactions, the most common and least severe of adverse events. Although specifics vary from medication to medication, the label usually describes the most common adverse reactions (>5% and at least twice the placebo rate) reported in RCTs submitted to the FDA. This report may be for adults, children, adolescents, or some combination of these groups.

In Table 11-5, common and less common adverse events for the 5 classes of group 1 medications are presented. Table 11-5 is based on, but not completely the same as, adverse reactions presented in FDA-approved labels. In addition, withdrawal symptoms are noted. Except for low-dose stimulants and fluoxetine, medications should be tapered to minimize withdrawal symptoms.

Monitoring Group 1 Medications

Frequency of monitoring may vary depending on a particular patient's health status, but, in general, it is more frequent during the initial phase of treatment with all group 1 medications. During this time, dosage is changing frequently as it is being titrated up to an effective and safe dose, and side effects often occur before benefit. Poor adherence is common, so monitoring for adherence is important to prevent unwarranted and potentially unsafe dose escalations in the child who is not adherent.

Table 11-5. Adverse Reactions Associated With Group 1 Psychotropic Medication Classes

Medication Class	Adverse Reactions[a]	Withdrawal Symptoms[b]
Stimulants Methylphenidate (Ritalin and others) Dexmethylphenidate (Focalin) Dextroamphetamine (Dexedrine and others) Amphetamine salts (Adderall and others)	*Common: insomnia, appetite suppression, headache, stomachache* Less common: cognitive dulling, irritability, exacerbation of tics **Monitor:** BP, pulse, height, weight, BMI	ADHD symptoms "worsen" at end of day when drug wears off. These are not considered withdrawal symptoms.
α₂-Adrenergic agonists Guanfacine (Tenex, Intuniv) Clonidine (Catapres, Kapvay)	*Common: somnolence* Less common: dry mouth, headache, nausea, decreased BP **Monitor:** BP, pulse	Elevated BP, nervousness, headache, confusion
Selective NRI Atomoxetine (Strattera)	*Common: dry mouth, insomnia, nausea, decreased appetite* Less common: increased HR, BP, palpitations, dizziness, sweating, dysuria, weight change **Monitor:** BMI, BP, HR	There are no reported withdrawal-induced adverse effects. Atomoxetine can be discontinued without tapering.

SSRIs Fluoxetine (Prozac) Sertraline (Zoloft) Escitalopram (Lexapro) Fluvoxamine (Luvox)	*Common: "activation" (restlessness, insomnia, impulsiveness, talkativeness [usually occur early in treatment]), GI upset, nausea, diarrhea* Less common: autonomic (eg, diaphoresis, mydriasis), cardio-vascular (eg, flushing, sinus tachycardia, hypertension), sexual (decreased libido, delayed ejaculation), akathisia **Monitor:** BMI; worsening of depression; emergence of suicidal thinking or behavior (especially with initiation or dose escalation); unusual changes in behavior, such as sleeplessness, agitation, or withdrawal from normal social situations	Especially for shorter half-life SSRIs such as sertraline: flu-like syndrome; dizziness (most common), nausea, vomiting, fatigue, headache, gait instability, insomnia, mood changes, myalgia. Tapering not needed for fluoxetine.
SNRI Duloxetine (Cymbalta)	*Common: nausea, dry mouth, somnolence, constipation, decreased appetite, hyperhidrosis*	Dizziness, headache, nausea, diarrhea, paresthesia, irritability, vomiting, insomnia, anxiety, hyperhidrosis, fatigue

Abbreviations: AACAP, American Academy of Child and Adolescent Psychiatry; ADHD, attention-deficit/hyperactivity disorder; BP, blood pressure; BMI, body mass index; FDA, US Food and Drug Administration; GI, gastrointestinal; HR, heart rate; NIH, National Institutes of Health; NRI, norepinephrine reuptake inhibitor; SNRI, serotonin-norepinephrine reuptake inhibitor; SSRI, selective serotonin reuptake inhibitor.

ᵃ Common adverse reactions in *italics*.

ᵇ Tapering suggested for all medications except fluoxetine.

Check for psychopharmacological medication updates from a reliable source, such as the National Library of Medicine or NIH, MedlinePlus "Drugs, Herbs and Supplements" (www.nlm.nih.gov/medlineplus/druginformation.html); FDA (www.fda.gov); or AACAP (www.aacap.org). "Practice Parameter on the Use of Psychotropic Medication in Children and Adolescents: The AACAP Practice Parameters" describe generally accepted practices. They are designed to assist physicians in providing high-quality assessment and treatment for children and adolescents consistent with best available scientific evidence and clinical consensus (http://download.journals.elsevierhealth.com/pdfs/journals/0890-8567/PIIS0890856709601568.pdf).

Finally, more frequent monitoring may be indicated for patients with certain medical conditions.

For stimulants, BP, HR, height, and weight should be monitored. In addition, patients taking stimulants should be observed for, and parents questioned about, tics. No specific laboratory studies are recommended. The recommendations for guanfacine, clonidine, and atomoxetine are similar.

Patients taking SSRIs should be monitored for several parameters during the first several weeks of treatment: emergence of suicidal thinking or behavior, worsening of depression, gastrointestinal symptoms (eg, pain, nausea, diarrhea), or the activation phenomenon (eg, agitation, insomnia, increased energy or activity). Over the longer term, height and weight, sexual dysfunction, and emergence of mania should be monitored. No specific laboratory tests are indicated, although thyroid function testing may be clinically indicated as part of the somatic evaluation for children and adolescents with new-onset depression or depression that does not respond to evidence-based treatment. Monitoring recommendations for duloxetine are similar to those for the SSRIs. In addition, pulse and BP monitoring are indicated.

Phases of Treatment

Medication treatment of ADHD, anxiety, or depression is often initiated during an acute clinical crisis, when the child's symptoms are at their worst. Thus, doses that are used in the immediate phase of illness and treatment may be higher than are needed later, during maintenance treatment. A decrease in dose is especially likely if the child and family are responsive to evidence-based psychosocial therapy that is initiated during the acute clinical crisis or shortly thereafter. Improved coping skills, more useful cognitive and behavioral constructs, reduced family tension, or successful behavioral feedback may reduce the need for medication either partially (eg, lower dose) or completely (eg, discontinuation). Over the longer term, doses may need to be increased in response to growth and maturation.

Adherence and Persistence

Obviously, medications that are not ingested are not effective.[24] The rate of nonadherence associated with pediatric psychopharmacology is not well studied or documented, except for stimulants, for which the data suggest high levels of nonadherence.[25] Parent reports of adherence to sustained-release stimulant preparations indicate about 10% to 25% nonadherence. Even more concerning, a retrospective comparison of the MTA Cooperative Group[9] showed that only 3% of caregivers reported that their children did not receive prescribed stimulant medication on the day of a study visit, whereas child saliva samples indicated that 25% of children were nonadherent.[26] Taken together, studies of parent reports and salivary samples indicate that nonadherence to stimulant medication is high and is underreported by caregivers.

Persistence refers to continuity of treatment. Because ADHD is a chronic disorder, relatively long-term treatment with stimulants would be expected, except for "drug holidays" or when they are discontinued because of unacceptable side effects or lack of adequate effect. However, data from community practice settings suggest that treatment is not persistent. In a study of more than 9,500 pharmacy and medical claims for 6- to 12-year-olds, the mean duration of stimulant treatment episodes was only about 145 days for immediate-release preparations and about 150 to 160 days for longer-acting preparations.[27] In a study using Medicaid claims for more than 40,000 5- to 20-year-olds, 27% to 50% were persistent for 12 months, allowing for a 1- or 3-month gap in use, respectively.[28] These and other studies suggest that a substantial proportion of children receiving stimulants may not receive them for more than 1 year.

Improving adherence and persistence is not a simple or easy task.[25] Discussing adherence and nonadherence in a nonjudgmental manner before prescribing a medication is important. It is important to establish a therapeutic approach through which children and parents feel that assessing adherence is part of the therapeutic process, helpful to clinical decision-making regarding dose changes and continuation of a medication, and not a negative judgment.

Procedures for improving adherence and persistence are described in the literature.[29] They include identification of barriers to adherence, application of motivational interviewing techniques, reminder and monitoring systems, and, when available, aids such as bubble packaging.

Prioritizing Medications

The following discussion regarding differences between various group 1 medications is offered as potentially useful information. It is not meant to protocolize or prohibit prescribing of any medication. An individualized decision regarding an individual medication for an individual patient is always the final responsibility of the individual prescriber.

Attention-deficit/Hyperactivity Disorder

Clinical guidance from the AAP and practice parameters from the AACAP[30] recommend starting with either a methylphenidate preparation or an amphetamine preparation. Also, the effect size, a measure of the magnitude of improvement relative to placebo, is greater for these stimulants than for the other medications approved for ADHD. In cases in which there are concerns about starting with a stimulant (eg, specific potential adverse events or parental preferences), guanfacine, clonidine, and atomoxetine are all secondary options and all have generally comparable effect sizes. As described previously, guanfacine and clonidine seem to have a favorable adverse-event profile compared with atomoxetine.

Anxiety

There are no data to suggest any differences in efficacy between fluoxetine, sertraline, fluvoxamine, and duloxetine for anxiety. Fluoxetine has a longer half-life and effect, which is an advantage if there are concerns about adherence but a disadvantage if there is a need to stop the medication because of adverse effects or drug interactions. Fluvoxamine inhibits cytochrome P450 isoenzymes that are different from those inhibited by fluoxetine or sertraline. Duloxetine has an FDA approval for GAD, which may be reassuring to patients and caregivers, but has more concerning warnings and precautions than SSRIs.

Depression

Fluoxetine has an FDA indication for treating depression in children and adolescents, while the indication for escitalopram is for adolescents only. There are no data to suggest any differences in efficacy for depression between fluoxetine and escitalopram. The potential advantages and disadvantages of fluoxetine for depression are the same as described previously for anxiety. An advantage of escitalopram is that it does not have any clinically significant interactions with cytochrome P450 isoenzymes.

Switching Medications

If the initial stimulant medication is not effective, data from published studies support switching[31] to a stimulant in the other category. Likewise, if the initial SSRI is not effective, switching to one of the other group 1 SSRIs may be successful.[32]

Multiple Medications

Many children treated in the pediatric primary care setting for ADHD, anxiety, or depression will need only 1 psychotropic medication. Some will need 2 (eg, children with ADHD, anxiety, and depression who require medication as part of the treatment plan). Fortunately, the medications for ADHD (methylphenidate, amphetamine, guanfacine, clonidine, and atomoxetine) can be used safely in combination with the medications for anxiety or depression (the SSRIs fluoxetine, sertraline, escitalopram, and fluvoxamine and the SNRI duloxetine).[33]

If 2 psychiatric medications do not effectively manage symptoms, advanced expertise in pediatric psychopharmacology or consultation with a child and adolescent psychiatrist is strongly advised. The PCC can, in either case, play an important role in monitoring the medications and in promoting a healthy lifestyle.

Group 2 Medications for Other Disorders: General Rationale

In addition to prescribing and monitoring group 1 medications, PCCs are ideally suited to collaborate with psychiatrists and other mental health specialists in the care of children with more severe or uncommon disorders. They may be asked to take on partial responsibility for monitoring the therapeutic and side effects of a variety of other medications, which are included in groups 2 and 3.

Group 2 medications can be monitored in primary care settings, but because they generally have a more serious safety profile or more complicated monitoring requirements than group 1 medications do, they are generally prescribed by specialists, that is, child psychiatrists, developmental-behavioral pediatricians, specialists in neurodevelopmental disabilities or adolescent medicine, pediatric neurologists, or adult psychiatrists with additional training in adolescent psychiatry. Depending on an individual PCC's skills and experience and availability of specialists for referral (or lack thereof, especially in rural and underserved areas), some PCCs with additional training in pediatric psychopharmacology may choose to prescribe group 2 medications.

Group 2 includes all FDA-approved medications for children with other disorders (ie, not ADHD, anxiety, or depression). Group 2 includes 7 second-generation antipsychotics (SGAs) (risperidone, aripiprazole, quetiapine, olanzapine, asenapine, paliperidone, and lurasidone) and lithium, a mood stabilizer. The SGAs are approved for treatment of psychosis in children with schizophrenia (all except asenapine); mania associated with bipolar I disorder (all except paliperidone and lurasidone); and irritability associated with ASD (only risperidone and aripiprazole). However, these medications are most commonly used off-label (ie, outside the FDA-approved indications) in children to treat behavioral problems, especially aggression.[34,35] Lithium is approved by the FDA for treatment of acute mania associated with bipolar I disorder; however, it also is used off-label to treat non–bipolar mood instability.

Group 2 Medications for Other Disorders: Specific Rationale

Antipsychotics

Antipsychotic medications can reduce the severity of various major psychiatric symptoms and have a variety of effects, including

▶ Antipsychotic effects for hallucinations, delusions, and disorganized thinking

▶ Mood-stabilizing effects for mania, irritability, and mood instability

▶ Calming effects for agitation and aggressive behavior

However, of all the psychotropic medications used in children and adolescents, SGAs generally have the most concerning adverse effects, including

▶ Sedation

▶ Weight gain

▶ Elevated glucose concentration and insulin resistance

▶ Elevated triglyceride levels and cholesterol level

▶ Abnormal movements (neurological)

▶ Others (Table 11-6)

Table 11-6. Group 2 Psychotropic Medications

Medication	Warnings, Precautions, and Adverse Events	Comments
Second-Generation Antipsychotics		
Risperidone *Indications:* schizophrenia (13–17 y), bipolar disorder mania (10–17 y), irritability associated with ASD (5–16 y) *Uses:* Schizophrenia, bipolar disorders, and irritability associated with ASD. Also, among many off-label uses: acute aggression, chronic irritability, tics, and other disorders not responsive to other medications. *Monitoring:* Height and weight. Fasting blood glucose and lipid profile. Abnormal involuntary movements.	*Boxed warnings:* none specifically applicable for pediatrics *Warnings and precautions:* neuroleptic malignant syndrome, tardive dyskinesia; metabolic changes (hyperglycemia/diabetes mellitus; dyslipidemia, weight gain): hyperprolactinemia; orthostatic hypotension; leukopenia, neutropenia, agranulocytosis; potential for cognitive and motor impairment; seizures *Adverse reactions:* in child and adolescent clinical trials (incidence ≥5% and twice placebo): somnolence, extrapyramidal syndrome, fatigue, nausea, akathisia, blurred vision, salivary hypersecretion, dizziness, tremor, sedation, increased appetite, drooling, vomiting, fever, decreased appetite, lethargy	Risperidone was the first SGA (other than clozapine, which is rarely used in children) approved by the FDA in 1993 for marketing in the United States. It is generally effective and safe for short-term use, but there are concerns about adverse effects of long-term use, such as obesity, diabetes, metabolic syndrome, and tardive dyskinesia. It can increase prolactin levels and is associated with gynecomastia and amenorrhea.
Aripiprazole *Indications:* schizophrenia (13–17 y), manic or mixed episodes (10–17 y), irritability associated with ASD (6–17 y), Tourette syndrome (6–17 y) *Uses:* same as risperidone *Monitoring:* same as risperidone	*Boxed warnings:* suicidality with antidepressants *Warnings and precautions:* same as risperidone excluding hyperprolactinemia and plus pathological gambling and other compulsive behaviors *Adverse reactions:* same as risperidone plus fever, headache, nasopharyngitis	Marketed since 2002, aripiprazole has a somewhat different mechanism of action than other SGAs. It is associated with less weight gain than other SGAs except for ziprasidone.

Table 11-6. Group 2 Psychotropic Medications (continued)

Medication	Warnings, Precautions, and Adverse Events	Comments
Second-Generation Antipsychotics		
Quetiapine *Indications:* schizophrenia (13–17 y), bipolar disorder mania (10–17 y) *Uses:* same as risperidone *Monitoring:* same as risperidone	*Boxed warnings:* suicidality with antidepressants *Warnings and precautions:* same as risperidone excluding hyperprolactinemia, cognitive and motor impairment, seizures and plus increased BP *Adverse reactions:* same as risperidone	Marketed since 1997, quetiapine is associated with more somnolence than other SGAs.
Olanzapine *Indications:* schizophrenia (13–17 y), manic or mixed episodes of bipolar I disorder (13–17 y) *Uses:* same as risperidone *Monitoring:* same as risperidone	*Boxed warnings:* none specifically applicable for pediatrics *Warnings and precautions:* suicide, neuroleptic malignant syndrome, drug reaction with eosinophilia and systemic symptoms, hyperglycemia, hyperlipidemia, tardive dyskinesia, orthostatic hypotension, leukopenia, neutropenia and agranulocytosis, seizures, potential for cognitive and motor impairment, hyperprolactinemia *Adverse events:* in adolescent clinical trials ($\geq$5% and at least twice that for placebo): somnolence, dizziness, fatigue, increased appetite, nausea, vomiting, dry mouth, tachycardia, weight gain	Marketed since 1996, olanzapine is associated with more weight gain and related metabolic side effects (adverse events) in adolescents than other SGAs.[a,b]
Asenapine *Indications:* bipolar disorder mania (10–17 y) *Uses:* same as risperidone *Monitoring:* same as risperidone	*Boxed warnings:* none specifically applicable for pediatrics *Warnings and precautions:* same as risperidone excluding hyperprolactinemia and plus QT prolongation *Adverse reactions:* somnolence, dizziness, dysgeusia, oral paresthesia, nausea, increased appetite, increased weight	Marketed since 2009 with pediatric indication since March 2015. Clinical experience in children and adolescents is currently limited. Drug must dissolve under tongue with no eating or drinking for subsequent 10 min.

Paliperidone

Indications: schizophrenia (12–17 y)

Uses: same as risperidone

Monitoring: same as risperidone

Boxed warnings: none specifically applicable for pediatrics

Warnings and precautions: neuroleptic malignant syndrome, QT prolongation, tardive dyskinesia, hyperglycemia and diabetes mellitus, hyperglycemia, dyslipidemia, weight gain, hyperprolactinemia, GI narrowing, orthostatic hypotension and syncope, leukopenia, neutropenia, agranulocytosis, potential for cognitive and motor impairment, seizures, suicide

Adverse events: Most common adverse reactions in adolescent clinical trials (≥5%) were somnolence, akathisia, tremor, dystonia, cogwheel rigidity, anxiety, weight increased, and tachycardia.

Because paliperidone is the major active metabolite of risperidone, it is very similar to risperidone in all respects.

Lurasidone

Indications: schizophrenia (13–17 y)

Uses: same as risperidone

Monitoring: same as risperidone

Boxed warnings: suicidal thoughts and behaviors

Warnings and precautions: same as risperidone excluding cognitive and motor impairment, and seizures

Adverse reactions: somnolence, nausea, akathisia, extrapyramidal symptoms, rhinitis (80 mg only), vomiting

Marketed since 2010 with pediatric indication since January 2017. Clinical experience in children and adolescents is currently limited. Must be taken with food ("at least 350 calories" in package insert) to facilitate absorption.

Table 11-6. Group 2 Psychotropic Medications (continued)

Medication	Warnings, Precautions, and Adverse Events	Comments
Mood Stabilizer		
Lithium *Class*: element of the alkali metal group (salt) *Indications*: mania associated with bipolar disorder (age >12 y) *Uses*: acute mania associated with and maintenance therapy for bipolar disorder; mood stabilization *Monitoring*: pregnancy testing, ECG, serum lithium levels, CBC, electrolyte levels, thyroid function, renal function	*Boxed warnings*: toxicity closely related to serum levels, can occur close to therapeutic dose levels *Warnings*: Very high risk for toxicity: significant cardiovascular or renal disease, severe debilitation, dehydration, sodium depletion, and taking diuretics or ACE inhibitors. Chronic use may lower renal concentrating ability and can present as nephrogenic diabetes insipidus, with polyuria/polydipsia. Encephalopathic syndrome (ie, weakness; lethargy; fever; tremulousness and confusion; leukocytosis; extrapyramidal symptoms; elevated serum enzyme levels, serum urea nitrogen level, and fasting blood glucose) may occur with lithium and a neuroleptic, often haloperidol. *Precautions*: hypothyroidism; impaired mental or physical abilities; any concomitant medications (ie, diuretics, ACE inhibitors, carbamazepine, fluoxetine) *Adverse events*: Mild: <1.5 mEq/L; mild/moderate: 1.5–2.5 mEq/L; and moderate/severe ≥2.0 mEq/L. <2.0 mEq/L: early signs of toxicity, including diarrhea, vomiting, drowsiness, muscular weakness, and lack of coordination; higher levels: giddiness, ataxia, blurred vision, tinnitus, and large output of dilute urine; and >3.0 mEq/L: complex clinically with multiple organs and organ systems.	Introduced in the United States in the early 1960s, it was the original mood stabilizer. Clear, documented evidence of effectiveness for immediate and maintenance treatment of mania and bipolar disorder in adults. No well-powered, placebo-controlled study for treatment of mania in children and adolescents, in large part because of the ethical and practical difficulties associated with conducting placebo-controlled studies. Evidence is mixed from several smaller studies.[c,d] Unpopular with children and adolescents because of common side effects and the need for repeated venipunctures for serum level monitoring.

Abbreviations: ACE, angiotensin-converting enzyme; ASD, autism spectrum disorder; CBC, complete blood cell count; ECG, electrocardiogram; FDA, US Food and Drug Administration; GI, gastrointestinal; SGA, second-generation antipsychotic.

[a] Correll CU, Manu P, Olshanskiy V, Napolitano B, Kane JM, Malhotra AK. Cardiometabolic risk of second-generation antipsychotic medications during first-time use in children and adolescents. *JAMA*. 2009;302(16):1765–1773.

[b] American Diabetes Association, American Psychiatric Association, American Association of Clinical Endocrinologists, North American Association for the Study of Obesity. Consensus development conference on antipsychotic drugs and obesity and diabetes. *Diabetes Care*. 2004;27(2):596–601.

[c] Geller B, Luby JL, Joshi P, et al. A randomized controlled trial of risperidone, lithium, or divalproex sodium for initial treatment of bipolar I disorder, manic or mixed phase, in children and adolescents. *Arch Gen Psychiatry*. 2012;69(5):515–528.

[d] Findling RL, Robb A, McNamara NK, et al. Lithium in the acute treatment of bipolar I disorder: a double-blind, placebo-controlled study. *Pediatrics*. 2015;136(5):885–894.

Many of the major adverse effects of SGAs, particularly weight gain, metabolic abnormalities, and involuntary movements, can develop into major health problems (eg, cardiovascular disease and its consequences, tardive dyskinesia) during long-term treatment and may not be reversible. Most disorders that may be treated with SGAs are chronic and generally require long-term treatment. Thus, weighing the benefit to risk trade-off is difficult when considering an SGA; input from the family or a consultant or both may be helpful.

There is no agreement about monitoring for weight and metabolic adverse events in children prescribed with SGAs. Neither the AAP nor the AACAP has issued formal guidelines or recommendations for monitoring.[36] The only available formal published guide is for adults; it is presented in Table 11-7.

The following discussion regarding differences between various group 2 medications is offered as potentially useful information. It is not meant to protocolize or prohibit prescribing of any medication. An individualized decision regarding an individual medication for an individual patient is always the final responsibility of the individual prescriber.

There are no useful data comparing effectiveness of the 7 group 2 SGAs in children. Paliperidone is the active metabolite of risperidone and seems similar to risperidone in efficacy and adverse-event profile. Perhaps the major difference is that risperidone has been in use longer (since 1993) than paliperidone (since 2006) and is available as a generic drug. Generally, clinically meaningful differences between SGAs focus on adverse events. Only a few relevant differences will be highlighted here. Olanzapine, in contrast to the other group 2 SGAs, is associated with more weight gain and metabolic adverse events. Aripiprazole is associated with the least weight gain and less severe metabolic adverse events. Risperidone is most likely to increase prolactin levels and is associated with gynecomastia and amenorrhea. Quetiapine seems to be the most sedating. Asenapine and lurasidone were recently approved for use in adolescents, in 2015 and 2017, respectively; there is less clinical experience with them than with the other SGAs. Detailed information regarding group 2 SGAs is presented in Table 11-6.

Lithium

Mood stabilizers (excluding antipsychotics) are used to treat mania, depression, irritability, and problematic mood swings or instability

Table 11-7. Monitoring Protocol for Adult Patients Taking Second-Generation Antipsychotics

	Baseline	4 Weeks	8 Weeks	12 Weeks	Quarterly	Annually	Every 5 Years
Personal and family history	X					X	
Weight (body mass index)	X	X	X	X	X		
Waist circumference	X					X	
Blood pressure	X			X		X	
Fasting plasma glucose	X			X		X	
Fasting lipid profile	X			X			X

Reprinted with permission from American Diabetes Association, American Psychiatric Association, American Association of Clinical Endocrinologists, North American Association for the Study of Obesity. Consensus Development Conference on Antipsychotic Drugs and Obesity and Diabetes. *Diabetes Care.* 2004;27(2):596–601.

associated with bipolar disorder and other mood disorders. There are 2 groups of mood stabilizers: traditional (lithium, valproic acid [divalproex sodium], and carbamazepine) and newer anticonvulsants (eg, lamotrigine). Use of mood stabilizers (excluding SGAs) in children seems to be decreasing. This decrease may result from one or more factors: available efficacy data are generally negative, regular monitoring of plasma levels is usually required, and the adverse event burden is substantial.

Lithium is the mood stabilizer included in group 2. It has an FDA indication for mania associated with bipolar disorder down to age 12 years, and available data for lithium, although limited, suggest efficacy for acute mania associated with bipolar I disorder.[37,38] Detailed information regarding lithium is presented in Table 11-6.

Group 3 Medications

The third group of medications (group 3) includes medications not approved by the FDA for children and thus not included in groups 1 or 2. There are a few other medications that have FDA indications for children, but these indications are based on premodern data (if there are any data) and were grandfathered in by the FDA years ago. Although the FDA has removed most of these grandfathered indications, a few remain. These remaining grandfathered approvals have been excluded from this conceptual framework because they were not subject to the same modern standards of evidence for safety and efficacy as medications included in groups 1 and 2.

For group 3 medications, 10 were selected for emphasis because they are commonly used and PCCs are likely to have patients for whom they have been prescribed. Table 11-8 summarizes available efficacy data and adverse-event profiles for these 10 medications. Other group 3 medications, which are less commonly prescribed, will not be discussed, but their adverse-event profiles can be accessed by electronic media (eg, Drugs@FDA, Epocrates, Micromedex).

Other Antidepressants

Four antidepressants (bupropion, citalopram, venlafaxine, and mirtazapine) are sometimes prescribed in children and adolescents. None has an FDA indication for use in children or adolescents.

Table 11-8. Group 3 Psychotropic Medications

Medication	Warnings, Precautions, and Adverse Events	Comments
Antidepressants		
Bupropion *Class:* atypical antidepressant; chemical structure like phenylethylamines, which are stimulants *Indications: adult:* MDD **Children and adolescents: none**[a,b] *Uses:* depression *Monitoring:* BP, HR, height, weight, suicidality	*Boxed warnings:* suicidality *Warnings and precautions:* seizures, hepatotoxicity, agitation and insomnia, psychosis and confusion, weight gain or loss, allergic reactions, hypertension *Adverse reactions:* agitation, dry mouth, insomnia, headache/migraine, nausea and vomiting, constipation, tremor	Because of its structural similarity to stimulants, bupropion is sometimes used to treat both depression and symptoms of ADHD.
Citalopram *Class:* SSRI *Indications: adult:* MDD **Children and adolescents: none** *Uses:* MDD *Monitoring:* same as other SSRIs (See Table 11-5.)	*Boxed warnings:* suicidality, ECG changes *Warnings and precautions:* similar to other SSRIs *Adverse reactions:* similar to other SSRIs	Offers no benefit over escitalopram, which is the group 1 therapeutically effective (S)-enantiomer of the racemic mixture citalopram. Also, citalopram has an FDA warning regarding maximum dose in adults because of the risk for QTc prolongation; relevant dosage maximum is not known in children and adolescents. Thus, the potential need to monitor with ECGs complicates treatment.

Table 11-8. Group 3 Psychotropic Medications (continued)

Medication	Warnings, Precautions, and Adverse Events	Comments
Antidepressants		
Venlafaxine *Class:* selective NRI *Indications: adult:* MDD **Children and adolescents: none** *Uses:* MDD *Monitoring:* BP, HR, height, weight, suicidality	*Boxed warnings:* suicidality *Warnings and precautions:* serotonin syndrome; sustained hypertension; mydriasis; discontinuation symptoms, especially anxiety and insomnia, decreased appetite and weight, height deceleration, activation of mania/hypomania, hyponatremia, seizures, increased risk for bleeding events, serum cholesterol level elevation, interstitial lung disease, eosinophilic pneumonia *Adverse reactions:* asthenia, sweating, nausea, constipation, anorexia, vomiting, somnolence, dry mouth, dizziness, nervousness, anxiety, tremor, blurred vision	Venlafaxine was compared with an SSRI in children and adolescents with depression who had not responded to initial treatment with an SSRI (TORDIA study[c]). The second SSRI and venlafaxine showed comparable efficacy; however, venlafaxine was associated with more adverse events and discontinuations.
Mirtazapine *Class:* tetracyclic *Indications: adult:* MDD **Children and adolescents: none** *Uses:* MDD *Monitoring:* BMI, WBC lipid panel, transaminase levels	*Boxed warnings:* suicidality *Warnings:* activation of mania/hypomania, agranulocytosis, serotonin syndrome, angle closure glaucoma *Precautions:* discontinuation symptoms; akathisia; hyponatremia; somnolence; dizziness; increased appetite; weight gain; cholesterol/triglyceride, transaminase elevations; seizures *Adverse reactions:* somnolence, increased appetite, weight gain, dizziness	Mirtazapine has both serotonergic actions and noradrenergic actions and is different from other class 1 and 2 antidepressants in its mechanism of action. It is generally more sedating and causes more weight gain than other antidepressants do.

Second-Generation Antipsychotic

Ziprasidone

Class: SGA

Indications: adult: schizophrenia, manic or mixed episodes associated with bipolar I disorder, adjunctive maintenance therapy for bipolar I disorder, agitation in schizophrenic patients (intramuscular injection)

Children and adolescents: none

Uses: same as risperidone

Monitoring: same as risperidone plus QTc prolongation on ECG

Boxed warnings: not applicable for pediatrics

Warnings and precautions: QT interval prolongation, neuroleptic malignant syndrome, tardive dyskinesia, hyperglycemia and diabetes mellitus, dyslipidemia, rash, orthostatic hypotension, leukopenia, neutropenia, agranulocytosis, seizures, potential for cognitive and motor impairment, suicide

Adverse events: most common adverse reactions in clinical trials (incidence ≥5% and twice placebo): somnolence, respiratory tract infection, extrapyramidal symptoms, dizziness, akathisia, abnormal vision, asthenia, vomiting, headache, nausea

Marketed since 2001, ziprasidone is associated with less weight gain than other SGAs. Because of potential to prolong the QT interval, ECG monitoring is needed.

Table 11-8. Group 3 Psychotropic Medications (continued)

Medication	Warnings, Precautions, and Adverse Events	Comments
Mood Stabilizer		
Valproic Acid *Class:* anticonvulsant mood stabilizer *Indications: adult:* therapy for complex partial seizures and simple and complex absence seizures **Children and adolescents: none for** psychiatric disorders *Uses:* mood stabilizer *Monitoring:* pregnancy testing; serum levels, CBC, liver function tests	*Boxed warnings:* Hepatotoxicity can be fatal, usually in first 6 mo of use in children <2 y; teratogenic; includes neural tube defects (eg, spina bifida), malformations, and decreased IQ; pancreatitis can be fatal, with hemorrhagic cases. *Warnings and precautions:* hepatotoxicity, birth defects and decreased IQ following in utero exposure, pancreatitis, suicidality, thrombocytopenia, multiorgan hypersensitivity reaction, hypothermia, hyperammonemia, hyperammonemic encephalopathy *Adverse reactions:* most common adverse reactions in clinical trials of mania (incidence ≥5%): abdominal pain, alopecia, amblyopia/blurred vision, amnesia, anorexia, asthenia, ataxia, bronchitis, constipation, depression, diarrhea, diplopia, dizziness, dyspepsia, dyspnea, ecchymosis, emotional lability, fever, flu-like syndrome, headache, increased appetite, infection, insomnia, nausea, nervousness, nystagmus, peripheral edema, pharyngitis, rhinitis, somnolence, abnormal thinking, thrombocytopenia, tinnitus, tremor, vomiting, weight gain, weight loss	Valproic acid to treat mania in adults is supported by substantial data. Supportive data are lacking in children. An industry-funded, multisite randomized controlled trial in children with mania and bipolar disorder did not show efficacy of valproic acid versus placebo.[d] In a comparison of valproic acid, lithium, and risperidone for bipolar disorder in children,[e] valproic acid had the lowest response rates, which were comparable to those for placebo in the industry-funded study.

Anxiolytics

Lorazepam

Class: benzodiazepine

Indications: adult: acute anxiety

Children and adolescents: none

Uses: acute anxiety

Monitoring: pregnancy testing

Boxed warnings: none

Warnings: worsening or emergence of depression, suicidality, respiratory depression, interference with cognitive and motor performance, physical and psychological dependence, risk of use in pregnancy, withdrawal symptoms

Precautions: paradoxical reactions (ie, behavioral disinhibition), should not be used with alcohol

Adverse reactions: In a sample of about 3,500 adult patients treated for anxiety, the most frequent adverse reaction was sedation (15.9%), followed by dizziness (6.9%), weakness (4.2%), and unsteadiness (3.4%).

Lorazepam is a short-acting benzodiazepine with a duration of effect of about 4–8 h. Primarily because of the possibility of physical and psychological dependence with prolonged use of benzodiazepines, lorazepam is generally recommended only for short-term use (days to a few weeks) for treatment of acute and severe anxiety following a trauma or preceding a medical procedure or while waiting for an SSRI or another anxiolytic to become effective.

Clonazepam

Class: benzodiazepine

Indications: adult: panic disorder

Children and adolescents: none

Uses: acute anxiety

Monitoring: pregnancy testing

Boxed warnings: none

Warnings: interference with cognitive and motor performance, suicidality, physical and psychological dependence, risk of use in pregnancy, withdrawal symptoms

Precautions: worsening of seizures, hypersalivation, should not be used with alcohol

Adverse reactions: somnolence, abnormal coordination, ataxia, depression

Clonazepam is similar to lorazepam, except for its longer half-life and once-daily dosing.

Table 11-8. Group 3 Psychotropic Medications (continued)

Medication	Warnings, Precautions, and Adverse Events	Comments
Sleep Aids		
Trazodone *Class:* serotonergic potentiator with un-clear specific mechanism of action *Indications: adult:* MDD **Children and adolescents: none** *Uses:* insomnia *Monitoring:* pregnancy testing	*Boxed warnings:* suicidality *Warnings and precautions:* serotonin syndrome, angle-closure glaucoma, activation of mania/hypomania, QT prolongation, orthostatic hypotension and syncope, abnormal bleeding, interaction with monoamine oxidase inhibitors, priapism, hyponatremia, potential for cogni-tive and motor impairment, discontinuation syndrome *Adverse reactions:* somnolence/sedation, dizziness, consti-pation, blurred vision	Trazodone is sometimes used as a sleep aid in low doses, generally 25 or 50 mg. Because of reports of priapism, its use in adolescent boys is limited.

Abbreviations: ADHD, attention-deficit/hyperactivity disorder; BMI, body mass index; BP, blood pressure; CBC, complete cell blood count; ECG, electrocardiogram; FDA, US Food and Drug Administration; HR, heart rate; MDD, major depressive disorder; NRI, norepinephrine reuptake inhibitor; SSRI, selective serotonin reuptake inhibitor; TORDIA, Treatment of SSRI-resistant Depression in Adolescents; WBC, white blood cell.

[a] Rynn MA, Riddle MA, Yeung PP, Kunz NR. Efficacy and safety of extended-release venlafaxine in the treatment of generalized anxiety disorder in children and adolescents: two placebo-controlled trials. *Am J Psychiatry.* 2007;164(2):290–300.

[b] Emslie GJ, Findling RL, Yeung PP, Kunz NR, Li Y. Venlafaxine ER for the treatment of pediatric subjects with depression: results of two placebo-controlled trials. *J Am Acad Child Adolesc Psychiatry.* 2007;46(4):479–488.

[c] Brent D, Emslie G, Clarke G, et al. Switching to another SSRI or to venlafaxine with or without cognitive behavioral therapy for adolescents with SSRI-resistant depression: the TORDIA randomized controlled trial. *JAMA.* 2008;299(8):901–913.

[d] Wagner KD, Redden L, Kowatch RA, et al. A double-blind, randomized, placebo-controlled trial of divalproex extended-release in the treatment of bipolar disorder in children and adolescents. *J Am Acad Child Adolesc Psychiatry.* 2009;48(5):519–532.

[e] Geller B, Luby JL, Joshi P, et al. A randomized controlled trial of risperidone, lithium, or divalproex sodium for initial treatment of bipolar I disorder, manic or mixed phase, in children and adolescents. *Arch Gen Psychiatry.* 2012;69(5):515–528.

Bupropion has a chemical structure similar to that of the phenylethy-lamines, which are stimulants. It is marketed for depression in adults and is sometimes used to treat comorbid depression and ADHD in children.

Although citalopram, an SSRI, is sometimes used for depression or anxiety in children, it offers no benefit over escitalopram, a group 1 medication, which is the therapeutically effective (S)-enantiomer of citalopram. Citalopram has an FDA warning regarding maximum dose in adults because of the risk for QTc prolongation; however, a relevant dosage maximum is not known in children and adolescents. Thus, the need to monitor with electrocardiograms complicates treatment in children.

Venlafaxine is an SNRI that acts like an SSRI at lower doses. It is used for anxiety or depression in children.[39,40] In children and adolescents, venlafaxine is associated with more adverse events than SSRIs are.[32] Industry-sponsored efficacy studies for depression and anxiety in children, although almost reaching statistical significance, have not demonstrated clear efficacy.[39,40]

Mirtazapine has a tetracyclic chemical structure that distinguishes it from other antidepressants. It is marketed for depression in adults. Mirtazapine is associated with more sedation and weight gain than other antidepressants are.

Other Antipsychotics

Ziprasidone is an SGA (marketed since 2001) that is approved in adults for psychosis associated with schizophrenia and mania associated with bipolar disorder. Ziprasidone has the advantage of generally being associated with less weight gain and fewer metabolic adverse events than other SGAs. Probably primarily because ziprasidone is associated with prolongation of QTc, it has not been approved by the FDA for children or adolescents.

Other Mood Stabilizers

Divalproex sodium (valproic acid), an anticonvulsant, is commonly prescribed to children as a mood stabilizer. Unfortunately, efficacy data for divalproex sodium suggest no difference from placebo[41] and less efficacy than comparators.[37] Monitoring requires venipunctures for drug levels.

Anxiolytics

Two benzodiazepine anxiolytics, that is, lorazepam (short-acting) and clonazepam (long-acting), are commonly prescribed in children and adolescents. Because dependence may develop with long-term benzodiazepine treatment, they are *only* for short-term use.

Benzodiazepines may be used before painful or stressful medical procedures. They can be used for short-term treatment of anxiety and distress following an acute traumatic incident or while waiting for an SSRI to have an effect. Also, benzodiazepines are used as an adjunctive treatment of schizophrenia.

Benzodiazepines are generally well tolerated. Sedation is the most common concerning adverse event. Daytime drowsiness can be dangerous when operating a motor vehicle or machinery. Other concerning side effects are unlikely if benzodiazepines are used short-term and at appropriately low doses.

Sleep Aids

Insomnia is a common concern of children with ADHD, anxiety, depression, and other psychiatric disorders. In general, treatment of the primary psychiatric disorders plus counseling or behavioral approaches to improving sleep hygiene will relieve the insomnia. If not, further evaluation is warranted. Although research data are lacking, various medications are used to treat insomnia in children and adolescents, especially those with ADHD or ASD associated with sleep problems. Two potential sleep aids, which are among the most commonly used in children, are included here.

Trazodone is an antidepressant approved for treatment of MDD in adults. It is sometimes used in low doses to treat insomnia in adolescents (and adults). Its mechanism of action is not well understood, but its major effect is thought to be on the serotonergic system. The adverse-effects profile of trazodone is similar to that of the SSRIs, but trazodone is also associated with priapism, which may limit its use in adolescent boys.

Melatonin is a hormone produced in the pineal gland that is available over the counter but not by prescription (and, therefore, is not included in Table 11-8). It can reduce initial insomnia. It is not recommended for long-term use. Studies, primarily in adults, indicate melatonin is effective for only 2 to 3 weeks.

Ramelteon, a relatively new FDA-approved sleep aid that is not commonly prescribed for children, is the first in a new class of sleep aids that are melatonin receptor agonists with high affinity for MT1 and MT2 receptors.

Individual State Programs for Improving Prescribing to Children and Adolescents

In response to recent federal guidelines, all states in the United States have developed or are developing programs to monitor psychotropic medications, primarily antipsychotics, prescribed to children and adolescents. Specific mandates require child welfare and Medicaid agencies to work collaboratively regarding children in foster care and state custody, for whom psychotropic medications are prescribed at disproportionately high rates. These programs range from consultation models promoting collaboration among providers to drug utilization review processes that restrict access when certain criteria are not met. These programs are too new to support a comprehensive assessment of their effect on children, families, and PCCs.

Disruptive Behavior and Aggression

This chapter has focused on the 3 common medication-responsive disorders identified by the AAP Task Force on Mental Health as potentially managed by PCCs independently. Symptoms of disruptive behavior and aggression also commonly present to PCCs and may be manifestations of oppositional defiant disorder, conduct disorder, disruptive mood dysregulation disorder, or other behavioral conditions. These disorders were not addressed in this chapter because they typically require comanagement with a mental health specialist and because there is considerable controversy regarding whether medication, targeted *only* at aggression or disruptive behavior, is an appropriate part of a comprehensive treatment plan.[34,35]

Summary

Because of the high prevalence of mental disorders, pediatric PCCs commonly encounter children whose care may involve assessment for, or treatment with, psychotropic medication. The AAP has released recommendations that pediatricians achieve competence in care of children with ADHD, anxiety, or depression, conditions that may, in some instances, benefit from medication. Moreover, pediatric PCCs may encounter children for whom psychotropic medications are prescribed by behavioral health or other specialty providers and who may require monitoring by pediatric PCCs for therapeutic benefit and potential side effects. Thus, an understanding of pediatric psychopharmacology is necessary for primary care pediatric practice. This chapter has proposed a conceptual framework and general guidance for decision-making about prescribing and monitoring psychotropic medications in pediatric primary care.

AAP Policy

American Academy of Pediatrics Committee on Psychosocial Aspects of Child and Family Health and Task Force on Mental Health. The future of pediatrics: mental health competencies for pediatric primary care. *Pediatrics.* 2009;124(1):410–421. Reaffirmed August 2013 (pediatrics.aappublications.org/content/124/1/410)

American Academy of Pediatrics Subcommittee on Attention-deficit/Hyperactivity Disorder and Steering Committee on Quality Improvement and Management. ADHD: clinical practice guideline for the diagnosis, evaluation, and treatment of attention-deficit/hyperactivity disorder in children and adolescents. *Pediatrics.* 2011;128(5):1007–1022 (pediatrics.aappublications.org/content/128/5/1007)

Cheung AH, Zuckerbrot RA, Jensen PS, Laraque D, Stein REK; GLAD-PC Steering Group. Guidelines for adolescent depression in primary care (GLAD-PC): II. Treatment and ongoing management. *Pediatrics.* 2018;141(3):e20174082 (pediatrics. aappublications.org/content/141/3/e20174082)

Zuckerbrot RA, Cheung AH, Jensen PS, Stein REK, Laraque D; GLAD-PC Steering Group. Guidelines for adolescent depression in primary care (GLAD-PC): Part I. Practice preparation, identification, assessment, and initial management. *Pediatrics.* 2018;141(3):e20174081. AAP endorsed (pediatrics.aappublications.org/content/141/3/ e20174081)

Suggested Reading

American Academy of Pediatrics. *Addressing Mental Health Concerns in Primary Care: A Clinician's Toolkit.* Elk Grove Village, IL: American Academy of Pediatrics; 2010

Riddle MA. *Pediatric Psychopharmacology for Primary Care.* Elk Grove Village, IL: American Academy of Pediatrics; 2016

References

1. Foy JM; American Academy of Pediatrics Task Force on Mental Health. Enhancing pediatric mental health care: report from the American Academy of Pediatrics Task Force on Mental Health. *Pediatrics.* 2010;125(suppl 3):S69–S159

2. American Psychiatric Association. *Diagnostic and Statistical Manual of Mental Disorders.* 5th ed. Arlington, VA: American Psychiatric Association; 2013

3. Foy JM; American Academy of Pediatrics Task Force on Mental Health. Enhancing pediatric mental health care: report from the American Academy of Pediatrics Task Force on Mental Health. Introduction. *Pediatrics.* 2010;125(suppl 3):S69–S74

4. Ginsburg GS, Riddle MA, Davies M. Somatic symptoms in children and adolescents with anxiety disorders. *J Am Acad Child Adolesc Psychiatry.* 2006; 45(10):1179–1187

5. Cohen JA, Kelleher KJ, Mannarino AP. Identifying, treating, and referring traumatized children: the role of pediatric providers. *Arch Pediatr Adolesc Med.* 2008;162(5):447–452

6. Ginsburg GS. Evidence-based treatments for children and adolescents. *J Clin Child Adolesc Psychol.* 2006;35(3):480–486

7. Weisz JR, Jensen-Doss A, Hawley KM. Evidence-based youth psychotherapies versus usual clinical care: a meta-analysis of direct comparisons. *Am Psychol.* 2006;61(7):671–689

8. Gleason MM, Egger HL, Emslie GJ, et al. Psychopharmacological treatment for very young children: contexts and guidelines. *J Am Acad Child Adolesc Psychiatry.* 2007;46(2):1532–1572

9. A 14-month randomized clinical trial of treatment strategies for attention-deficit/ hyperactivity disorder. The MTA Cooperative Group. Multimodal Treatment Study of Children with ADHD. *Arch Gen Psychiatry.* 1999;56(12):1073–1086

10. Walkup JT, Albano AM, Piacentini J, et al. Cognitive behavioral therapy, sertraline, or a combination in childhood anxiety. *N Engl J Med.* 2008;359(26):2753–2766

11. March J, Silva S, Petrycki S, et al; Treatment for Adolescents With Depression Study Team. Fluoxetine, cognitive-behavioral therapy, and their combination for adolescents with depression: Treatment for Adolescents With Depression Study (TADS) randomized controlled trial. *JAMA.* 2004;292(7):807–820

12. American Academy of Pediatrics Committee on Psychosocial Aspects of Child and Family Health and Task Force on Mental Health. The future of pediatrics: mental health competencies for pediatric primary care. *Pediatrics.* 2009;124(1):410–421

13. Olfson M, Blanco C, Wang S, Laje G, Correll CU. National trends in the mental health care of children, adolescents, and adults by office-based physicians. *JAMA Psychiatry.* 2014;71(1):81–90

14. Birmaher B, Axelson DA, Monk K, et al. Fluoxetine for the treatment of childhood anxiety disorders. *J Am Acad Child Adolesc Psychiatry.* 2003;42(4):415–423

15. Fluvoxamine for the treatment of anxiety disorders in children and adolescents. The Research Unit on Pediatric Psychopharmacology Anxiety Study Group. *N Engl J Med.* 2001;344(17):1279–1285

16. Hammad TA, Laughren T, Racoosin J. Suicidality in pediatric patients treated with antidepressant drugs. *Arch Gen Psychiatry.* 2006;63(3):332–339

17. Bridge JA, Iyengar S, Salary CB, et al. Clinical response and risk for reported suicidal ideation and suicide attempts in pediatric antidepressant treatment: a meta-analysis of randomized controlled trials. *JAMA.* 2007;297(15):1683–1696

18. Julious SA. Efficacy and suicidal risk for antidepressants in paediatric and adolescent patients. *Stat Methods Med Res.* 2013;22(2):190–218

19. Mannuzza S, Klein RG, Truong NL, et al. Age of methylphenidate treatment initiation in children with ADHD and later substance abuse: prospective follow-up into adulthood. *Am J Psychiatry.* 2008;165(5):604–609

20. Wilson JJ. ADHD and substance use disorders: developmental aspects and the impact of stimulant treatment. *Am J Addict.* 2007;16(suppl 1):5–11

21. Biederman J, Monuteaux MC, Spencer T, Wilens TE, Macpherson HA, Faraone SV. Stimulant therapy and risk for subsequent substance use disorders in male adults with ADHD: a naturalistic controlled 10-year follow-up study. *Am J Psychiatry.* 2008;165(5):597–603

22. Wilens TE, Adler LA, Adams J, et al. Misuse and diversion of stimulants prescribed for ADHD: a systematic review of the literature. *J Am Acad Child Adolesc Psychiatry.* 2008;47(1):21–31

23. Aptensio XR [package insert]. Coventry, RI: Rhodes Pharmaceuticals LP; 2017

24. World Health Organization. *Adherence to Long-term Therapies: Evidence to Action.* Geneva, Switzerland: World Health Organization; 2003

25. Case BG. Nonadherence: the silent majority. *J Am Acad Child Adolesc Psychiatry.* 2011;50(5):435–437

26. Pappadopulos E, Jensen PS, Chait AR, et al. Medication adherence in the MTA: saliva methylphenidate samples versus parent report and mediating effect of concomitant behavioral treatment. *J Am Acad Child Adolesc Psychiatry.* 2009;48(5):501–510

27. Olfson M, Marcus S, Wan G. Stimulant dosing for children with ADHD: a medical claims analysis. *J Am Acad Child Adolesc Psychiatry.* 2009;48(1):51–59

28. Winterstein AG, Gerhard T, Shuster J, et al. Utilization of pharmacologic treatment in youths with attention deficit/hyperactivity disorder in Medicaid database. *Ann Pharmacother.* 2008;42(1):24–31

29. Charach A, Fernandez R. Enhancing ADHD medication adherence: challenges and opportunities. *Curr Psychiatry Rep.* 2013;15(7):371

30. Pliszka S; American Academy of Child and Adolescent Psychiatry Work Group on Quality Issues. Practice parameter for the assessment and treatment of children and adolescents with attention-deficit/hyperactivity disorder. *J Am Acad Child Adolesc Psychiatry.* 2007;46(7):894–921

31. Elia J, Borcherding BG, Rapoport JL, Keysor CS. Methylphenidate and dextro-amphetamine treatments of hyperactivity: are there true nonresponders? *Psychiatry Res.* 1991;36(2):141–155

32. Brent D, Emslie G, Clarke G, et al. Switching to another SSRI or to venlafaxine with or without cognitive behavioral therapy for adolescents with SSRI-resistant depression: the TORDIA randomized controlled trial. *JAMA.* 2008;299(8):901–913

33. Abikoff H, McGough J, Vitiello B, et al; RUPP ADHD/Anxiety Study Group. Sequential pharmacotherapy for children with comorbid attention-deficit/hyperactivity and anxiety disorders. *J Am Acad Child Adolesc Psychiatry.* 2005;44(5):418–427

34. Knapp P, Chait A, Pappadopulos E, Crystal S, Jensen PS; T-MAY Steering Group. Treatment of maladaptive aggression in youth: CERT guidelines I. Engagement, assessment, and management. *Pediatrics.* 2012;129(6):e1562–e1576

35. Rosato NS, Correll CU, Pappadopulos E, Chait A, Crystal S, Jensen PS. Treatment of maladaptive aggression in youth: CERT guidelines II. Treatments and ongoing management. *Pediatrics.* 2012;129(6):e1577–e1586

36. Correll CU, Manu P, Olshanskiy V, Napolitano B, Kane JM, Malhotra AK. Cardiometabolic risk of second-generation antipsychotic medications during first-time use in children and adolescents. *JAMA.* 2009;302(16):1765–1773

37. Geller B, Luby JL, Joshi P, et al. A randomized controlled trial of risperidone, lithium, or divalproex sodium for initial treatment of bipolar I disorder, manic or mixed phase, in children and adolescents. *Arch Gen Psychiatry.* 2012;69(5): 515–528

38. Findling RL, Robb A, McNamara NK, et al. Lithium in the acute treatment of bipolar I disorder: a double-blind, placebo-controlled study. *Pediatrics.* 2015; 136(5):885–894

39. Rynn MA, Riddle MA, Yeung PP, Kunz NR. Efficacy and safety of extended-release venlafaxine in the treatment of generalized anxiety disorder in children and adolescents: two placebo-controlled trials. *Am J Psychiatry.* 2007;164(2):290–300

40. Emslie GJ, Findling RL, Yeung PP, Kunz NR, Li Y. Venlafaxine ER for the treatment of pediatric subjects with depression: results of two placebo-controlled trials. *J Am Acad Child Adolesc Psychiatry.* 2007;46(4):479–488

41. Wagner KD, Redden L, Kowatch RA, et al. A double-blind, randomized, placebo-controlled trial of divalproex extended-release in the treatment of bipolar disorder in children and adolescents. *J Am Acad Child Adolesc Psychiatry.* 2009;48(5): 519–532

CHAPTER 12

Transitioning Adolescents With Mental Health Conditions to Adult Care

Gary Maslow, MD, MPH; Laura Hart, MD; and
Nicole Heilbron, PhD

> "For young people with mental health conditions, there is both an acute need to make sure they are receiving appropriate care in the moment and a long-term need to make sure they are connected to ongoing care."

Introduction

Each year in the United States, an estimated 500,000 adolescents with special health care needs turn 18 years of age.[1] Although this is the legal age of majority, many of these young adults struggle to become fully independent adults.[2] The health care needs of young adults with chronic mental and physical health conditions as they transition into adult care are often unmet, and the system of care is fragmented, disorganized, and ill prepared to support new generations of these young adults.[3,4]

While improving this health care transition is important to the health of all young adults graduating from pediatric practices, there is a pressing need to address this issue for young adults with mental health conditions. Analysis of data from the Great Smoky Mountains Study found that only 20% of young adults (aged 18–21) with fourth edition of *Diagnostic and Statistical Manual of Mental Disorders* (commonly known as *DSM-IV*) conditions were receiving any mental health services, as compared with more than 50% of adolescents (aged 13–17).[5] This large drop-off in service use is especially troubling given that many mental health conditions worsen during adolescence. Moreover, it is concerning given that many patients with the most disabling psychiatric conditions, such as schizophrenia, first present during this time period. A prospective study from the United Kingdom examining transfer from the child to adult mental health system found that out of 154 patients who were eligible to be referred to adult services, only 61 attended a first appointment and only 41 remained in care long-term.[6] Less than one-third of young people ages 13 to 24 who had been cared for by the child mental health system were successfully transferred to the adult system. Because they see patients for annual health supervision visits and acute medical needs and often have the opportunity to remain connected to their patients as young adults, pediatric primary care clinicians (PCCs) (pediatricians, family physicians, internists, nurse practitioners, and physician assistants who provide frontline, longitudinal health care to children and adolescents) can play a role in helping their patients successfully navigate the adult mental health care system.

The purpose of this chapter is to outline the challenges facing young adult patients with mental health difficulties and their PCCs around the transition from pediatric to adult care. The child and adult mental health systems are distinct, and even PCCs who understand the child mental health system may struggle to identify appropriate adult providers for their patients. There are 2 groups to focus on: patients whose mental health problems have been managed only in pediatric primary care (eg, those with attention-deficit/hyperactivity disorder [ADHD], some with depression or anxiety) and patients whose mental health conditions have been cared for in the child mental health system. Special consideration is given to the health care transitions of patients with both primary physical conditions (eg, diabetes) and comorbid mental health conditions and of patients with developmental disabilities.

General Considerations for Transition of Patients With Special Physical and Mental Health Care Needs

The transition to adult care entails high stakes for young people with childhood-onset chronic physical illness or with childhood-onset mental illness or with both, because early adulthood is a period of particular health vulnerability for these patients and many face a worsening of their health during this time.[7-13] Despite recognition of the importance of promoting a smooth transition, few of them receive even the most basic education about this health care transition. The 2005–2006 National Survey of Children with Special Health Care Needs found that only 42% of preadolescents and adolescents aged 12 to 17 years had been counseled regarding 4 basic aspects of the health care transition: seeing adult providers, future adult health care needs, changes in health insurance, and the need to take increased responsibility for their conditions.[2] Lack of counseling may be caused partly by a lack of evidence of best practices for promoting successful health care transitions.[14]

Recognition that a smooth, planned, and purposeful transition from pediatric to adult medical care could prevent future health and psychosocial problems has led to recommendations from the American Academy of Pediatrics, the Society of Adolescent Health and Medicine (SAHM), and the Maternal and Child Health Bureau.[15-17] SAHM defines this transition as "the purposeful, planned movement of adolescents and young adults with chronic physical and medical conditions [including mental health conditions] from child-centered to adult-oriented health-care systems."[18] Healthy People 2010 contains a broader statement on the transition of youths with special health care needs (YSHCN), recognizing that the health care transition is one of many transitions that youths are experiencing as they enter young adulthood.[19] Transition continues to be a point of emphasis in the Healthy People 2020 goals, with an aim for a 10% improvement in the number of YSHCN getting transition services.[20]

There is agreement on the key barriers to a successful health care transition, which are similar for patients with physical and mental health conditions.[12,21-25] These include barriers related to patients, pediatric clinics, adult providers and clinics, and the broader health system. At the individual and clinic levels, adolescents and families report being reluctant to leave the familiar pediatric setting and may be distrustful of adult clinics.[1,3,26,27] Like adolescents and parents, pediatric PCCs may be distrustful of the adult medical system.[1,26,28,29] Adult clinics are often reluctant to take on young adults with chronic medical conditions or developmental disabilities because adult providers may lack experience with what was previously considered a disease or disorder of childhood, such as cystic fibrosis, congenital heart disease, or autism spectrum disorder (ASD).[30] In addition, adult medical clinics are set up to focus on individual patients and do not follow the pediatric model of family-centered care.

The financing of health care also influences the transition between pediatric care and adult care. Many adolescents with chronic illness are eligible for Medicaid prior to their 19th birthdays, but they do not qualify after that time.[31] For Medicaid-enrolled children in foster care, who disproportionately experience mental health problems and often lack family support during their transitions to adulthood, this loss of insurance is particularly problematic. Prior to the passage of the Affordable Care Act (ACA) in 2010, more than 20% of young adults with disabilities who were older than 18 years were uninsured and 10% of preadolescents and adolescents aged 11 to 18 years were uninsured.[31] While the ACA has improved coverage, especially for young adults, many of these patients continue to lack coverage.[32] Lack of health insurance results in lapses in medical and mental health care, including missed appointments and inability to adhere to medication therapies.

Health Care Transition Tools for Pediatric Primary Care

Transition tools (www.gottransition.org) have been created to help pediatric PCCs implement best practices around health care transition for their patients. A standardized approach created by the Center for Health Care Transition Improvement consists of 6 core elements (Box 12-1).

1. Transition policy: The first step in preparing patients for a successful transition is to develop a clinic-level policy for the pediatric medical home. This policy should be agreed on by staff and clinicians and then distributed to patients and families by sharing the policy during a visit and posting the policy in the waiting area and other general areas of the office. This communication is critical so there is a shared understanding of the time frame for transition.

Box 12-1. Six Core Elements of Health Care Transition From Adolescence to Adulthood

1. Transition policy
2. Tracking and monitoring
3. Transition readiness
4. Transition planning
5. Transfer of care
6. Transition completion

Adapted from Six Core Elements of Health Care Transition 2.0. GotTransition.org. http://www.gottransition.org/providers/index.cfm. Accessed February 7, 2018.

2. Tracking and monitoring: Got Transition recommendations include establishing a registry, which can serve as a valuable tool enabling the pediatric PCC to track patients as they move through the transition process, identify patients who are behind on transition steps, and ensure transfer occurs in a timely fashion for those who have completed the steps of transition that are needed prior to transfer to adult care. Such tracking and monitoring is crucial to ensuring that all patients get their transitional care needs addressed. (See Chapter 3, Office and Network Systems to Support Mental Health Care, for a full discussion of practice preparations for monitoring YSHCN.)

3. Transition readiness: For individual patients, assessment of transition readiness by the pediatric PCC should begin in early adolescence. It is important to begin evaluating a patient's knowledge of his or her condition and readiness to take on self-management and health care navigation. This evaluation can be part of an annual checkup using a standardized scale or can be a brief part of any chronic care follow-up.

4. Transition planning: Transition preparation is a critical step. Adolescents need education regarding their condition and how to navigate the adult system. Parents also need training and support in how to navigate the adult system and support their young adult in taking on more responsibility for self-management. As part of transition preparation, the pediatric PCC can facilitate development of a written care plan for each patient. This plan can serve as a succinct medical care summary and emergency care plan for accepting providers.

5. Transfer of care: A process through which the pediatric PCC can track the transfer process and ensure that patients do not drop out of care during this time is critically important. This process should include contact with accepting providers prior to transfer and ensuring that accepting providers have the care summary prior to the first appointment with the transferring patient.

6. Transition completion: In the transfer completion step, pediatric PCCs are encouraged to follow-up with patients and families about the transition and transfer process to get feedback about how to improve it. They can also follow up with accepting providers to address any questions or concerns that have come up as transferred patients are getting established in adult care.

Transition of Patients With Mental Health Conditions

In many cases, children and adolescents receive treatment for psychiatric symptoms only in the primary care setting. In other cases, children and adolescents receive psychiatric care through specialized mental health services. The following sections outline health care transition considerations for both these groups.

Transition of Patients Receiving Care Only in the Primary Care System

Case Example and Discussion

Case Example 1

John is a 22-year-old man who has been seen by his pediatric PCC since birth. He was diagnosed at age 7 years as having ADHD and did well with a long-acting formulation of methylphenidate. He had several trials off the medication in high school and then in college, and it seemed clear that he benefited from treatment and still had symptoms of ADHD while off the medication. Overall, he has thrived and is now preparing to graduate from college. His pediatric PCC has continued to prescribe his ADHD medication and see him when he is back from school on break. He comes in for a visit and is excited to share with his PCC that he got a job across the country and will be moving there soon after he graduates. This is likely his last visit with his pediatric PCC. He asks if his PCC can continue to prescribe the stimulant, even though he is going to be living across the country.

The case example provides a relatively common patient care issue faced by many pediatric PCCs, who are routinely providing mental health care and prescribing medications, including stimulants and selective serotonin reuptake inhibitors (commonly known as SSRIs), to young adults.[33] Up to 80% of pediatric patients who are on psychotropic medication receive prescriptions for these medications from a pediatrician or general practitioner.[34,35] For this reason, the most common type of transition involving a young adult with a diagnosed mental health condition will involve transition from the pediatric PCC who has been prescribing his or her medication to another primary care provider, rather than from the pediatric PCC to an adult mental health specialist. Consequently, it is of particular importance to consider the plan for transferring care of young adults who receive psychotropic medication from a pediatric office, including not only those with ADHD but also those with other conditions commonly treated by pediatric PCCs, including anxiety and depression.

In John's case, he has experienced symptom relief from ADHD medication and has felt supported by his long-standing pediatric provider. Attention-deficit/hyperactivity disorder has historically been thought of as a condition that diminishes with age or doesn't require treatment in adulthood; however, newer evidence suggests that anywhere from 15% to 65% of adults require treatment of ADHD in adulthood.[36] Despite this increased recognition of the need for long-term treatment, pediatric PCCs often report difficulties finding providers to assume care of adults with any number of pediatric-onset conditions, including ADHD.[37] Studies have shown relatively high rates of psychiatric comorbidities in adults with ADHD, such as depression, anxiety, and substance use,[38] making treatment of ADHD more complicated for those patients. While psychiatrists are comfortable treating adults with ADHD, even in the setting of psychiatric comorbidities, patients may be reluctant to seek care from psychiatrists because of stigma or costs. A lack of psychiatrists may also present a barrier, particularly in rural settings.[39]

Data specific to facilitating transition for this population are generally targeted toward transition from pediatric mental health services to adult mental health services, rather than from pediatric primary care to adult-oriented primary care.[12,39–40] For this population, then, pediatric PCCs should deliver their transitional care services according to the general guidance for transitional care that is currently available.

Approach to Health Care Transition

Transition Policy

It is important to set clear guidelines that will inform transition planning for patients and families. These guidelines should communicate the practice's expectations regarding timing of the patient's transfer to adult care, practice procedures for protecting patient confidentiality and autonomy upon reaching the age of majority, the practice's approach to the transition process throughout adolescence, and condition-specific details such as how frequently a patient should be seen for the practice to continue refilling prescriptions. Similarly, policies related to the limits of patient confidentiality and privacy, including how to support a patient's decision-making and about granting parents access to information after the adolescent reaches the age of majority, are key considerations. Finally, it is helpful to provide an overview of the expected transition process for patients. This explicit transition policy should be readily available to patients and families. In the case example earlier in this chapter, many of John's questions would have been previously addressed if such a policy had been in place.

The following issues are specific to the care of patients who have ADHD and should also be considered when setting guidelines:

▶ If and when pediatric providers plan to screen for substance use and misuse of stimulant medications

▶ That adult providers are likely to screen for substance use and misuse of stimulant medications and may require a contract for continued prescribing of stimulant medications

▶ For patients going away to college, the importance of keeping medications locked up and the options for receiving prescription refills closer to where they live

Tracking and Monitoring

Ideally, patients like John would be included in a transition registry once they reached middle school. Some practices start registries at older ages (eg, age 16 years or once patients start college), but in each of these scenarios, putting younger patients on a transition registry allows for discussion of their needs in preparation for transfer to adult care. This step also ensures that discussion of all those needs is not limited to one last visit, before a young adult moves across the country.

Transition Readiness

The transition readiness step includes assessing the patient's readiness and educating patients and families about both the adult health system and the tasks patients will be expected to complete independently once they reach the adult health care system.

Multiple assessment forms are available. Got Transition offers a transition readiness assessment for providers. The American College of Physicians incorporated this assessment into their transition toolkit in 2016, so some adult care physicians may be familiar with it. This form rates overall confidence and completion of skills, rather than monitoring improvement in skills over time. With younger patients, who would not be expected to have mastered skills, findings from this kind of tool can be difficult to interpret; rather, a tool that shows gradual change over time (from no skill, to some skill, to mastery) could be more useful for tracking progress with skills, such as the TRAQ (Transition Readiness Assessment Questionnaire) and the STAR$_x$ Questionnaire (Self-Management and Transition to Adulthood with R$_x$ Questionnaire).[41,42] See Appendix 2, Mental Health Tools for Pediatrics, for more information. Such tools may take a bit longer to complete than those assessing completion of skill acquisition.

Education of patients and parents about the adult health system is critical. The adult health system tends to be stricter about enforcing privacy policies and has higher expectations regarding patients' initiative. Accordingly, many young adults entering adult care will now be expected to take over the responsibility for many aspects of their care (eg, scheduling their own medical appointments, calling for and picking up prescriptions themselves, talking with clinic staff and providers, and navigating the adult health system [which is generally less well integrated than the pediatric health system]). This change may present a particular challenge for young people with both a chronic physical illness and a mental health problem, as they will need to navigate both adult medical systems and adult mental health systems. Also, parents may need to continue to play an active supporting role, particularly if their young person has a significant learning disability or intellectual disability. Additionally, pressures may be coming from the young person and, at times, the parents for the young person to become fully independent when he or she reaches a certain age. Requiring young people to function more or less independently should be based on skills, rather than chronological age, so pediatric PCCs may have to engage with patients and families about ensuring a balance of autonomy and safety for young adults.

Patients and parents should also be made aware that while educational supports are available in college, young adults will need to be proactive to access and maintain them. Patients and parents will need to plan and talk with colleges early to ensure that services are in place when classes start.

Suggested areas to focus on as part of transition readiness include

▶ Encourage patients and parents to talk with the college office on disability services as early as possible.

▶ Consider referral to the office on vocational rehabilitation when concerns about holding a job arise.

▶ Assist with navigation when specific types of treatment or support are needed (eg, bipolar disorder treatment, substance use treatment, eating disorder therapy).

▶ Directly discuss potential stigma that can be a barrier to seeking treatment.

Transition Planning

For young people with mental health conditions who are transferring from pediatric care, pediatric PCCs may be able to ensure a smooth transfer to a mental health provider prior to transitioning them out of pediatric primary care. It is important as part of transition planning to map out the medical team of providers caring for a patient and to identify the timing of transfer for each of these providers. Transition planning should also take into account changes in insurance and changes in living situation that may be coming (eg, if the patient goes away to college). Written documentation of a transition plan that is shared with the patient and family is one way to facilitate this process. Several "transition passports" have been created to facilitate transition planning.[43]

Transition planning should also include development of a transfer letter to be sent to new providers. This letter should include a succinct summary of the patient's history, a list of current medical and mental health conditions and associated medications, a list of allergies, vaccination records, and a current emergency care plan. Ideally, this letter should also include contact information for the pediatric practice, so adult care providers can reach out if questions or concerns arise. Pediatric providers are encouraged to maintain a current emergency care plan with a succinct medical summary for their patients, as this documentation often makes the writing of a transfer letter more streamlined.

Transfer of Care

To facilitate the process of transitioning patients from pediatric care to adult care providers, pediatric PCCs are encouraged to maintain information about adult care providers in the area who are comfortable treating mental health conditions in a primary care setting. Pediatric providers can remain involved throughout the transfer and ensure that the transfer goes smoothly. In fact, one of the reasons to have a registry system, as recommended earlier, is to prevent loss to follow-up during the transfer of care.

Transition Completion

The transition process does not end for the patient at the first adult appointment; nor should it end for the pediatric PCC at the first adult appointment. By reaching out to patients after the first appointment in adult care, pediatric PCCs have the opportunity to follow up on questions not previously addressed with the patient, as well as to elicit feedback from patients and families on how to improve the transition process. Pediatric PCCs can also follow up with accepting providers to assist with any questions that they may have.

Although the transition process as outlined in this chapter may seem onerous, cases like John's highlight its importance. He is experiencing many changes in his life, including graduation from college, a new job, and a move across the country, and will now also have to manage a transfer to a new provider, specifically, a transition for which little planning has yet been done. With a more systematic approach as described in this chapter, pediatric PCCs can set up patients for success after "graduating" from pediatric care.

Transition of Patients Receiving Care in the Child Mental Health System

Case Example and Discussion

Case Example 2

Stacy is a 20-year-old woman who has been receiving treatment of severe depression since early adolescence. She is seen by a local child psychiatrist for medication management and receives weekly psychotherapy from a clinical social worker at a nearby child mental health clinic. Her pediatric PCC has worked collaboratively with the child psychiatrist and a pediatric endocrinologist over the years to support Stacy in the management of her other health conditions, including type 1 diabetes and obesity. She recently lost her job and no longer has health insurance to cover the costs associated with her mental health treatment. She presents to her pediatric PCC asking for assistance because she has become increasingly depressed and hopeless.

It is widely acknowledged that there is a precipitous decline in the treatment of psychiatric conditions as young people like Stacy, described in Case Example 2, transition from specialized pediatric mental health services to adult mental health services. As noted previously, many factors contribute to this decrease in mental health service use, including the loss of eligibility for public mental health care, a lack of access to adult providers who are trained to address the specific needs of transition-aged patients (eg, daily living skills), and a lack of perceived relevance of treatment.[44-46] On the basis of a growing recognition of these problems, SAMHSA (Substance Abuse and Mental Health Services Administration) has created grant programs to incentivize and support communities in developing transition services. Some state and local mental health systems have developed transition programs that include care managers, peer navigators, and other strategies. Where such programs exist, it is important for the pediatric team to become familiar with them and provide appropriate referrals of transitioning patients.

During transition, the role of the pediatric PCC in the care of a patient like Stacy is to provide a safety net. Pediatric PCCs are often called on to refill medications or continue treatments when patients are transitioning between mental health services or from the hospital to home. This is not an ideal situation, and it speaks to the need for pediatric health care professionals to develop collaborative relationships with mental health providers. Integrated behavioral health strategies in which mental health personnel are embedded in or partnered with primary care or subspecialty pediatric offices are one way to provide additional supports to pediatric clinicians and patients.

There may be adolescents with mental health conditions such as bipolar disorders, schizophrenia, and substance use disorders who receive services in the pediatric mental health system and, unlike Stacy, rarely use primary care services. Even when they seek primary care, these adolescents and their parents may not disclose their mental health histories because of stigma, confidentiality concerns, or the perception that their mental health conditions are not a primary care concern. Pediatric practices are encouraged to put a system into place to gather information, proactively and routinely, about mental health services that children and adolescents are receiving elsewhere. (See Chapter 3, Office and Network Systems to Support Mental Health Care.) Any contact with a pediatric practice (eg, acute care visit, visit to monitor a chronic medical condition, request for a job physical examination, completion of a college entry form) is an opportunity to check in and see whether a patient is engaged in mental health care.

Patients with chronic medical conditions are a particular challenge in transition. They are more likely than other adolescents and young adults to have mental health problems, such as depression. Furthermore, their mental health comorbidity may compound their risk for poor medical outcomes. For example, up to one-third of young people who have had a kidney transplant lose the kidney graft following the transfer from pediatric to adult care,[47] and young people with sickle cell disease have increased mortality after the age of 18 years.[48] While further study is needed to examine the intersection between mental health illness and chronic physical illness during the transition from pediatric to adult care, there are studies of this issue in patients like Stacy, who have diabetes. Data from a longitudinal study of patients with type 1 diabetes showed that depression in adolescence predicted medical complications and hospitalization in young adulthood.[49] Another longitudinal study of patients with type 1 diabetes, with a median follow-up of 10 years and controlling for age of onset of diabetes, showed that depression in adolescence was associated with worse retinopathy.[50] These studies have raised the question of whether screening for and treating depression in children and adolescents with physical illness could improve young adult outcomes.

Pediatric PCCs, together with any involved pediatric subspecialists, need to plan collaboratively for the medical transition of patients with chronic physical conditions. If a patient also has an identifiable mental health condition, it is critical that the transition team incorporate the patient's mental health specialist or specialists as well. It is important to consider the specific types of neuropsychological challenges that patients with chronic physical illness face and to consider what these challenges will mean for them as they transition to adulthood. For example, patients with neurological conditions such as epilepsy and patients who have survived brain tumors are at elevated risk for having ADHD or learning disabilities. For this group of patients, planning for transition should include consideration of relevant educational and vocational supports, not just finding an adult provider to prescribe a stimulant.

Patients With Developmental Disabilities

Young people with developmental disabilities, including ASD, and their families face several additional challenges during the transition to adult-focused health care.[51] For example, findings suggest that youths with ASD are significantly less likely to receive health care transition services than are YSHCN generally.[25,52] This suggestion is particularly concerning because these patients and their families may need to address numerous transition-related issues, including the issue of guardianship and decision-making and the issue of financial planning, and will likely need much support navigating the transition from school support services to the services available to support adults with disabilities. Moreover, it is widely acknowledged that there is a relative paucity of knowledge about ASD and other developmental disabilities among adult health care providers.[53-55]

Approach to Health Care Transition

Transition Policy

It is important as part of the primary care clinic policy to include that transition planning will address all aspects of health care, including physical and mental health. For patients like Stacy with special health care needs (eg, chronic physical illnesses, developmental disabilities), there is a need for PCCs to work collaboratively with both pediatric specialists and mental health providers. The policy should also include information regarding whether, how, and how long the practice will be able to continue to prescribe medications. This information is of particular importance as young people move away to pursue job opportunities or further education.

Tracking and Monitoring

For patients with developmental disabilities, early initiation of tracking and monitoring of transition is especially important. Many school systems begin to address student and family post–high school goals in middle school or early in high school. By starting the medical transition process around the same time, patients and families can be in a position to consider the effects of health on postsecondary education plans and how certain postsecondary education plans may affect health. Using a tracking system, pediatric PCCs can also ensure that other needs, such as insurance, guardianship (if needed), and estate planning are considered before adolescents reach the age of 18 years and are legally adults.

Transition Readiness

In the transition readiness domain, pediatric clinicians should assess a patient's transition readiness, as well as educate patients and families about the adult health care system.

Transition assessments come in a variety of forms. Some assessments are specific to a particular illness or issue, such as cystic fibrosis or transplants, and require involvement of subspecialists, whereas others are applicable to a variety of conditions and lend themselves to use in primary care.[56] Two of the tools that are not specific to a particular condition are the TRAQ and the STAR$_x$ Questionnaire. These tools have been validated with populations of youths with a number of chronic illnesses and disabilities.[41,42,57,58]

These tools are self-assessments that are completed by patients independently; therefore, they can often be done while a patient is waiting to be seen. They ask about a variety of aspects of transition readiness, including medical knowledge, self-management skills such as medication management, and advocacy skills such as speaking to providers about medical needs. This level of detail allows providers to target transition education and preparation to the needs of a specific patient. The scoring systems of these tools also allow for tracking of improvement in transition readiness over time.

Got Transition has also developed a transition readiness assessment for providers (accessible at www.gottransition.org). This readiness assessment was incorporated into the transition toolkit developed by the American College of Physicians in 2016 for internists seeking to address transition, so it may be familiar to adult-oriented providers. This form rates overall confidence and completion of skills, rather than monitoring improvement in skills over time, so it may have more utility with older patients than with younger ones, who may not be expected to have mastered many skills.[59]

For young people with intellectual disabilities or developmental disabilities (or both), it is important to include specific assessment of capacity, including the issues of decision-making and guardianship, as part of the transition assessment.[27] It may be as simple as asking for documentation of guardianship or health care proxy from parents of young adults with intellectual disabilities. This information can influence the degree to which the target of transition planning is the young adult's ability to care for himself or herself vs the parents' or guardians' readiness to transition to a different medical setting.

Education of patients and parents around the adult health system is critical. In particular, transitioning patients need to learn about how to make their appointments and navigate the adult health system. This challenge may present a particular challenge for young people with both a chronic physical illness and a mental health problem, as they may need to navigate both the adult medical systems and the adult mental health systems. Also, parents may need to continue to play an active role in supporting their young adults as they navigate this system, particularly if those young adults have a significant learning disability or intellectual disability. In addition, the mental health system is challenging for young people to navigate. Experienced and trained parents or young adults can be used to help provide this education. Each state has a Family Voices program (www.familyvoices.org), which can assist patients and families in finding and working with peer supports. In some communities, additional transition services are offered by the public mental health system.

Transition Planning

For patients with both a chronic physical illness and a mental health condition, pediatric PCCs may want to consider ensuring that these young people have had a smooth mental health transfer prior to transitioning them out of pediatric primary care. It is important as part of transition planning to map out the medical team of providers caring for a patient and to identify the timing of transfer for each of these providers. Transition planning should also take into account changes in insurance and changes in living situation that may be coming. The timing of transfer may be related to a patient's moving to college or a family's moving to another city: in this case, the planning should be expedited. Written documentation of a transition plan that is shared with the patient and family is one way to facilitate this process. Several transition passports have been created to help facilitate transition planning.[43]

Transition planning should also include development of a transfer letter to be sent by the pediatric PCC to new providers. This letter should include a succinct summary of the patient's history, a list of current mental health and medical problems and medications, a list of allergies, and vaccination records. Ideally, this letter should also include the pediatric practice's contact information, so adult providers can reach out to pediatric providers if questions or concerns arise. Providers are encouraged to keep a current emergency care plan with a succinct medical summary for their patients, as this documentation often makes the writing of a transfer letter more streamlined.

Transfer of Care

The process of providing transition care for young people with chronic physical and mental health problems or developmental disabilities (or both) is complex. It is truly a longitudinal process that begins by identifying adolescents with these conditions and working to ensure a smooth transfer for the range of medical and mental health care that they receive. Pediatric PCCs can stay involved throughout the transfer of specialty care and ensure that the transfer in each domain, including mental and behavioral health, goes smoothly prior to transferring them out of primary care.

For patients with chronic physical illness and comorbid mental health conditions, a registry system or another way to monitor transfer completion can help prevent these patients from dropping out of care.

Transition Completion

After the transfer of care is complete, pediatric PCCs should follow up with patients and families and with accepting providers. Follow-up with patients and families ensures that concerns or questions that have come up since the last pediatric visit can be addressed. It also allows pediatric PCCs to get feedback about the transition process, so it can be improved for future patients. Follow-up with accepting providers ensures that accepting providers can ask any questions that come up. This opportunity can be especially helpful when transferring young people with developmental disabilities, whose needs may be less familiar to adult-oriented providers. Pediatric PCCs should continue to be available to answer questions for accepting providers so that young adults with mental health conditions can be well situated in adult care.

Summary

Pediatric primary care clinicians can play a critical role in supporting the transition from pediatric to adult care for patients with a wide range of mental health and developmental conditions. For young people like John and Stacy, described in the brief vignettes in this chapter, there is both an acute need to make sure they are receiving appropriate care in the moment and a long-term need to make sure they are connected to ongoing care. A systematic approach is needed by pediatric PCCs and other pediatric health care professionals and their practices to ensure that young adult patients with mental health problems do not fall through the cracks and drop out of care.

AAP Policy

American Academy of Pediatrics, American Academy of Family Physicians, American College of Physicians, Transitions Clinical Report Authoring Group. Supporting the health care transition from adolescence to adulthood in the medical home. *Pediatrics.* 2011;128(1):182–200. Reaffirmed August 2015 (pediatrics.aappublications. org/content/128/1/182)

American Academy of Pediatrics Council on Foster Care, Adoption, and Kinship Care and Committee on Early Childhood. Health care of youth aging out of foster care. *Pediatrics.* 2012;130(6):1170–1173. Reaffirmed July 2017 (pediatrics.aappublications. org/content/130/6/1170)

References

1. Reiss J, Gibson R. Health care transition: destinations unknown. *Pediatrics.* 2002;110(6, pt 2):1307–1314
2. Lotstein DS, Ghandour R, Cash A, McGuire E, Strickland B, Newacheck P. Planning for health care transitions: results from the 2005–2006 National Survey of Children with Special Health Care Needs. *Pediatrics.* 2009;123(1):e145–e152
3. Gray WN, Resmini AR, Baker KD, et al. Concerns, barriers, and recommendations to improve transition from pediatric to adult IBD care: perspectives of patients, parents, and health professionals. *Inflamm Bowel Dis.* 2015;21(7):1641–1651

4. Okumura MJ, Saunders M, Rehm RS. The role of health advocacy in transitions from pediatric to adult care for children with special health care needs: bridging families, provider and community services. *J Pediatr Nurs.* 2015;30(5):714–723

5. Copeland WE, Shanahan L, Davis M, Burns BJ, Angold A, Costello EJ. Untreated psychiatric cases increase during the transition to adulthood. *Psychiatr Serv.* 2015;66(4):397–403

6. Singh SP, Paul M, Ford T, Kramer T, Weaver T. Transitions of care from child and adolescent mental health services to adult mental health services (TRACK study): a study of protocols in Greater London. *BMC Health Serv Res.* 2008;8(1):135

7. Scal P, Davern M, Ireland M, Park K. Transition to adulthood: delays and unmet needs among adolescents and young adults with asthma. *J Pediatr.* 2008;152(4): 471–475.e1

8. Hersh A, von Scheven E, Yelin E. Adult outcomes of childhood-onset rheumatic diseases. *Nat Rev Rheumatol.* 2011;7(5):290–295

9. Northam EA, Lin A, Finch S, Werther GA, Cameron FJ. Psychosocial well-being and functional outcomes in youth with type 1 diabetes 12 years after disease onset. *Diabetes Care.* 2010;33(7):1430–1437

10. British Cardiac Society Working Party. Grown-up congenital heart (GUCH) disease: current needs and provision of service for adolescents and adults with congenital heart disease in the UK. *Heart.* 2002;88(suppl 1):i1–i14

11. Webb GD, Williams RG. Care of the adult with congenital heart disease: introduction. *J Am Coll Cardiol.* 2001;37(5):1166

12. Swift KD, Hall CL, Marimuttu V, Redstone L, Sayal K, Hollis C. Transition to adult mental health services for young people with attention deficit/hyperactivity disorder (ADHD): a qualitative analysis of their experiences. *BMC Psychiatry.* 2013;13(1):74

13. McGorry PD, Purcell R, Hickie IB, Jorm AF. Investing in youth mental health is a best buy. *Med J Aust.* 2007;187(7)(suppl):S5

14. Freed GL, Hudson EJ. Transitioning children with chronic diseases to adult care: current knowledge, practices, and directions. *J Pediatr.* 2006;148(6):824–827

15. American Academy of Pediatrics, American Academy of Family Physicians, American College of Physicians, Transitions Clinical Report Authoring Group. Supporting the health care transition from adolescence to adulthood in the medical home. *Pediatrics.* 2011;128(1):182–200

16. Rosen DS, Blum RW, Britto M, Sawyer SM, Siegel DM. Transition to adult health care for adolescents and young adults with chronic conditions: position paper of the Society for Adolescent Medicine. *J Adolesc Health.* 2003;33(4):309–311

17. American Academy of Pediatrics, American Academy of Family Physicians, American College of Physicians-American Society of Internal Medicine. A consensus statement on health care transitions for young adults with special health care needs. *Pediatrics.* 2002;110(6, pt 2):1304–1306

18. Blum RW, Garell D, Hodgman CH, et al. Transition from child-centered to adult health-care systems for adolescents with chronic conditions. A position paper of the Society for Adolescent Medicine. *J Adolesc Health.* 1993;14(7):570–576

19. Maternal Child Health Bureau. *Achieving Success for All Children and Youth With Special Healthcare Needs: A 10-Year Action Plan to Accompany Healthy People 2010.* Washington, DC: Maternal Child Health Bureau; 2001

20. Office of Disease Prevention and Health Promotion. Barriers to health care. HealthyPeople.gov Web site. https://www.healthypeople.gov/2020/topics-objectives/objective/dh-5. Accessed February 7, 2018

21. Tuchman LK, Schwartz LA, Sawicki GS, Britto MT. Cystic fibrosis and transition to adult medical care. *Pediatrics.* 2010;125(3):566–573

22. Treadwell M, Telfair J, Gibson RW, Johnson S, Osunkwo I. Transition from pediatric to adult care in sickle cell disease: establishing evidence-based practice and directions for research. *Am J Hematol.* 2011;86(1):116–120

23. Nakhla M, Daneman D, Frank M, Guttmann A. Translating transition: a critical review of the diabetes literature. *J Pediatr Endocrinol Metab.* 2008;21(6):507–516

24. McDonagh JE. Young people first, juvenile idiopathic arthritis second: transitional care in rheumatology. *Arthritis Rheum.* 2008;59(8):1162–1170

25. Cheak-Zamora NC, Yang X, Farmer JE, Clark M. Disparities in transition planning for youth with autism spectrum disorder. *Pediatrics.* 2013;131(3):447–454

26. Reiss JG, Gibson RW, Walker LR. Health care transition: youth, family, and provider perspectives. *Pediatrics.* 2005;115(1):112–120

27. Cheak-Zamora NC, Teti M. "You think it's hard now ... It gets much harder for our children": Youth with autism and their caregiver's perspectives of health care transition services. *Autism.* 2015;19(8):992–1001

28. Sawyer SM, Blair S, Bowes G. Chronic illness in adolescents: transfer or transition to adult services? *J Paediatr Child Health.* 1997;33(2):88–90

29. Burke R, Spoerri M, Price A, Cardosi AM, Flanagan P. Survey of primary care pediatricians on the transition and transfer of adolescents to adult health care. *Clin Pediatr (Phila).* 2008;47(4):347–354

30. Kennedy A, Sloman F, Douglass JA, Sawyer SM. Young people with chronic illness: the approach to transition. *Intern Med J.* 2007;37(8):555–560

31. Fishman E. Aging out of coverage: young adults with special health needs. *Health Aff (Millwood).* 2001;20(6):254–266

32. Berger A. Did the Affordable Care Act affect insurance coverage for young adults? *Integr Health Interview Serv.* 2015;2:1–13

33. Goodwin R, Gould MS, Blanco C, Olfson M. Prescription of psychotropic medications to youths in office-based practice. *Psychiatr Serv.* 2001;52(8): 1081–1087

34. Rushton JL, Clark SJ, Freed GL. Pediatrician and family physician prescription of selective serotonin reuptake inhibitors. *Pediatrics.* 2000;105(6):e82

35. Harpaz-Rotem I, Rosenheck RA. Prescribing practices of psychiatrists and primary care physicians caring for children with mental illness. *Child Care Health Dev.* 2006;32(2):225–238

36. Faraone SV, Biederman J, Mick E. The age-dependent decline of attention deficit hyperactivity disorder: a meta-analysis of follow-up studies. *Psychol Med.* 2006;36(2):159–165

37. Okumura MJ, Kerr EA, Cabana MD, Davis MM, Demonner S, Heisler M. Physician views on barriers to primary care for young adults with childhood-onset chronic disease. *Pediatrics.* 2010;125(4):e748–e754

38. Kessler RC, Adler L, Barkley R, et al. The prevalence and correlates of adult ADHD in the United States: results from the National Comorbidity Survey Replication. *Am J Psychiatry.* 2006;163(4):716–723

39. Young S, Murphy CM, Coghill D. Avoiding the 'twilight zone': recommendations for the transition of services from adolescence to adulthood for young people with ADHD. *BMC Psychiatry.* 2011;11(1):174

40. Paul M, Street C, Wheeler N, Singh SP. Transition to adult services for young people with mental health needs: a systematic review. *Clin Child Psychol Psychiatry.* 2015;20(3):436–457

41. Sawicki GS, Lukens-Bull K, Yin X, et al. Measuring the transition readiness of youth with special healthcare needs: validation of the TRAQ—Transition Readiness Assessment Questionnaire. *J Pediatr Psychol.* 2011;36(2):160–171

42. Ferris M, Cohen S, Haberman C, et al. Self-management and transition readiness assessment: development, reliability, and factor structure of the STAR$_x$ Questionnaire. *J Pediatr Nurs.* 2015;30(5):691–699

43. Amaria K, Stinson J, Cullen-Dean G, Sappleton K, Kaufman M. Tools for addressing systems issues in transition. *Healthc Q.* 2011;14(3):72–76

44. Pullmann MD, Heflinger CA, Satterwhite Mayberry L. Patterns of Medicaid disenrollment for youth with mental health problems. *Med Care Res Rev.* 2010;67(6):657–675

45. Pottick KJ, Bilder S, Vander Stoep A, Warner LA, Alvarez MF. US patterns of mental health service utilization for transition-age youth and young adults. *J Behav Health Serv Res.* 2008;35(4):373–389

46. Davis M, Vander Stoep A. The transition to adulthood for youth who have serious emotional disturbance: developmental transition and young adult outcomes. *J Ment Health Adm.* 1997;24(4):400–427

47. Watson AR. Non-compliance and transfer from paediatric to adult transplant unit. *Pediatr Nephrol.* 2000;14(6):469–472

48. Mathias MD, Zhang S, Rogers ZR, Buchanan GR, Nero AC, McCavit TL. Survival into adulthood in sickle cell disease from the Dallas Newborn Cohort. *Blood.* 2014;124(21):559

49. Stewart SM, Rao U, Emslie GJ, Klein D, White PC. Depressive symptoms predict hospitalization for adolescents with type 1 diabetes mellitus. *Pediatrics.* 2005;115(5):1315–1319

50. Kovacs M, Mukerji P, Drash A, Iyengar S. Biomedical and psychiatric risk factors for retinopathy among children with IDDM. *Diabetes Care.* 1995;18(12):1592–1599

51. Walsh C, Jones B, Schonwald A. Health care transition planning among adolescents with autism spectrum disorder. *J Autism Dev Disord.* 2017:1–12

52. Cheak-Zamora NC, Farmer JE, Mayfield WA, et al. Health care transition services for youth with autism spectrum disorders. *Rehabil Psychol.* 2014;59(3):340–348

53. Bruder MB, Kerins G, Mazzarella C, Sims J, Stein N. Brief report: the medical care of adults with autism spectrum disorders: identifying the needs. *J Autism Dev Disord.* 2012;42(11):2498–2504

54. Golnik A, Ireland M, Borowsky IW. Medical homes for children with autism: a physician survey. *Pediatrics.* 2009;123(3):966–971

55. Heidgerken AD, Geffken G, Modi A, Frakey L. A survey of autism knowledge in a health care setting. *J Autism Dev Disord.* 2005;35(3):323–330

56. Zhang LF, Ho JS, Kennedy SE. A systematic review of the psychometric properties of transition readiness assessment tools in adolescents with chronic disease. *BMC Pediatr.* 2014;14:4

57. Wood DL, Sawicki GS, Miller MD, et al. The Transition Readiness Assessment Questionnaire (TRAQ): its factor structure, reliability, and validity. *Acad Pediatr.* 2014;14(4):415–422

58. Cohen SE, Hooper SR, Javalkar K, et al. Self-management and transition readiness assessment: concurrent, predictive and discriminant validation of the STAR$_x$ Questionnaire. *J Pediatr Nurs.* 2015;30(5):668–676

59. American College of Physicians. ACP Pediatric to Adult Care Transitions initiative: condition-specific tools. American College of Physicians Web site. https://www.acponline.org/clinical-information/high-value-care/resources-for-clinicians/pediatric-to-adult-care-transitions-initiative/condition-specific-tools. Accessed February 7, 2018

Pediatric Care of Children With Common Mental Health Concerns, Signs, and Symptoms

Agitation, Suicidality, and Other Psychiatric Emergencies

Heather J. Walter, MD, MPH, and David R. DeMaso, MD

"In the face of increasingly frequent psychiatric emergencies, such as those outlined in this chapter, it is critical for pediatric primary care clinicians to establish collaborative partnerships with mental health specialists who can perform urgently needed psychiatric assessments and involve the primary care clinician in care planning and follow-up."

Pediatric primary care clinicians (PCCs)—that is, pediatricians, family physicians, internists, nurse practitioners, and physician assistants who provide frontline, longitudinal care to children and adolescents—increasingly face psychiatric emergencies in their daily work. They are being asked to assess levels of risk in crisis situations and determine whether immediate intervention is indicated and to have systems in place to ensure that mental health evaluations will be completed. This chapter provides a solid foundation for understanding psychiatric emergencies in general as well as evidence-based approaches to 4 specific emergency situations: suicidality, acute agitation, acute psychosis, and disaster exposure.

Nature and Scope of Psychiatric Emergencies

The number of visits for psychiatric problems by youths (in this chapter, unless otherwise specified, *patient* and *youth(s)* refer to children and adolescents aged 6–18 years) to both pediatric primary care settings and emergency department (ED) settings has increased dramatically; such visits now account for up to 25% to 50% of primary care and 5% of ED visits.[1] Compared with other pediatric ED visits, psychiatric visits are longer, more frequently triaged to urgent evaluation, and more likely to result in patient admission or transfer.[2]

Several factors contribute to the apparent increase in psychiatric emergencies.[3] Among these is the high prevalence of adolescent risk behaviors likely to result in emergency psychiatric assessment (Box 13-1). Another factor is the unavailability of mental health services at both ends of the treatment spectrum. Community and outpatient mental health services and inpatient psychiatric beds and lengths of stay have been steadily eroded by efforts at cost containment by the government and the private sector. Available services are further constrained by the extreme shortage of mental health specialists across disciplines, including child and adolescent psychiatry, child psychology, and child-trained clinical social work and mental health counseling, and by a shortage of training in evidenced-based approaches to treatment. As a result, untreated or undertreated youths accumulate across the spectrum of care, and pediatric clinicians often face patients in crisis without readily accessible mental health specialty resources.

The judgment of what constitutes a psychiatric emergency derives from several sources, including the perceptions of a caregiver, a teacher, a

---

Box 13-1. Prevalence of Selected Risk Factors for Psychiatric Emergencies in High School Students

- 22.6% of students had been in a physical fight 1 or more times
- 4.1% of students carried a weapon on school property
- 6.0% of students had been threatened or injured with a weapon on school property
- 20.2% of students had been bullied on school property
- 15.5% of students had been electronically bullied
- 5.6% of students were afraid to go to school because of safety concerns
- 6.7% of students had been physically forced to have sexual intercourse
- 17.7% of students had seriously considered attempting suicide
- 8.6% of students had attempted suicide
- 17.7% of students had had 5 or more drinks of alcohol in a row
- 2.1% to 32.8% of students (depending upon the substance) had used potentially intoxicating substances

From Kann L, McManus T, Harris WA, et al. Youth Risk Behavioral Surveillance—United States, 2015. *MMWR Surveill Summ.* 2016;65(6):1–174. https://www.cdc.gov/healthyyouth/data/yrbs/pdf/2015/ss6506_updated.pdf. Published June 10, 2016. Accessed February 8, 2018. Reproduced with permission.

police officer, and a PCC and of a youth himself or herself. Rarely does an emergency occur without warning. Almost invariably, the acute event has been preceded by a long period of instability on the part of the youth and impaired relationships within the family or community. Accordingly, a youth in crisis represents a family and community in crisis.[3]

Adolescents account for most psychiatric emergencies in youths. Data suggest a preponderance of females among emergency visits, perhaps because females in crisis are more often perceived to have a psychiatric problem, while males are perceived to have a delinquency problem. Although varying by community, most psychiatric emergency visits are for suicidal threats or behavior, followed by assaultive, destructive, or otherwise violent behavior. Additional commonly encountered psychiatric emergencies are anxiety states (often combined with physical concerns or school refusal) and acute mental status changes, including intoxication, psychosis, and delirium.

General Emergency Psychiatric Assessment Considerations

Child psychiatric emergencies are characterized by severe symptoms, functional impairment, significant distress, and a sense of danger and urgency. Because a youth's mental health highly depends on the functioning of the family, school, and community in which she lives, any disturbance in the functioning of these systems has the potential to precipitate a crisis. It is therefore critical to answer the questions, "Who is concerned about the youth? Why now?"

Whether information is obtained in a primary care clinic visit or in a telephone call from a caregiver, PCCs need to determine whether they can manage the situation themselves or if the problem is sufficiently severe to require emergency assessment by a mental health specialist. Threats of harm to self or others, severe out-of-control behavior, and acute mental status changes such as psychosis or delirium all require immediate mental health specialty evaluation. Overwhelming caregiver distress, acute change in overall functioning, or significant symptom exacerbation are examples of circumstances warranting urgent (within 48–72 hours), but not necessarily immediate, evaluation. When immediate evaluation is indicated, PCCs must have a system in place to obtain an emergency assessment in the mental health specialty system; Figure 13-1 presents an

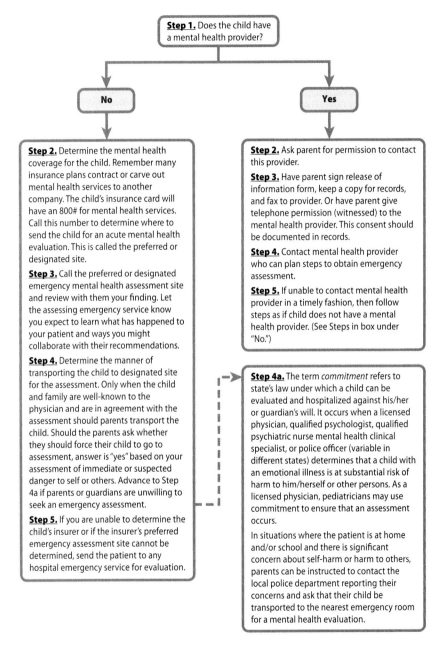

Figure 13-1. Algorithm for accessing an emergency assessment.

From Children's Hospital Boston, Blue Cross Blue Shield of Massachusetts. *Rapid Mental Health Triage for Children and Adolescents: A Practical Guide for Clinicians.* Boston, MA: Blue Cross Blue Shield of Massachusetts; 2007. Reproduced with permission.

algorithm for accessing this level of care. Whenever possible, the PCC should request parental consent for release of information from the mental health facility to obtain feedback about the findings from the evaluation and treatment recommendations.

Elements of Emergency Psychiatric Assessment

The critical elements of an emergency psychiatric assessment are outlined in Box 13-2.[3] Although the requirement to obtain consent for assessment and treatment is generally waived in emergency situations, reasonable attempts should be made to obtain and document consent from the patient's legal guardian[4] and document their permission for bidirectional

---

Box 13-2. Elements of an Emergency Psychiatric Assessment

- Obtain each informant's account of the crisis from his or her point of view.
- Develop a working alliance with the patient and other involved parties around assessment and disposition.
- Obtain a focused history of the patient, including present illness, stressors, psychiatric treatment, and medical, school, developmental, social, and family elements.
- Perform a Mental Status Examination, with close attention to suicidal or homicidal ideation and other mental status abnormalities (eg, hallucinations, delusions, thought disorder, disorientation or confusion, rage, humiliation, anxiety, hopelessness, agitation, impulsivity, impaired communication or cognition, impaired judgment or insight).
- Assess the characteristics of the family relevant to crisis intervention and disposition planning, including the presence of firearms in the home.
- Perform a focused medical assessment as indicated by history and physical signs or symptoms.
- Develop a differential diagnosis, including a formulation of predisposing, precipitating, and perpetuating factors.
- Arrive at a judgment of probable danger to self or others.
- Develop and implement a crisis intervention plan.
- Plan and implement an appropriate disposition.
- Communicate assessment findings to relevant parties, including the PCC.

Abbreviation: PCC, primary care clinician.

Derived in part from King RA. Practice parameters for the psychiatric assessment of children and adolescents. *J Am Acad Child Adolesc Psychiatry*. 1995;34(10):1386–1402.

exchange of information between the mental health professional and PCC. State laws vary regarding the age at which a minor may self-consent to mental health assessment and treatment. Before the mental health professional begins an assessment, the limits of confidentiality should be reviewed with the patient and his caregivers. Confidentiality of the patient's disclosures to the clinician should not be maintained in circumstances in which the youth presents a danger to himself or others. All professionals are required by federal law to report suspected abuse or neglect. The federal Child Abuse Prevention and Treatment Act[5] sets forth broad guidelines for defining child abuse and neglect; states vary regarding whether there must be knowledge of abuse or merely suspicion of abuse to initiate a report. A searchable database of state statutes is available online through the Child Welfare Information Gateway (www.childwelfare.gov/topics/systemwide/laws-policies/state). Although consent from the patient's guardian may be a prerequisite for exchanging clinical information with collateral informants, the identification of the situation as emergent can supersede confidentiality protections.

The physical setting for the emergency assessment should reflect the severity of the encountered problem. Some presentations (eg, suicidality, assaultiveness, unmanageable dangerous behavior, acute mental status changes) generally require the full spectrum of evaluative and stabilization services available in the hospital ED setting. As outlined in Figure 13-1, in cases with which there is likelihood of serious harm, transport by ambulance may be required to ensure safety, using involuntary commitment procedures if necessary. In these situations, the assessment setting should be secluded from other patients and safeguarded by removing any potentially dangerous personal possessions, clothing, furniture, medical equipment, and medications. Assistance should be readily available in the event of escalating unmanageability.

Other, less urgent, presentations may be suitable for assessment in less restrictive settings. In these cases, the parent may be able to safely transport the patient to the assessment venue; alternatively, in some states mental health emergency service providers (ESPs) or mobile mental health crisis teams may be able to provide assessment in the community (at home, at school, or in the primary care office). It would be helpful for PCCs to inquire about the availability of ESPs or crisis teams in their local area and to verify the requirements for accessing this service.

Obtaining a full and accurate diagnostic picture requires gathering information from diverse sources, including (as relevant) the family; the PCC; school staff; prior and current mental health treatment providers; representatives from social services, child welfare, and juvenile justice agencies; and police officers. At a minimum, the assessment should include an interview of the patient and any accompanying adults. If the caregivers are not present, every effort must be made to contact them for inclusion in the assessment.

Informants may differ in their access to relevant information. Caregivers or school staff may be quick to report the youth's disruptive, aggressive behavior or angry mood, but they may be less aware of the youth's sadness, worries, or fears. Caregivers may be unaware of how discord within the family system or other traumatic exposure can precipitate a mental health crisis in the youth. The interviewer should be aware that vague or sketchy responses to queries, from the caregivers or the patient, or minimization of clear problems can signal a patient or family secret, such as physical or sexual abuse, domestic violence, illegal activity, or parental impairment.[3]

In contrast to a routine mental health assessment, of which several sessions may be required to reach a comfort level with the interviewer, an emergency assessment requires that the interviewer gather salient information expeditiously, thereby precluding systematic relationship building. Nonetheless, the interviewer must make every effort to put the patient at ease. A useful strategy is to emphasize an interest in the patient's perspective of the events leading to the crisis.

The emergency assessment includes a careful physical examination and laboratory tests when indicated by history and physical signs or symptoms, including evidence of a physical illness, prescribed medication use, or substance use that may cause altered mental status.

A key outcome of the emergency assessment is achieving consensus among the caregiver, the PCC or other referring party, and the patient on the nature of the encountered problem, its precipitants, and realistic solutions to the problem. Lack of consensus bodes poorly for the success of crisis intervention and disposition plans. Conversely, caregivers and referral sources as well as youths who are able to recognize recurrent patterns and their role in those patterns may be more likely to successfully transition from emergency intervention to treatment and eventually to health.

Caregivers reassuming the care of their children after emergency assessment must be capable of adhering to, safeguarding, and monitoring disposition recommendations.

Disposition of the patient requires 2 primary decisions: Does the patient present imminent and substantial danger to himself or others? What is the most appropriate level of care? Empirically derived risk factors for inpatient level of care include suicidal or aggressive presentation, increasing age, presentation during the school year, and substance use by the patient or a family member. Disposition decision-making is complicated by the constraints of the mental health care delivery and reimbursement systems. In general, there has been a decline in available psychiatry inpatient beds and fewer days of inpatient care for children and adolescents. When youths needing a higher level of care are discharged to community or outpatient settings (where there is often a long wait to first visit and between subsequent visits), the stage is set for recurrent crisis presentations. After a psychiatric hospitalization, it is critical that the PCC receive detailed information about discharge medications, monitoring requirements, follow-up treatment plans, and access to ongoing psychiatric consultation. Where procedures are not in place to convey this information routinely from the discharging facility to PCCs, system improvements are critical to preventing recurrent crises and readmissions.

Specific Emergent Presentations
Suicidality

Presentation

Patients with suicidality present on a dimensional spectrum ranging from thoughts about causing intentional self-injury or death (suicidal ideation) to acts that cause intentional self-injury (suicide attempt) or death (completed suicide). The intent to harm oneself, which may be explicit and strong or ambiguous and vague, is the defining characteristic of suicidal behavior, complicated by variations in the construct of intentionality from early childhood to late adolescence. Suicide is rare before age 10 years. Teenaged and young adult American Indian and Alaska Native as well as non-Hispanic white males have the highest rates of suicide completions, and teenaged Hispanic females have the highest rates of suicide attempts. Firearms and ingestion are the most commonly used methods of completing suicide for males and females, respectively. Ingestion is the most commonly used method of attempting suicide. Attempters who have made prior suicide attempts, who used a method other than ingestion, and who still want to die are at increased risk of completed suicide. Table 13-1 outlines several important risk factors for youth suicide.

Table 13-1. Risk Factors for Youth Suicide	
Risk Factors	**Comment**
Suicidal ideation	~ 33% of youths with suicidal ideation make a suicide plan.
Prior history of a suicide attempt	Increases the risk of suicide nearly 90-fold; is strongest predictor
Psychiatric disorder	~ 90% of youths who complete suicide have a psychiatric disorder at the time of death. Most common among these youths are mood disorders, including major depressive disorder and bipolar disorders, followed by substance use, anxiety, and behavioral disorders.
Multiple psychiatric disorders	>70% have multiple psychiatric disorders.
Lack of psychiatric treatment	Large proportion of youths completing suicide had not received treatment.
Personality characteristics	Mood instability, impulsiveness, perfectionism, aggression, odd thinking, or introversion
Neurotransmitter dysregulation	Especially serotonergic systems
Neuroendocrine dysregulation	Especially the hypothalamic-pituitary-adrenal axis
Disordered sleep architecture	Chronobiological studies suggest a role.
High rates of cumulative stressors	Such as family losses, family discord and violence, parental incapacity, physical or sexual abuse, sexual orientation, immigrant status, living outside the home, not working or attending school, having academic difficulties, bullying, early physical trauma (prenatal, perinatal, or postnatal), and chronic medical illness
Social maladjustment	Poor interpersonal relationships with family, teachers, or counselors resulting in lack of available empathic adults who could offer guidance and support
Cognitive distortions	Perceived inadequacies, catastrophic thinking, or hopelessness. Hopeless feelings in particular impair the youth's ability to manage strong feelings, solve problems, and cope with adversity.

Evaluation

Assessment of suicidal ideation should be a part of every presentation of a youth in crisis, especially those with depressed mood, signs of substance use, or altered mental status. All suicidal ideation and attempts should be taken seriously and require a thorough assessment to evaluate the youth's current state of mind, underlying psychiatric conditions, and ongoing risk of harm. Gathering information from multiple sources and by varied culturally and developmentally sensitive techniques is essential in evaluating suicidal risk factors.

Suicidal ideation can be assessed by a series of questions such as those in Box 13-3. Several self-report instruments can be helpful in screening for suicidal ideation; however, they tend to be oversensitive and underspecific. Using 2 scales with different foci simultaneously (eg, the Suicidal Ideation Questionnaire and the Child-Adolescent Suicidal Potential Index) may provide better coverage of key predictive constructs. (See Appendix 2, Mental Health Tools for Pediatrics.) All positive results on a screening instrument must be followed by a thorough assessment.

The assessment of suicidal attempts should include a detailed exploration of the hours immediately preceding the attempt, to identify precipitants, as well as the circumstances of the attempt itself, to identify intent and potential lethality. A series of relevant topics to address is listed in

---

Box 13-3. Questions to Elicit Suicidal Ideation or Behavior

- Did you ever feel so sad or upset that you wished you were not alive or wanted to die?
- Have you ever thought that you or your family would be better off if you were dead?
- Did you ever do something that you knew was so dangerous that you could get hurt or killed by doing it?
- Have you ever thought about killing yourself?
- Did you ever make a plan to kill yourself? If so, what was the plan?
- Did you ever try to kill yourself? What was the method?
- Did you ever try to kill yourself and not tell anyone?

Box 13-4. Developmental considerations should guide the interview. Thus, young children are susceptible to unintentional suicide through imitation or suggestion. Preadolescents may have difficulty with the construct of intentionality. In adolescents, lethality is not necessarily related to the severity of the attempt; adolescents with serious intent, for example, may think that a small number of over-the-counter analgesic pills can be lethal.

Acute changes in mental status (eg, intoxication, agitation, psychosis, disorientation) increase the risk of suicidality and require physical examination to rule out a medical etiology for the change. Physical examination may provide evidence of physical or sexual abuse, prior suicide attempts, or other self-harm, or a physical illness that could cause altered mental status. Laboratory studies should be considered when suggested by the physical findings (eg, urine toxicology screening, a pregnancy test).

Box 13-4. Topics to Explore for a Suicide Attempt

- Why was the method chosen?
- What were the expectations from the attempt (did the patient think the attempt was going to kill him)?
- How reversible was the attempt?
- Did the circumstances permit the patient to change her mind about the attempt?
- Does the patient demonstrate ambivalence about living?
- How strong was the patient's intent to die?
- Was there evidence of premeditation, including preparations and precautions against discovery?
- Did the patient tell anyone about the attempt, particularly responsible caregivers?
- What did the patient do immediately after the attempt?
- Did the patient seek help or simply disregard the danger of the attempt?
- Did the patient acknowledge the attempt or try to hide or deny the attempt?
- Is the patient relieved or disappointed that he survived the attempt?

Management

The assessment of suicidality culminates in answers to 2 basic questions: Is the patient at current risk for attempted or completed suicide? Are the patient and family able to adhere to recommendations regarding supervision, safeguarding, and follow-up care? Management should be embedded within the pediatric medical home, where the PCC is informed and aware of the management plan. Follow-up visits in the pediatric setting support mental health management.

Psychiatric hospitalization is indicated when the youth actively voices suicidal intent.[6] Intent can be explicitly stated ("I want to die") or implied ("I can't see any reason to go on living"). These youths typically have frequent thoughts about suicide that occur over long periods of time. They describe specific plans that are not only well conceived and potentially lethal but also feasible in their environments. Concern is heightened if the youth has known risk factors for suicidality (especially a previous attempt, untreated depression, or substance use) or if the youth is aware of another youth (with whom he can identify) or a family member who has completed suicide. Medical hospitalization may follow a suicide attempt. When the youth is medically stable, but remains potentially dangerous, a transfer to a psychiatric facility should be arranged.

Hospitalization is also indicated in the context of altered mental status, a history of psychiatric disorder unsuccessfully treated in outpatient or day-hospital settings, active substance use, and caregiver incapacity. Caregivers of a suicidal youth must believe that their relationship with their child is sufficiently close that their child will disclose suicidal thoughts, should they occur in the future. Caregivers must be able to supervise their child closely during the immediate phase of assessment and treatment, to safeguard the home by removing access to potentially lethal methods of suicide (eg, firearms, prescribed and over-the-counter medications), and to adhere to all follow-up assessment and treatment recommendations.

The primary goal of hospitalization is to keep the youth safe from self-harm. Other goals are to clarify psychiatric diagnoses and develop a comprehensive treatment plan with individual, family, and environmental (eg, school, community) interventions. Pharmacotherapy may be initiated in the presence of moderate to severe psychopathology. Youths typically remain hospitalized until active intent to die has abated and a safe and secure discharge plan to which caregivers can adhere is in place.

A referral for psychiatric outpatient follow-up may be appropriate if the youth has suicidal ideation without intent or plan, has an intact mental status, has few to no other risk factors for suicidality, is willing and able to participate in outpatient treatment, and has caregivers able to provide emotional support, supervision, safeguarding, and adherence to follow-up. Other considerations are systems related, including the availability of urgent outpatient appointments, qualified mental health providers, and evidence-based treatment modalities.

Primary care clinicians should be aware that the rate of completed psychiatric outpatient referrals is known to be very poor. Moreover, approximately one-third of referred youths attend only 1 or 2 sessions, and one-quarter appear only 3 or 4 times. Several factors influence likelihood of follow-through, including a history of previous hospitalization, severe symptoms of psychiatric disorders, and the lethality of the attempt.[7] Primary care clinicians can help educate the patient and family about the causes and treatment of suicidality, and the risks of failing to treat. The likelihood of a completed referral can also be increased by making sure that the family secures a specific appointment day and time at the time of the emergency psychiatric assessment.

The goals of psychiatric outpatient treatment are to successfully treat the underlying psychiatric disorders and to prevent further suicidality. Optimal treatment will consist of evidence-based approaches, including individual psychotherapy and pharmacotherapy, family therapy, and group therapy. Although no specific treatment modalities have been shown in rigorous studies to prevent suicidality, several psychotherapies have been shown to be promising, including dialectical behavioral therapy,[8] cognitive behavioral therapy (CBT) for suicide prevention,[9] family interventions,[10] and mentalization-based treatment[11] (Table 13-2).

If the psychiatric disorder underlying suicidality is depression, antidepressant medication can be considered as part of a comprehensive treatment plan. In a pilot study among adolescent suicide attempters with depression, combination treatment (antidepressant medication and CBT) resulted in improvements in depressive symptoms similar to those demonstrated in other studies among nonsuicidal depressed adolescents.[12] Clinicians must be aware of the association between antidepressant medications and suicidal thoughts and the need to closely monitor patients who are prescribed these medications.

Table 13-2. Psychotherapies for Suicidality	
Psychotherapy Type	**Description**
Dialectical behavioral therapy	Designed for individuals with deficits in emotional regulation; focus is both on mindfulness and acceptance (derived from Asian philosophy) and on skills building (derived from CBT). Uses 4 skills modules to address emotion regulation, interpersonal effectiveness, mindfulness, and distress tolerance.
CBT for suicide prevention	Designed for youths who have made a suicide attempt; detailed chain analysis identifies proximal risk factors (eg, emotional, cognitive, behavioral, family) active just before and after the attempt. These factors include deficits in the youth's ability to regulate emotions, resolve problems, tolerate distress, and address negative thoughts such as worthlessness or hopelessness. A core feature of the treatment is the development of an individualized case conceptualization that identifies problem areas to be targeted and specific interventions to be used during periods of acute emotional distress.
Family interventions	Designed to enhance parent and family strengths; can include managing parental stress, understanding adolescence, promoting communication, and enhancing attachment
Mentalization-based treatment	Designed to foster the capacity to understand actions of thoughts and feelings so as to enhance self-control

Abbreviation: CBT, cognitive behavioral therapy.

Acute Agitation

Presentation

Acute agitation encompasses a psychological state (feeling of inner tension or arousal) as well as a motor state (eg, pacing, hand-wringing, fidgeting). It can occur in the context of many psychiatric, general medical, and substance-induced conditions, as outlined in Box 13-5. The critical first step is to determine whether the acute agitation is caused by a general medical condition, substance- or medication-induced condition, or primary psychiatric disorder.

Acute agitation caused by a general medical or substance- or medication-induced condition is characterized by disturbances in consciousness

Box 13-5. Disorders Commonly Associated With Agitation

General Medical Conditions
- Delirium related to direct effect of physical illness
- Acute drug intoxication

Psychiatric Disorders
- Neurodevelopmental disorders
  - Intellectual disability
  - Autism spectrum disorder
  - Attention-deficit/hyperactivity disorder
- Disruptive behavioral and impulse control disorders
  - Oppositional defiant disorder
  - Intermittent explosive disorder
  - Conduct disorder
- Anxiety disorders
  - Separation anxiety disorder
  - Panic disorder
  - Generalized anxiety disorder
- Depressive and bipolar disorders
  - Major depressive disorder
  - Bipolar I and bipolar II disorders
  - Disruptive mood dysregulation disorder
- Obsessive-compulsive disorder
- Trauma- and stressor-related disorders
  - PTSD
  - Acute stress disorder
- Psychosis
  - Schizophrenia
  - Other psychoses
- Substance-related disorders
  - Intoxication or withdrawal states

Parent-Child Relational Problem

Abuse and Neglect

Abbreviation: PTSD, post-traumatic stress disorder.

(reduced clarity of awareness of environment) and changes in cognition over a short period of time. Consistent with the diagnosis of delirium, this type of agitation is often accompanied by cognitive changes (eg, memory deficit, disorientation, inattention, language disturbance), mood changes (eg, irritability), and perceptual disturbances (eg, acute illusions, hallucinations, or delusions). In contrast, agitation in patients with primary psychiatric disorders is generally not accompanied by the acute disturbances in consciousness or cognition. Agitation in patients with autism spectrum disorder can be associated with underlying physical illnesses that cannot be readily communicated by the patient to others or with environmental changes that unsettle the needed consistent daily routines.

Evaluation

A youth with acute agitation must be thoroughly assessed for underlying medical, medication, or substance use causes using physical examination and laboratory and radiologic tests as indicated (Box 13-6). This process must be completed before assuming a psychiatric cause for a patient's agitation. In the case of suspected delirium, serial assessments are required because of the fluctuating nature of the disorder. Various screening instruments are used to diagnose delirium and assess symptom severity. Among the most widely used instruments for youths is the Delirium

---

Box 13-6. Selected Tests to Be Considered for the Medical Evaluation of Agitation

Hematologic

Complete blood cell count

Chemistry

Electrolyte levels, glucose level, serum urea nitrogen, creatinine level, total protein level, liver function tests, calcium level, magnesium level, phosphorus level, thyroid function tests, and kidney function tests

Other Laboratory

Pregnancy test, heavy metals, vitamin B_{12} level, folate level, lupus erythematosus cell test, antinuclear antibody titers, urine porphyrin concentrations, ammonia level, erythrocyte sedimentation rate, HIV test, urine toxicology screening, serum drug concentrations, and arterial blood gas analysis

Radiologic

Chest radiography, computed tomography, magnetic resonance imaging, echocardiography, and endoscopy

Other

Electroencephalography, electrocardiography, and lumbar puncture

Rating Scale,[13] which has versions for children and adolescents. Table 13-3 outlines the differential diagnosis of pediatric delirium using the mnemonic "I WATCH DEATH."

Management

For all cases of agitation, the most effective treatment addresses the underlying cause. In the interim, the clinician treats the acute agitation to ease the distress of the patient and family, reduce the potential for unintentional harm, and improve the medical outcome (if relevant). Box 13-7 outlines nonpharmacological approaches for the clinician presented with a youth with acute agitation. If these initial interventions are ineffective,

Table 13-3. Differential Diagnosis of Pediatric Delirium: The "I WATCH DEATH" Mnemonic	
Infection	Encephalitis,[a] meningitis,[a] syphilis, human immuno-deficiency virus, or sepsis[a]
Withdrawal	Alcohol, barbiturates, or sedative-hypnotics[a]
Acute metabolic	Acidosis, alkalosis, electrolyte disturbance,[a] hepatic failure, or renal failure
Trauma	Closed-head injury,[a] heatstroke, postoperative,[a] or severe burns[a]
Central nervous system pathology	Abscess, hemorrhage, hydrocephalus, subdural hematoma, infection,[a] seizures,[a] stroke, tumors, metastases, or vasculitis[a]
Hypoxia	Anemia, carbon monoxide poisoning, hypotension, pulmonary failure, or cardiac failure
Deficiencies	Vitamin B_{12}, folate, niacin, or thiamine
Endocrinopathies	Hyper/hypoadrenocorticism, hyper/hypoglycemia, myxedema, or hyperparathyroidism
Acute vascular	Hypertensive encephalopathy, stroke, arrhythmia, or shock[a]
Toxins or drugs	Medications,[a] illicit drugs, pesticides, or solvents
Heavy metals	Lead, manganese, or mercury[a]

[a] More commonly seen in pediatric delirium.
From Wise MG, Brandt G. Delirium. In: Hales RE, Yudofsky SC, eds. *American Psychiatry Press Textbook of Neuropsychiatry.* 2nd ed. Washington, DC: American Psychiatric Press; 1992:302. Copyright 1992 American Psychiatric Press, Inc. Used with permission.

Box 13-7. Nonpharmacologic Approaches to the Youth With Acute Agitation

Educate

- Explain to the patient and caretaker your understanding of the cause of the acute agitation and that it is a time-limited consequence of an underlying disorder.

- Because of interference with cognitive ability, explanations or statements to the patient should be short, succinct, and focused (eg, "You must calm down…we will be giving you medicine to help you stay safe…you can have the medicine by mouth or by injection").

- Outline the needed intervention, which may include physical and medication restraints. Explain that this is an emergency situation that will require intervention to protect the patient as well as others.

- If possible, obtain consent from the caretaker regarding the intervention plan.

Calming Interventions

- If you are feeling alarmed, this is an indication that patient is "out of control."

- Do not take anger personally, but do take into consideration your own safety.

- Clearly introduce yourself to patient.

- Use simplified language, soft voice, and slow movements.

- Explain what will happen in the outpatient setting, the emergency department, or the medical/surgical floor.

- Reassure the patient that you are there to keep him safe.

- Have someone familiar provide frequent, repeated reassurance and reorientation to help decrease fear and confusion.

- Do not leave the patient alone; instead, the patient should remain in the company of a family member or clinical staff.

- Tell the patient how you plan to honor her reasonable requests.

- Understand the patient's goal, and link cooperation to the goal.

- Offer food or drink.

- Reduce environmental stimulation (eg, reduce lighting and number of people).

- Remove access to breakable objects or equipment.

- Find things for the patient to control.

- If appropriate, offer distracting toys or sensory modalities.

- Limiting staff changes and involving relatives in care often eliminates the need for medication.

- If the patient does not respond to verbal reassurance, it may be necessary to provide a "show of force" to convey a message to the patient that external control will be placed on his behavior to protect him as well as others. Hospital security staff or police in the community can effectively deter acting-out behaviors simply by being visible in sufficient numbers.

From Department of Psychiatry, Boston Children's Hospital. 2017.

clinicians should consider the use of pharmacological interventions or seclusion or restraint, if necessary, to prevent harm to self or others. States vary in their regulations on the use of emergency pharmacological interventions and seclusion or restraint for out-of-control behavior. Box 13-8 presents considerations in the assessment of youths for emergency medication treatment, and Box 13-9 presents national guidelines for the use of seclusion and restraint.[14]

Special treatment considerations pertain to the youth with delirium. Environmental intervention is particularly important. Frequent and repeated reassurance and reorientation by someone familiar helps

---

Box 13-8. Considerations in Assessment of Children for Emergency Medication Treatment

1. Benefits of treatment and risks of withholding treatment.

2. Benefits and potential risks of proposed medication.

3. Route of medication administration: Is oral administration possible? If not, does the patient have alternative routes already in place such as intravenous access or a gastric tube, or would the medication have to be administered rectally or intramuscularly and potentially be more traumatic?

4. Necessity of physical restraint to administer medication.

5. Patient age: A mature minor may be able to consent to treatment. Efforts should be made to document that the physician has communicated with the patient before giving the medication. The younger the child, the less input she will have regarding treatment.

6. Level of anxiety: A mild panic attack episode characterized by hyperventilation and tremors may not require any immediate intervention, whereas a severe attack associated with acute agitation (eg, pulling out intravenous or nasogastric tubes or removing an oxygen mask) constitutes a higher level of urgency.

7. Level of agitation: A mild episode characterized by restlessness may not require any immediate intervention, whereas severe agitation associated with significant threat of harm to others would constitute a higher level of urgency.

From Ibeziako P, Bourne R, Shaw RJ, DeMaso DR. Legal and forensic issues. In: Shaw RJ, DeMaso DR, eds. *Textbook of Pediatric Psychosomatic Medicine: Mental Health Consultation With Physically Ill Children*. Washington, DC: American Psychiatric Press Inc; 2010:47–62. Reproduced with permission.

Box 13-9. Guidelines for the Use of Seclusion and Restraint With Children and Adolescents

Restraint or seclusion must be used only when a patient is at imminent risk of harm to self or others and less restrictive interventions have been unsuccessful or determined to be ineffective or inappropriate.

1. The physician primarily responsible for the patient's ongoing care orders the use of restraint or seclusion in a manner consistent with hospital policy.

2. The attending physician is consulted as soon as possible if he or she did not order the restraint or seclusion.

3. The physician primarily responsible for the patient's ongoing care conducts an in-person evaluation of the patient within 1 h of initiation.

4. The in-person evaluation by the physician includes an evaluation of the patient's immediate situation, the patient's reaction to the intervention, the patient's medical and behavioral condition, and the need to continue or terminate the restraint or seclusion.

5. Orders are time limited and may be renewed within 2 h for children and adolescents aged 9–17 y, and within 1 h for children younger than 9 years, for a maximum of 24 consecutive hours.

6. At least every 24 h, the physician must evaluate the patient before writing a new order for restraint or seclusion.

7. Patients in seclusion or restraint must be continuously monitored.

8. Seclusion and restraint must be documented in the patient's medical record in a manner consistent with hospital policy.

Derived from Joint Commission Resources. *2017 Comprehensive Accreditation Manual for Hospitals.* Oakbrook Terrace, IL: Joint Commission Resources; 2016.

decrease fear and confusion. Limiting staff changes; providing a safe and uncluttered environment, but with orienting objects (eg, clocks, calendars, pictures of family and home, familiar objects from home); minimizing excess ambient noise; and providing good day lighting and low night lighting all facilitate orientation. If pharmacological interventions are needed to maintain safety, antipsychotic medications can be very beneficial for the agitated patient with perceptual disturbances, sleep-wake cycle abnormalities, and behavioral dyscontrol. Haloperidol has been favored because it has few metabolites, a safe parenteral form, few anticholinergic and hypotensive adverse effects, and relatively less sedation than other agents. The intravenous route should be considered if rapid acute control of agitation is required. Care should be taken to monitor anticholinergic (eg, acute dystonia) and cardiac (eg, prolongation of the QTc interval) adverse effects.

Agitation derived from causes other than delirium can be treated with medication according to guidelines presented in Tables 13-4 and 13-5 and Box 13-10.[15]

Acute Psychosis

Presentation

Psychotic symptoms include delusions, hallucinations, disorganized thinking (as manifested in disorganized speech), disorganized behavior, and "negative" symptoms (eg, diminished emotional expressiveness,

Table 13-4. Psychotropic Medication Management of Acute Agitation in Children and Adolescents

Medication Considerations for Moderate Agitation

Moderate agitation can be defined as raising voice/yelling/screaming, verbally aggressive behavior, threatening posture (eg, clenched fists), pacing, rocking, throwing small objects without aiming at people, and self-injuring that does not break skin (eg, scratching, light self-hitting, brief head banging).

Parameter	Child (25–50 kg)	Adolescent (>50 kg)
Preferred agent(s)	Diphenhydramine **or** lorazepam	Diphenhydramine **or** lorazepam
Administration route	By mouth	By mouth
Initial dosing	Diphenhydramine 25 mg **or** Lorazepam 0.25 mg	Diphenhydramine 50 mg **or** Lorazepam 0.5 mg
Repeat dosing (60 min after initial dose if ineffective)	Diphenhydramine 25 mg **or** Lorazepam 0.25 mg	Diphenhydramine 25 mg **or** Lorazepam 0.5 mg
Subsequent re-dosing frequency	Every 4–6 h Not to exceed 100 mg of diphenhydramine **or** 2 mg of lorazepam in 24 h	Every 4–6 h Not to exceed 150 mg of diphenhydramine **or** 4 mg of lorazepam in 24 h

Table 13-5. Psychotropic Medication Management of Acute Severe Agitation in Children and Adolescents

Medication Considerations for Severe Agitation

Severe agitation can be defined as imminent risk to self or others (eg, attempts to strangle or cut self, deep scratches, forceful or prolonged head banging), combative behavior, assault toward others, moving or throwing large objects, and destroying property.

Parameter	Child (25–50 kg)	Adolescent (>50 kg)
Preferred agent(s)	Olanzapine[a] **or** Haloperidol[b] **and** diphenhydramine[c]	Olanzapine[a] **or** Haloperidol[b] **and** diphenhydramine[c]
Administration route	By mouth (oral disintegrating tablet for olanzapine) or IM	By mouth (oral disintegrating tablet for olanzapine) or IM
Initial dosing	Olanzapine 2.5 mg **or** Haloperidol 2 mg **and** diphenhydramine 25 mg	Olanzapine 5 mg **or** Haloperidol 5 mg **and** diphenhydramine 50 mg
Repeat dosing (45 min after initial dose if ineffective)	Olanzapine 2.5 mg **or** Haloperidol 2 mg **and** diphenhydramine 25 mg	Olanzapine 5 mg **or** Haloperidol 2.5 mg **and** diphenhydramine 25 mg
Subsequent re-dosing frequency	Every 4 h Do not exceed: 10 mg of olanzapine in 24 h 5 mg of haloperidol in 24 h 100 mg of diphenhydramine in 24 h	Every 4 h Do not exceed: 15 mg of olanzapine in 24 h 10 mg of haloperidol in 24 h 150 mg of diphenhydramine in 24 h

Abbreviations: IM, intramuscular; IV, intravenous.

[a] Do NOT use olanzapine within 4 h of administering IM/IV lorazepam because of risk of cardiopulmonary depression.

[b] Use of haloperidol is contraindicated if the patient is taking citalopram, escitalopram, or fluoxetine.

[c] Use of diphenhydramine with haloperidol is preferred to haloperidol alone to avoid risk of acute dystonic reactions.

Lorazepam, diphenhydramine, and haloperidol are available in an oral liquid form. Olanzapine is available in a dissolvable tablet form. All can be given IM.

If pharmaceutical interventions are not effective, patients at risk for self-harm or harming others may require physical restraints.

Box 13-10. Medication Monitoring Requirements and Administration Considerations

Monitoring Requirements

- When the patient is calm/cooperative, acute medication monitoring includes vital signs and blood pressure along with observation of the development of extrapyramidal side effects (eg, akathisia, dystonic reactions) and respiratory depression.

- When clinically appropriate (eg, prior to/after first time use of antipsychotic), obtain an EKG to assess QT interval.

Administration Considerations

- Both first-generation (typical) and second-generation (atypical) antipsychotics have evidence supporting their utilization for acute agitation. To date, neither type has been proven superior to the other. Each medication has its own individual side effects, which should be considered for each patient. These medication guidelines are only for acute situations.

- Medication can be given in an emergency situation without parental (or legal guardian) consent when there is danger to self or others.

- Show of force (eg, security or other personnel) when administering medication can be helpful, if medication is resisted by patient.

- Prepare both by mouth and intramuscular formulations so that either can be given.

- Use a time frame (eg, you have 5 minutes to take this medication by mouth; otherwise, we will need to give you the medication as a shot).

Abbreviations: EKG, electrocardiogram.

From Department of Psychiatry, Boston Children's Hospital. 2017.

---

decreased motivation). Hallucinations can be auditory, visual, tactile, olfactory, or gustatory, and they occur in the absence of identifiable external stimuli.

Evaluation

New-onset psychotic psychiatric disorders are uncommon before adolescence; psychotic symptoms occur more commonly in the context of an underlying medical illness or substance-related conditions. The differential diagnosis of medical causes of acute psychosis is broad (Box 13-11). As with the evaluation of acute agitation, a thorough history and physical

Box 13-11. Differential Diagnosis of Medical Causes of Acute Psychosis

Drugs (Prescribed and Illicit)

Trauma

Organ Failure

- Cardiopulmonary
- Hypertensive encephalopathy
- Renal azotemia
- Hepatic encephalopathy

Electrolyte Abnormalities

Neurologic

- Stroke
- Lupus cerebritis
- Multiple sclerosis
- Seizures
- Huntington disease or chorea

Endocrine

- Diabetic ketoacidosis
- Addison disease
- Cushing disease
- Thyroid disease
- Pituitary disease

Hematologic

Paraneoplastic

Acute Intermittent Porphyria

Structural

- Chronic subdural hematoma
- Intracranial aneurysm or intracranial angioma
- Normal-pressure hydrocephalus
- Cerebral neoplasm
- Cerebral abscess

Toxins

- Plants
- Carbon monoxide
- Heavy metals or industrial toxins

Box 13-11. Differential Diagnosis of Medical Causes of Acute Psychosis (*continued*)

Infections

- Sepsis

- AIDS encephalopathy

- Pneumonia

- Meningitis or encephalitis

- Rocky Mountain spotted fever

- Legionnaire disease

- Lyme disease

- Acute rheumatic fever

Vitamin Deficiencies

Anoxia or Hypoxia

---

examination are crucial investigatory tools, and laboratory and radiologic workup can narrow the differential (see Box 13-6).

If a medical cause for acute psychosis can be ruled out, psychiatric etiologies can be considered. The differential diagnosis for hallucinations comprises a broad range of psychiatric disorders, including diagnoses in which hallucinations are not the hallmark feature but may be viewed as associated symptoms (eg, post-traumatic stress disorder [PTSD], nonpsychotic mood disorders, disruptive behavioral disorders), diagnoses that are defined by psychotic features (eg, brief psychotic disorder, schizophrenia, major depressive disorder or bipolar disorder with psychotic features), and at-risk clinical states (eg, poor reality testing).

In youths with nonpsychotic hallucinations, the symptom cluster of psychosis (delusions, disorganized thoughts and behavior, and negative symptoms) is absent. Nonpsychotic hallucinations commonly occur in the context of severe traumatic stress, developmental delays or disability, social-emotional deprivation, caregivers whose own psychopathology promotes a breakdown in the youth's sense of reality, cultural beliefs in mysticism, unresolved mourning, and normal development (magical thinking).

Management

The underlying condition will determine the type of treatment needed. Nonpsychotic hallucinations suggest the need for disorder-specific psychotherapy (eg, trauma-focused cognitive behavioral therapy [TF-CBT] for PTSD, parent management training for behavioral disorders) and perhaps adjunctive medication (eg, an antidepressant for depression or anxiety, or a brief course of antipsychotic medication). Psychotic hallucinations may be an indication for antipsychotic medication. Hallucinations from intoxication or physical illness typically resolve in parallel with the underlying condition.

Disaster Exposure

Presentation

A disaster is a sudden and severe ecological and psychosocial disruption that greatly exceeds the coping capacity of the community. Youths may experience a spectrum of psychological effects across the disaster timeline that vary according to developmental stage (Box 13-12). Transient moderate psychological distress may be a normative reaction to traumatic exposure. More severe symptoms in the first month may qualify for a diagnosis of acute stress disorder; symptoms persisting longer than 1 month may qualify for a diagnosis of PTSD.

Risk Factors

Several factors can mediate the effect of disaster exposure on youths.[16] These include the specific nature of the traumatic exposure (eg, type of disaster, intensity, duration, physical proximity, injury, loss of loved ones, loss of possessions, exposure to media coverage), individual factors (eg, age and developmental stage, gender, preexisting academic function, premorbid psychiatric or medical illnesses, post-trauma exposure or grief experiences, adaptive coping skills, resilience, positive emotions), family factors (eg, good parent-child relationships, parental harmony, positive family ambience, extended family support, cultural identification), and community factors (eg, secondary stressors, traumatic reminders, social support, school and religious affiliations).

Most individuals who experience life-threatening events manifest symptoms immediately. However, only around one-third tend to manifest enduring symptomatology after the first month. Female gender, previous

> **Box 13-12. General Trauma Reactions of Children and Adolescents**
>
> <u>Younger Children</u>
> - Clinging and dependent behaviors
> - Phobic reactions
> - Sleep and appetite disturbances
> - Nightmares
> - Loss of bladder and bowel control
> - Tantrums
> - Hyperactivity
>
> <u>Older Children</u>
> - Reenacting the trauma through play
> - Sleep and appetite disturbances
> - Somatic concerns
> - Concentration difficulties
> - Irritability
> - Hyperactivity
> - Decline in school performance
>
> <u>Adolescents</u>
> - Hyperarousal
> - Avoidance
> - Numbing
> - Anxiety, including panic
> - Depressed mood
> - Social withdrawal
> - Suicidal ideation and behavior
> - Flight into pseudoindependence
> - Belligerence
> - Risky behaviors (eg, sex, drugs, violence)
> - Interpersonal conflict

trauma exposure, multiple traumas, greater exposure to the index trauma, presence of a preexisting psychiatric disorder (particularly an anxiety disorder), parental psychopathology, and lack of social support are risk factors for a youth's developing PTSD after trauma exposure.[17] Conversely, parental support, lower levels of parental PTSD, and resolution of other parental trauma-related symptoms have been found to predict lower levels of PTSD symptoms in youths. Increased television viewing of disaster-related events, delayed evacuation, extreme panic symptoms, or having felt that one's own or a family member's life was in danger have each been found to be independently and significantly associated with the development of PTSD. Untreated PTSD is associated with significant morbidity. Despite some studies showing "natural recovery," other studies have shown that PTSD symptoms in youths can persist over many years, affecting function in multiple domains.

Assessment

Psychological screening of disaster survivors facilitates intervention by identifying those with the greatest need. The appropriate timing of screening remains in debate because of the nearly ubiquitous distress that accompanies disasters. Screening is often conducted in school settings using instruments to screen trauma exposure as well as internalizing and externalizing reactions to the exposure. A limitation of standardized screening is the wide variety of emotional and behavioral responses to trauma exhibited by youths.

For youths with clinically significant symptoms, formal clinical assessment should ensue, including a personal interview with the youth and caregivers supplemented by information from other sources. The parent interview should clarify the nature, severity, and duration of the youth's and family's disaster exposure and experience; identify the inventory of current stressors; examine the spectrum of symptoms in the youth; document the youth's psychiatric, developmental, school, and family history; and enumerate important contextual mediators. Youths should be asked directly about their experience of and reactions to traumatic exposure. In most instances, youths are able to recount their experience in words or to use nonverbal means (eg, play, drawing) to relate what occurred. It is important that the interviewer provide the youth with the opportunity to describe his experiences in whatever medium he chooses and support the youth by explaining emotional reactions, cognitive distortions, and maladaptive behaviors.

The diagnosis of both acute stress disorder and PTSD requires exposure to actual or threatened death, serious injury, or sexual violation in one of the following ways: directly experiencing the event; witnessing, in person, the event as it occurred to others; learning that the event (which must be violent or unintentional) occurred to a close family member or close friend; and, in the context of work (eg, first responders), experiencing repeated or extreme exposure to aversive details of the event. If the trauma exposure criterion has been satisfied, diagnosis requires meeting the specified number of symptoms for the disorder, along with duration, distress, and impairment criteria.

In individuals with acute stress disorder, the disturbance persists for at least 3 days to 1 month; for PTSD, the disturbance persists for more than 1 month. A diagnosis of PTSD requires 1 or more symptoms of intrusion (eg, recurrent, distressing memories or dreams; dissociative reactions; physiologic reactions to internal or external cues related to the event); 1 or more symptoms of avoidance (eg, of distressing memories or external reminders of the event); 2 or more symptoms of negative cognition or mood (eg, inability to remember an important aspect of the event, persistent negative emotional state, diminished interest in significant activities); and 2 or more symptoms of hyperarousal (eg, irritable, reckless, or self-destructive behavior; hypervigilance; sleep disturbance).

A separate set of symptom clusters (not presented) pertains to children younger than 6 years. The major differences in the PTSD criteria for very young children include the requirement for only 1 or more avoidance or negative cognition and mood symptoms, the elimination of symptoms requiring reflective cognitive ability, and the expression of intrusion symptoms in play rather than verbally.

Treatment

Recovery from a disaster occurs across several distinct phases.[16] In the impact phase (immediate aftermath), efforts focus on restoring youths' and families' sense of safety and security (eg, provision of basic needs, including food, water, and shelter). In the short-term adaptation phase (first 3 months), efforts focus on limiting the youth's ongoing exposure to the trauma and decreasing negative psychological reactions to the trauma. In both phases, interventions may be provided in a broad range of venues (eg, emergency shelters, family assistance centers, medical and pediatric health care settings, schools, community agencies) by a broad range of personnel (eg, trained volunteers, PCCs, school and community agency personnel). In the medium- to long-term recovery phase (3 months or longer), efforts focus on facilitating controlled reexposure to the traumatic event, emotional and cognitive reparative reprocessing of the event in a safe setting, and the development of coping skills. These interventions are typically provided in mental health settings.

Psychological first aid is the primary intervention used during the impact phase of a disaster. Several organizations, including the National Child Traumatic Stress Network (NCTSN), the National Center for Posttraumatic Stress Disorder (commonly known as NCPTSD), and the American Red Cross, have developed modular approaches to psychological first aid for use by mental health responders in diverse settings under diverse conditions. Psychological first aid focuses on establishing contact, reducing physiologic hyperarousal, offering and mobilizing support and psychosocial assistance, providing accurate and timely information about disaster reactions and available resources, and conducting ongoing assessments of functional status with triage and referral as indicated.

Beyond psychological first aid, specific clinical approaches in the aftermath of a disaster include family outreach and psychoeducation as well as anxiety reduction. Caregivers often underestimate the negative effects of disaster on their children; thus, family outreach is an important first step in the recovery process. Once contact is established, psychoeducation is used to normalize disaster reactions, correct distortions and misperceptions, enhance the youth's sense of control, encourage use of family and social supports, promote adaptive coping, and assess risk and protective factors. Specific psychoeducational advice that can be given to parents of youths of different ages is presented in Box 13-13. Several organizations, including the American Academy of Child and Adolescent Psychiatry (www.aacap.org), the American Red Cross (www.redcross.org/services/disaster), FEMA (www.fema.gov), the National Association of School Psychologists (www.nasponline.org), and the NCTSN (www.nctsnet.org/nccts), publish psychoeducational fact sheets and other useful information about coping with disaster events.

The management of anxiety, which dominates the clinical presentation in the aftermath of a disaster, is an essential aspect of the therapeutic response. Recent data have suggested that panic symptoms in the immediate aftermath of trauma exposure are predictive of the development of PTSD. Maintaining routines to the extent possible should help allay anxiety. Specific anxiety reduction techniques include relaxation strategies

Box 13-13. Psychoeducation Guidelines for Caregivers

Infants and Toddlers

- Provide reassurance.
- Return to normal activities as soon as possible.
- Provide soothing activities.
- Avoid unnecessary separation from caregivers.
- Maintain calm among caregivers.
- Avoid television exposure.

Preschool-aged Children

- Provide reassurance.
- Return to normal activities as soon as possible.
- Provide explanations using simple language.
- Expect and tolerate regressed behavior.
- Expect and tolerate repetitive play about the event.
- Avoid media exposure.
- Censor adult conversations about the trauma.
- Give honest answers (OK to say, "I don't know").

School-aged Children

- Maintain routines.
- Expect and tolerate repetitive play and retelling of the event.
- Give the child control over choices.
- Provide clear and honest answers.
- Allow the child to discuss the event at her own pace.
- Check with school and other caregivers to assess the child's functioning.
- Limit media exposure.

Adolescents

- Be flexible around routines.
- Discuss family, work, and school changes.
- Reassure and normalize strong emotions.
- Try to delay any major changes.
- Encourage involvement in enjoyable activities.
- Provide access for conversations, but do not push.
- Limit media exposure.

such as deep breathing and muscle relaxation and cognitive behavioral strategies such as positive self-talk, problem-solving, and scheduling enjoyable activities.

Trauma-focused cognitive behavioral therapy has received the most empirical support for the clinical treatment of PTSD.[17] To the patient with TF-CBT, the clinician teaches stress management skills in preparation for the exposure-based interventions that are aimed at providing mastery over trauma reminders. The usual components of TF-CBT are presented in Box 13-14.

Box 13-14. Components of Trauma-Focused Cognitive Behavioral Therapy

- Psychoeducation
  - Educating the child and parent about the nature of the traumatic event and expected trauma reactions.

- Parenting skills
  - Use of effective parenting interventions (contingency management).

- Relaxation skills
  - Focused breathing, progressive muscle relaxation, and positive imagery.

- Affective modulation skills
  - Identification of feelings, use of positive self-talk and thought interruption, and enhancing safety, problem-solving, and social skills; recognizing and self-regulating negative affective states.

- Cognitive coping and processing
  - Recognizing relations between thoughts, feelings, and behaviors; changing inaccurate and unhelpful thoughts.

- Trauma narrative
  - Creating a narrative of the child's experience of the trauma, correcting cognitive distortions, and placing the experience in the context of the child's whole life.

- In vivo mastery of trauma reminders
  - Graduated exposure to feared trauma-related stimuli.

- Conjoint child-caregiver sessions
  - Child shares trauma narrative with caregiver; other family issues are addressed.

- Enhancing future safety and development
  - Prevention of future trauma and return to normal developmental trajectory.

Evidence derived from one study suggests that intervening early after a traumatic event with brief caregiver-and-child dyadic therapy can significantly reduce trauma-related symptoms.[18] Early intervention focuses on education about normalizing the child's symptoms in the context of trauma, teaching relaxation techniques to address anxiety, and teaching coping strategies to address intrusive thoughts (eg, guided imagery, thought stopping, distraction techniques). See also Chapter 14, Anxiety and Trauma-Related Distress.

Conclusion

In the face of increasingly frequent psychiatric emergencies, such as those outlined in this chapter, it is critical for PCCs to establish collaborative partnerships with mental health specialists who can perform urgently needed psychiatric assessments and involve the PCC in care planning and follow-up. These partnerships can provide pediatric clinicians with consultative, educational, and case-management services that are important to ongoing patient care. Such partnerships are crucial to having a responsive pediatric medical home wherein the physical and emotional needs of youths and their families are fully addressed.

References

1. Chun TH, Katz ER, Duffy SJ. Pediatric mental health emergencies and special health care needs. *Pediatr Clin North Am.* 2013;60(5):1185–1201

2. Case SD, Case BG, Olfson M, Linakis JG, Laska EM. Length of stay of pediatric mental health emergency department visits in the United States. *J Am Acad Child Adolesc Psychiatry.* 2011;50(11):1110–1119

3. Thomas LE, King RA. Child and adolescent psychiatric emergencies. In: Martin A, Volkmar FR, eds. *Lewis's Child and Adolescent Psychiatry—A Comprehensive Textbook.* 4th ed. Philadelphia, PA: Lippincott Williams & Wilkins; 2007:900–909

4. Fortunati FG, Zonana HV. Legal considerations in the child psychiatric emergency department. *Child Adolesc Psychiatr Clin N Am.* 2003;12(4):745–761

5. *The Child Abuse Prevention and Treatment Act.* Washington, DC: US Dept of Health and Human Services; 2003. https://www.acf.hhs.gov/programs/cb/laws_policies/cblaws/capta03/capta_manual.pdf. Accessed February 8, 2018

6. Giles LL, Martini DR. Psychiatric emergencies. In: Dulcan MK, ed. *Dulcan's Textbook of Child and Adolescent Psychiatry.* 2nd ed. Arlington, VA: American Psychiatric Association Publishing Inc; 2016:621–635

7. Spirito A, Lewander WJ, Levy S, Kurkjian J, Fritz G. Emergency department assessment of adolescent suicide attempters: factors related to short-term follow-up outcome. *Pediatr Emerg Care.* 1994;10(1):6–12

8. Rathus JH, Miller AL. Dialectical behavior therapy adapted for suicidal adolescents. *Suicide Life Threat Behav.* 2002;32(2):146–157

9. Stanley B, Brown G, Brent DA, et al. Cognitive-behavioral therapy for suicide prevention (CBT-SP): treatment model, feasibility, and acceptability. *J Am Acad Child Adolesc Psychiatry.* 2009;48(10):1005–1013

10. Pineda J, Dadds MR. Family intervention for adolescents with suicidal behavior: a randomized controlled trial and mediation analysis. *J Am Acad Child Adolesc Psychiatry.* 2013;52(8):851–862

11. Rossouw TI, Fonagy P. Mentalization-based treatment for self-harm in adolescents: a randomized controlled trial. *J Am Acad Child Adolesc Psychiatry.* 2012;51(12):1304–1313

12. Vitiello B, Brent DA, Greenhill LL, et al. Depressive symptoms and clinical status during the Treatment of Adolescent Suicide Attempters (TASA) study. *J Am Acad Child Adolesc Psychiatry.* 2009;48(10):997–1004

13. Turkel SB, Braslow K, Tavaré CJ, Trzepacz PT. The delirium rating scale in children and adolescents. *Psychosomatics.* 2003;44(2):126–129

14. Joint Commission Resources. *2017 Comprehensive Accreditation Manual for Hospitals.* Oakbrook Terrace, IL: Joint Commission; 2016

15. Hilt RJ, Woodward TA. Agitation treatment for pediatric emergency patients. *J Am Acad Child Adolesc Psychiatry.* 2008;47(2):132–138

16. American Academy of Child and Adolescent Psychiatry (AACAP) Official Action. Practice parameter on disaster preparedness. *J Am Acad Child Adolesc Psychiatry.* 2013;52(11):1224–1238

17. Cohen JA, Bukstein O, Walter H, et al. Practice parameter for the assessment and treatment of children and adolescents with posttraumatic stress disorder. *J Am Acad Child Adolesc Psychiatry.* 2010;49(4):414–430

18. Berkowitz SJ, Stover CS, Marans SR. The Child and Family Traumatic Stress Intervention: secondary prevention for youth at risk of developing PTSD. *J Child Psychol Psychiatry.* 2010;52(6):676-685

CHAPTER 14

Anxiety and Trauma-Related Distress

Lawrence S. Wissow, MD, MPH

> *"Although…there are several distinct forms of anxiety and stress-related disorders, they often co-occur, sharing core symptoms and approaches to initial treatment."*

Introduction

Symptoms of anxiety affect many children, including a large number whose symptoms do not rise to the level of a disorder. At some life stages and in some circumstances, a certain level of anxiety is developmentally appropriate (eg, stranger anxiety in late infancy or anxiety in anticipation of a painful medical procedure). However, from 6% to 20% of children and adolescents will meet diagnostic criteria for an anxiety disorder at some time before adulthood,[1] with approximately half experiencing impairment of daily functioning.[2] Anxiety disorders (generalized anxiety disorder, panic disorder, separation anxiety disorder, agoraphobia, social phobia, obsessive-compulsive disorder [OCD], and specific phobias) (Table 14-1)

Table 14-1. General Overview of Anxiety and Anxiety-Related Disorders	
Type	**Description[a]**
Anxiety	
Generalized anxiety disorder	Excessive anxiety and worry about a number of events or activities. Children tend to worry excessively about their competence or the quality of their performances at school or in sporting events.
Panic disorder	Recurrent, unexpected, abrupt surge of intense fear or discomfort that reaches a peak within minutes and includes symptoms such as sweating, trembling, palpitations, and dizziness
Separation anxiety disorder	Developmentally inappropriate and excessive fear or anxiety concerning separation from those to whom the individual is attached

Table 14-1. General Overview of Anxiety and Anxiety-Related Disorders (*continued*)

Type	Description[a]
Agoraphobia	Marked fear or anxiety in using public transportation, being in open or enclosed spaces, standing in line or being in a crowd, or being outside the home alone
Social phobia	Marked fear or anxiety about ≥1 social situation in which the individual is exposed to possible scrutiny by others. In children, the anxiety must occur in peer settings and not just during interactions with adults.
Specific phobias	Marked fear or anxiety about a specific object or situation (eg, insects, heights, storms, needles, airplanes, loud sounds, costumed characters). In children, the fear or anxiety may be expressed by crying, tantrums, freezing, or clinging.
Obsessive-Compulsive Disorder	
OCD	Presence of obsessions or compulsions. Obsessions are recurrent and persistent thoughts, urges, or images that are experienced as intrusive and unwanted. Compulsions are repetitive behaviors or mental acts that an individual is driven to perform, often in response to an obsession or rigidly applied rules.
Trauma- and Stressor-Related Disorders	
PTSD	Changes in mood, arousal, sense of reality, or behavior, or experience of intrusive thoughts or dreams, related to a trauma after a traumatic event that is directly experienced, witnessed, or experienced vicariously; manifestations in young children may not seem to be directly linked to the trauma and may not seem to be distressing. Onset may not necessarily be immediately after the event.
Adjustment disorder	The presence of emotional or behavioral symptoms in response to ≥1 identifiable stressor occurring within 3 mo of the onset of the stressor (can be predominantly anxious or a mixture of anxiety, depression, and a change in behavior)
Acute stress disorder	Changes in mood, arousal, sense of reality, or behavior, or experience of intrusive thoughts or dreams, related to a trauma, occurring from 2 d–1 mo after a traumatic event that is directly experienced, witnessed, or experienced vicariously

Abbreviations: OCD, obsessive-compulsive disorder; PTSD, post-traumatic stress disorder.
[a] For all disorders, the symptoms interfere with function in ≥1 important area, including at school, at work, at home, and among peers.
Derived from American Psychiatric Association. *Diagnostic and Statistical Manual of Mental Disorders.* 5th ed. Arlington, VA: American Psychiatric Association; 2013.

are among the most common mental disorders in children and adolescents (collectively called *children* in the remainder of this chapter unless otherwise specified).[2] Anxiety-like symptoms are a frequent response to trauma (physical or psychological), and they can be features of post-traumatic stress disorder [PTSD], acute stress disorder, and adjustment disorder. Anxiety disorders often occur concomitantly with chronic medical conditions, affecting children's use of medical resources through frequent emergency department visits and hospitalizations,[3] and with other psychiatric disorders, especially depression.[4] Medical "trauma," including painful procedures, diagnoses evoking fears of death, disfigurement, or separation from loved ones, can also be associated with stress-related conditions. Anxious children often have an anxious or a depressed parent whose care is an integral part of helping the child.

The guidance in this chapter applies to the care of children presenting with symptoms of anxiety in any pediatric clinical setting. Its audience is therefore all pediatric clinicians: primary care pediatricians, pediatric subspecialists, family physicians, internists, nurse practitioners, and physician assistants who provide health care to children. In several places the chapter calls out pediatric primary care clinicians (ie, clinicians in frontline, longitudinal relationships with children and families), abbreviated PCCs, for their specific role in the care of children experiencing anxiety.

Although, as noted previously, there are several distinct forms of anxiety and stress-related disorders, they often co-occur, sharing core symptoms and approaches to initial treatment. Thus, the pediatric clinician may want to start building competence in this area by learning about anxiety and stress-related problems in general before trying to further differentiate the various disorders.

The following guidance is based on the work of the World Health Organization, whose recommendations may be updated annually. The most up-to-date information can be found at www.who.int/mental_health/publications/mhGAP_intervention_guide/en.

Findings Suggesting Anxiety

Symptoms of anxiety vary by age and severity. Children may experience developmentally normal fears; they may have fears that are exaggerated or persistent beyond norms for their ages; and they may have fear-associated behaviors and physical symptoms that impair their functioning at school, at home, or with peers. Box 14-1 provides a summary of the symptoms and clinical findings that suggest anxiety. These may be elicited from either parents or youths (children and adolescents aged 6–18 years). Parents and youths often disagree on the severity of anxiety symptoms; however, agreement is much better if the discussion is about whether there are symptoms at all, regardless of severity or effect on function. Agreement at this level may facilitate further discussion of how to approach the problem.

Box 14-2 summarizes symptoms and clinical findings that suggest a response to trauma.

Box 14-1. Symptoms and Clinical Findings Suggesting Anxiety

- Normal fears (eg, strangers, dark, separation, new social situations, unfamiliar animals or objects, public speaking) are exaggerated or persistent.

- Fears are keeping child from developmentally appropriate experiences (eg, school refusal, extreme shyness or clinging, refusal to sleep alone).

- Tantrum, tearfulness, acting-out behavior, or another display of distress occurs when child is asked to engage in feared activity.

- Child worries about harm coming to self or loved ones or fears something bad is going to happen.

- Somatic features accompany worries: palpitations, stomachaches, headaches, breathlessness, difficulty getting to sleep, nausea, feeling wobbly ("jelly legs"), butterflies.

- *Panic attacks* occur in response to feared objects or situations, or they happen spontaneously. These are unexpected and repeated periods of intense fear, dread, or discomfort along with symptoms such as racing heartbeat, shortness of breath, dizziness, light-headedness, feeling smothered, trembling, sense of unreality, or fear of dying, losing control, or losing one's mind. Panic attacks often develop without warning and last minutes to hours.

Box 14-2. Symptoms and Clinical Findings Suggesting Trauma Response

The following behavior changes after a traumatic experience, such as abuse, witness to violence, loss of a loved one, or medical trauma, suggest trauma response:

- **Infants and toddlers:** Crying, clinging, change in sleep or eating habits, regression to earlier behavior (eg, bed-wetting, thumb-sucking), repetitive play or talk.

- **3- to 5-year-olds:** Separation fears, clinging, tantrums, fighting, crying, withdrawal, regression to earlier behavior (eg, bed-wetting, thumb-sucking), sleep difficulty. May have repetitive play or other interaction that reenacts the trauma with or without apparent distress. May have new onset of frightening dreams or fears that do not have content with obvious links to the trauma.

- **6- to 9-year-olds:** Anger, fighting, bullying, irritability, fluctuating moods, fear of separation or of being alone, fear that traumatic events will recur, withdrawal, regression to earlier behavior, physical concerns (eg, stomachaches, headaches), school problems (eg, avoidance, academic difficulty, difficulty concentrating).

- **10- to 12-year-olds:** Crying, aggression, irritability, bullying, resentment, sadness, social withdrawal, fears that traumatic events will recur, suppressed emotions or avoidance of situations or discussions that evoke memories of the traumatic event, sleep disturbance, concern about physical health of self or others, academic problems or decline related to lack of attention.

- **13- to 18-year-olds:** Numbing, reexperiencing, avoidance of feelings (or situations or discussions that evoke memories of the traumatic event), resentment, loss of trust or optimism about future, depression, withdrawal, mood swings, irritability, anxiety, anger, exaggerated euphoria, acting out, substance use, fear of similar events, appetite and sleep changes, physical concerns, academic decline, school refusal.

Tools to Assist With Identification

Because many children do not spontaneously disclose their symptoms, standardized psychosocial screening instruments may be used to identify children with symptoms of anxiety. See Appendix 2, Mental Health Tools for Pediatrics, for descriptions of tools in common use. Several instruments have versions to collect information directly from the youth or from parents or teachers. Table 14-2 provides a synopsis of screening

Table 14-2. General Psychosocial Screening/Results Suggesting Anxiety and Post-traumatic Stress

Screening Instrument	Score Suggesting Anxiety
PSC-35	• Total score ≥24 for children aged ≤5 y. • ≥28 for those 6–16 y. • ≥30 for those aged ≥17 y. *and* • Further discussion of items related to anxiety confirms a concern in that area.
PSC-17	• Internalizing subscale is ≥5. *and* • Further discussion of items related to anxiety confirms a concern in that area.
SDQ	• Total symptom score of >19. • Emotional symptom score of 7–10 (see instructions at www.sdqinfo.com). • Impact scale score of 1 (medium impairment) or ≥2 (high impairment). *and* • Further discussion of items related to anxiety confirms a concern in that area.
Screening Instrument	**Score Suggesting Trauma Response**
ASC-Kids	All items are scored as 0-1-2 (with 2 items reverse scored). An item rated as *2* (very or often true) is considered to be a positive item when assessing presence of diagnostic criteria. Generates a continuous severity score (sum of 19 symptom items).
SCARED Brief Assessment of PTS Symptoms	• Score of ≥3 suggests clinical level of anxiety. • Score of ≥6 suggests PTSD.

Abbreviations: ASC, Acute Stress Checklist for Children; PSC, Pediatric Symptom Checklist; PTS, post-traumatic stress; PTSD, post-traumatic stress disorder; SCARED, Screen for Child Anxiety Related Disorders; SDQ, Strengths and Difficulties Questionnaires.

results suggesting that anxiety may be present. Use of additional instruments, such as the Spence Children's Anxiety Scale or Screen for Child Anxiety Related Disorders (commonly known as SCARED), can help confirm findings of the initial screening, and use of a functional assessment tool, such as the Strengths and Difficulties Questionnaires (SDQ) or

Columbia Impairment Scale (commonly known as CIS), will assist in determining whether the child is significantly impaired by the symptoms. Use of a tool to assess the effect of the child's problem on other members of the family may also be helpful; the Caregiver Strain Questionnaire (commonly known as CGSQ) is an example. (See Appendix 2, Mental Health Tools for Pediatrics, for further details about each of these instruments.)

It is important to differentiate the use of these tools as screening instruments at routine visits from their use to refine concerns that have already been raised. When used as screening tools, they tend to have relatively low sensitivity and positive predictive value. That is, positive results need further discussion to understand the meaning of the result, and negative results may not be reassuring if the parent or youth is truly concerned. When used to follow up on existing concerns, results still need discussion with families, but they are more likely be a fair indicator of the nature and severity of the youth's problems.

Assessment

Assessment begins by differentiating the child's symptoms from normal behavior. Some children have a temperament that is, from the outset, marked by having more difficulty with change and wariness of new situations or individuals. Children who have difficulty reading others' emotions or interpreting their behavior are also at a higher risk of developing anxiety problems, especially problems related to social interactions. Recognizing that these are long-standing traits can help parents promote active coping skills, avoid misinterpreting the child's behavior as oppositional, and possibly seek a more specific treatment (eg, a social skills support program).

Symptoms may take on different significance in the setting of trauma. Knowing that there may be a trauma antecedent can trigger exploration for some of the other symptoms associated with trauma exposure (reexperiencing, avoidance, hyperarousal, and dissociation).

Anxiety is a universal experience, and it can occur predictably at particular stages of life or in particular situations. When anxiety persists outside of these stages and situations, or when its severity is disruptive, further assessment and treatment may be warranted. Anxieties may normally emerge in the following stages:

▶ **Infancy at 8 to 9 months:** Peak of stranger anxiety.

▶ **Toddlerhood and early school age:** Development of separation anxiety (fear of new people, places, or being away from trusted caregivers), usually ends by age 2 to 3 years. Depending on their temperaments, toddlers and young children may have greater or lesser tolerance of changes to routine or to expectations or of novel experiences (which can include new clothing and foods). Fears of the dark (or of unseen monsters) are common and exacerbated by other stresses and exposure to frightening media.

▶ **Childhood at 5 to 8 years:** During this period, many children experience an increase in worry about harm to parents or attachment figures. Worries may be triggered by illness in or death of family members, by the child's own illness, or by world events.

▶ **School age at any age:** Many children experience anxiety and distress at the time of high-stakes testing, as well as initial reluctance to socialize in new situations.

▶ **Adolescence:** Previously resolved anxiety issues often occur again in early adolescence, sometimes associated with concerns about appearance, new social situations, and school performance.

Children with anxiety disorders have fear and distress that interferes with functioning in response to everyday situations. Verbal older children and adolescents are usually able to describe their fears ("worries" may be a more understandable concept), but evaluating reports of younger children's anxiety may be challenging, especially if the parent giving information is also anxious; therefore, it is important to communicate directly with children about these symptoms and to observe or obtain the child's report of physiologic symptoms (eg, increased heart rate, shortness of breath, numbness, tingling). Sometimes, children will display anxiety through repetitive play that acts out their concerns, for example, crashing toy cars or having violent or tragic things happen to dolls, or through drawings that they make in response to simple requests to "draw something." Bad behavior can also be a masked presentation of anxiety. Children at any age may become irritable or oppositional in the face of situations, imminent or anticipated, that they fear. Depression or bereavement may mimic or co-occur with anxiety, so at least some exploration of other emotional symptoms and of current stressors is always warranted. When children of any age are anxious, it is always important to ask about stressors in the family environment, for example, serious illness (including anxiety and depression) in a family member, economic problems, or marital discord. It may be necessary to ask parents privately about these issues; often, they will have avoided talking about them in front of their children and believe that their children are not aware. In fact, children are sensitive to changes in parents' behavior and mood, and anxiety is readily communicated nonverbally.

Anxiety, like depression, may also occur in multiple family members. When children are found to be anxious, it is not unusual to find that one or more close family members are anxious as well. Helping parents manage their own anxiety can be important, especially, as discussed in the following text, when trying to use modeling as a form of treatment. Table 14-3 provides a summary of conditions that frequently co-occur with anxiety.

Children with anxiety sometimes have panic attacks, which are episodes of autonomic arousal that occur suddenly, often (but not always) cued by thoughts of a feared situation. People experiencing panic attacks usually report sudden onset of shortness of breath, palpitations, trembling, diaphoresis, and, often, a feeling of faintness, dread, or impending doom. The attacks usually subside by themselves over the course of several minutes, but it is not unusual, especially among teenagers, for some of the symptoms to be prolonged and result in a call for emergency medical assistance. Differentiating panic attacks from hypoglycemia, asthma exacerbations, or cardiac conditions may in itself help with their treatment; often, they will improve as other aspects of anxiety are treated. As noted in the following text, they can sometimes be suppressed with medication if their frequency is causing disability; in this situation medication can facilitate treatment of the underlying anxiety problem.

Treatment of anxiety generally involves identifying the specific situations in which it is triggered and helping individuals learn how to reduce anxious or avoidant feelings when they occur. The goal is to gradually become tolerant of the triggers until anxious responses either are no longer evoked or remain manageable (with or without consciously using coping mechanisms such as deep breathing or visualization). Treatment is

Table 14-3. Conditions That May Co-occur With Anxiety

Condition	Rationale
Learning problems or disabilities	If symptoms of anxiety are associated with problems of school attendance or performance, the child may be experiencing academic difficulties. (See Chapter 21, Learning Difficulty, for more information.)
Attention problems	Anxiety in school can make it seem that a child cannot stay focused on his or her work, and difficulty focusing or negative feedback from peers and teachers associated with ADHD can make children anxious. (See Chapter 20, Inattention and Impulsivity, for more information.)
Somatic concerns	Anxious children may present with a variety of somatic concerns (eg, GI symptoms, headaches, chest pain). These may elicit medical workups if they are not recognized. Conversely, acute or chronic medical conditions or pain syndromes may cause anxiety. (See Chapter 24, Medically Unexplained Symptoms, for more information.)
Depression	Depression can be very difficult to distinguish from anxiety. Depression coexists in half or more of anxious children. Marked sleep disturbance, disturbed appetite, low mood, or tearfulness in the absence of direct anxiety provocation could indicate that a child is depressed. (See Chapter 22, Low Mood, for more information.)
Bereavement	Most children will experience the death of a family member or friend sometime in childhood. Other losses may also trigger grief responses, for example, separation or divorce of parents, relocation, change of school, deployment of a parent in military service, breakup with a girlfriend or boyfriend, or remarriage of a parent. Such losses are traumatic. They may result in feelings of insecurity and anxiety immediately following the loss or exacerbate existing anxiety. Furthermore, they may make the child more susceptible to impaired functioning at the time of subsequent losses.
Pervasive developmental disorders, including ASD and Asperger syndrome	Children who have these difficulties also have problems with social relatedness (eg, poor eye contact, preference for solitary activities), language (often stilted), and range of interest (persistent and intense interest in an activity or a subject). They will often have rigid expectations for routine or parent promises and become anxious or angry if these expectations are not met.

Table 14-3. Conditions That May Co-occur With Anxiety (*continued*)	
Condition	**Rationale**
Exposure to ACEs (eg, acute or chronic stress or trauma)	Children who have experienced or witnessed trauma, violence, a natural disaster, separation from a parent, parental divorce or separation, parental substance use, neglect, or physical, emotional, or sexual abuse are at high risk of developing emotional difficulties such as adjustment disorder or PTSD. Determination of the temporal relationship between the trauma and onset of anxiety symptoms is essential. Denial of trauma symptoms does not mean trauma did not occur; questions about ACEs should be repeated as a trusting relationship is established.
Psychosis	Symptoms associated with psychosis, such as hallucinations or delusions, may occur in children with PTSD. They may also occur infrequently with adolescent onset of a bipolar disorder and are features of schizophrenia, which may also have its onset in adolescence. The teen may manifest fear without disclosing the hallucinations or delusions.
Physical illness	Medical issues that can mimic or provoke anxiety symptoms include thyroid disease, hypoglycemia, harmful side effects of medications (eg, bronchodilators), and endocrine tumors (pheochromocytoma). Drug withdrawal or alcohol withdrawal is a consideration for teens (the latter, potentially a medical emergency).
Selective mutism	Consider selective mutism if a child who has had normal language development suddenly stops talking in certain situations (most often in school and with adults outside the home). This disorder can be confused with children making a language transition (eg, a child raised speaking Spanish who is suddenly placed in an English-speaking class.)

Abbreviations: ACE, adverse childhood experience; ADHD, attention-deficit/hyperactivity disorder; ASD, autism spectrum disorder; GI, gastrointestinal; PTSD, post-traumatic stress disorder.

usually tailored to the specific triggering situation, often through carefully supported increasing exposure to the trigger coupled with practice of a variety of cognitive, somatic, and social coping strategies. Treatment of OCD and PTSD involves these same elements, but the etiologic origin of the disorders takes on a role (whereas in the treatment of other anxiety disorders, less emphasis is placed on how the problem began and more on how to get it to remit). For OCD, that obsessions and compulsions develop without particular triggers (although they can be worsened by other stresses) plays an important role in children's and families' understanding of the condition. For PTSD, linking what may be nonspecific symptoms to a past trauma can be an important part of treatment. In particular, when the trauma has gone undisclosed or invalidated, or is something that is stigmatized, acknowledgement of the trauma-symptom link can help on many levels.

▶ **Consider OCD in the presence of marked rituals or compulsive behaviors.** Most children have phases of ritualized behavior that can usually be distinguished from OCD by the degree of distress caused if a ritual is interrupted. Individuals with OCD usually report, or, after discussion, will admit, that the symptoms have a major effect on how they plan their activities or interact with others and that attempts to stop the thoughts or actions have been difficult to carry out or even contemplate. School-aged children will often, once the symptoms can be openly discussed, admit being aware that there is something objectively out of proportion about their concerns, even though having these concerns remains difficult to resist. The most common concerns center on contamination such as fears of touching things that may be dirty or the need to repetitively wash or bathe. Other common difficulties are a need to check that something has been done (usually related to security [eg, doors locked, stove turned off]) or a need to have one's personal possessions in a particular order or place.

▶ **Consider acute stress disorder, adjustment disorder, and PTSD if the onset of anxiety was preceded by an extremely distressing experience,** such as witnessing violence, losing a loved one, undergoing medical trauma, or experiencing sexual or physical abuse. Parents may be unaware of exposures to trauma, such as bullying at school or in the community, and there may be major traumas in the family (eg, serious illness in a parent, pending divorce) that are similarly not discussed or disclosed; consequently, pediatric clinicians may need to interview children and parents separately to elicit a complete history. It is important to note that the triggering circumstances need only be traumatic in the eye of the child. Most antecedents have in common situations in which the child felt that there was risk to her life or to that of someone close to her. The hallmark symptoms of anxiety in the wake of trauma are *reexperiencing* (often repetitive play in young children; intrusive thoughts and nightmares; and extreme reactions to reminders of the trauma), *avoidance* of memories or situations that recall the trauma, and *hypervigilance* (eg, increased worry about safety, startling or anxiousness at unexpected sounds or events) (may involve irritability, aggression, recklessness, and problems concentrating). Avoidance can take the form of changing the subject or acting inappropriately when subjects related to trauma are brought up in conversation. Post-traumatic symptoms may also be accompanied by symptoms that mimic depression, including expressions of guilt, feelings of detachment from others, constricted emotions, and lack of interest in previously pleasurable activities. Children most at risk for developing PTSD following trauma or loss are those with preexisting mental health conditions; those whose caregivers are experiencing emotional difficulties; those facing preexisting or consequent family life stressors, such as divorce or loss of job; those with previous loss or trauma experiences; those repeatedly exposed to media coverage of traumatic events; and those with a limited support network.[4] Clinicians can provide the child with a safe and comfortable environment to express her feelings and allow the child to control the interview, taking breaks or discontinuing as needed. Even children with limited symptoms of PTSD after a trauma can benefit from treatment. For further guidance in caring for children exposed to trauma, see the *Feelings Need Check Ups Too* toolkit at www.aap.org/en-us/advocacy-and-policy/aap-health-initiatives/Children-and-Disasters/Pages/Feelings-Need-Checkups-Too-Toolkit.aspx and the National Child Traumatic Stress Network Web site at www.nctsn.org.

Plan of Care for Children With Anxiety and Trauma-Related Distress

The care of a child experiencing anxiety can begin in the primary care or pediatric subspecialty setting from the time symptoms are recognized, even if the child's symptoms do not rise to the level of a disorder and regardless of whether referral to a mental health specialist is ultimately part of the care plan. Both children and parents may, by temperament, be more or less socially outgoing and more or less open to new or unexpected experiences. Helping parents appreciate their own areas of comfort and discomfort, and how these may differ from those of their child, can be a first step toward treatment. Regardless of parent or child temperament, parents can be taught ways to help their child gain better emotional regulation.

Engaging Child and Family in Care

Without engagement, most families will not seek or persist in care. The process may require multiple visits.[5]

Reinforce strengths of the child and family (eg, good relationships with at least one parent or important adult, prosocial peers, concerned or caring family, help seeking, connection to positive organizations) as a method of engagement, and identify any barriers to addressing the problem (eg, stigma, family conflict, resistance to treatment). Use "common factors" techniques[6] (represented by the HELP mnemonic, Box 14-3) to build trust and optimism, reach agreement on incremental next steps, develop a plan of care, and collaboratively determine the role of the PCC. Regardless of other roles, the pediatric clinician can encourage a positive view of treatment on the part of the child and family.

Remember that it is in many ways normal for people with anxiety problems to initially shy away from treatment, because most people cope with anxiety through avoidance, and initiating treatment means that one has to start thinking about the situations that trigger the anxious feelings. Many people have been led to feel ashamed or weak about their anxieties, or they have worked hard over a long time to hide them. People who have experienced trauma may be particularly wary of discussing their feelings. Their greatest fear may be of the unknown: what will happen after disclosure, what might happen during examinations, or whether there will be retribution from a perpetrator. Clinicians can keep in mind that individuals who have experienced trauma are, by definition, survivors, and their survival has depended on maintaining a delicate equilibrium between their adaptive skills and ongoing, dangerous feelings and situations. To engage in

---

Box 14-3. Common Factors Mnemonic: HELP Build a Therapeutic Alliance
H = Hope
E = Empathy
L^2 = Language, Loyalty
P^3 = Permission, Partnership, Plan

Adapted with permission from American Academy of Pediatrics. *Addressing Mental Health Concerns in Primary Care: A Clinician's Toolkit.* Elk Grove Village, IL: American Academy of Pediatrics; 2010. For the fully annotated mnemonic, please refer to Appendix 5.

treatment, individuals who have experienced trauma need to feel that they can begin to shift the equilibrium in ways and at a pace with which they feel safe and comfortable. They need to feel assured of both the clinician's expertise and the clinician's willingness to help them on their own terms.

Providing Psychoeducation

Tell the family a little bit about anxiety and trauma; much of the material discussed previously in this chapter could be useful. Emphasize that anxiety is a normal human emotion, that anxiety problems are very common, and that they can be addressed. For some children and families, it can be helpful to talk about variations in temperament or personal style that make some people more or less anxious in new situations or more or less responsive to threats. Again, acknowledge that these are traits we are born with and not to be ashamed of. The clinician can also say that anxiety has nothing to do with bravery or accomplishment, noting that many famous performers and athletes experience serious degrees of stage fright and yet, with support and encouragement, have become very successful (usually by working hard to prepare themselves). It can be helpful to point out that one can greatly enjoy and be good at things but still experience anxiety when having to do them in front of others or in particularly high-stakes circumstances.

Psychoeducation on trauma starts with empathy and a lack of assumptions. Initially, clinicians may know little of the details of what has happened and perhaps even less about what the patient or family is actually experiencing. The "education" may consist more of acknowledging that, regardless of what happened, various kinds of help are available; that the clinician will stand by the family to secure that help; and that the clinician will, when asked or when appropriate, offer choices and help the family decide what seems best for them. With permission, clinicians can talk about the possible major categories of responses to trauma (reexperiencing, avoidance, mood and behavior changes, and hypervigilance) and that there is a growing understanding of why our brains and bodies respond in this way.

Addressing Security and Normalcy

In many situations involving trauma, and sometimes for patients with anxiety, there are ongoing threats to safety and security. The actual traumatic threat may still be present (eg, an abuser, a bully) or there may have been disruptions to safety and routines caused by trauma (eg, family members are separated, families must leave their homes, children have to change schools). Ask about what has changed and what it is feared might change in the course of disclosure and treatment, and make a plan to help restore or maintain security and normalcy to the extent possible. Acknowledge that trauma to one family member may be felt by others who were not directly affected, and offer to help assess this effect and provide support or referral as needed. Ask particularly about siblings and include them in plans for support.

Encouraging Healthy Habits

Encourage exercise, outdoor play, balanced and consistent diet, sleep (critically important to mental health), special time with parents, frequent acknowledgment of the child's strengths, and open communication with a trusted adult about worries. Children, particularly younger ones, should be shielded from certain types of media, such as television (TV) news, when there are violent or disturbing images or stories. Likewise, some TV shows and video games, even some cartoons, may contribute to a child's feeling anxious. For preteens and teens, media messages about unattainable body images and social media exchanges may contribute to or exacerbate anxiety.

Reducing Overall Stress

Consider the child's social environment (eg, family social history, parental depression screening, results of any family assessment tools administered, reports from child care or school). Questions to raise might include

▶ **Is the family experiencing a particular stress** (related to illness, finances, or a confluence of demands) for which there might be a form of help aside from treating the child (eg, assistance with bills or housing stability)?

▶ **Is an external problem causing the child to be anxious** (eg, bullying at school, academic difficulties, disruption at home)? Take steps to address the problem.

▶ **Is the child exposed to frightening electronic media?** Sometimes, this exposure results from unsupervised access to TV or Internet content, but it may also occur during shared family activities (eg, movies, TV, video games) when parents or other family members underestimate or fail to recognize how frightened the child has become. Limiting these exposures, and providing reassuring explanations if they occur, can be an important part of reducing anxiety, especially among younger children.

▶ **Is the child's worry about a parent's welfare legitimate because of a serious illness, domestic violence, or parent impairment?** Address environmental issues, enlisting the help of school personnel or social services as appropriate to the situation.

▶ **Is the parent anxious or depressed or impaired because of substance use? Has the parent experienced trauma or loss?** Anxious children often have an anxious or a depressed parent. Advise parents to minimize their own displays of fear or worry when the child is present. A referral to adult mental health services might also be appropriate.

Offering Initial Interventions to Address the Anxiety Symptoms

Children with developmentally expected anxiety problems will usually respond to empathy, assistance with active coping, and modeling and rewarding brave behavior. Children vary in their temperaments and some may choose longer adaptations to their fears (such as sleeping with a light on) that help them stay within a range of normal functioning. In contrast, children with anxiety disorders have fear and distress that interferes with functioning despite attempts at coping and provision of adult assistance.

The strategies described in the following text are common elements of evidence-based psychosocial interventions for anxiety disorders. They are applicable to the care of children with mild or emerging anxiety symptoms and to those with impairing symptoms that do not rise to the level of a disorder. They can also be used as initial treatment of children with anxiety disorders and while readying children for referral or awaiting access to specialty care. Medications can be helpful, especially to speed suppression of panic and OCD symptoms or when time-limited and severe stressors need to be faced, but, in the absence of psychosocial therapies, symptoms may recur as the medications are discontinued. Interpreting the results of a medication trial can also be problematic, because the severity of anxiety problems is often cyclic. Families may seek care as symptoms are peaking. If medication is started at this point, it often cannot be determined whether the condition improved on its own or improved with medication. Thus, starting with a carefully administered psychosocial therapy plan may be a reasonable first step until the severity and natural history of the anxiety concerns are better understood.

Guide parents in managing their child's fears. Help the parents identify their child's fear or fears, and reach consensus with the child and family on the goal of reducing symptoms and on a way to do it. Steps could include teaching the child and parents cognitive behavioral strategies to improve coping skills at times when the child feels anxious. Examples of these skills include deep breathing, muscle relaxation, positive self-talk, thought stopping, and thinking of a safe place. The child and family may also benefit from reading material or participating in a Web course, as appropriate to their literacy levels.

Gradually increase exposure. One of the best validated approaches to anxiety and phobias is to gradually increase a child's exposure to feared objects or experiences. The eventual goal is for the child to master rather than avoid feared things. To do this, the parent might start the child out with brief exposure to the feared object or activity and gradually lengthen the exposure. First, the parent helps the child imagine or talk about the feared object or activity or look at pictures; then, the child learns to tolerate a short exposure with support from the parent, proceeds to tolerate a longer exposure in a group or with the parent or another coach, and, finally, tolerates the feared activity alone (when that is appropriate) but with a chance to get help if needed. During these trials, parents need to stay as calm and confident as possible; if they become distressed, it will be a cue for the child to become distressed.

Manage school phobia. For some children who are vulnerable to anxiety, it is necessary to return the child promptly to the anxiety-producing situation. School phobia is an example. For a child who is afraid at school or resists going to school, rule out bullying, trauma, learning difficulties, and medical conditions that may be contributing to stress and fear. The PCC can partner with school personnel to manage the child's return to school and gently, but firmly, insist that the child attend, in addition to providing positive feedback and calm support. If absence becomes prolonged or parents are reluctant to support the child's return, referral to a mental health specialist will be necessary.

If anxiety is secondary to environmental stress, support the parents' efforts to protect the child, buffer stress, and help the child master his anxiety. Help the child rename the fear (ie, "annoying worry") and assist the child to become the boss of the worry. It is also helpful to reward brave behavior (Table 14-4).

Children with marked symptoms in the wake of trauma will likely be referred for specialty care (see the Involving Specialists section later in this chapter). A first-line response, however, can include

▶ Gently challenging negative thoughts about shame, guilt, and hopelessness (and inquiring about thoughts of self-harm)

▶ Encouraging self-care and ways of seeking a feeling of security when symptoms are not prominent

▶ When symptoms are prominent, using distraction and relaxation and having a plan for seeking supportive company

▶ Getting permission to ask about triggering situations and, if the child is willing to discuss them, making plans to avoid or manage them in a more active, open, and empowered way

Attend to overall parenting style. Children can become anxious if parents are inconsistent about rules and expectations. Determine whether consequences for failure are catastrophic ("I know Dad will get angry if I bring home a bad grade...."). Explore the child's sense of responsibility for the family's stresses ("I know that the only reason Mom and Dad work hard is so I can go to a better school, so I'm afraid that if don't do well...").

Treat panic attacks. Early treatment, including psychosocial and psychopharmacological therapy, is useful and may prevent progression to

Table 14-4. Tips for Reward System	
Reward Systems for Brave Behavior	**Guidelines for Use**
Small rewards	Include positive feedback.
Star charts	• Focus on only 1 or 2 behaviors at a time. • Have 1 star chart per behavior. • Negotiate rules for the star chart (eg, sleeping in own bed for 1 night = 1 star; 4 stars = trip to the pool). • Ignore mistakes and failures; do not mark them on the star chart. • Continue awarding stars when they are earned.

agoraphobia and other problems such as depression and substance use.[7] When children are aware of the triggers for their attacks, developing alternative responses to those triggers can diminish the frequency of attacks. When attacks appear without apparent triggers, referral for pharmacological treatment may be most effective.

Providing Resources

The American Academy of Pediatrics and its chapters have developed a number of resources to help parents deal with their child's anxiety: *Helping Your Child Cope With Anxiety* (www.ohioaap.org/wp-content/uploads/2013/07/Helping-Your-Child-Cope-with-Anxiety.pdf), *Helping Your Child Cope With Life* (patiented.solutions.aap.org), "How to Ease Your Child's Separation Anxiety" (www.healthychildren.org/English/ages-stages/toddler/Pages/Soothing-Your-Childs-Separation-Anxiety.aspx), *Stressed?* (patiented.solutions.aap.org), and *Tips for Parenting the Anxious Child* (www.brightfutures.org/mentalhealth/pdf/families/mc/tips.pdf). Provide the family with contact numbers and resources in case of emergency.

Monitoring the Child's Progress Toward Therapeutic Goals

Child care, preschool, or school reports can be helpful in monitoring progress. Screening instruments that gather information from multiple reporters (youth, parent, and teacher), such as the SDQ, can be helpful in monitoring progress with symptoms and functioning.

It is important for PCCs to work with the family to understand that it is not uncommon for treatment to be successful for a period of time and then seem to lose effectiveness. This setback can happen when there are new stresses or demands or when, after a period of success, there has been a letup on treatment. If troubleshooting existing treatment and ways of dealing with new stresses does not help get function back to baseline, new treatments or new diagnoses need to be considered. In particular, as school demands increase, learning issues may need to be considered, even if they were not seen as contributing problems in the past.

Involving Specialists

Involve one or more specialists if the child does not respond to initial interventions or if the following clinical circumstances exist:

► Child has severe functional impairments at school, at home, or with peers, for example, if anxiety threatens to interfere with academic progress or other developmentally important goals.

► Multiple symptoms of anxiety occur in many domains of life (eg, fearful of new situations, reluctant to do things in public, trouble separating, worries a lot).

► The child or parent is very distressed by the symptom or symptoms.

► There are co-occurring behavioral problems. (The combination of shyness, anxiety, and behavioral problems is thought to be particularly risky for future behavioral problems of a more serious nature.)

► The anxiety was preceded by serious trauma or symptoms suggesting PTSD, acute stress disorder, or adjustment disorder.

► The child seems to have panic disorder or OCD, both of which require specialized treatment.

► The anxiety occurs in a child with autism spectrum disorder (ASD). Anxiety about normal childhood issues (eg, weather, animals), as well as the orderliness and predictability of daily routines, is relatively common among higher-functioning children who display ASD symptoms, including stereotyped interests and poor social perceptions and skills.

When specialty care is needed, ensure that it is evidence informed and assist the family in accessing it. A variety of evidence-based and evidence-informed psychosocial interventions, and some pharmacological interventions, are available for the treatment of anxiety disorders in children and adolescents. Ideally, those referred for care in the mental health specialty system would have access to the safest and most effective treatments. Recommended psychosocial interventions are summarized in Table 14-5 and are based on current evidence and updated biannually at www.aap. org/mentalhealth. Box 14-4 summarizes psychopharmacological interventions approved at the time of this book's publication by the US Food and Drug Administration for treatment of anxiety and trauma-related disorders in children and adolescents.

Youths referred for mental health specialty care complete the referral process only 61% of the time, and significantly fewer persist in care.[8] Approaches to improving the referral process include making sure that the family is ready for this step in care, has some idea of what the specialty

Table 14-5. Psychosocial Therapies for Anxiety and Trauma-Related Distress: Evidence Base as of April 2018					
Problem Area	Level 1 – Best Support	Level 2 – Good Support	Level 3 – Moderate Support	Level 4 – Minimal Support	Level 5 – No Support
Anxious or Avoidant Behaviors	CBT, CBT and Medication, CBT for Child and Parent, CBT with Parents, Education, Exposure, Modeling	Assertiveness Training, Attention, Attention Training, CBT and Music Therapy, CBT and PMT, CBT with Parents Only, Cultural Storytelling, Family Psychoeducation, Hypnosis, Mindfulness, Relaxation, Stress Inoculation	Contingency Management, Group Therapy	Behavioral Activation and Exposure, Biofeedback, Play Therapy, PMT, Psychodynamic Therapy, Rational Emotive Therapy, Social Skills	Assessment/Monitoring, Attachment Therapy, Client Centered Therapy, EMDR, Peer Pairing, Psychoeducation, Relationship Counseling, Teacher Psychoeducation
Traumatic Stress	CBT, CBT with Parents, EMDR	Exposure	None	Play Therapy, Psychodrama, Relaxation and Expression	Advice/Encouragement, Client Centered Therapy, CBT and Medication, CBT with Parents Only, Education, Expressive Play, Interpersonal Therapy, Problem Solving, Psychodynamic Therapy, Psychoeducation, Relaxation, Structured Listening

Abbreviations: CBT, Cognitive Behavior Therapy; EMDR, Eye Movement Desensitization and Reprocessing; PMT, Parent Management Training; Level 5 refers to treatments whose tests were unsupportive or inconclusive. This report updates and replaces the "Blue Menu" originally distributed by the Hawaii Department of Health, Child and Adolescent Mental Health Division, Evidence-Based Services Committee from 2002–2009.

Excerpted from PracticeWise Evidence-Based Child and Adolescent Psychosocial Interventions, created for the period October 2017—April 2018, using the PracticeWise Evidence-Based Services Database, available at www.practicewise.com. See Appendix 6 for the full table and details on background and evidence. For biannual updates go to www.aap.org/en-us/documents/crpsychosocialinterventions.pdf.

Box 14-4. US Food and Drug Administration–Approved Psychopharmacological Interventions for Children and Adolescents (as of March 12, 2018)[a,b]	
Diagnostic Area	**Psychopharmacological Intervention**
Anxiety disorders	The only psychopharmacological interventions approved by the FDA for children and adolescents are the SSRIs fluoxetine, sertraline, and fluvoxamine; the TCA clomipramine for the treatment of OCD; and the SNRI duloxetine for GAD. Currently, no psychopharmacological interventions have been approved for other anxiety disorders, although a number of randomly controlled clinical trials suggest their efficacy and safety. Fluoxetine is approved for treatment of major depression in children aged ≥8 y and escitalopram for those aged ≥12 y. Depression often occurs along with anxiety, and treatment may effectively target symptoms of both disorders.
Trauma-related disorders	Approved medication may be helpful for co-occurring conditions as an adjunct to non-medication treatment focused on response to trauma. The SSRIs sertraline and paroxetine are approved for treatment of PTSD in adults.

Abbreviations: FDA, US Food and Drug Administration; GAD, generalized anxiety disorder; OCD, obsessive-compulsive disorder; PTSD, post-traumatic stress disorder; SNRI, serotonin and norepinephrine reuptake inhibitor; SSRI, selective serotonin reuptake inhibitor; TCA, tricyclic antidepressant.

[a] For up-to-date information about FDA-approved interventions, go to www.fda.gov/ScienceResearch/SpecialTopics/PediatricTherapeuticsResearch/default.htm.

[b] See also Chapter 11, Psychotropic Medications in Primary Care, for guidance in primary care prescribing.

care will involve, and understands what the referring clinician's ongoing role may be. If the specialty appointment is not likely to occur shortly, the child's PCC can work with the child and family on a plan to manage the problem in the meantime.

Note that not all evidence-based interventions may be available in every community. If a particular intervention is not available, this lack of intervention becomes an opportunity to collaborate with others in the community to advocate on behalf of children. Increasingly, states offer both telepsychiatry services and consultation and referral support "warm-lines" that help PCCs provide initial treatment and locate resources. The availability of the latter form of help is tracked at www.nncpap.org.

Reach agreement on respective roles in the child's care. If the child is referred to mental health specialty care for an anxiety disorder, the PCC may be responsible for initiating medication or adjusting doses, monitoring response to treatment, monitoring adverse effects, engaging and encouraging the child's and family's positive views of treatment, and coordinating care provided by parents, school, medical home, and specialists. In fact, the child may improve just knowing that the PCC is involved and interested.

Acknowledgments: The author and editor wish to acknowledge the contributions of Linda Paul, MPH, manager of the American Academy of Pediatrics Mental Health Leadership Work Group.

AAP Policy

American Academy of Pediatrics Section on Complementary and Integrative Medicine and Council on Children With Disabilities. Sensory integration therapies for children with developmental and behavioral disorders. *Pediatrics*. 2012;129(6):1186–1189 (pediatrics.aappublications.org/content/129/6/1186)

Thurber CA, Walton E; American Academy of Pediatrics Council on School Health. Preventing and treating homesickness. *Pediatrics*. 2007;119(1):192–201. Reaffirmed May 2012 (pediatrics.aappublications.org/content/119/1/192)

References

1. Connolly SD, Bernstein GA; Work Group on Quality Issues. Practice parameter for the assessment and treatment of children and adolescents with anxiety disorders. *J Am Acad Child Adolesc Psychiatry*. 2007;46(2):267–283
2. Merikangas KR. Vulnerability factors for anxiety disorders in children and adolescents. *Child Adolesc Psychiatr Clin N Am*. 2005;14(4):649–679
3. Bernal P. Hidden morbidity in pediatric primary care. *Pediatr Ann*. 2003;32(6):413–418
4. Williamson DE, Forbes EE, Dahl RE, Ryan ND. A genetic epidemiologic perspective on comorbidity of depression and anxiety. *Child Adolesc Psychiatr Clin N Am*. 2005;14(4):707–726
5. Foy JM; American Academy of Pediatrics Task Force on Mental Health. Enhancing pediatric mental health care: algorithms for primary care. *Pediatrics*. 2010;125(suppl 3):S109–S125
6. Wissow LS, Gadomski A, Roter D, et al. A cluster-randomized trial of mental health communication skills for pediatric generalists. *Pediatrics*. 2008;121(2): 266–275
7. Creswell C, Waite P, Cooper PJ. Assessment and management of anxiety disorders in children and adolescents. *Arch Dis Child*. 2014;99(7):674–678
8. Chisolm DJ, Klima J, Gardner W, Kelleher KJ. Adolescent behavioral risk screening and use of health services. *Adm Policy Ment Health*. 2009;36(6):374–380

CHAPTER 15

Disruptive Behavior and Aggression

Lawrence S. Wissow, MD, MPH

> *"Usually, what parents are hoping to hear is a combination of reassurances that the behavior will improve over time and concrete plans that will work toward improvement in the short term."*

Disruptive and aggressive behaviors are common among children from toddlerhood through adolescence. They may be transient, that is, influenced by temperament and environmental factors, or they may be persistent, rising to the level of oppositional defiant disorder (ODD) or conduct disorder (CD) and causing significant impairment in the child's and family's functioning. Oppositional defiant disorder affects 1% to 16% of children, depending on the population studied; CD affects 1.5% to 3.4%. Male to female ratio varies with age and diagnosis from a 3.2:1 ratio to a 5:1 ratio.[1] Some children progress from ODD to CD. They can be extremely challenging to treat and, if untreated, experience an increased risk of school failure, difficulty with legal authorities, substance use, and, ultimately, underemployment as adults. Those who go on to develop CD may be dangerous to themselves and others and, in some instances, require emergent treatment. All children and adolescents (collectively called *children* in the remainder of this chapter unless otherwise specified) manifesting disruptive or aggressive behaviors require intervention, education, support from parents and teachers, and careful monitoring.

There is accumulating evidence that some behavioral problems can be prevented. Effective strategies include population-based interventions,[2] supporting parents' moods and reducing exposure to stresses, helping parents learn to both read and help modulate infant emotions, and helping parents learn ways to stimulate and have positive interactions with their infants and young children. As children get older, pediatric primary care clinicians (PCCs)—pediatricians, family physicians, internists, nurse practitioners, and physician assistants who provide frontline, longitudinal care to children—can offer anticipatory guidance about predictable parenting issues, referrals to parenting workshops, and written or online parenting materials. See, for example, the "Child Development: Positive

Parenting Tips" Web page at www.cdc.gov/ncbddd/childdevelopment/ positiveparenting/index.html, "Everybody Gets Mad: Helping Your Child Cope With Conflict" Web page at www.healthychildren.org/English/ healthy-living/emotional-wellness/Pages/Everybody-Gets-Mad-Helping-Your-Child-Cope-with-Conflict.aspx, *Parents' Roles in Teaching Respect* handout at www.brightfutures.org/mentalhealth/pdf/families/mc/parent_ role.pdf, and *Play Nicely* video at www.playnicely.org. The American Academy of Pediatrics has published guidelines for effective discipline.[3]

The guidance in this chapter applies to the care of children presenting with symptoms of disruptive behavior or aggression in any pediatric clinical setting. Its audience is, therefore, all pediatric clinicians—PCCs, as well as pediatric subspecialists. In several places the chapter calls out PCCs for their specific role in the care of children experiencing disruptive behavior or aggression. The guidance in this chapter is based on the work of the World Health Organization, whose recommendations may be updated annually. The most up-to-date information can be found at www.who.int/ mental_health/publications/mhGAP_intervention_guide/en.

Findings Suggesting Disruptive Behavior or Aggression

Manifestations of disruptive behavior and aggression vary by age. In younger children, they include tantrums, defiance, fighting, and bullying. In older children and adolescents, they may include serious lawbreaking such as stealing, damage to property, or assault. A summary of the symptoms and clinical findings that suggest disruptive behavior and aggression can be found in Box 15-1. These may be elicited from parents, teachers, others familiar with the child or adolescent, and youths (children and adolescents aged 6–18 years) themselves. Children, youths, and even parents may minimize problems, and parents and teachers may be unaware of conduct problems that happen when the child is out of their direct supervision. Thus, tactful but persistent discussion and comparing notes among observers may be required to get a full picture of the child's behavioral issues.

Tools to Assist With Identification

Because some children and parents do not spontaneously disclose their symptoms to their PCCs, standardized psychosocial screening instruments

Box 15-1. Symptoms and Clinical Findings Suggesting Disruptive Behavior and Aggression

Indications of Disruptive Behavior and Aggression

- In younger children, marked tantrums, defiance, fighting, and bullying.

- In older children and adolescents, serious lawbreaking such as stealing, damage to property, or assault.

- Repetitive, persistent, excessive aggression or defiance; behaviors out of keeping with the child's development level, norms of peer group behavior, and cultural context indicating a disorder rather than a phase or transitional disruption.

- Aggression may be impulsive and associated with intense emotional states, or it may be predatory and premeditated. It is important to distinguish which pattern of aggression the child is showing.

Behaviors Characteristic of Oppositional Defiant Disorder

- Symptoms may be confined only to school, home, or the community.

- Angry outbursts.

- Loss of temper.

- Refusal to obey commands and rules.

- Destructiveness.

- Hitting.

- Intentional annoyance of others but without the presence of serious lawbreaking.

Behaviors Characteristic of Conduct Disorder

- Vandalism

- Cruelty to people and animals (including sexual and physical violence)

- Bullying

- Lying

- Stealing

- Truancy

- Drug and alcohol use

- Criminal acts

- All the features of ODD

Abbreviation: ODD, oppositional defiant disorder.

may be used to identify children with symptoms of disruptive behavior or aggression. Several instruments have versions to collect information from youths, parents, and teachers. For more information about these tools, see Appendix 2, Mental Health Tools for Pediatrics. Table 15-1 provides examples of general psychosocial screening results suggesting that a child has disruptive behavior or aggression. Use of additional instruments, such as the NICHQ Vanderbilt attention-deficit/hyperactivity disorder (ADHD) assessment scales (developed for children 6–12 years of age) and the Modified Overt Aggression Scale (developed for adults but sometimes used with adolescents), can help confirm findings of the initial screening; the use of a functional assessment tool, such as the Strengths and Difficulties Questionnaires (SDQ) or Columbia Impairment Scale, will help the pediatric clinician determine whether the child is significantly impaired by the symptoms. For adolescents, consider assessing the extent of substance use. Use of a tool to assess the effect of the child's problem on other members of the family may also be helpful; the Caregiver Strain Questionnaire is one example of such a tool. All these instruments require consideration of their results in the context of other clinical information obtained in the process of discussing the results with the child or youth and the family members. (See Appendix 2, Mental Health Tools for Pediatrics, for further details about each of these instruments.)

Assessment

Assessment begins by differentiating the child's or adolescent's symptoms from normal behavior. All children are defiant at times, and it is a normal part of adolescence to, at times, do or at least consider doing the opposite of what one is told. A problem or disorder may be present if the behaviors interfere with family life, school, or peer relationships, or put the child or others in danger. Children with disruptive behavior or aggression tend to exhibit repetitive and excessive aggression or defiance out of keeping with developmental and social norms. The behaviors persist, rather than appearing briefly as part of adaptation to a new situation or developmental period. Aggression may be impulsive and associated with intense emotional states, or it may be predatory and premeditated. It is important to distinguish which pattern of aggression the child is showing.

Some conditions, such as depression (with prominent irritability), anxiety (with a desire to avoid feared situations), ADHD, or sleep deprivation, can

Table 15-1. General Psychosocial Screening/Results Suggesting Disruptive Behavior and Aggression

Screening Instrument	Score
PSC-35	• Total score ≥24 for children aged ≤5 y. • ≥28 for those 6–16 y. • ≥30 for those aged ≥17 y. *and* • Further discussion of items related to disruptive behavior and aggression confirms a concern in that area.
PSC-17	• Externalizing subscale is ≥7. *and* • Further discussion of items related to disruptive behavior and aggression confirms a concern in that area.
SDQ	• Total symptom score of >19. • Conduct problem score of 5–10 (see instructions at www.sdqinfo.com). • Impact scale (back of form) score of 1 (medium impairment) or ≥2 (high impairment). *and* • Further discussion of items related to disruptive behavior and aggression confirms a concern in that area.
ASQ:SE-2	• Cutoff score varies by age-specific questionnaire.
ECSA	• Total score of ≥18. *and* • Thorough emotional and behavioral history, family history, and close follow-up. • Regardless of the total score, any items with a + circled should be explored further. These +'s correlate with a child's emotional or behavioral problems, although, in some cases, parental reassurance is all that is necessary. *Parent score* • A score of 1 or 2 on questions 39 and 40 identify depression in adult primary care settings. • Scores >0 on items 37 and 38 should be further investigated for maternal distress.

Abbreviations: ASQ:SE, Ages & Stages Questionnaires: Social-Emotional, Second Edition; ECSA, Early Childhood Screening Assessment; PSC, Pediatric Symptom Checklist; SDQ, Strengths and Difficulties Questionnaires.

mimic or co-occur with lesser degrees of disruptive behavior and aggression. Substance use may play a role in both minor forms and more severe forms of behavioral problems. Having witnessed or experienced trauma, or currently living in a stressful or an anxiety-provoking situation, may also provoke disruptive behavior. Table 15-2 summarizes these conditions.

In addition, perceptions of the child's symptoms may vary among caregivers or as a particular caregiver's circumstances change. A child whose

Table 15-2. Conditions That May Mimic or Co-occur With Disruptive Behavior and Aggression	
Condition	**Rationale**
ADHD	ADHD is a common comorbidity. Association of ODD and ADHD confers a poorer prognosis, and children tend to be more aggressive, have more behavioral problems that are more persistent, experience peer rejection at higher levels, and have more significant academic underachievement. See also Chapter 20, Inattention and Impulsivity.
Sleep deprivation	Sleep problems can cause irritability and contribute to outbursts of anger and poor impulse control. See Chapter 28, Sleep Disturbances.
Learning problems or disabilities	Unidentified learning difficulties can contribute to frustration and oppositional behavior. If disruptive or aggressive behavior is associated with problems of school performance, the child may have a learning disability. See Chapter 21, Learning Difficulty, to explore this possibility.
Developmental problems	Children with overall intellectual or social limitations may experience frustration and poor impulse control.
Exposure to ACEs	Children who have experienced or witnessed trauma, violence, a natural disaster, separation from a parent, parental divorce or separation, parental substance use, neglect, or physical, emotional, or sexual abuse are at high risk of developing emotional difficulties such as adjustment disorder or PTSD and may manifest outbursts of disruptive or aggressive behavior; this possibility should always be borne in mind because PTSD requires specific trauma-focused interventions. The clinician should tactfully explore the possibility that harsh physical or emotional punishment is related to the child's behavioral problem or that tensions might escalate to that point. Denial of trauma symptoms does not mean trauma did not occur; questions about ACEs should be repeated as a trusting relationship is established. See Chapter 14, Anxiety and Trauma-Related Distress.

Table 15-2. Conditions That May Mimic or Co-occur With Disruptive Behavior and Aggression (*continued*)

Condition	Rationale
Bereavement	Most children will experience the death of a family member or friend sometime in childhood. Other losses may also trigger grief responses, for example, separation or divorce of parents, relocation, change of school, deployment of a parent in military service, breakup with a girlfriend or boyfriend, or remarriage of parent. Such losses are traumatic. They may result in feelings of sadness, despair, insecurity, anger, or anxiety immediately following the loss and, in some instances, more persistent anxiety or mood problems, including PTSD or depression. In some children, such losses trigger aggressive or disruptive behavior. See also Chapter 22, Low Mood.
Anxiety	Many children with disruptive or aggressive behaviors have anxiety. When faced with demands that make them anxious, they use oppositional behavior to manage their anxiety or avoid the expectations that triggered their anxiety. See Chapter 14, Anxiety and Trauma-Related Distress.
Depression or bipolar disorders	Marked sleep disturbance, disturbed appetite, irritability, low mood, or tearfulness could indicate that a child is depressed. Symptoms of depression rapidly alternating with cycles of agitation may suggest bipolar disorder. Common symptoms of pediatric bipolar disorder include explosive or destructive tantrums, dangerous or hypersexual behavior, aggression, irritability, bossiness with adults, driven creativity (sometimes depicting graphic violence), excessive talking, separation anxiety, chronic depression, sleep disturbance, delusions, hallucinations, psychosis, and talk of homicide or suicide. See Chapter 22, Low Mood.
Substance use	All children exhibiting disruptive or aggressive behavior should be screened for substance use and use disorder, because drug effects or withdrawal from drugs may cause irritability and reduced self-control. See Chapter 30, Substance Use 1: Use of Tobacco and Nicotine, and Chapter 31, Substance Use 2: Use of Other Substances.
ASD	Children with this developmental pattern also have problems with social relatedness (eg, poor eye contact, preference for solitary activities), language (often stilted), and range of interest (persistent and intense interest in a particular activity or subject). They will often have very rigid expectations for routine or parent promises and become anxious or angry if these expectations are not met.

Abbreviations: ACE, adverse childhood experience; ADHD, attention-deficit/hyperactivity disorder; ASD, autism spectrum disorder; ODD, oppositional defiant disorder; PTSD, post-traumatic stress disorder.

behavior is perfectly acceptable in one setting may be seen as problematic in another where there are greater dangers or constraints or where a caregiver may be experiencing other stressors. Recognizing the influence of context can be therapeutic by itself and can lead to development of a more holistic approach to intervention engaging the child, the primary caregiver, and others who support them.

Plan of Care for Children With Disruptive Behavior or Aggression

Suicidal or homicidal intent is an emergency requiring immediate treatment and close supervision of the youth at all times. Other emergencies may involve parents who feel that they can no longer tolerate the child's behavior, parents who have considered expelling the child from the home or feel that they could harm the child, or situations in which the child's behavior is related to past or ongoing trauma. Community social service agencies often have crisis services that may be of help in these situations and that can provide either respite care or emergency in-home intervention.

The care of a child exhibiting disruptive behavior or aggression can begin in the primary care setting from the time symptoms are recognized, even if the child's symptoms do not rise to the level of a disorder or if referral to a mental health specialist is ultimately part of the care plan.

Engaging the Child and Family in Care

Without engagement, most families will not seek or persist in care. The process may require multiple visits.[4]

Reinforce strengths of the child and family (eg, good relationships with at least one parent or important adult, prosocial peers, concerned or caring family, help seeking, connection to positive organizations) as a method of engagement, and identify any barriers to addressing the problem (eg, stigma, family conflict, resistance to treatment). Use "common factors" techniques[5] to build trust and optimism, reach agreement on incremental next steps, develop a plan of care, and collaboratively determine the role of the pediatric clinician. These techniques can be represented by the HELP mnemonic, Box 15-2.

Box 15-2. Common Factors Mnemonic: HELP Build a Therapeutic Alliance

H = Hope

E = Empathy

L^2 = Language, Loyalty

P^3 = Permission, Partnership, Plan

Adapted from American Academy of Pediatrics. *Addressing Mental Health Concerns in Primary Care: A Clinician's Toolkit.* Elk Grove Village, IL: American Academy of Pediatrics; 2010. For the fully annotated mnemonic, please refer to Appendix 5.

Regardless of other roles, the pediatric clinician can encourage a positive view of treatment on the part of the youth and family. To do this, the clinician will likely have to manage visits in which strong negative emotions are expressed. Parents and youths may accuse each other of instigating problems, or they may make derogatory remarks about each other. Either party may express hopelessness about improving the situation, and youths, in particular, may refuse to speak or otherwise collaborate in care. Techniques for making the best of these encounters include avoiding taking sides, acknowledging the legitimacy of feelings, acknowledging the frequency with which these problems occur, reminding that strong feelings often occur when people care about each other, and offering to have separate conversations with the youth and parents so as to give both a chance to be fully heard.

One particular problem in families with oppositional children is that parents can become chronically angry and depressed, perpetuating a cycle of opposition. It may be necessary to talk with the parent or parents alone, empathizing with their difficulties (which often extend beyond problems with this particular child) and helping them find openings to appreciate their child and find hope that the situation will improve. At a moment when parents are feeling less vulnerable and more empowered (not usually at the beginning of care), linking them to services that support them or address their own mood issues may be helpful.

Providing Psychoeducation

Families can be assured that behavioral problems are common and something for which the clinician is well prepared to offer help. By the time families seek help, they are often discouraged and both angry and fearful of being criticized. Clinicians can help by emphasizing the great variation among children's temperaments and personalities, families' constantly evolving circumstances and stressors, and how these factors can combine to form challenges for any parent. Psychoeducation can often be tailored to a given situation by asking parents what they think are the causes of the child's behavioral problems. Clinicians can acknowledge the validity of these beliefs and, to the extent necessary, begin to sketch out a range of other possible contributing factors that can be explored as treatment progresses. Usually, what parents are hoping to hear is a combination of reassurances that the behavior will improve over time and concrete plans that will work toward improvement in the short term.

Encouraging Healthy Habits

Encourage exercise, outdoor play, balanced and consistent diet, sleep (critically important to mental health), avoidance of exposure to frightening or violent media, limits on cell phone use and on television and video games, positive and consistent (not punitive) experiences with parents, praise for good behavior, and reinforcement of strengths. This advice may extend to the parent; if the parent thinks that his or her ability to carry out normal activities is restricted by the child's behavior, it may be appropriate to see if there are ways the parent can feel freer to do routine or enjoyable activities.

Reducing Stress

Consider the environment (eg, family social history, parental depression screening, results of any family assessment tools administered, reports from child care or school). Questions to raise might include

▶ **Is stress on the parent or parents from causes other than the child leading to parental irritability or low mood, drinking, or greater demands for the child to behave? Are there ways for parents to get more support for themselves?** Explore parents' readiness to seek and accept help.

▶ **Do inconsistencies or differing beliefs about parenting among caregivers (eg, parents, grandparents) undermine attempts to create rules, limits, or consequences? Can caregivers agree on priority behavioral problems and how to address them?** Explore conflicts; seek agreement on common beliefs and achievable steps to help the child.

▶ **Are nonacademic issues such as the presence of bullying contributing to the behavior? Are there other social or behavioral challenges in school?** Collect information directly from the school to explore these issues.

If problems are mainly or exclusively at school, parents should request that the school assess the child for special educational needs and develop a plan to monitor behavior while at school. Pediatric clinicians can often provide support in these situations by communicating to the school the degree to which the parents are actively engaged in finding help for their child's problems.

Offering Initial Interventions

The strategies described in the following text are common elements of evidence-based and evidence-informed psychosocial interventions for disruptive behavior and aggression. They are applicable to the care of children with mild or emerging problems with disruptive behavior and aggression and to the care of those with impairing symptoms that do not rise to the level of a disorder. They can also be used as initial treatment of children with CD or ODD while readying them for referral or awaiting access to specialty care.

Promote daily positive joint activities between parents and the child or teen. The clinician can counsel parents to reinforce adherent, prosocial behavior using parental attention ("Catch 'em being good" [Ed Christopherson]). In addition, parents can encourage, praise, and reward specific, agreed-on, and desired (target) behaviors; both parents and clinicians can be reminded that positive reinforcement is a more powerful tool for behavior change than punishment. If appropriate, positive behaviors can be monitored with a chart. Parents can negotiate rewards with the child, remembering that positive regard from the parent is usually the most powerful. Change target behaviors every 2 to 6 weeks; change rewards more frequently. The choice of target behaviors and the time intervals for rewards should be developmentally appropriate. Parents can be encouraged to focus discipline on priority areas. Some minor unwanted behaviors can be ignored; often they will stop as the main focus of child-parent conflict improves. What is most important is that parents find a way to reduce the overall negative tone of interaction and find as many successes as possible about which to comment.

Encourage parents to focus on prevention. There are several ways for parents to do this. They can reduce positive reinforcement of disruptive behavior by not responding to negative bids for attention and by not engaging in discussion with the child when delivering a request or consequence. In contrast, when children seek attention in a prosocial way, parents should make every attempt to respond positively, even if the response is brief. When possible, parents can try to reorganize the child's day to prevent situations in which the child cannot control himself. Examples include asking a neighbor to look after the child while the parent goes shopping, ensuring that activities are available for long car journeys or other potentially boring activities, and arranging activities in separate rooms for siblings who are prone to fight. In addition, parents can monitor the whereabouts of adolescents by telephoning the parents of friends whom they say they are visiting. All children appreciate age-appropriate notice of what will be expected of them and opportunities to make choices about how to meet those expectations.

Parents can also determine ways to limit contact with friends who have behavioral problems and promote contact with friends who are a positive influence. If parents suspect the child's behavior may be caused or exacerbated by a learning problem, they can request that the school evaluate the child for learning problems.

Encourage parents to be calm and consistent. The clinician can suggest the following strategies to parents:

▶ Set clear house rules and give short, specific commands about the desired behavior, not prohibitions about undesired behavior (eg, "Please walk slowly," rather than "Don't run").

▶ Prioritize issues and target only a few key behaviors until things improve. Within these areas of behavior, make initial targets easily achievable.

▶ Provide consistent and calm consequences for misbehavior. Consequences should not be drastic or, in the case of young children, go on for so long that the child is likely to forget what he or she originally did wrong. Time-out should be brief (the rule of thumb for preschoolers is 1 minute per year of age); consequences for older children can involve brief loss of privileges or parental attention. Ideally, these punishments are mirrored by inverse responses for good behavior, especially more parental attention.

▶ Find a way for children to make reparation for a negative behavior (eg, doing something nice for a sibling they have struck, cleaning up a mess they made while in a tantrum), followed by praise.

▶ When enforcing a rule, avoid getting into arguments or explanations, because this action merely provides additional attention for the misbehavior; defer negotiations until periods of calm. If one parent has trouble staying calm when enforcing rules, make that parent the "rule maker" and another adult the "rule enforcer." The rule maker can point out the problem but defer action until the enforcer is present.

▶ If the behavior is taking place in public, quietly advise the child or youth that the problem has been noted but, if possible, defer a response until home or in a less public place.

▶ Consider parenting classes. Many parents find individual, group, written, or online support for parenting to be helpful, although for many getting referred to "parenting" feels as if they are getting remedial training and feels stigmatizing. Framing the referral as something tailored to the needs of a particular child, or as a way for the parent to spend some positive time with his or her own peers, may overcome the potential stigma.

▶ See also the suggestions in Chapter 20, Inattention and Impulsivity, including Box 20-3, Strategies for Working Constructively With a Child's School, and Guidelines for Homework Battles.

Create a safety and emergency plan. When behavioral problems are severe or involve threats of violence or running away, a care plan should be developed jointly with the family, including a listing of telephone numbers to call for emergencies. This listing can include hotlines, the on-call telephone number for the practice, or area mental health crisis response team contact information, according to community protocol. The clinician should also instruct the family to proactively remove weapons from the home and monitor for situations that trigger outbursts.

In many communities, it has become customary when children are deemed to be "out of control" to either bring them to an emergency department (ED) or call the police. Both of these are problematic responses with major risks. Children brought to EDs often face long waits for mental health evaluations; when police arrive, they have been known to handcuff even school-aged children. When oppositional behavior escalates to running away, throwing things, or seizing potentially dangerous objects and threatening others, calling non–mental health emergency responders may seem like an immediate path to safety. Parents should be counseled to think carefully whether these actions are truly being taken for safety reasons and not just as a more extreme form of punishment. Telling young children that the police may be called may make them frightened and further escalate their behaviors.

It is, of course, best to practice de-escalation techniques prior to these interventions being needed. These techniques include noticing when a child is starting to get agitated (there may be changes to body language or tone of voice), asking all involved adults to remain calm, and staging a quiet "show of force" (responsible adults gather, keep their distances, and calmly suggest that the child be calm as well so that whatever issues are at hand can be worked out). Resolution of these issues, unless emergent, should be delayed until everyone feels more relaxed. It may be best to have the discussion at the pediatric or mental health office, where everyone can feel supported by a neutral, trusted party.

Providing Resources

Offer the child and parents educational resources to assist them with self-management. See the introduction to this chapter for examples. Provide the family with contact numbers and resources in case of an emergency.

Monitoring the Child's Progress Toward Therapeutic Goals

Child care, preschool, or school reports can be helpful in monitoring progress. Screening instruments that gather information from multiple reporters (eg, youth, parent, and teacher), such as the SDQ and Pediatric Symptom Checklist, can be helpful in monitoring progress with symptoms and functioning.

It is important for the clinician to help the family understand that it is not uncommon for treatment to be successful for a period and then seem to lose effectiveness. This setback can happen when there are new stresses or demands or when, after a period of success, there has been a letup on treatment. If troubleshooting existing treatment and ways of dealing with new stresses do not help get function back to baseline, new treatments, or new diagnoses, need to be considered. In particular, as school demands increase, learning issues may need to be considered, even if they were not seen as contributing problems in the past.

Involving Specialists

Consider involving one or more specialists if the child does not respond to initial interventions or if indicated by the following clinical circumstances:

► Child is younger than 5 years and problems go beyond what is expected developmentally. Parents will likely need professional advocacy if their child is told that he or she may not return to a child care or preschool facility because of behavioral problems.

► Family is not able to maintain a calm, consistent, or safe environment.

► Child's behaviors are injurious to other children or animals.

► Child has comorbid depression.

► Child is experiencing severe dysfunction in any domain.

► Child has comorbid anxiety. (The combination of shyness, anxiety, and behavioral problems is thought to be particularly risky for future behavioral problems of a more serious nature.)

► An adolescent has co-occurring problems with substance use.

► Problems at school are interfering with academic achievement or relationships.

► Child or adolescent is involved with legal authorities. (This situation requires coordination with probation officers and understanding the terms of probation; simply reminding the adolescent and family of the consequences of violating probation can help promote participation in treatment or changes to lifestyle.)

When specialty care is needed, ensure that it is evidence informed and assist the family in accessing it. A variety of evidence-based and evidence-informed interventions are available for the treatment of emotional problems in young children and for CD and ODD in school-aged children and adolescents. Ideally, those referred for care in the mental health specialty system would have access to the safest and most effective treatments. Table 15-3 lists programs targeting young children and their families. Recommended psychosocial interventions are summarized in Table 15-4, based on current evidence and updated biannually at www.aap.org/mentalhealth. Box 15-3 summarizes psychopharmacological interventions approved at the time of this book's publication by the US Food and Drug Administration for treatment of aggression in children and adolescents.

Table 15-3. Evidence-Based Parenting Programs

Cluster Area	Parenting Program
For disruptive behavioral problems	• The Incredible Years (www.incredibleyears.com) • Triple P – Positive Parenting Program (www.triplep.net) • Parent-Child Interaction Therapy (http://pcit.phhp.ufl.edu) • "Helping the Noncompliant Child" parent training program (www.guilford.com/books/Helping-the-Noncompliant-Child/McMahon-Forehand/9781593852412)
For high-risk pregnant women (If first-time mother, refer before 28 weeks' gestation.)	• Nurse-Family Partnership (www.nursefamilypartnership.org)
For children in foster care	• Attachment and Biobehavioral Catch-up (www.infantcaregiverproject.com) • Multidimensional Treatment Foster Care Program for Preschoolers (www.tfcoregon.com) • Parent-Child Interaction Therapy (www.pcit.org)
For parent-child relationship disturbances and high-risk parenting situations	• Circle of Security (www.circleofsecurity.net) • Promoting First Relationships (www.pfrprogram.org) • Parents as Teachers (www.parentsasteachers.org) • Child-Parent Psychotherapy (http://childtrauma.ucsf.edu/child-parent-psychotherapy-training)
For children exposed to trauma, including sexual abuse or domestic violence	• Child-Parent Psychotherapy • TF-CBT (http://tfcbt.musc.edu)

Abbreviation: TF-CBT, trauma-focused cognitive behavioral therapy.

Approaches to improving the referral process include making sure that the family is ready for this step in care, that they have some idea of what the specialty care will involve, and that they understand what the clinician's ongoing role may be. If the specialty appointment is not likely to occur in the near future, the clinician can work with parents on a plan to manage the problem as well as possible in the meantime.

Table 15-4. Psychosocial Therapies for Disruptive Behavior and Aggression: Evidence Base as of April 2018					
Problem Area	Level 1 – Best Support	Level 2 – Good Support	Level 3 – Moderate Support	Level 4 – Minimal Support	Level 5 – No Support
Delinquency and Disruptive Behavior	Anger Control, Assertiveness Training, CBT, Contingency Management, Multisystemic Therapy, PMT, PMT and Problem Solving, Problem Solving, Social Skills, Therapeutic Foster Care	CBT and PMT, CBT and Teacher Training, Communication Skills, Cooperative Problem Solving, Family Therapy, Functional Family Therapy, PMT and Classroom Management, PMT and Social Skills, Rational Emotive Therapy, Relaxation, Self Control Training, Transactional Analysis	Client Centered Therapy, Moral Reasoning Training, Outreach Counseling, Peer Pairing	CBT and Teacher Psychoeducation, Exposure, Physical Exercise, PMT and Classroom Management and CBT, PMT and Self-Verbalization, Stress Inoculation	Behavioral Family Therapy, Catharsis, CBT with Parents, Education, Family Empowerment and Support, Family Systems Therapy, Group Therapy, Imagery Training, Play Therapy, PMT and Peer Support, Psychodynamic Therapy, Self Verbalization, Skill Development, Wraparound

Abbreviations: CBT, Cognitive Behavior Therapy; PMT, Parent Management Training; Level 5 refers to treatments whose tests were unsupportive or inconclusive. This report updates and replaces the "Blue Menu" originally distributed by the Hawaii Department of Health, Child and Adolescent Mental Health Division, Evidence-Based Services Committee from 2002–2009.

Excerpted from PracticeWise Evidence-Based Child and Adolescent Psychosocial Interventions, created for the period October 2017—April 2018, using the PracticeWise Evidence-Based Services Database, available at www.practicewise.com. See Appendix 6 for the full table and details on background and evidence. For biannual updates go to www.aap.org/en-us/documents/crpsychosocialinterventions.pdf.

Box 15-3. US Food and Drug Administration–Approved Psychopharmacological Interventions (as of March 12, 2018)[a,b]	
Diagnostic Area	**Psychopharmacological Intervention**
Aggression	The FDA has no approved indications for aggression in children and adolescents apart from irritability-associated aggression in children with ASD (risperidone and aripiprazole). In other populations, recent federally supported evidence-based reviews suggest efficacy for some psychotherapeutic agents.

Abbreviations: ASD, autism spectrum disorder; FDA, US Food and Drug Administration.

[a] For up-to-date information about FDA-approved interventions, go to www.fda.gov/ScienceResearch/SpecialTopics/PediatricTherapeuticsResearch/default.htm.

[b] See also Chapter 11, Psychotropic Medications in Primary Care, for guidance in primary care prescribing.

Note that not all evidence-based interventions may be available in every community. If a particular intervention is not available, this lack of intervention becomes an opportunity to collaborate with others in the community to advocate on behalf of children. Increasingly, states offer both telepsychiatry services and consultation and referral support "warmlines" that help PCCs provide initial treatment and locate resources. The availability of the latter form of help is tracked at www.nncpap.org.

Reach agreement on respective roles in the child's care. If the child is referred to mental health specialty care, the PCC may be responsible for monitoring response to treatment through use of parent and teacher reports and communication with referral sources or agencies involved in care; engaging and encouraging a positive view of treatment; coordinating care provided by parents, school, medical home, and specialists; and observing for comorbidities.

Acknowledgments: The author and editor wish to acknowledge the contributions of Linda Paul, MPH, manager of the American Academy of Pediatrics Mental Health Leadership Work Group.

References

1. Loeber R, Burke JD, Lahey BB, Winters A, Zera M. Oppositional defiant and conduct disorder: a review of the past 10 years, part I. *J Am Acad Child Adolesc Psychiatry*. 2000;39(12):1468–1484

2. World Health Organization. *The World Report on Violence and Health*. Geneva, Switzerland: World Health Organization; 2002

3. American Academy of Pediatrics Committee on Psychosocial Aspects of Child and Family Health. Guidance for effective discipline. *Pediatrics*. 1998;101(4, pt 1): 723–728

4. Foy JM; American Academy of Pediatrics Task Force on Mental Health. Enhancing pediatric mental health care: algorithms for primary care. *Pediatrics*. 2010;125(suppl 3):S109–S125

5. Wissow LS, Gadomski A, Roter D, et al. A cluster-randomized trial of mental health communication skills for pediatric generalists. *Pediatrics*. 2008;121(2):266–275

CHAPTER 16

Eating Abnormalities

Marcie Schneider, MD, and Martin Fisher, MD

> *"...there may be no clinical condition encountered in pediatric and adolescent medicine in which medical and mental health care are as closely intertwined as is true in the diagnosis, evaluation, and management of eating abnormalities and disorders."*

Introduction

Eating abnormalities are a frequently encountered occurrence in pediatric practice. Pediatric clinicians—primary care clinicians (PCCs) (pediatricians, family physicians, internists, nurse practitioners, and physician assistants who provide frontline care to children and adolescents), as well as pediatric subspecialists—are called on to provide counseling and management for a wide variety of eating concerns, ranging from picky eating in younger children to severe eating disorders in older children and adolescents. In many cases, especially for younger children, simple guidance and reassurance may be all that is required. In some cases, especially in older children and adolescents, the presence of an eating disorder requires complex medical and mental health care. In fact, there may be no clinical condition encountered in pediatric and adolescent medicine in which medical and mental health care are as closely intertwined as is true in the diagnosis, evaluation, and management of eating abnormalities and disorders.

Accordingly, this chapter will focus on the eating abnormalities and disorders that are encountered in pediatric practice. As was made clear in the fifth edition of the *Diagnostic and Statistical Manual of Mental Disorders* (*DSM-5*), published by the American Psychiatric Association in 2013,[1] this includes both the classic eating disorders that are associated with body-image concerns (anorexia nervosa [AN], bulimia nervosa [BN], and their various subtypes) and the more recently described eating disorder not associated with body-image concerns (avoidant/restrictive food intake disorder [ARFID]).

Definitions

For more than 20 years, the diagnostic criteria for the eating disorders were based on the fourth edition (and fourth edition text revision) of the *Diagnostic and Statistical Manual of Mental Disorders* (*DSM-IV* and *DSM-IV-TR*).[2] The publication of the *DSM-5* in May 2013 has resulted in significant changes in the definition of the major eating disorders, which have, in turn, resulted in improved diagnostic accuracy.[1] Whereas more than 50% of pediatric and adolescent patients with eating disorders were receiving diagnoses of "eating disorders not otherwise specified" (commonly known as EDNOS) using the *DSM-IV* criteria, almost all children and adolescents with eating disorders are now receiving specific diagnoses using the new *DSM-5* criteria.[3]

The 4 major eating disorders in the *DSM-5* are AN, BN, binge-eating disorder (BED), and the more newly described diagnosis referred to as ARFID.

Anorexia nervosa, per the *DSM-5,* is defined by the restriction of dietary intake, which results in a low body weight compared to what is expected in the context of the patient's age, sex, pubertal stage, and physical health. Additionally, there is an intense fear of gaining weight and a distortion in body image. Patients are also categorized as having restricting or bingeing and purging subtypes of AN. To describe patients who start out as overweight and then develop eating disorder thoughts and behaviors, but who have normal weight or still are overweight, the *DSM-5* added a diagnosis of atypical AN under a category entitled "Other Specified Eating and Feeding Disorder."

Bulimia nervosa, per the *DSM-5,* is defined by binge eating and participating in repeated behaviors to prevent weight gain (vomiting, use of laxatives or diuretics, use of diet pills, restricting food, or overexercise, or any combination of those behaviors) at least once a week over a 3-month period. Patients with BN feel overly influenced by the appearance of their bodies. A new diagnosis, purging disorder (PD), has been added to the "Other Specified Eating and Feeding Disorder" category in the *DSM-5* to describe patients who purge but do not binge, which is a more common phenomenon in adolescents than it is in adults.

Binge-eating disorder, per the *DSM-5,* is defined by binge eating at least once a week for 3 months without any compensatory behaviors and marked distress about bingeing.

Avoidant/restrictive food intake disorder, per the *DSM-5,* is defined as a problem with eating that causes significant weight loss or lack of expected gain, a decline in social functioning, and possible dependence on nutritional supplements, all of which are not caused by a medical reason or lack of available nutrition. Importantly, no body-image distortion is present, as is found in patients with AN.

Epidemiology

Anorexia Nervosa

Conservatively, AN occurs in 0.5% to 1.0% of girls and young women and 0.2% of boys and young men.[4,5] A bimodal peak of onset occurs during the adolescent and young adult years at 14.5 and 18 years of age.[6] Increasingly, the onset of AN has been seen in both prepubertal children and adults.[7] Mortality is higher than in any other psychiatric illness, up to 5% per decade after the onset of the eating disorder.[8,9] With the introduction of the new diagnosis of atypical AN, preliminary data indicate that among adolescents with AN, the ratio of patients with AN to those with atypical AN is 3:2.[3]

Bulimia Nervosa

Up to 15% of adolescents report binge eating, purging, or both.[10,11] However, only 2.0% of female adolescents and 0.3% of male adolescents actually meet full diagnostic criteria for BN.[5,12,13] The peak prevalence of lifetime BN is reported to be 2% to 4% among white Western girls and women aged 17 to 25 years,[13,14] with a modal age of onset of 18 to 19 years.[15,16] Bulimia nervosa occurs in patients younger than 14 years, but this situation is very rare.[17] There is minimal data so far on the epidemiology of the new diagnosis of PD. In one of our own programs, the ratio of patients with BN to those with PD was 2:1.[3]

Avoidant/Restrictive Food Intake Disorder

There are no epidemiological data available yet to indicate the prevalence of ARFID as a diagnosis in the general population of children and adolescents. What is known to date is that among patients who present to adolescent medicine eating disorder programs, approximately 15% to 20% have a diagnosis of ARFID, and the ratio of girls to boys is in the 70:30 range, in contrast to the 90:10 range for both AN and BN.[3,18,19] It has not yet been determined how many of these patients have a shorter-term diagnosis (ie, those who decreased their eating recently because of a fear of choking or vomiting or gastrointestinal [GI] symptoms) and how many have a longer-term diagnosis (ie, those who have had restricted eating for many years). And among this latter group it is not yet clear how many children and adolescents can be classified as having an eating abnormality that is not affecting their growth or psychosocial functioning in a meaningful way and how many are at the level of having a diagnosis of ARFID.

Etiology

Several factors most likely converge in the development of an eating disorder. The adolescent who is culturally primed, biologically at risk, and psychologically vulnerable may begin dieting or vomiting in response to a particular precipitant (often an insult by family or friends, exposure to another individual who has an eating disorder, or a stressful situation). The positive psychological feedback that initially accompanies a perceived improved appearance and the biochemical changes that occur in response to decreased nutrition may serve to perpetuate the behavior.

Genetic factors have been linked to AN and BN.[20,21] There may be pubertal activation of these factors. Additionally, there is evidence of interplay between genetic and environmental factors.[22] Leptin and endocrine abnormalities in the hypothalamic-pituitary-adrenal axis have been linked to eating disorders.[23,24] Dieting itself is an important risk factor for developing an eating disorder.[25] More recently, the predilection of many in society to eat "healthy diets" can lead to dietary restrictions that cause weight loss and the onset of an eating disorder.

Risk Factors

A family history of eating disorders increases the risk for having an eating disorder by 7- to 12-fold.[26] A greater prevalence of eating disorders in monozygotic vs dizygotic twins is present, and 54% to 83% of the variance in BN can be accounted for by genetic factors.[26] Twin studies have shown AN to be heritable in 33% to 84% of cases and BN to be heritable in 28% to 83%.[21] Molecular genetic research studies on several genes, including the most recent study on estrogen-related receptor α (*ESRRA*) and histone deacetylase 4 (*HDAC4*) mutations,[27] provide a new and exciting area of study aimed at gaining an understanding of the genetics of these disorders. In addition to the genetic risk factors for the development of eating disorders discussed previously, other risk factors considered in the literature are presented in Box 16-1.

Comorbid Psychiatric Conditions

It is exceedingly common for patients with eating disorders to have comorbid psychiatric conditions. These conditions most prominently include depression, anxiety, and obsessive-compulsive disorder (OCD).[28] Depression can be both a cause of the initiation of an eating disorder and a result of the malnutrition that develops as part of AN. In terms of anxiety and OCD, the diagnoses of AN and BN and the diagnosis of ARFID all involve anxiety, as well as obsessive thoughts, about food and weight. And it has been shown that patients with a diagnosis of anxiety or OCD (or both) have a higher propensity for the development of eating disorders, of all types, than those in the general population.[29,30] Family studies have also shown that first-degree relatives of those with eating disorders are at higher risk for the presence of depression, anxiety, and OCD, as well as the development of an eating disorder. In the case of BN, it is established that patients are prone to other externalizing behaviors (including high-risk behaviors such as smoking, drinking, and substance use, and self-harm behaviors, including cutting and suicidal ideation) and are more commonly diagnosed as having a bipolar disorder or borderline personality disorder or as having a history of sexual abuse (or both).

Box 16-1. Risk Factors for the Development of an Eating Disorder

Risk Factors for Anorexia Nervosa

- Low self-esteem
- Perfectionism
- Obsessiveness
- Family history of eating disorders
- Family dieting
- Focus on weight in the family
- Preterm and small for gestational age
- Possible links to chromosomes 1, 2, 4, and 13 and to serotonergic or dopaminergic genes

Risk Factors for Bulimia Nervosa

- Dieting
- Links to chromosomes 10 and 14 genes
- Early menarche
- Early sexual experiences in both females and males
- Early or late puberty
- Obesity
- Parental obesity
- Urbanization
- Childhood sexual abuse
- Premorbid negative self-evaluation
- Parental alcohol use
- Low parental contact
- High parental expectations
- Family history of mood disorders or eating disorders
- High levels of family conflict
- Inadequate expression of emotions
- Lack of parental warmth and care
- Impulsivity

Risk Factors for Avoidant/Restrictive Food Intake Disorder

- Anxiety
- Sensitivity to textures
- Autism spectrum disorder

Findings Suggesting an Eating Abnormality

The patient who has an eating abnormality may seek medical care in a variety of ways. Some patients visit their PCC or an adolescent specialist because of concern about weight loss, vomiting, or abnormal eating attitudes noticed by family, friends, or school authorities; others visit a gynecologist or pediatric endocrinologist because of the menstrual irregularities that characteristically accompany the disorder; still others visit a pediatric gastroenterologist because of GI symptoms or weight loss. Many patients are seen first by a psychiatrist, psychologist, or social worker; others may be seen for the first time in an emergency department because of dehydration or other medical complications. Some patients may be seen within weeks of the disorder's onset; others avoid medical care for months or even years. Being brought in for an initial evaluation against one's will is common for many patients, although some may seek help willingly. Many patients who have mild to moderate eating disorders, either AN and BN, avoid medical care altogether by hiding or denying their illness.[10] Patients with restricted eating and longer-term ARFID may be followed for many years before psychosocial or growth difficulties begin to emerge as a child reaches the preadolescent or adolescent years.

In cases of AN, it may be the PCC who first notices a falloff in weight, or sometimes in height, that indicates the presence of an eating disorder, or, more often, in cases of either AN or BN, it is the PCC who is the first person a family brings their child or adolescent to when they, or their school, suspect there is an eating disorder. In the case of ARFID, it is the PCC who follows children who are eating poorly throughout the childhood years and it is the PCC who is most likely called on to determine when it is something that requires attention. This determination generally involves making the distinction between an eating abnormality that may require only primary care intervention and an eating disorder that will require a full diagnostic workup and multidisciplinary treatment. Symptoms and clinical findings that suggest the presence of an eating disorder are presented in Box 16-2.

Box 16-2. Symptoms and Clinical Findings That Suggest Disordered Eating

Physical symptoms of AN or ARFID may include

- Cold hands and feet
- Dry skin
- Alopecia or thinning hair
- Constipation
- Fatigue
- Amenorrhea
- Dizziness
- Easy bruising

Social manifestations of AN or ARFID may include

- Socially withdrawn personality
- Asexual orientation
- Avoidance of eating with anyone
- Increased irritability
- Family dysfunction or family difficulties or both
- Possibly a decline in school performance

Physical symptoms of BN may include

- Fullness
- Constipation
- Fatigue
- Menstrual changes
- Heartburn

Social symptoms of BN include

- Secretive eating
- Frequent bathroom use

Abbreviations: AN, anorexia nervosa; ARFID, avoidant/restrictive food intake disorder; BN, bulimia nervosa.

Initial Assessment

When the pediatric clinician is called on to evaluate a child or an adolescent who presents with symptoms suggesting an eating disorder, she or he first needs to know what the child or adolescent is eating. The initial assessment is then focused on 3 sets of questions.

1. Has the child's or adolescent's eating changed? (If so, why?)

2. Are there decreases in weight, height, or body mass index (BMI), or any combination of those measurements, either in real-time measurements or as reflected in the growth curve?

3. Are there abnormal behaviors such as purposeful vomiting; use of diet pills, laxatives, or diuretics; periods of fasting or starvation; or excessive exercise?

In the assessment of the child or adolescent who has mildly abnormal eating patterns, such as those who are picky eaters, the answers to all these questions will be no. For those children and adolescents, even those who eat a minimal range of foods, as long as there are neither changes in eating patterns nor decreases in weight or BMI curves, watchful waiting may well be the most appropriate approach.

Among those with changes in eating or changes in weight or both, diagnoses of ARFID or AN should be considered. For those who do not have body-image concerns, including those who have almost always eaten poorly and are now falling off their growth curves, or those who have decreased their eating for other reasons (such as fear of choking or vomiting, anxiety, or GI symptoms), a diagnosis of ARFID is made and a workup is begun. For those with body-image concerns, the diagnosis is in the AN category, either the more classic AN in those who are underweight or the newer diagnosis of atypical AN for those who have normal weight or still are overweight despite a significant and unhealthy weight loss.

And last, for those with abnormal eating behaviors (eg, vomiting, laxatives) a diagnosis of BN or PD is made. According to the results of the initial assessment just described, an initial set of intervention steps are begun (Box 16-3).

Box 16-3. Initial Interventions for Children With Eating Abnormalities

- Present and explain the presumptive diagnosis or the diagnoses under consideration.

- Outline the steps that will be required in the evaluation.

- Provide dietary recommendations (for those with less concerning eating abnormalities or milder eating disorders) or a referral to a registered dietician (for those who require more detailed nutritional counseling).

- Discuss options for further evaluation and management of the mental health aspects of care (which can include a recommendation for psychotherapy or a referral to a psychiatrist or both).

- Plan for a follow-up visit or an eating disorder/adolescent medicine program referral.

Differential Diagnosis

The differential diagnosis of the eating disorders described in this chapter includes possible medical causes of weight loss or vomiting and other psychiatric causes of poor appetite. Included in the differential diagnosis are malignancies and central nervous system tumors; GI problems, including malabsorption, celiac disease, and inflammatory bowel disease; endocrinologic problems such as diabetes mellitus, hyperthyroidism, and hypopituitarism; chronic illnesses and chronic infections; and superior mesenteric artery syndrome. The history, physical examination, and baseline laboratory tests should help rule out most of these diagnoses; further testing may be necessary if the weight loss or vomiting cannot be explained adequately. Magnetic resonance imaging (MRI) of the brain, endoscopy, or other tests may be considered in some cases for patients who claim to be eating well or not vomiting on purpose. In some instances, a patient may show obvious pleasure in the weight loss or vomiting brought on by another disorder; however, this circumstance must not be confused with a positive diagnosis of AN or BN.

Psychiatric causes of weight loss can include depression, OCD, and psychosis (especially schizophrenia). The patient who refuses to eat because of a desire to lose weight must be differentiated from the patient who cannot eat because of depression or the patient who will not eat because of delusional fears (eg, that the food is poisoned). Although patients may have concomitant depression or psychosis with AN or BN, separate criteria must be used to establish each entity. A full psychosocial history must be obtained as part of the initial evaluation to establish both the diagnosis and the psychosocial severity of the disorder. (See Chapter 6, Iterative Mental Health Assessment.) The patient's functioning in the family, in school, and among peers must be evaluated, and possible psychiatric symptoms such as sleep disorders, hallucinations, delusions, or obsessions should be elicited. Almost all patients with an eating disorder exhibit psychosocial changes with the onset of the illness. These changes generally include fighting with the family, withdrawing from friends, and performing less optimally in school, although some patients paradoxically report improved school performance as they withdraw from friends and family. If additional psychiatric symptoms are found, the possibility of an additional diagnosis should be pursued.

Evaluation

Application of the specific diagnostic criteria for eating disorders listed in the *DSM-5* serves to both elucidate the diagnosis and determine the severity of the illness. Distortion of body image, a hallmark in the diagnosis of AN, may be evaluated by exploring the patient's views of initial, current, and desired weights. Establishing the patient's eating and exercise patterns and use of vomiting or medications designed to promote weight loss (including diet pills, laxatives, diuretics, and ipecac) provides hints to both the diagnosis and the possibility of medical complications. Care must be taken to avoid being misled by the patient who is not completely forthright; the results of the physical examination and laboratory tests often suggest the true extent of the patient's disorder.

Anorexia Nervosa and ARFID

History

Initial evaluation of the patient with weight loss includes a determination of the diagnosis and its severity, an evaluation of other possible causes of weight loss and the effects of malnutrition, an analysis of the psychological context of the illness, and a decision about treatment. Relevant history includes the patient's recollection of height, maximum weight, minimum weight, current weight, and desired weight. Additionally, evaluation for a distortion in body image, a history of bingeing or purging, and a history of overexercising is necessary. On the review of systems, symptoms of malnutrition, including alopecia, cold hands and feet, dry skin, constipation, fatigue, and amenorrhea, may be present. For girls, a full menstrual history should be obtained, including age at menarche, last normal menstrual period, usual length of menses, heaviness of flow, presence of dysmenorrhea, and regularity of menses. A comprehensive nutrition history should be obtained, both in patients suspected of having AN and in those suspected of having ARFID, with a focus on changes in eating patterns over time.

Physical Examination

The first steps in the physical examination of the patient who is thought to have AN or ARFID include measuring height, weight, and vital signs; plotting the height, weight, and BMI on the patient's growth curve; and calculation of the percentage below ideal body weight (IBW). The percentage below IBW, which may be calculated by comparing the patient's current weight with the average weight expected for height, age, and sex (as determined by standard pediatric growth charts), serves both as one of the diagnostic criteria and as a gross estimate of the degree of malnutrition. For patients with either AN or ARFID, body weight more than 25% below IBW represents severe malnutrition, body weight 20% below IBW represents moderate malnutrition, and body weight not yet 20% below IBW represents mild malnutrition. However, for patients with atypical AN, who start out as overweight and are not yet technically considered underweight at presentation, the degree of malnutrition must be determined by comparing the patient's current weight with both the patient's highest weight and the patient's IBW for height. Pediatric growth charts (www.cdc.gov/growthcharts) are needed to evaluate patients with AN, atypical AN, or ARFID; these charts are especially important for premenarchal girls and growing boys in order to determine previous heights and weights as a way to establish appropriate weight goals for achievement of expected adult height. Plotting height, weight, and BMI on the patient's growth curve gives perspective to the current weight and the current height. For older children and younger adolescents with AN, it can be a change in pattern on the growth curve that may be the first indication of the presence of an eating disorder; for patients with ARFID, it is often growth curve changes that distinguish between children or young adolescents who are just picky eaters and those who have developed a clinical diagnosis.

Vital signs provide further evidence of the degree of malnutrition because chronic malnutrition associated with each of the eating disorder diagnoses is accompanied by declines in blood pressure, pulse, and electrocardiographic (ECG) voltage.[31] Other cardiovascular changes can include sinus bradycardia, prolonged QTc, orthostatic hypotension, increased vagal tone, poor myocardial contractility, mitral valve prolapse, pericardial effusion, and decreased left-ventricular mass.[32] So the patient's orthostatic changes can be documented accurately, the patient's blood pressure and pulse should be checked in the sitting position, followed by standing for 2 minutes. An increase of 20 beats/min in pulse, a decrease of 20 mm Hg in systolic blood pressure, or a decrease of 10 mm Hg in diastolic blood pressure is considered significant.[33] Other physical findings associated with malnutrition include scaphoid abdomen, muscle wasting, acrocyanosis, decreased subcutaneous fat, lanugo hair similar to that seen on newborns, ecchymoses, diminished reflexes, and dry skin. The physical findings and medical complications of AN and BN are outlined in Box 16-4.

Laboratory Evaluation

Laboratory tests further elucidate the severity of the illness. Most patients who have AN or ARFID have normal laboratory results initially, although all organ systems are probably affected by the malnutrition. The laboratory abnormalities found on routine testing are related generally to the individual's particular nutritional pattern. Thus, the patient who is chronically malnourished may have leukopenia, thrombocytopenia (occasionally), and, in rare cases, severe anemia (being protected for some time from iron-deficiency anemia by the concomitant amenorrhea). The patient who restricts fluid intake may show evidence of dehydration (including an elevated sodium or serum urea nitrogen concentration), whereas the patient who drinks excessive fluids to satisfy hunger or the physician's scale may show signs of hyponatremia and dilute urine. Conversely, the patient who vomits or uses laxatives may show evidence of hypokalemia, which is often severe in people who use both methods of weight control. Nutrient values, including levels of zinc, calcium, magnesium, copper,

Box 16-4. Physical Findings and Medical Complications of Anorexia Nervosa and Bulimia Nervosa

Anorexia Nervosa

- Acrocyanosis
- Alopecia
- Dry skin
- Lanugo hair
- Ecchymosis
- Fatigue
- Hypothermia
- Muscle wasting
- Bloating
- Postprandial fullness
- Decreased subcutaneous fat
- Decreased deep tendon reflexes
- Constipation
- Delayed gastric emptying
- Delayed gastric motility
- Orthostatic hypotension
- Bradycardia
- Mitral valve prolapse
- Pericardial effusion
- ECG abnormalities, including prolonged QT interval
- Decreased left-ventricular mass and contractility
- Psychomotor retardation
- Growth delay
- Pubertal delay
- Amenorrhea or menstrual irregularity
- Osteopenia and osteoporosis
- Cortical atrophy on MRI
- Electrolyte abnormalities from water loading or purging
- Hypercholesterolemia without hyperlipidemia
- Euthyroid sick syndrome
- Low levels of LH, FSH, and estradiol
- Elevated cortisol level
- Low IGF-1 level
- Low leptin level

> **Box 16-4. Physical Findings and Medical Complications of Anorexia Nervosa and Bulimia Nervosa (*continued*)**
>
> <u>Bulimia Nervosa</u>
> - Hypertension or hypotension
> - Electrolyte abnormalities, including hypokalemia, hypochloremia, and elevated serum bicarbonate level
> - Dehydration
> - Erosion of dental enamel
> - Calluses on the dorsum of the hand
> - Parotid enlargement
> - Acute pancreatitis
> - Acute gastric dilatation or rupture
> - Mallory-Weiss tears
> - Gastroesophageal irritation
> - Gastroesophageal bleeding
> - GERD
> - Barrett esophagus
> - Aspiration pneumonia
> - Diarrhea, constipation, steatorrhea
> - Emetine cardiomyopathy
> - Menstrual irregularity
> - PCOS
> - Osteopenia and osteoporosis
>
> ---
>
> Abbreviations: ECG, electrocardiographic; FSH, follicle-stimulating hormone; GERD, gastroesophageal reflux disease; IGF-1, insulinlike growth factor 1; LH, luteinizing hormone; MRI, magnetic resonance image; PCOS, polycystic ovarian syndrome.

vitamin B_{12}, and folate, may all be altered in the malnourished patient, but they are usually normal. Hormonal testing may produce evidence of dysfunction in the endocrine system.[34] Development of a relative hypothyroidism caused by a combination of euthyroid sick syndrome and decreased production on a hypothalamic basis is believed to be an adaptive response to inadequate nutrition. Hypothyroidism is generally evident by low-normal levels of triiodothyronine, thyroxine, thyrotropin, or any combination of those hormones. Amenorrhea, or menstrual irregularity, may develop and is accompanied by low levels of luteinizing hormone (LH) and follicle-stimulating hormone (FSH). Hypercortisolemia with loss of diurnal variation, low levels of insulinlike growth factor 1 (IGF-1) and leptin, increased ghrelin level, and increased peptide Y level are seen in patients with AN, although these tests need not be performed in most patients.[35,36]

In general, the initial laboratory workup of patients with AN or ARFID includes a complete blood cell count (CBC), evaluation of levels of serum electrolytes, liver and thyroid function tests, and evaluation of levels of LH, FSH, estradiol, and prolactin in patients who have amenorrhea. Obtaining a urinalysis result for specific gravity and ketonuria is often helpful. An ECG is obtained for people with bradycardia. This battery of tests is generally sufficient to provide a barometer of current status, a baseline to monitor further changes, and screening for other possible causes of weight loss. Data have demonstrated that patients who have eating disorders, especially those whose amenorrhea is prolonged because of malnutrition, show evidence of osteopenia on bone-density studies.[37] Initial studies have shown that this effect may not be preventable, even with calcium supplementation or hormonal replacement, or completely reversible, even after patients regain their normal weight.[38] A 3-fold increase in the long-term risk for fracture development has been seen in patients with a history of AN.[39] Studies are underway to determine the possible causes of osteopenia, including hypoestrogenemia, hypercortisolemia, and decreased IGF-1 level. Bone-density values in patients with AN are correlated with BMI, age at onset, and duration of illness.[40] Bone densitometry, using dual energy x-ray absorptiometry, has become a common determination in the evaluation of patients who have eating disorders and amenorrhea of at least 6 to 12 months' duration.[41] Evidence of abnormalities may be found on computed tomography and MRI of the brain, but these tests are generally reserved for evaluating other possible causes when the diagnosis is in question. Magnetic resonance image changes in the brain, including gray-matter deficits and increased ventricular volume, seem to be reversible with weight recovery.[42,43] Additionally, delayed gastric emptying and decreased GI motility can be seen in patients with AN. Gastric emptying studies can be done to evaluate these abnormalities, if necessary. The initial laboratory evaluation workup of patients with suspected eating disorders is presented in Box 16-5.

Box 16-5. Initial Laboratory Workup of Patients With Symptoms Suggesting an Eating Disorder

- CBC
- Evaluation of levels of serum electrolytes
- Liver function tests
- Thyroid function tests
- Evaluation of levels of LH, FSH, estradiol, and prolactin if patient is amenorrheic
- Evaluation of testosterone level for male patients (optional)
- Urinalysis for specific gravity and ketones
- ECG if patient is bradycardic
- Bone density determination considered for female patients with amenorrhea of ≥6 mo

---

Abbreviations: CBC, complete blood cell count; ECG, electrocardiogram.

Bulimia Nervosa and Purging Disorder

History

Initial evaluation of a patient with BN or PD includes determining the diagnosis and its severity and evaluating other causes of the symptoms. Relevant history includes frequency of bingeing; frequency of purging behaviors, including laxative, diuretic, diet pill, or ipecac use; and frequency of vomiting or exercising. History of maximum, minimum, and usual weights is also obtained. Similar to patients with AN, patients with BN or PD may have symptoms of malnutrition, including cold hands and feet, hair loss, and irregular menses. Symptoms related to purging, which include heartburn, hematemesis, constipation, and diarrhea, should be explored.

Physical Examination

Patients with BN or PD may be underweight, overweight, or normal weight. Specific abnormalities on the physical examination are rarely found; therefore, subtler changes in vital signs, the complete physical examination findings, and laboratory test results should be sought. Vital signs will vary depending on the substances used to control weight. For example, people using diet pills may have tachycardia, hypertension, or both, whereas those using substances that cause dehydration, such as stimulant laxatives or diuretics, may have tachycardia, hypotension, or both. Vomiting can cause hypovolemia and, in turn, tachycardia and hypotension. For people who exercise excessively, resting heart rates may show significant bradycardia. Thus, the initial physical examination generally begins with measurements of weight, height, blood pressure, and pulse. If dehydration needs to be ruled out, then measuring blood pressure for orthostatic changes as previously described is needed. Hands should be examined for Russell sign (ie, irritation on the dorsum of the joints of the fingers used to induce vomiting), teeth should be examined for erosion of enamel caused by vomiting, and parotid enlargement from vomiting may also be seen.

Laboratory Evaluation

Blood tests include a CBC with differential, electrolytes, lipid studies, liver function tests, and serum chemistries. Amylase levels and urinary pH may be elevated in some patients who have BN or PD. The urinalysis may reveal an elevated specific gravity associated with dehydration, ketones associated with starvation, increased pH in the presence of vomiting, or any combination of those findings. A hormonal workup is performed if menstrual periods are problematic; these tests include thyroid function tests, as well as assessments of LH, FSH, estradiol, and prolactin (if the patient is amenorrheic). If potassium levels are abnormal or if a history of ipecac use exists, an ECG should be obtained. If patients are oligomenorrheic or amenorrheic, a bone-density assessment looking for osteopenia should be pursued. In general, the laboratory abnormalities found in patients with BN or PD are caused almost solely by purging or by laxative or diuretic use (or by both those behaviors), rather than malnutrition or the binging behaviors, so the laboratory tests' results do not differ for patients with BN vs those with PD.

Treatment of Eating Disorders

Team Approach

The combination of medical and psychological interventions required in the treatment of eating disorders makes the task of being proficient in all aspects of care difficult for any single professional.[44] No single individual can be totally responsible for any patient's care beyond the initial evaluation or for the most straightforward of cases.[44,45] Rather, a team approach is most often used. The team may consist of a PCC; a psychiatrist, psychologist, or social worker; and a nutritionist, with the exact combination determined by local expertise, availability, and preference. The team of providers must be able to communicate with each other regularly. The medical provider can be the PCC, if he/she feels comfortable in this position. If not, the PCC should refer to another medical provider, such as an adolescent medicine–trained specialist, to evaluate and set up treatment goals for medically related issues, which can then be followed by either the PCC or adolescent medicine specialist. Clinicians can use the following general referral guidelines (Box 16-6) if the patient is medically stable and open to therapy.

Generally, each team member manages specific aspects of care, and team meetings and discussions are held frequently to prevent miscommunication that can sabotage the treatment.

Box 16-6. When to Involve One or More Specialists in Treating an Eating Disorder

- Refer to a psychotherapist if the patient is unable to attain goals set by the PCC, even if the patient is resistant.

- Refer to a dietitian to reinforce the PCC's nutritional recommendations or to set a nutritional plan with the patient if the PCC does not have the time or expertise.

- Refer for psychopharmacological evaluation if both the PCC and the therapist believe that the patient might benefit from medication (if the patient is bingeing and open to medication or if obsessive-compulsive symptoms are interfering with treatment).

- Refer to an adolescent medicine specialist if the PCC is not comfortable with treating the patient or does not have the time to do so or if the patient does not adhere to the PCC's treatment plan.

- Refer patients with ARFID to a speech/swallow specialist if there is any suspicion of a swallowing difficulty or to a behavioral therapist for exposure and response therapy to enhance patient acceptance of a wider range of foods.

- Refer to other subspecialists deemed appropriate by the treatment team.

Abbreviations: ARFID, avoidant/restrictive food intake disorder; PCC, primary care clinician.

Medical and Nutritional Rehabilitation

Determination of the treatment setting as inpatient, outpatient, or in a day program is made by the evaluating provider. The malnutrition that accompanies AN is directly responsible for most, if not all, of the physical abnormalities noted in the disorder, as well as for some of the mental deterioration. Accordingly, medical and nutritional rehabilitation is crucial in the treatment of the patient who has AN. Restoration of body weight, generally to within 10% of IBW, with restoration of menses if the patient is amenorrheic, should be among the main goals of treatment. For many patients whose malnutrition is mild to moderate (15%–25% below IBW), this task may be accomplished on an outpatient basis; patients who have moderate to severe malnutrition (>25% below IBW) can rarely accomplish the required weight gain without hospitalization (see Box 16-7). Medical treatment includes management of electrolyte abnormalities, cardiovascular issues, endocrine disorders, and other organ system dysfunction. These aspects of care are managed simultaneously with and are abetted by nutritional rehabilitation, which is generally achieved through oral feedings. Whether in the inpatient or outpatient setting, a daily intake of 3 substantial meals and 3 to 4 snacks is usually sufficient to bring about required weight gain and improvement of medical parameters. On inpatient units, meals are generally provided as part of a strict regimen, and snacks generally consist of high-calorie supplements, available as liquids or puddings in various brands and flavors. Care is taken to avoid overfeeding patients whose malnutrition is severe, because a too-rapid weight gain has been associated with severe metabolic abnormalities (ie, the refeeding syndrome) in some patients.[46] Slow refeeding and phosphorus supplementation are required in patients with severe malnutrition to prevent this syndrome, which may result in heart failure, hemolysis, coma, and death.

For patients with BN or PD, the medical rehabilitation is focused on treating the patient's physical symptoms or laboratory abnormalities and stopping, or at least decreasing, the patient's participation in risky behaviors, including bingeing, vomiting, and laxative, diuretic, or diet pill use, while the nutritional rehabilitation is focused on normalizing eating patterns and ensuring balanced nutrition. For patients with atypical AN, the medical and nutritional goals of treatment are to stop ongoing weight loss and to return eating patterns to normal. Although these patients are not

Box 16-7. When to Admit

Anorexia Nervosa

- <75% ideal body weight or ongoing weight loss despite intensive management
- Refusal to eat
- Body fat <10 %
- Heart rate <45 beats/min daytime; <40 beats/min nighttime
- Systolic pressure <90 mm Hg
- Orthostatic changes in pulse (>20 beats/min) or blood pressure (>10 mm Hg)
- Temperature <96°F
- Arrhythmia
- Failure to respond to outpatient treatment

Bulimia Nervosa

- Syncope
- Serum potassium concentration, ≤3.2 mmol/L
- Serum chloride concentration <88 mmol/L
- Esophageal tears
- Cardiac arrhythmias including prolonged QTc
- Hypothermia
- Suicide risk
- Intractable vomiting
- Hematemesis
- Failure to respond to outpatient treatment

technically underweight, most patients with AN require some amount of weight gain to restore both physiologic function and psychological function to a normal state. The amount of weight gain that is required in patients with atypical AN can be variable; it is generally to a weight that is partway between initial weight and the weight at presentation, but usually closer to the latter. Studies have shown that patients with atypical AN generally require a weight that is above IBW for return of menses.

For patients with ARFID, the medical and nutritional goals of treatment depend on the specific behaviors of each patient. For those who have stopped eating because of fear of vomiting or choking, a return to premorbid baseline eating patterns is the goal. For those who have had restricted diets for many years, the first goal of treatment is to ensure sufficient nutrition intake to accomplish appropriate growth, in both weight and height. A second goal, which is often more difficult to achieve, is to have patients broaden their food choices over time.

Dietary Plan

In the outpatient setting, an appropriate meal pattern may be developed according to the patient's and the family's prior eating habits or to a specific dietary plan offered by the physician or a nutritionist or by the parents if they are in family-based treatment. The dietary plan should be specific to prevent ambiguities that can lead to family fighting; it should provide approximately 2,000 to 3,000 cal/d. Some of these calories may be supplied in the form of high-calorie supplements. The plan should be well-balanced and include foods from each of the major food groups. For patients with AN, outpatient gains should be 0.5 to 1.0 kg/wk (1–2 lb/wk),[47] whereas inpatient gains may be 1.0 to 2.0 kg/wk (2–4 lb/wk).[48] For older children and younger adolescents with ARFID, a weight gain of 0.5 to 1.0 kg/wk (1–2 lb/mo) may suffice. Adherence to the dietary regimen may be evaluated by having the patient keep a diet diary; however, many patients do not always keep these records accurately and honestly.

A similar dietary plan but without the high-calorie supplements may be offered to patients at a healthy weight who have BN or PD because these patients generally require nutritional adjustment rather than nutritional rehabilitation. Caloric requirements for people with BN or PD will depend on the need for weight gain, loss, or maintenance. Because caloric restriction may often spark binge-eating episodes, the implementation of a nonrestrictive, well-balanced diet is warranted. If hospitalization is necessary for uncontrolled binge or purge cycles, abnormal levels of electrolytes, or unstable vital signs, then supervision after meals, locked bathrooms, and restricted access to food are often necessary.

Menses Restoration in Those With Amenorrhea

Menses restoration generally requires an estradiol level of 30 to 50 mg/dL.[49] Resumption and presence of menses have been linked to improved cognitive function in patients with AN.[50] Researchers are exploring other treatments, such as recombinant human IGFs, dehydroepiandrosterone, bisphosphonates, testosterone, and a combination of recombinant human IGF-1 (commonly known as rhIGF-1) and oral estrogen,[50-52] in an effort to find ways to protect the bones of patients with eating disorders. Oral estrogen-progesterone combination pills are not effective in increasing bone density. Physiologic estrogen replacement in the form of a transdermal patch along with cyclic progesterone has been found to possibly increase the rate of bone accrual in adolescents with AN in one recent study.[53] Still, regaining weight is the only definitive treatment to bring about the return of menses.

Treatment Settings

Inpatient and Residential Settings

Patients are admitted to inpatient hospitals for the reasons previously outlined, which are either medically or psychiatrically emergent. They are put on protocols to ensure weight gain and to guard against refeeding syndrome. Many units begin with food, moving to oral supplements or nasogastric feedings if meals are not consistently consumed. In fact, there is some evidence that using nasogastric tubes at the time of admission can increase the rate of weight gain.[54,55]

After patients are stabilized, they are often transferred to residential programs, which have less medical monitoring and more psychological support. Various behavioral approaches may be used, including several phases of treatment, with patients moving from one phase to another on the basis of achievement of progressively higher weight goals or improved behaviors or attitudes. Each phase incorporates additional privileges into the patient's daily activities (eg, food choices, food preparation, passes for outings with family).

Day Programs and Intensive Outpatient Programs

After patients are ready to leave the residential setting, they are stepped down to a day program, which generally runs 5 days a week, providing 2 to 3 meals and snacks daily. Following this program, it is ideal to step down again to an intensive outpatient program (IOP), which generally runs 3 hours per day, 3 days a week, providing a meal and an individual or group therapy session. In both settings, patients still live at home, and with the IOPs, patients can attend school. Often, IOP and day programs are used as a step-up from a general outpatient setting, in an effort to prevent the next higher level of care.

Outpatient Settings

This least intensive option often includes medical monitoring, nutritional support, psychiatric treatment, and therapy, which may include individual, family, or group therapy, or any combination of those therapies. In fact, most patients with eating disorders, of all types (AN, atypical AN, BN, PD, and ARFID), are treated solely in the outpatient setting. Less than 10% to 15% of patients presenting to eating disorder programs require the higher levels of care previously outlined.

Psychosocial Therapy Options

Individual therapy, cognitive behavioral therapy (CBT), dialectical behavioral therapy (commonly known as DBT), and family-based treatment (FBT) are the most commonly used modalities for patients with eating disorders. Individual therapy is varied and difficult to study for this reason. Family-based therapy is considered to be a particularly useful modality for younger patients with AN.[56]

Cognitive behavioral therapy was formulated by Fairburn in 1981.[57] Use of CBT for eating disorders is aimed at decreasing nutritional restriction, normalizing eating, developing skills for coping with situations that trigger binge eating or purging (or both), and changing perceptions over concern with body weight and shape. Cognitive behavioral therapy is the treatment of choice for adults with BN or BED. Both CBT and FBT have also been studied for adolescents with BN and found to be effective.

Psychopharmacological Therapy

Pharmacological treatment of the eating disorders has concentrated on psychoactive medications, especially the selective serotonin reuptake inhibitor (SSRI) antidepressants. Two specific lines of reasoning have guided the use of these medications. In patients who are diagnosed as having an eating disorder along with, or as part of, another psychiatric diagnosis, medication for the associated diagnosis is offered with the expectation that the eating disorder will improve as other psychiatric symptoms are relieved. Alternatively, more recent evidence has demonstrated that use of these medications diminishes the urge to binge and purge in patients who have BN and helps treat obsessive-compulsive symptoms in patients with either AN or BN.[58]

Only clinicians who are familiar with the use of psychopharmacological agents should prescribe these medications as part of the treatment, given the recent concerns about the potential for SSRI medications to increase the risk for suicide among some children and adolescents treated for depression. The SSRI medications have not been shown to be effective in promoting weight gain in patients with AN or treating symptoms of depression or OCD when body weight is low; some questions remain about whether they may be effective in preventing relapse in patients initially treated successfully for AN.[58] Atypical antipsychotic agents at low doses can improve weight gain and treat symptoms of depression and obsessional thoughts in patients with severe eating disorders, including both AN and BN. Both SSRIs and atypical antipsychotic medications have been used in patients with ARFID who are afraid to eat because of fear of choking or vomiting or because of overwhelming anxiety. These medications have shown some success in these groups of patients, but they are generally not used in patients with ARFID who have had long-term restrictions in dietary intake.[59-62]

Outcome and Prognosis

Eating disorders must be viewed as a chronic illness, similar to other medical or psychiatric chronic illnesses. A wide range of outcomes can be expected.[63] Adolescents who have severe AN have a protracted disease course, yet recovery estimates 10 to 15 years later vary from 24% to 76%.[64,65] Although many different approaches are used to evaluate outcome, at least an estimated 50% of patients do well long-term, 30% show varying degrees of improvement, and 20% do poorly despite adequate treatment. Patients who are younger, as well as those whose forms of the disease are milder, seem to have a better prognosis than these general numbers indicate.[66] Follow-up of patients with BN has recently been reviewed and has improved in studies done after 2004 compared with those done before 2004. Approximately 70% of these patients recover, 20% experience relapse, and 10% continue to meet the full criteria for BN 5 years after diagnosis.[66-68] Numerous personal, family, and treatment factors may predict the outcome of an eating disorder; none of these factors may be predictive for an individual patient. For instance, a poorer outcome of AN has been associated with factors such as older age, vomiting, and premorbid personality problems, yet any particular patient who has this constellation of findings may do well with treatment. Furthermore, no specific treatment has been shown by controlled studies to be more effective than others, in general or for any particular type of patient. There are not yet any studies delineating the course or outcome of patients with ARFID, nor are there any data yet on differences in prognosis for patients with atypical AN compared with those with typical AN.

Prevention

Although a focus on both primary prevention and secondary prevention has increased of late, the best strategies for the prevention of eating disorders remain unclear.[69] There is increasing evidence that eating disorders and obesity may be related, with dieting, weight-related teasing, and body dissatisfaction as risk factors[70]; therefore, using an integrated approach to prevention is sensible. To date, several programs geared toward both teenaged boys and teenaged girls, primarily in school settings, have been implemented. These programs generally provide factual information and are aimed at maintaining a healthy body image, healthy eating, and promoting self-esteem without relation to weight, and they appear to succeed in increasing awareness of and knowledge about eating disorders.[71] However, whether these programs prevent or actually promote eating-disordered behaviors is debatable.[72,73] The concept of preventing eating disorders through more generic programs focused on building self-esteem is currently being explored. In keeping with this effort, the concept of a comprehensive school-based approach has been advocated.[74] This approach would include classroom interventions, staff training throughout the school, informal discussions between staff and students, integration of material about eating issues into the curriculum, more intensive work with students at high risk, changes within the school with respect to cafeteria food and physical education, and referrals and outreach, both within the school and to the community. A recent meta-analysis of prevention studies found that multiple interactive sessions targeted at those at risk and older than 15 years were the most likely to succeed.[75] Early case detection remains the most effective preventive measure currently available. For most patients, the earlier an eating disorder is treated, the easier the treatment will be and the less entrenched the disease becomes. Therefore, families, friends, school personnel, and health care professionals must be vigilant for the signs and symptoms of an eating disorder so that early treatment can be initiated.

AAP Policy

Rosen DS; American Academy of Pediatrics Committee on Adolescence. Identification and management of eating disorders in children and adolescents. *Pediatrics.* 2010;126(6):1240–1253. Reaffirmed November 2014 (pediatrics.aappublications.org/content/126/6/1240)

References

1. American Psychiatric Association. *Diagnostic and Statistical Manual of Mental Disorders.* 5th ed. Arlington, VA: American Psychiatric Association; 2013
2. American Psychiatric Association. *Diagnostic and Statistical Manual of Mental Disorders.* 4th rev ed. Arlington, VA: American Psychiatric Association; 2000
3. Fisher M, Gonzalez M, Malizio J. Eating disorders in adolescents: how does the *DSM-5* change the diagnosis? *Int J Adolesc Med Health.* 2015;27(4):437–441
4. Lucas AR, Beard CM, O'Fallon WM, Kurland LT. 50-year trends in the incidence of anorexia nervosa in Rochester, Minn.: a population-based study. *Am J Psychiatry.* 1991;148(7):917–922
5. Carlat DJ, Camargo CA Jr, Herzog DB. Eating disorders in males: a report on 135 patients. *Am J Psychiatry.* 1997;154(8):1127–1132
6. Halmi KA, Casper RC, Eckert ED, Goldberg SC, Davis JM. Unique features associated with age of onset of anorexia nervosa. *Psychiatry Res.* 1979;1(2):209–215
7. Beck D, Casper R, Andersen A. Truly late onset of eating disorders: a study of 11 cases averaging 60 years of age at presentation. *Int J Eat Disord.* 1996;20(4):389–395
8. Sullivan PF. Mortality in anorexia nervosa. *Am J Psychiatry.* 1995;152(7):1073–1074
9. Campbell K, Peebles R. Eating disorders in children and adolescents: state of the art review. *Pediatrics.* 2014;134(3):582–592
10. French SA, Leffert N, Story M, Neumark-Sztainer D, Hannan P, Benson PL. Adolescent binge/purge and weight loss behaviors: associations with developmental assets. *J Adolesc Health.* 2001;28(3):211–221
11. Stice E, Killen JD, Hayward C, Taylor CB. Age of onset for binge eating and purging during late adolescence: a 4-year survival analysis. *J Abnorm Psychol.* 1998;107(4):671–675
12. Kaltiala-Heino R, Rimpelä M, Rissanen A, Rantanen P. Early puberty and early sexual activity are associated with bulimic-type eating pathology in middle adolescence. *J Adolesc Health.* 2001;28(4):346–352
13. Flament M, Ledoux S, Jeamet P, et al. A population study of bulimia nervosa and subclinical eating disorders in adolescence. In: Steinhausen HC, ed. *Eating Disorders in Adolescence: Anorexia and Bulimia Nervosa.* New York, NY: De Gruyter; 1995
14. McCallum K. Eating disorders. *Curr Opin Psychiatry.* 1993;6:480–485
15. Fairburn CG, Cooper PJ. The clinical features of bulimia nervosa. *Br J Psychiatry.* 1984;144:238–246
16. Fairburn CG, Beglin SJ. Studies of the epidemiology of bulimia nervosa. *Am J Psychiatry.* 1990;147(4):401–408
17. Stein S, Chalhoub N, Hodes M. Very early-onset bulimia nervosa: report of two cases. *Int J Eat Disord.* 1998;24(3):323–327
18. Fisher MM, Rosen DS, Ornstein RM, et al. Characteristics of avoidant/restrictive food intake disorder in children and adolescents: a "new disorder" in *DSM-5.* *J Adolesc Health.* 2014;55(1):49–52

19. Ornstein RM, Rosen DS, Mammel KA, et al. Distribution of eating disorders in children and adolescents using the purposed *DSM-5* criteria for feeding and eating disorders. *J Adolesc Health.* 2013;53(2):303–305

20. Bulik CM. Exploring the gene-environment nexus in eating disorders. *J Psychiatry Neurosci.* 2005;30(5):335–339

21. Trace SE, Baker JH, Peñas-Lledó E, Bulik CM. The genetics of eating disorders. *Annu Rev Clin Psychol.* 2013;9:589–620

22. Mazzeo SE, Bulik CM. Environmental and genetic risk factors for eating disorders: what the clinician needs to know. *Child Adolesc Psychiatr Clin N Am.* 2009;18(1): 67–82

23. Chamay-Weber C, Narring F, Michaud PA. Partial eating disorders among adolescents: a review. *J Adolesc Health.* 2005;37(5):417–427

24. Hebebrand J, Muller TD, Holtkamp K, Herpertz-Dahlmann B. The role of leptin in anorexia nervosa: clinical implications. *Mol Psychiatry.* 2007;12(1):23–35

25. Neumark-Sztainer D, Wall M, Guo J, Story M, Haines J, Eisenberg M. Obesity, disordered eating, and eating disorders in a longitudinal study of adolescents: how do dieters fare 5 years later? *J Am Diet Assoc.* 2006;106(4):559–568

26. Klump KL, Kaye WH, Strober M. The evolving genetic foundations of eating disorders. *Psychiatr Clin North Am.* 2001;24(2):215–225

27. Cui H, Moore J, Ashimi SS, et al. Eating disorder predisposition is associated with *ESRRA* and *HDAC4* mutations. *J Clin Invest.* 2013;123(11):4706–4713

28. Salbach-Andrae H, Lenz K, Simmendinger N, Klinkowski N, Lehmkuhl U, Pfeiffer E. Psychiatric comorbidities among female adolescents with anorexia nervosa. *Child Psychiatry Hum Dev.* 2008;39(3):261–272

29. Godart NT, Flament MF, Lecrubier Y, Jeammet P. Anxiety disorders in anorexia nervosa and bulimia nervosa: co-morbidity and chronology of appearance. *Eur Psychiatry.* 2000;15(1):38–45

30. Milos G, Spindler A, Ruggiero G, Klaghofer R, Schnyder U. Comorbidity of obsessive-compulsive disorders and duration of eating disorders. *Int J Eat Disord.* 2002;31(3):284–289

31. Fisher M. Medical complications of anorexia and bulimia nervosa. *Adolesc Med.* 1992;3(3):487–502

32. Katzman DK. Medical complications in adolescents with anorexia nervosa: a review of the literature. *Int J Eat Disord.* 2005;37(suppl):S52–S59

33. Engstrom JW, Aminoff MJ. Evaluation and treatment of orthostatic hypotension. *Am Fam Physician.* 1997;56(5):1378–1384

34. Newman MM, Halmi KA. The endocrinology of anorexia nervosa and bulimia nervosa. *Endocrinol Metab Clin North Am.* 1988;17(1):195–212

35. Misra M, Aggarwal A, Miller KK, et al. Effects of anorexia nervosa on clinical, hematologic, biochemical, and bone density parameters in community-dwelling adolescent girls. *Pediatrics.* 2004;114(6):1574–1583

36. Misra M, Klibanski A. Neuroendocrine consequences of anorexia nervosa in adolescents. *Endocr Dev.* 2010;17:197–214

37. Wong JC, Lewindon P, Mortimer R, Shepherd R. Bone mineral density in adolescent females with recently diagnosed anorexia nervosa. *Int J Eat Disord.* 2001;29(1):11–16

38. Bachrach LK, Katzman DK, Litt IF, Guido D, Marcus R. Recovery from osteopenia in adolescent girls with anorexia nervosa. *J Clin Endocrinol Metab.* 1991;72(3): 602–606

39. Lucas AR, Melton LJ III, Crowson CS, O'Fallon WM. Long-term fracture risk among women with anorexia nervosa: a population-based cohort study. *Mayo Clin Proc.* 1999;74(10):972–977

40. Castro J, Lázaro L, Pons F, Halperin I, Toro J. Predictors of bone mineral density reduction in adolescents with anorexia nervosa. *J Am Acad Child Adolesc Psychiatry.* 2000;39(11):1365–1370

41. Grinspoon S, Thomas E, Pitts S, et al. Prevalence and predictive factors for regional osteopenia in women with anorexia nervosa. *Ann Intern Med.* 2000;133(10): 790–794

42. Katzman DK, Zipursky RB, Lambe EK, Mikulis DJ. A longitudinal magnetic resonance imaging study of brain changes in adolescents with anorexia nervosa. *Arch Pediatr Adolesc Med.* 1997;151(8):793–797

43. Chui HT, Christensen BK, Zipursky RB, et al. Cognitive function and brain structure in females with a history of adolescent-onset anorexia nervosa. *Pediatrics.* 2008;122(2):e426–e437

44. American Academy of Pediatrics Committee on Adolescence. Identifying and treating eating disorders. *Pediatrics.* 2003;111(1):204–211

45. Becker AE, Grinspoon SK, Klibanski A, Herzog DB. Eating disorders. *N Engl J Med.* 1999;340(14):1092–1098

46. Fisher M, Simpser E, Schneider M. Hypophosphatemia secondary to oral refeeding in anorexia nervosa. *Int J Eat Disord.* 2000;28(2):181–187

47. American Psychiatric Association Work Group on Eating Disorders. Practice guideline for the treatment of patients with eating disorders (revision). *Am J Psychiatry.* 2000;157(1) (suppl):1–39

48. Howard WT, Evans KK, Quintero-Howard CV, Bowers WA, Andersen AE. Predictors of success or failure of transition to day hospital treatment for inpatients with anorexia nervosa. *Am J Psychiatry.* 1999;156(11):1697–1702

49. Golden NH, Jacobson MS, Schebendach J, Solanto MV, Hertz SM, Shenker IR. Resumption of menses in anorexia nervosa. *Arch Pediatr Adolesc Med.* 1997;151(1):16–21

50. Gordon CM, Grace E, Emans SJ, et al. Use of DHEA to prevent osteoporosis in patients with anorexia nervosa. *J Adolesc Health.* 1998;22(2):176

51. Miller KK, Grieco KA, Klibanski A. Testosterone administration in women with anorexia nervosa. *J Clin Endocrinol Metab.* 2005;90(3):1428–1433

52. Misra M, Klibanski A. Anorexia nervosa and osteoporosis. *Rev Endocr Metab Disord.* 2006;7(1–2):91–99

53. Misra M, Klibanski A. Anorexia nervosa and bone. *J Endocrinol.* 2014;221(3): R163–R176

54. Agostino H, Erdstein J, Di Meglio G. Shifting paradigms: continuous nasogastric feeding with high caloric intakes in anorexia nervosa. *J Adolesc Health.* 2013;53(5):590–594

55. Silber TJ, Robb AS, Orrell-Valente JK, Ellis N, Valadez-Meltzer A, Dadson MJ. Nocturnal nasogastric refeeding for hospitalized adolescent boys with anorexia nervosa. *J Dev Behav Pediatr.* 2004;25(6):415–418

56. Katzman DK, Peebles R, Sawyer SM, Lock J, Le Grange D. The role of the pediatrician in family-based treatment for adolescent eating disorders: opportunities and challenges. *J Adolesc Health.* 2013;53(4):433–440

57. Fairburn CG, Jones R, Peveler RC, Hope RA, O'Connor M. Psychotherapy and bulimia nervosa. Longer-term effects of interpersonal psychotherapy, behavior therapy, and cognitive behavior therapy. *Arch Gen Psychiatry.* 1993;50(6):419–428

58. Walsh BT, Kaplan AS, Attia E, et al. Fluoxetine after weight restoration in anorexia nervosa: a randomized controlled trial. *JAMA.* 2006;295(22):2605–2612

59. Barbarich NC, McConaha CW, Gaskill J, et al. An open trial of olanzapine in anorexia nervosa. *J Clin Psychiatry.* 2004;65(11):1480–1482

60. La Via MC, Gray N, Kaye WH. Case reports of olanzapine treatment of anorexia nervosa. *Int J Eat Disord.* 2000;27(3):363–366

61. Powers PS, Santana CA, Bannon YS. Olanzapine in the treatment of anorexia nervosa: an open label trial. *Int J Eat Disord.* 2002;32(2):146–154

62. Bissada H, Tasca GA, Barber AM, Bradwejn J. Olanzapine in the treatment of low body weight and obsessive thinking in women with anorexia nervosa: a randomized, double-blind, placebo-controlled trial. *Am J Psychiatry.* 2008;165(10):1281–1288

63. Fisher M. The course and outcome of eating disorders in adults and in adolescents: a review. *Adolesc Med.* 2003;14(1):149–158

64. Strober M, Freeman R, Morrell W. The long-term course of severe anorexia nervosa in adolescents: survival analysis of recovery, relapse, and outcome predictors over 10-15 years in a prospective study. *Int J Eat Disord.* 1997;22(4):339–360

65. Eckert ED, Halmi KA, Marchi P, Grove W, Crosby R. Ten-year follow-up of anorexia nervosa: clinical course and outcome. *Psychol Med.* 1995;25(1):143–156

66. Steinhausen HC. Outcome of anorexia nervosa in the younger patient. *J Child Psychol Psychiatry.* 1997;38(3):271–276

67. Keel PK, Mitchell JE. Outcome in bulimia nervosa. *Am J Psychiatry.* 1997;154(3):313–321

68. Keel PK, Brown TA. Update on course and outcome in eating disorders. *Int J Eat Disord.* 2010;43(3):195–204

69. Rosen DS, Neumark-Sztainer D. Review of options for primary prevention of eating disturbances among adolescents. *J Adolesc Health.* 1998;23(6):354–363

70. Haines J, Neumark-Sztainer D. Prevention of obesity and eating disorders: a consideration of shared risk factors. *Health Educ Res.* 2006;21(6):770–782

71. Story M, Neumark-Sztainer D. Promoting healthy eating and physical activity in adolescents. *Adolesc Med.* 1999;10(1):109–123

72. Mann T, Nolen-Hoeksema S, Huang K, Burgard D, Wright A, Hanson K. Are two interventions worse than none? Joint primary and secondary prevention of eating disorders in college females. *Health Psychol.* 1997;16(3):215–225

73. Neumark-Sztainer D, Butler R, Palti H. Eating disturbances among adolescent girls: evaluation of a school-based primary prevention program. *J Nutr Educ.* 1995;27(1):24–31

74. Neumark-Sztainer D. School-based programs for preventing eating disturbances. *J Sch Health.* 1996;66(2):64–71

75. Stice E, Shaw H, Marti CN. A meta-analytic review of eating disorder prevention programs: encouraging findings. *Annu Rev Clin Psychol.* 2007;3:207–231

Emotional or Behavioral Disturbance in Children Younger Than 5 Years

Mary Margaret Gleason, MD

"A child's relationship with caring and nurturing adults is the most critical factor in developing resilience to the normative stresses of childhood and in buffering a child from the adverse effects of toxic stresses."

Young children's emotional patterns are common foci of pediatric primary care visits. Box 17-1 summarizes the wide range of concerning symptoms and signs that may come to the attention of pediatric primary care clinicians, hereafter referred to as PCCs, including pediatricians, family physicians, nurse practitioners, and physician assistants who

---

Box 17-1. Symptoms and Clinical Findings Suggesting Social-Emotional Problems in Children Younger Than 5 Years

Concerns About the Child's Behavior or Emotions

- Regulatory difficulties evidenced by difficulty calming, irregular sleep or feeding patterns, or excessive sensitivity to sensory experiences.

- Difficulty organizing behaviors and demonstrates extreme aggression or severe or persistent tantrums that involve injury or damage to objects.

- Significant difficulty adjusting to child care or preschool or has been expelled from child care or preschool.

- Activity and impulsivity levels are excessive for developmental age and impair typical activities for age.

- Mood is unhappy, irritable, or lacking in true joy more frequently than the average child.

- More anxiety than others his age, especially related to specific triggers or traumatic reminders, separation from caregiver, or experiencing new situations.

- Inability to talk in public, even with reassurance.

- Excessively rigid behavioral patterns or "habits" that interfere with typical functioning.

Box 17-1. Symptoms and Clinical Findings Suggesting Social-Emotional Problems in Children Younger Than 5 Years (*continued*)

Concerns About Caregiver

- Difficulties considering the child's strengths, becomes disorganized or rambling when talking about the child, or talks about the child using only a negative tone

- Trouble anticipating a child's need for comfort or does not offer appropriate comfort in new situations or times of distress, such as immunizations or physical examinations

- Excessive protection of child and does not allow developmentally appropriate exploration (eg, observed in the office or by history in other settings)

- Past or current abusive or neglectful patterns (eg, involvement with child protective services)

Concerns About Caregiver-Child Relationship

- Child does not or cannot elicit comfort or reassurance effectively from caregiver in times of distress (eg, immunizations or separations).

- Child (older than 9 months' developmental age) does not look to caregiver in novel situations or to share joy or excitement.

- Child does not manifest age-appropriate stranger anxiety.

- Child has not met appropriate social milestones related to social reciprocity, peer interactions, adult interactions, or focused attachment (comfort-seeking) behaviors with a primary caregiver.

- Child's relationship with caregiver has been disrupted (eg, foster care, military deployment of parent, death of parent).

Risk Factors for Increased Susceptibility

- History of maltreatment or significant caregiving disruption (such as is seen in children in foster care, those who have been adopted, or those with other caregiving disruptions)

- Family stressors (eg, poverty, divorce, single parenting, unemployment, limited access to health care, lack of safe and affordable housing or food, social isolation, community violence, community or natural disaster, chronic or extreme medical events)

- History of ACE in parents

- Parental substance use, mental disorder, or domestic violence

Abbreviation: ACE, adverse childhood experience.

provide frontline, longitudinal care to infants and children younger than 5 years of age.

The clinical approach to these symptoms and signs requires a wide lens of assessment, with awareness that, although the child is the patient, the PCC must remain vigilant that the child's behavior, particularly with respect to social-emotional problems, may reflect difficulty or dysfunction within the child's caregiving context. This chapter outlines the PCC's role in preventing, identifying, and addressing social-emotional problems in young children, a role that is critical because of the numerous associated adverse outcomes, including child and family suffering, school failure, mental and physical illnesses, and fractured social networks throughout the life span. This chapter focuses on infants and children in the first 5 years of life (hereafter called simply *children* unless otherwise specified) using the term *social-emotional problems* to describe the full range of behavioral difficulties, emotional disturbances, and relationship difficulties that may occur in early childhood, especially in the context of adverse childhood experiences. These problems may also be defined as mental health problems or, sometimes, psychiatric disorders. This chapter will refer to the child's primary caregiver as the parents, who may be biological parents, grandparents, foster parents, or other guardians.

Background and Epidemiology

During early childhood, social-emotional health develops through a complex interaction of a child's genetic makeup, temperament, and social and physical environments, particularly through parent-child relationships. Previously, biological risks were not thought to be easily modifiable. However, recent research demonstrates that complex interactions among a child's biological factors, including genetic and epigenetic factors, and the caregiving environments shape social-emotional development. The early childhood period is particularly sensitive to environmental exposures. Synaptogenesis occurs at rates more than 700 synapses per second, meaning that even relatively minor changes in the environment influence outcomes substantially. Similarly, experience can also shape neural circuitry through pruning, by which neural circuitry and synapses not used during this period are lost.[1] Adversity, such as developmental, behavioral, economic, social, educational, biological, or family stresses, can overwhelm the child's ability to cope, alter the brain's architecture, and lead to impaired social functioning and impulse control.[1] Specific examples of adversity include child maltreatment, violence exposure, family disruptions, parent impairment through mental disorders or substance use disorders or both, disasters, and medical trauma.[2-4] The effect of these stressors on children can vary greatly depending on their developmental stages, their social supports, and the type, intensity, frequency, and duration of their stressors. There is an additive effect of multiple stressors or risk factors, with more adverse events related to increased risk of adverse outcomes, likely through the disruption of developmentally normative experiences or the repeated activation of the physiologic trauma responses.[4,5] Therefore, it is important to identify and ameliorate sources of traumatic stress as early as possible. A study by Egger and Angold demonstrated rates of psychopathology among very young children similar to rates among older children.[6] These disorders can persist and interfere with future development and school readiness.[7-10]

A child's relationship with caring and nurturing adults is the most critical factor in developing resilience to the normative stresses of childhood and in buffering a child from the adverse effects of toxic stresses. Interventions that support the development of positive parent-child interactions can positively influence a young child's brain development, intelligence, and central nervous system hormonal patterns.[11,12] Specifically, these interventions focus on ensuring that a child experiences sensitive caregiving, through which a caregiver anticipates and responds to a child's unique physical and emotional needs and responds to a child's positive and negative behaviors consistently, persistently, and contingently. Beginning in infancy and continuing through childhood and into adolescence, parents and other caregivers can support their child's development in emotional regulation by providing a safe environment, modeling regulated emotional responses to everyday challenges, and reinforcing positive behaviors in their child and by helping their child organize emotions in response to challenging situations.

Role of the Primary Care Clinician
At the Community Level

The PCC can collaborate with local community partners such as developmental-behavioral pediatricians, early childhood mental health professionals, Early Intervention professionals, early childhood educators in child care and schools, child advocates, and public health agencies to promote and strengthen protective factors by identifying supports for children at high risk for social-emotional problems. A summary of approaches for screening strategies and interventions can be found on the American Academy of Pediatrics (AAP) Early Brain and Child Development Web site (www.aap.org/en-us/advocacy-and-policy/aap-health-initiatives/EBCD/Pages/default.aspx). Such approaches may include advocating for the creation of safe outdoor spaces for children's exploration, for domestic violence shelters, for evidence-based home visiting programs, for increased access to quality early childhood caregiving environments, or for appropriate access to prenatal care and postnatal nutrition.

At the Practice Level

Universal screening and other preventive approaches also occur within the primary care practice. By addressing strengths and risks in the caregiving environment for all children, PCCs can create an environment in which parents feel comfortable raising their own questions about emotional or behavioral concerns. For example, implementing the AAP-recommended universal maternal depression screening at the infant's 1-, 2-, 4-, and 6-month visits can open the conversation about caregiver well-being. (See Chapter 23, Maternal Depression.) The Bright Futures/AAP *Recommendations for Preventive Pediatric Health Care* (periodicity schedule) also includes recommendations for psychosocial and behavioral assessment at every visit (described as "family centered [and possibly including] an assessment of child social-emotional health, caregiver depression, and social determinants of health"); developmental surveillance at regular intervals throughout childhood; formal developmental screening at 9 months, 18 months, and 2½ years; and formal autism spectrum disorder screening at 18 months and 2 years.[13] Boxes 1-8 and 1-9, in Chapter 1, Integrating Preventive Mental Health Care Into Pediatric Practice, summarize additional surveillance and screening recommendations for children and families with enhanced risks for social-emotional problems. Primary care clinicians can promote wellness and open communication by including information about social-emotional well-being in routine anticipatory guidance and through posters and literature in the waiting room. Structured universal approaches, such as partnering with an early childhood mental health consultant or implementing a program such as the Video Interaction Project, can also be useful in expanding the conversations that will promote early childhood well-being.[14,15]

For children with clinical level social-emotional concerns, PCCs are often the first professionals to address the problem. Supporting parents to focus on the child as a person with emotional symptoms rather than a "bad" child is an important intervention. Even before a more extensive assessment, PCCs can apply "common factors" skills (see Box 17-2, the HELP mnemonic, and Chapter 5, Effective Communication Methods: Common Factors Skills) to ensure effective communication that will reduce parents' stress and enhance referral success when applicable.

Findings Suggesting Social-Emotional Problems or Risk Factors for Problems

The symptoms that suggest social-emotional problems in children younger than 5 years can be identified in the child, the caregiver, or the relationship between the child and caregiver, as summarized in Box 17-1. Any of these findings triggers the need for further assessment.

Tools to Assist With Identification

Validated, standardized screening instruments may be used to identify children at high risk for having social-emotional problems, because of either parent-reported symptoms or the caregiving environment. Table 17-1 provides examples of nonproprietary general psychosocial screening instrument results that may suggest a child has social-emotional problems. Negative screening results indicate that a child is within a lower-risk group, and they can be an opportunity for positive feedback or may guide anticipatory guidance. A negative screening result should not override clinical judgment if a PCC has concerns caused by history or observations. With all parent report measures, but especially

---

Box 17-2. Common Factors Mnemonic: HELP Build a Therapeutic Alliance

H = Hope

E = Empathy

L^2 = Language, Loyalty

P^3 = Permission, Partnership, Plan

Adapted from American Academy of Pediatrics. *Addressing Mental Health Concerns in Primary Care: A Clinician's Toolkit.* Elk Grove Village, IL: American Academy of Pediatrics; 2010. For the fully annotated mnemonic, please refer to Appendix 5.

Table 17-1. General Psychosocial Screening Results Suggesting Social-Emotional Problems

Screening Area	Screening Instrument	Score
Child	Ages & Stages Questionnaires: Social-Emotional	Each age range has a developmentally specific questionnaire and score cutoff. Parent concern is factored into the total score.
	Baby Pediatric Symptom Checklist (irritability, inflexibility, and difficulties in parenting)	A score of ≥3 is considered positive.
	Preschool Pediatric Symptom Checklist (internalizing, externalizing, attention, and parenting challenges)	A score of ≥9 is considered positive.
	Early Childhood Screening Assessment (emotional and behavioral development in young children 18–60 months of age and maternal distress)	A score of ≥18 on items 1–36 indicates a higher than usual risk of disorder. A score >1 on 37 or 38 may reflect parenting stress. A score of ≥1 on items 39 or 40 suggests risk of caregiver depression.
	Brief Early Childhood Screening Assessment	A score of ≥9 on items 1–24 represents a positive screening result. Same parent scoring for adult items.
Environment	Edinburgh Postnatal Depression Scale	Score of ≥12 is considered positive.
	Patient Health Questionnaire-2	Any positive response is considered positive.
	Abuse Assessment Screen	A positive response to any question indicates high risk of interpersonal violence.
	Safe Environment for Every Kid	Positive responses suggest presence of family stressors.
	Caregiver Strain Questionnaire	Score of ≥7 suggests high level of caregiver strain.
	Bright Futures surveillance questions	Answers suggest social-emotional stressors.
	Parenting Stress Index	Results suggest high levels of stress associated with parenting or within the parent-child relationship.

in early childhood mental health, it is particularly important to recognize that a parent report reflects that parent's perception of the child's behaviors. Positive screening results may indicate that the child has a mental health problem, that the parent is experiencing extreme distress (because of the child or another cause), or that there is a problem within the relationship between the parent and the child. All 3 possibilities have implications for the child's development and warrant clinical attention. Therefore, a positive screening result should be followed by further assessment to determine more about the clinical concern.

Assessment

Assessment begins by differentiating the child's symptoms from normal behavior. Children vary in temperament and in their capacity to self-regulate and adapt. Virtually all young children exhibit challenging behaviors at times, especially during periods of adjustment to new environmental circumstances, such as birth of a sibling, a move, a new child care arrangement, or a family crisis. Children with social-emotional problems may experience more severe and persistent emotional or behavioral reactions to these normative stresses or even in the absence of an acute stressor. Clinical level problems cause impairment in the child's functioning or extreme adaptations by caregivers to accommodate to the child's patterns (eg, leaving a job because a child has extreme separation distress). Also, some conditions may mimic or co-occur with social-emotional problems of young children. Table 17-2 provides a summary of these conditions. Extreme tantrums or emotional or behavioral responses to small events such as limit setting can reflect a range of clinical issues. Figure 17-1 provides categories of possible child, parent, or relationship difficulties that should be considered when a parent reports concerns about the child's emotional or behavioral development. Importantly, PCCs can help parents recognize that a maladaptive behavior such as aggression often represents the only tool a child has to cope with an overwhelming emotion, such as anxiety, frustration (with self or other), or distress. It is critically important to address parental concern about social, emotional, or behavioral patterns, even if the PCC does not identify atypical development, because these perceptions drive how the parent interacts with and thinks about the child. Providing parental support around parenting stresses; wondering about alternative attributions for behavior; strategizing around safe, consistent, nurturing responses to difficult behaviors; and close follow-up all may be helpful.

Table 17-2. Differential Diagnosis of Extreme Emotional or Behavioral Dysregulation

Domain	Differential Diagnosis	Rationale
Typical development	None	Extreme responses to normal limits, fatigue, hunger, or new situations are part of typical development in the third and fourth years after birth.
Developmental delays as well as frustration	Cognitive and language disabilities	Children with language deficits may experience frustration expressing their needs and desires and may therefore exhibit symptoms of social-emotional problems. Children with intellectual disabilities may function at a level younger than their chronological age and size. This gap between their ability and adult expectations for their behaviors can lead to frustration for the child and caregiver, and limited expressive skills can produce aggressive or otherwise disruptive behaviors during times of frustration.
	Hearing or vision problems	All children who are manifesting atypical development or behavior should be screened for sensory deficits. All young children with delay in language development should undergo a complete hearing assessment.
	ASD	Children with ASD have problems with social relatedness (eg, poor eye contact, preference for solitary activities, lack of joy in sharing with others, lack of empathy), problems with language (delayed expressive language or unusual syntax or prosody), limitations in their range of interest (persistent and intense interest in a particular activity or subject), or atypical mannerisms that can interfere with their ability to function. They may have a need for routine and can become anxious or angry if a routine is disrupted. Accordingly, these children may manifest symptoms of social-emotional problems. In addition, children with ASD are also at higher than usual risk of comorbid psychiatric disorders that may present in early childhood.

Table 17-2. Differential Diagnosis of Extreme Emotional or Behavioral Dysregulation *(continued)*

Domain	Differential Diagnosis	Rationale
Regulatory problem	Sleep problems	Sleep deprivation caused by bedtime struggles, night waking, or obstructive sleep apnea can cause irritability and behavioral problems; conversely, social-emotional problems can cause sleep difficulties.
	Feeding disorders	Difficulties with feeding, that is, either refusal, sensitivities, or overeating, can cause disruptive or distressed patterns in an infant or a toddler, which can occur in a mutually escalating cycle with parental distress around the eating patterns.
Child disruptive behavioral problem	ADHD	High levels of impulsivity, as well as inattentiveness and distractibility, may be seen in very young children with ADHD. It is especially important to assess whether the symptoms occur in multiple settings (as required in ADHD) or whether they are specific to a context or relationship, a pattern that would likely represent an adjustment to that situation. Because of the range of normal activity levels of very young children, ADHD must be distinguished from developmentally inappropriate expectations for young children and from parental depression that may make normal child behaviors less tolerable. Children with exposure to traumatic events may present with patterns that may mimic ADHD but sometimes can be linked temporally to exposure to traumatic events or reminders. Other anxiety and mood symptoms may be encountered with symptoms that must be distinguished from ADHD. In addition, symptoms suggestive of ADHD should be distinguished from those of lead toxicity and from effects of medications such as steroids or sympathomimetics. First-line therapy of ADHD in young children is psychosocial therapy that includes child and caregiver.
	Disruptive behavioral disorders (oppositional defiant disorder and conduct disorder)	Disruptive behaviors in young children may present with extreme oppositional behaviors or conduct disordered symptoms, including aggression. These can occur when a child experiences an inconsistent or coercive caregiving environment.

Child mood symptoms	Depression	Very young children can present with all the symptoms of major depressive disorder, and this diagnosis should be considered in children with extreme sadness or irritability. Associated symptoms include sleep and appetite changes, play or talk centered around death and dying, decreased joy in playing, and concentration difficulties. The validity of the diagnosis of bipolar disorders in preschool has not been established.
Child anxiety	Anxiety disorders	Preschoolers may present with general anxiety, extreme separation anxiety, school avoidance behaviors, and selective mutism, all often accompanied by extreme distress in the face of the trigger. Anxiety in young children can present with hypervigilant and disorganized behaviors, as well as extreme dysregulation, although it can also present with more typical inhibited symptoms. Very young children with obsessive-compulsive behaviors may present with disruptive behavior patterns when asked to interrupt a compulsive behavior.
	PTSD and other trauma-related symptoms	Children who have experienced traumatic events may exhibit a set of symptoms similar to the presentation of PTSD seen in older children (reexperiencing the trauma in thoughts, speech, play, and dreams; emotional and physiologic hyperarousal to reminders of the trauma; avoidance of reminders of the trauma; and numbing symptoms). The symptoms must be elicited with careful interview. It is not uncommon for children who have experienced traumatic events to present with disruptive behaviors, perhaps related to their own inability to organize their reactions or because of less consistent parenting after the traumatic event.

Table 17-2. Differential Diagnosis of Extreme Emotional or Behavioral Dysregulation (*continued*)

Domain	Differential Diagnosis	Rationale
Parent-child relationship disturbances	Parental mental health problems, substance use problems, or severe cognitive limitations	Young children who experience unpredictable or inconsistent parenting, especially if it includes neglectful or dangerous experiences, may present with inconsistent and sometimes dangerous behaviors. Treatment of parents and consideration of child protective services involvement is critical in addressing these clinical scenarios. Depression or other mental disorder, psychological factors, bereavement, substance use, cognitive disability, or disadvantaged socioeconomic circumstances may prevent a child's caregivers from nurturing the child effectively and may contribute to social-emotional problems in the child.
	Disordered attachment or parent-child relationship difficulties	The bond between a child and his caregiver can be affected by characteristics of the child or caregiver or by temperamental "goodness of fit" between child and caregiver. Manifestations of a suboptimal parent-child relationship that increases the risk of attachment problems may include ineffective or inconsistent soothing, nurturing, or disciplinary behaviors of the caregiver, or lack of responsiveness of the child to his caregiver's soothing and nurturing efforts. A parent's own history of unsafe relationships (as a child or in romantic relationships) may shift how a parent thinks about herself in the intimate relationship of parenting and how the parent experiences the child's behaviors and needs. Relationship difficulties may be encountered in the clinic with a parent who experiences the needs of her child as excessive or troublesome, with a child who develops a pattern of maladaptive ways of engaging the parent's attention, or with a child who does not seem to make any attempts to engage the parent, even when he might be expected to need comforting.

Abbreviations: ADHD, attention-deficit/hyperactivity disorder; ASD, autism spectrum disorder; PTSD, post-traumatic stress disorder.

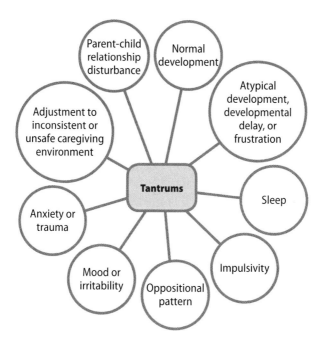

Figure 17-1. Differential diagnosis of emotional or behavioral dysregulation.

The special circumstance of a chronic or significant medical problem should be considered, as it may trigger social-emotional problems in a range of domains. Young children with chronic medical problems are more likely to experience developmental delays and traumatic experiences in the form of medical procedures and separations from parents, and they may be viewed as particularly vulnerable by their parents because of their medical condition. They may also take medications that may affect mood regulation (eg, steroids) or have primary central nervous system lesions that interfere with emotional, behavioral, or developmental regulation. Similarly, although all children with growth failure should be evaluated for underlying medical problems, psychosocial growth failure can occur in the context of an inadequate caregiving environment, and the role of the caregiving environment as a protective or risk factor should be considered in all cases of growth failure. (See Figure 17-1.)

If a child or caregiver seems to be experiencing symptoms, the PCC can further assess for problems by collecting further information, refer the child to an appropriate specialist, or review diagnostic criteria for symptoms. The *DC:0–5; Diagnostic Classification of Mental Health and*

Developmental Disorders of Infancy and Early Childhood, which defines the diagnostic criteria of disorders of very young children, was recently published and offers useful information, especially about very young children.[16]

The PCC can elicit information from other caregivers, child care staff, and preschool staff about eating, sleeping, irritability, and aggression with peers, using behavior or food diaries or validated, structured measures, such as the Baby Pediatric Symptom Checklist (BPSC), Preschool Pediatric Symptom Checklist (PPSC), or Early Childhood Screening Assessment. See Appendix 2, Mental Health Tools for Pediatrics, for details.

Referral may be to a developmental-behavioral pediatrician, a mental health professional with expertise in assessment of young children and their families, or an Early Intervention agency, or varying combinations thereof, depending on the resources in the community and the child's specific needs. To be able to develop a plan with the parents, it is useful for PCCs to be aware of the child-serving professionals in the community, including developmental services professionals, developmental-behavioral pediatricians, psychotherapists, and agencies that provide parent mental health services, and to address basic needs such as food insecurity. (See Appendix 4, Sources of Key Mental Health Services.) Children are best served when their PCCs are familiar with the appropriate evidence-based services for early childhood mental health problems and prepared to refer and comanage effectively with other providers.[15]

Plan of Care for Children With Social-Emotional Problems

The care of a child experiencing social-emotional problems can begin in the primary care setting. Universal screening or active surveillance for social-emotional problems can create an environment in which families feel comfortable discussing social-emotional issues. It is critical that the PCC or the medical home team is prepared to address positive screening results or surveillance with first-line approaches described in Chapter 2, Pediatric Care of Children and Adolescents With Mental Health Problems. The role of the PCC always includes providing support and a promise of an ongoing relationship with the family. Other specifics of the PCC's role vary with circumstances: for mild clinical problems and when a family is not ready to seek specialty care, the role will include providing support, ongoing education, and first-line approaches; for more impairing problems and after a family has been successfully engaged in help seeking, the PCC's role will include referral and comanagement with specialty care providers. Without engagement, most families will not seek or continue in specialty mental health care. The process of engagement may require multiple primary care visits and application of common factors skills to address barriers. See Box 17-2, the HELP mnemonic, and Chapter 5, Effective Communication Methods: Common Factors Skills.

Following are the elements of providing care to a child with social-emotional problems identified in the primary care setting.

Celebrating the Strengths and Engaging Child and Family in Care

Primary care clinicians can engage families by recognizing and reinforcing the strengths of both child and family and by acknowledging the distress and emotional costs of the social-emotional concern. The PCC can acknowledge and reinforce protective factors (eg, good relationships with at least 1 parent or important adult, prosocial peers, concerned or caring family, help seeking, or connection to positive organizations). Most parents whose child has impairing emotional or behavioral patterns have heard from family and strangers that they are not meeting their child's needs, so recognizing strengths is an important engagement approach. In fostering engagement, it can be useful to use the HELP mnemonic to build trust and optimism, including reaching agreement on incremental next steps and, ultimately, therapeutic goals; developing a plan of care (see the following clinical guidance); and determining the role of the PCC.

Promoting Safety

Families whose children experience social-emotional difficulties are at particularly high risk of exposure to unsafe situations. These may include family partner violence, child abuse, or community exposure to violence. In addition, some families may experience safety risks related to housing conditions or a child's access to potentially dangerous medications (eg, diabetes medications, sleeping medications, antihypertensive medications). Assessment for other risks, including weapons in the home, is an important role of the PCC.

Addressing Basic Needs

Identifying families' basic needs is perhaps the most important universal intervention for all children with social-emotional problems. Family distress may be reduced by addressing unmet basic needs such as housing, child care, or access to food and a safe place to live. Without addressing these needs, it is unlikely that mental health referrals will be successful.

Supporting Parental Mental Health

Whether a parent is experiencing a clinical-level problem or distress related to sleep deprivation, it is important for a parent to experience clinical interactions with the PCC as supportive. Even when there are concerns about specific parenting approaches, families will consider changing their behaviors only if they feel that the clinical approach is helpful and that their perspective is respected. Discussion of parental clinical mental health issues such as depression or substance use, including those identified by screening, may be an important clinical step toward addressing the child's emotional needs. It can be helpful to focus these discussions on the parent's desire to be the best parent he can be and the interference that sleep deprivation, stress, or clinical problems cause in reaching this nearly universal goal.

Reframing the Child's Behaviors

When a parent seems to perceive a child as overwhelmingly negative or interprets developmentally typical behaviors as intentionally disruptive to the parent, it can be helpful to offer a new lens or to reframe the behaviors in a way that may allow the parent to experience the same behaviors differently. For example, reframing "clingy and needy" behaviors in toddlers as a demonstration of using a parent for emotional support as they begin to venture out to explore their environment may be helpful. Using handouts such as those found on the AAP Early Brain and Child Development Web site or the Circle of Security handout (http://circleofsecurity.org) or video (www.youtube.com/user/CircleOfSecurity) may be helpful and efficient ways to inform parents about children's basic emotional needs. It is important to note that telling a parent that the child's behavior is "normal" without putting it into a developmental or emotional context may be experienced as rejection by parents who are worried about their child.

Encouraging Consistency in Child's Caregiving Environment

No matter what the clinical concern, children will benefit from predictable, consistent, and safe responses to both prosocial behaviors and negative behaviors. The PCC can encourage the primary caregivers to reflect on and enhance their own consistency. In addition, the PCC can assist the primary caregivers in developing strategies to increase the consistency that the child experiences across caregivers, including mother, father, grandparents, babysitters, and child care providers.

Exploring Opportunities for Positive Parent-Child Interactions

Whether a clinical problem seems to be located primarily within the child, the parent, or their relationship, it is likely that all family members are experiencing less joy and fulfillment from their interactions than they would like. Assisting a parent in identifying a child's strengths and positively reinforcing positive behaviors, or efforts toward positive behaviors, can be a useful first step toward healing. "Time in," as little as 5 minutes a day of interactive playtime with the child, can be a way for parents to delight in their child, feel competent, and feel appreciated and for the child to enjoy the parent. If a caregiver's own history of problematic relationships or mental health problems is affecting her relationship with the child, it can be useful to explore her readiness to address these problems as part of helping the child. Handouts on www.HealthyChildren.org and parent handouts and resources at www2.tulane.edu/som/tecc may offer valuable supports.

Encouraging Healthy Habits and Activities

The PCC can encourage healthy child and family habits that will provide a sound foundation for ongoing development. These healthy habits can include opportunities for active play, good nutrition, media-free family meals, regular bedtime routines, and adequate sleep. Discussions of media exposure and the dangers of frightening or violent media can be especially important for parents of children with anxiety, aggressive behaviors, or a history of trauma exposure. Additionally, the AAP recommended limits to screen time can promote healthy brain development, increase interactive and exploratory time, and reduce the potential for exposure to adult content or violence.[17]

The PCC can direct the parent toward high-quality early childhood care and education such as Head Start and programs accredited by the NAEYC (National Association for the Education of Young Children). The PCC can also encourage communication between child care or preschool personnel and home, and coach them to praise progress and effort, not just outcomes. The AAP Early Brain and Child Development resources can be shared with parents to give to child care providers to promote consistency across a child's environments.

Offering Initial Interventions

Evidence-based psychosocial interventions for social-emotional problems include several common elements amenable to implementation in the primary care setting. Table 17-3 provides strategies that the PCC can suggest to the family.

Providing Resources

Examples of materials that are helpful in counseling parents include *Connected Kids* at https://patiented.solutions.aap.org, "Everybody Gets Mad: Helping Your Child Cope With Conflict" at www.healthychildren. org/English/healthy-living/emotional-wellness/Pages/Everybody-Gets-Mad-Helping-Your-Child-Cope-with-Conflict.aspx, and *Parents' Roles in Teaching Respect* at www.brightfutures.org/mentalhealth/pdf/families/mc/parent_role.pdf.

Monitoring Progress

Symptoms can be tracked using screening measures described in Table 17-1 or disorder-specific measures. General measures such as the BPSC and PPSC and the Early Childhood Screening Assessment, or the Strengths and Difficulties Questionnaires, are useful in monitoring symptoms over time. Symptom-specific measures such as the Eyberg Child Behavior Inventory (disruptive behaviors) and the Preschool Feelings Checklist (depression) are valuable and validated measures that provide more specific information about a child's course. Child care or preschool reports can be helpful in monitoring progress. Attention-deficit/hyperactivity disorder (ADHD) can be tracked (but not diagnosed) using measures validated on older children, such as the NICHQ Vanderbilt ADHD assessment scales and the Conners 3. More extensive measures, such as the Child Behavior Checklist/1½-5, are validated in screening of children as young as 18 months of age but are longer than a

Table 17-3. Strategies for Building Child's Social-Emotional Skills and Resilience and in Addressing Behavioral Problems

Strategy	Advice to Caregivers
Reduce family stress.	• Enlist support of extended family, friends, faith group, or involved agency to relieve parent of some stresses and provide emotional support.
Promote daily positive joint activities between parents and child.	• Educate about the importance of smiling with and talking and cooing to infants, attending to vocalizations or speech, and reading and playing at all ages. • Assist with recognizing a child's cues by labeling the child's behaviors and needs in the office and supporting the parent in responding sensitively. • Increase parent's one-on-one time with child (eg, interacting, feeding, reading, playing). Daily routines around mealtime and bedtime, for example, can ensure that these activities are well integrated into family life. • Promote resilience at every visit by using the anticipatory guidance of Bright Futures or the AAP EBCD Web site (www.aap.org/en-us/advocacy-and-policy/aap-health-initiatives/EBCD/Pages/default.aspx) and by emphasizing individual strengths.
Apply positive parenting principles to toddlers and preschoolers (positive attention for positive behaviors, removing attention for low-level behaviors, and safe, consistent, calm consequences for unacceptable or unsafe behaviors).	• Reinforce desired behaviors using parental attention (eg, "Catch them being good"). • Help the child develop vocabulary to describe feelings. • Encourage praise and reinforcement ("rewards") for specific, desired (target) behaviors. The choice of target behaviors and the time intervals for reinforcements should be developmentally appropriate and sustainable. • Teach parents to reduce attention to ("ignore") minor, provocative behaviors. "Pick battles" and focus discipline on priority areas. • Reduce positive reinforcement of disruptive behavior (eg, laughing when a child curses or uses adult language). • When possible, reorganize the child's day to prevent trouble by avoiding situations in which the child cannot control herself. Examples include asking a neighbor to look after the child while the parent goes shopping, ensuring that activities are available for long car journeys, and arranging activities in separate rooms for siblings who are prone to fighting. • Talk with the child care center or preschool staff and suggest that similar principles be applied.

Table 17-3. Strategies for Building Child's Social-Emotional Skills and Resilience and in Addressing Behavioral Problems (*continued*)	
Strategy	**Advice to Caregivers**
Teach relaxation and anxiety management.	• Teach parents to recognize the child's anxiety, expose the child only to manageable anxiety-provoking situations, provide support around unavoidable anxiety-provoking situations, and praise the child's management of her feelings. • For high stress families, teach relaxation exercises such as breathing or muscle relaxation.
Encourage parents to be calm and consistent.	Suggest that parents • Set clear house rules agreed on by the primary caregivers. • Give short, specific commands about the desired behavior, not prohibitions about undesired behavior (eg, "Please walk slowly," rather than, "Don't run"). • Provide consistent and calm consequences for misbehavior. Consequences should not be dangerous, drastic, or of extreme duration. • Use natural consequences, such as the child cleaning up a mess she has created. • When enforcing a rule, avoid getting into arguments or explanations, reduce additional attention for the misbehavior, and defer negotiations until periods of calm. • Consider parenting classes or community support.

Abbreviations: AAP, American Academy of Pediatrics; EBCD, Early Brain and Child Development.

PCC can regularly use. See Appendix 2, Mental Health Tools for Pediatrics, for more information about these instruments.

Involving Specialists

Involvement of a specialist may be considered appropriate under the following circumstances:

► A child younger than 5 years has symptoms of social-emotional problems causing functional impairment or distress. For example,

– The child has symptoms of anxiety, sadness, or irritability that limit participation in family interactions, child care experiences, or other normative experiences.

– The child has behaviors that are disruptive in the home or in out-of-home settings or that limit participation in developmentally appropriate experiences.

- The child does not use the caregiver effectively for emotional support or is indiscriminate in social interactions with strangers.

- The child exhibits sleep or eating problems that are not responsive to primary care interventions.

▶ The parent is very negative toward child, compromised by physical or mental disorder, disengaged, inconsistent in providing nurturing, or unresponsive to primary care guidance.

▶ The parent has difficulty allowing a child to have developmentally appropriate opportunities for exploration.

▶ The family is not able to maintain a calm, consistent, or safe environment. (In this instance, also consider reporting to child protective services.)

When mental health specialty care is needed, a PCC should recommend evidence-informed treatment.

A variety of evidence-based and evidence-informed psychosocial interventions are available for the treatment of social-emotional problems in children younger than 5 years.[15] See Table 17-4 and Box 17-3.

The PCC and mental health specialists should clarify roles in the child's care. The PCC's role may, for example, include engaging and encouraging the family's positive view of interventions or referral and serving as the

Table 17-4. Psychosocial and Psychopharmacological Therapies for Social-Emotional Problems in Young Children	
Evidence-Based Parenting Programs	
Cluster Area	**Parenting Program**
For disruptive behavioral problems	• The Incredible Years (www.incredibleyears.com) • Triple P – Positive Parenting Program (www.triplep.net) • Parent-Child Interaction Therapy (www.pcit.org) • "Helping the Noncompliant Child" parent training program (www.guilford.com/books/Helping-the-Noncompliant-Child/McMahon-Forehand/9781593852412)
For first-time pregnant, low-income women prior to 28 weeks' gestation	• Nurse-Family Partnership (www.nursefamilypartnership.org)

Table 17-4. Psychosocial and Psychopharmacological Therapies for Social-Emotional Problems in Young Children (*continued*)	
Evidence-Based Parenting Programs	
Cluster Area	**Parenting Program**
For children in foster care	• Attachment and Biobehavioral Catch-up (www.infantcaregiverproject.com) • Multidimensional Treatment Foster Care Program for Preschoolers (www.tfcoregon.com) • Parent-Child Interaction Therapy[a]
For parent-child relationship disturbances and high-risk parenting situations	• Promoting First Relationships (http://pfrprogram.org) • Parents as Teachers (http://parentsasteachers.org) • Child-Parent Psychotherapy (http://nctsn.org/sites/default/files/assets/pdfs/cpp_general.pdf)
For children exposed to trauma, including sexual abuse or domestic violence	• Child-Parent Psychotherapy (http://www.cebc4cw.org/program/child-parent-psychotherapy/detailed) • CBT[b-d] (http://www.cebc4cw.org/program/preschool-ptsd-treatment/detailed)

Abbreviation: CBT, cognitive behavioral therapy.
Updates are available at www.aap.org/mentalhealth.
[a] Chaffin M, Funderburk B, Bard D, Valle LA, Gurwitch R. A combined motivation and parent-child interaction therapy package reduces child welfare recidivism in a randomized dismantling field trial. *J Consult Clin Psychol*. 2011;79(1):84–95.
[b] Cohen JA, Mannarino AP. Factors that mediate treatment outcome of sexually abused preschool children: six- and 12-month follow-up. *J Am Acad Child Adolesc Psychiatry*. 1998;37(1):44–51.
[c] Cohen JA, Mannarino AP. A treatment study for sexually abuse preschool children: outcome during a one-year follow-up. *J Am Acad Child Adolesc Psychiatry*. 1997;36(9):1228–1235.
[d] Scheeringa MS, Weems CF, Cohen JA, Amaya-Jackson L, Guthrie D. Trauma-focused cognitive-behavioral therapy for posttraumatic stress disorder in three-through six year-old children: a randomized clinical trial. *J Child Psychol Psychiatry*. 2011;52(8):853–860.

medical home hub, coordinating care provided by parents, child care and preschool staff, medical home professionals, Early Intervention agency, and specialists. Either a mental health specialist or the PCC may monitor the child's and family's progress and observe for and address any comorbidities that may develop. Whatever their assigned roles, each provider should share findings with the others.

AAP Policy

American Academy of Pediatrics Council on Early Childhood, Committee on Psychosocial Aspects of Child and Family Health, and Section on Developmental and Behavioral Pediatrics. Addressing early childhood emotional and behavioral

Box 17-3. US Food and Drug Administration-Approved Psychopharmacological Interventions (as of March 12, 2018)[a,b]	
Diagnostic Area	**Social-Emotional Problems in Young Children**
Psychopharmacological intervention	Limited evidence supports psychopharmacological intervention in this age-group. Available are a single multisite, placebo-controlled, randomized trial of methylphenidate and another focused on atomoxetine as a treatment of ADHD in preschoolers. Both showed that the medication was more effective than placebo but less effective than in older children and was associated with a higher rate of adverse effects.[c,d]

Abbreviations: ADHD, attention-deficit/hyperactivity disorder; FDA, US Food and Drug Administration.

[a] For up-to-date information about FDA-approved interventions, go to www.fda.gov/ScienceResearch/SpecialTopics/PediatricTherapeuticsResearch/default.htm.

[b] See also Chapter 11, Psychotropic Medications in Primary Care, for guidance in primary care prescribing.

[c] Kratochvil CJ, Vaughan BS, Stoner JA, et al. A double-blind, placebo-controlled study of atomoxetine in young children with ADHD. *Pediatrics.* 2011;127(4):e862–e868.

[d] Greenhill L, Kollins S, Abikoff H, et al. Efficacy and safety of immediate-release methylphenidate treatment for preschoolers with ADHD. *J Am Acad Child Adolesc Psychiatry.* 2006;45(11):1284–1293.

problems. *Pediatrics.* 2016;138(6):e20163023 (pediatrics.aappublications.org/content/138/6/e20163023)

Garner AS, Shonkoff JP; American Academy of Pediatrics Committee on Psychosocial Aspects of Child and Family Health; Committee on Early Childhood, Adoption, and Dependent Care; and Section on Developmental and Behavioral Pediatrics. Early childhood adversity, toxic stress, and the role of the pediatrician: translating developmental science into lifelong health. *Pediatrics.* 2012;129(1):e224–e231. Reaffirmed July 2016 (pediatrics.aappublications.org/content/129/1/e224)

Gleason MM, Goldson E, Yogman MW; American Academy of Pediatrics Council on Early Childhood, Committee on Psychosocial Aspects of Child and Family Health, and Section on Developmental and Behavioral Pediatrics. Addressing early childhood emotional and behavioral problems. *Pediatrics.* 2016;138(6):e20163025 (pediatrics.aappublications.org/content/138/6/e20163025)

References

1. Shonkoff JP, Garner AS; American Academy of Pediatrics Committee on Psychosocial Aspects of Child and Family Health; Committee on Early Childhood, Adoption, and Dependent Care; and Section on Developmental and Behavioral Pediatrics. The lifelong effects of early childhood adversity and toxic stress. *Pediatrics.* 2012;129(1):e232–e246

2. Felitti VJ, Anda RF, Nordenberg D, et al. Relationship of childhood abuse and household dysfunction to many of the leading causes of death in adults: the Adverse Childhood Experiences (ACE) Study. *Am J Prev Med.* 1998;14(4):245–258

3. Substance Abuse and Mental Health Services Administration. *Transforming Mental Health Care in America: The Federal Action Agenda: "A Living Agenda."* Washington, DC: US Dept of Health and Human Services; 2008

4. Sameroff A, ed. *The Transactional Model of Development: How Children and Contexts Shape Each Other.* Washington, DC: American Psychological Association; 2009

5. Felitti VJ, Anda RF. The relationship of adverse childhood experiences to adult medical disease, psychiatric disorders and sexual behavior: implications for healthcare. In: Lanius RA, Vermetten E, Pain C, eds. *The Impact of Early Life Trauma on Health and Disease: The Hidden Epidemic.* New York, NY: Cambridge University Press; 2010:77–87

6. Egger HL, Angold A. Common emotional and behavioral disorders in preschool children: presentation, nosology, and epidemiology. *J Child Psychol Psychiatry.* 2006;47(3–4):313–337

7. Scheeringa MS, Zeanah CH, Myers L, et al. Predictive validity in a prospective follow-up of PTSD in preschool children. *J Am Acad Child Adolesc Psychiatry.* 2005;44(9):899–906

8. Kim-Cohen J, Arseneault L, Newcombe R, et al. Five-year predictive validity of *DSM-IV* conduct disorder research diagnosis in 4 (1/2)-5-year-old children. *Eur Child Adolesc Psychiatry.* 2009;18(5):284–291

9. Lahey BB, Pelham WE, Loney J, et al. Three-year predictive validity of *DSM-IV* attention deficit hyperactivity disorder in children diagnosed at 4-6 years of age. *Am J Psychiatry.* 2004;161(11):2014–2020

10. Dougherty LR, Smith VC, Bufferd SJ, et al. Preschool irritability: longitudinal associations with psychiatric disorders at age 6 and parental psychopathology. *J Am Acad Child Adolesc Psychiatry.* 2013;52(12):1304–1313

11. Nelson CA, Bosquet M. Neurobiology of fetal and infant development: implications for infant mental health. In: Zeanah CH, ed. *Handbook of Infant Mental Health.* New York, NY: Guilford; 2000:37–59

12. Dozier M, Peloso E, Lewis E, et al. Effects of an attachment-based intervention on the cortisol production of infants and toddlers in foster care. *Dev Psychopathol.* 2008;20(3):845–859

13. American Academy of Pediatrics. Recommendations for pediatric preventive health care. American Academy of Pediatrics. AAP.org. Web site. https://www.aap.org/en-us/Documents/periodicity_schedule.pdf. Updated February 2017. Accessed February 8, 2018

14. Mendelsohn AL, Valdez PT, Flynn V, et al. Use of videotaped interactions during pediatric well-child care: impact at 33 months on parenting and on child development. *J Dev Behav Pediatr.* 2007;28(3):206–212

15. Gleason MM, Goldson E, Yogman MW, et al. Addressing early childhood emotional and behavioral problems. *Pediatrics.* 2016;138(6):e20163025

16. Zero to Three Diagnostic Classification Task Force. *Diagnostic Classification of Mental Health and Development Disorders of Infancy and Early Childhood; DC:0-5.* Washington, DC: Zero to Three Press; 2016

17. Hill D, Ameenuddin N, Reid Chassiakos Y, et al. Media and young minds. *Pediatrics.* 2016;138(5):e20162591

CHAPTER 18

Family Dysfunction

Mary Iftner Dobbins, MD, and Sandra Vicari, PhD, LCPC

> "*For the primary care clinician, attention to family functioning is inextricably linked to practice, providing many opportunities for supporting the development of healthy families as well as for addressing problems as they may arise.*"

Introduction

Theories of child development have long recognized that children in modern Western cultures require approximately 2 decades after birth to achieve the self-sufficiency necessary for separation from their families. Because of this relatively prolonged dependency and because adverse childhood experiences negatively affect the developing brain and long-term health outcomes,[1-4] the functioning of the family is of utmost importance for optimal development and well-being of the child.

Complex sociocultural changes continue to redefine the family, with fewer "traditional" households that historically have consisted of 2 married biological parents located near extended family members for support.[5,6] Single, divorced, remarried, same-gender, foster, and adoptive parents are commonplace. Children and adolescents (collectively called simply *children* in this chapter) may also experience multiple, changing parental figures if grandparents assume their care or if biological parents move on to new partners. Many children have half-, step-, or foster siblings. Particularly in times of economic hardship, families may move in together or experience frequent changes in composition.

In the case of separation or divorce, children often live between 2 different households. Children may also be separated from a caregiver for prolonged periods because of parental employment, illness, or incarceration. The mobility of Western society has resulted in the geographic isolation of many nuclear families from extended family support. Oftentimes, nonrelatives assume the roles of extended family members.

Many children have a family that changes dramatically over time. As a result, family may be defined less by composition and more by functional relationships. In fact, the American Academy of Family Physicians (AAFP) states, "The family is a group of individuals with a continuing legal, genetic and/or emotional relationship."[7] The AAFP additionally asserts, "Society relies on the family group to provide for the economic and protective needs of individuals, especially children and the elderly." When children are involved, the most important function of the family is to provide a safe and caring environment in which the child can grow and develop into a healthy adult.

Family Characteristics

Families function in complex and multifaceted ways, with family members tending to assume various roles that interplay.[8] Changes in the functioning of an individual member affect the family unit, and changes in the family unit affect the individual members and their interactive roles. As a result, a variety of internal and external factors may influence the functioning of a family, and some families are more adaptable and resilient than others.

Healthy families have well-defined roles (ie, parent or child). Members freely ask for and provide attention, but boundaries are respected. Rules tend to be explicit and remain consistent, but with some flexibility to adapt to the individual. Communication is encouraged, and emotional expression is accepted. Security in relationships allows individuals to explore their own interests, and individuation is encouraged. As individual members grow and develop, the family as a unit adapts, also experiencing ongoing intrinsic growth and development over time, which is a sign of health.

All families experience misunderstandings, conflicts, and stressors at some time. Stressors may be internal (eg, illness, change in composition) or external (eg, financial insecurity, relocation). Healthy families cope with difficulties and maintain a sense of connectedness, which fosters a sense of security, self-worth, and competence in their children.

Parent Characteristics

For the child, the most critical characteristic of a healthy family is an adult who functions as caregiver. In fact, the most important contributory factor regarding children's resilience is the presence in their lives of at least 1 consistent, caring adult.[9,10] This adult not only addresses safety and basic needs but also shares an emotional connection with the child, conveying the sense that she has intrinsic value and is loved.

When 2 (or more) caregivers are involved, the relationship between them is exceptionally important. A supportive and flexible partnership fosters good parenting. Even those with very different backgrounds, knowledge, and attitudes can provide a consistent and united approach without undermining each other.

Specific parental practices do not have to be perfect. Although some are more intuitive than others, people with a variety of abilities, personal backgrounds, and personality types can be good parents. However, there are certain characteristics of maturity that are necessary for optimal caregiving—the ability to care for oneself, a sense of self-worth, the ability to emotionally connect with another person, a sense of responsibility, and a degree of selflessness.[8] Healthy parents do not desire a child to fix something in their own lives or relationships.

Parenting styles depend on many factors, including the parent's emotional health, experience in his or her own family of origin, and experience in the parental role, as well as the influence of or compromise with other adults assuming a co-parenting role, culture, and socioeconomic factors. Some traits are more enduring, but parenting styles may be dynamic because of these changeable influences.[11,12] The needs and temperament of a particular child may also result in variations in parenting. Conversely, children may vary in their responses to parenting styles because of their developmental stages, temperaments, and degrees of resilience.

A parent who can maintain a healthy caregiver role helps the child develop a sense of self-worth and competence, learn to maintain appropriate interpersonal relationships, and plan for her independent future.

Effects of Parenting Styles

Certain parenting styles are characteristic of healthy families. A caring yet authoritative parent will be attentive to the child and responsive to his needs, yet set consistent and developmentally appropriate expectations. Emphasis is placed on the parent-child relationship and communication, and discipline is provided in a constructive fashion that fosters the child's learning and self-control. Growing up in a context of guided yet growing autonomy, these children demonstrate more academic mastery, social and moral maturity, self-regulation, and sense of self-worth as they reach adulthood.[9]

Conversely, some parenting styles may have less favorable outcomes. Authoritarian parents satisfy their own need for control by granting little autonomy while also remaining less interpersonally involved with the child. Expectations for behavior give poor consideration to the needs or developmental abilities of the child, who learns over time that approval and affection may be conditional and unpredictable. Consequently, these children typically have poor self-esteem, are withdrawn and anxious, lack in resourcefulness, and are easily frustrated.[9] They reach adulthood with much less mastery, and often exhibit dependent or aggressive behaviors as adults. These children not only are at high risk for maltreatment but also are at high risk for perpetuating the cycle of maltreatment when they have children of their own.[13–15]

Alternatively, parents may relinquish their authoritative parental role if they are distracted by their own needs or insecure in their parent-child relationships. The resultant permissiveness, whether arising through inattentiveness or overindulgence, grants the child developmentally inappropriate autonomy, adversely affecting his ability to delay gratification and work to meet his own needs. These children enter adulthood with less academic and interpersonal mastery, resulting in less self-control and more demanding and disruptive social behavior.[9]

Parents may also be relatively uninvolved, either from their own emotional detachments or from being overwhelmed by the stressors of their own lives. In the extreme form, this may present as true neglect, and the child may have developmental delays in a variety of areas, including interpersonal attachment. Growing up with little support or discipline, these children often reach adulthood with little emotional, academic, or interpersonal mastery, demonstrating poor self-esteem and antisocial behaviors.[9]

Family Dysfunction

Difficult life circumstances may stress family functioning. If these circumstances are short-lived or less severe, healthier families adjust and persevere in their developmental tasks. When families become overwhelmed, composition is unstable, individual members are emotionally unhealthy, roles and boundaries are blurred, or communication is impaired, families may function in variations of chronically maladaptive patterns. When a parent figure fails to maintain a healthy parent role, the child's emotional health and development suffer, with potentially lifelong consequences.

Dysfunction can be subtle or severe. However, consequences of these problems affect almost all aspects of a child's life, including relationships, emotions, behavior, learning, the acquisition of coping skills, and psychological development.[1-4,16] Instead of developing a sense of self-worth and competence, the child incorporates self-doubt and insecurity. The child has difficulty developing trust and the balanced give-and-take of healthy relationships.[17,18] In severe cases, chronic disappointment and frustration lead to hopelessness and limited expectations for the future.[19]

Patterns of Dysfunction

Parental dysfunction typically exists in certain core areas. The parent who lacks the desire or ability to emotionally connect with and appreciate the child causes the child to feel devalued and unlovable, undermining the development of healthy attachment. The insecure parent may be overcontrolling in an effort to demonstrate her authority, be permissive in an attempt to ensure the child's love, prioritize a partner over caring for the child, or use the child to meet her own needs. The parent who cannot consistently care for herself cannot consistently care for the child, resulting in the child's feeling insecure and frustrated. In severe cases, the roles may become reversed, with the child becoming "parentified." These characteristics may manifest themselves in many circumstances, but are especially predictable in certain patterns.[8,9]

Uninvolved Parent

The uninvolved or "inaccessible" parent may be preoccupied with his career, relationships, or community status. As our culture continues to change, even very committed parents may fall into routines that allow less time for their children. They may become caregivers for their own parents or seek new educational or employment opportunities. Families may easily become overscheduled, being "together" disproportionately in a social context rather than as a family unit. In addition, technology frequently replaces, rather than enhances, true interpersonal interaction and communication.

Over-involved Parent

Conversely, parents may become over-involved for multiple reasons. Commonly, parents attempt to relive their own youths through their children's activities and status, and may allow little individuation or have unhealthy expectations. Additionally, societal factors have resulted in an extreme focus on achievement, and many children grow up in a culture of extreme competition. Even the possibility of failure may be perceived as an unbearable threat to self-worth, despite the fact that optimal development depends on the child's learning by trial and error. Less secure parents may become overprotective and try to lessen either the risks or the consequences for their children. As a result, the child tends to become less self-reliant, have unrealistically entitled expectations for life independent of the family, blame others rather than learn personal responsibility, paradoxically develop a decreased sense of competency, and consider self-worth to be conditional rather than intrinsic.[8,9]

Divided Loyalties

When power struggles exist in the family, the child may be put in the middle of the conflict. This is especially true in cases of divorce, in which the parents or extended family members may harbor a great deal of unresolved hurt and animosity. The child, now especially vulnerable and insecure as the family restructures, may be considered a trophy, used as a conduit of information, or forced to choose sides. Children tend to blame themselves for the parents' divorce, and often learn to consider love and relationships as conditional. Frequently, they live with unresolved grief. If parents cannot model appropriate conflict resolution, children often become bullies or victims of bullying.[8,9]

Blurred Roles or Boundaries

If a parent becomes vulnerable (ie, from illness, addiction, financial insecurity, loss of a relationship, or interpersonal violence), the child also becomes vulnerable. The child not only has lost a degree of support but often takes on a degree of worry about the parent. If stigma is associated with parental impairment (ie, addiction or mental illness), the child may receive little information or guidance to deal with her confusion, fear, and shame over the parent's circumstances. Many children are unable to develop close relationships because of feelings of loneliness and helplessness.[8,9,20,21]

Blurred parent-child roles or boundaries may occur in a variety of circumstances. When a parent is significantly impaired or when a child loses a parent through death or divorce, the child may become parentified, taking on tasks, concerns, and family roles more appropriately associated with an adult caregiver. This typically results in a tremendous amount of stress and can interfere with her developmental tasks.[8]

Presentations in the Primary Care Setting

Clinicians caring for children should be mindful of family functioning, as it affects the well-being of the children both physically and emotionally. This is especially true in the setting of the medical home, where a primary care clinician (PCC) (ie, a pediatrician, family physician, internist, nurse practitioner, or family physician who has an ongoing relationship with the child and family) coordinates continuity of care. The American Academy of Pediatrics (AAP) Task Force on Mental Health has recommended that children's health supervision visits routinely include psychosocial screening of the family, as well as the child.[22–25] However, any encounter provides an opportunity for assessment and intervention as indicated.

Family dysfunction may present in a wide variety of ways in the primary care setting. The appropriateness of physical care is typically more obvious, as the PCC assesses safety, growth and development, general health, and medical care. The family who has trouble keeping appointments or completing treatment may be showing signs that the parent is overwhelmed or that there are other barriers to care.[26]

The child in a struggling family often develops signs of stress, which may manifest physically (eg, frequent somatic concerns) or emotionally (eg, mood or behavior changes). Changes in sleep, appetite, energy, motivation, self-care, school achievement, recreational pursuits, or social interactions are cause for some degree of further exploration. Often, parents are unaware of the child's internal distress until external behavioral problems (eg, irritability, aggression, school failure, drug use, self-injury) arise.[27,28]

When family disturbance is severe, maltreatment may occur. Primary care clinicians receive formal training in the detection of child abuse and neglect and are uniformly considered to be mandated reporters for child welfare agencies. However, families (including the victim) often conceal abuse or neglect, necessitating a high index of suspicion. Chronic maltreatment, especially sexual abuse, may only be detected by specific investigation.[14,23]

The growing tendency of families to use emergency departments and urgent care centers in addition to (or instead of) a medical home setting (or even the practice of seeing more than one clinician within a clinic) undermines continuity of care, and may also mask the degree of dysfunction. The use of multiple clinicians should alert the PCC to increase vigilance. Appropriate documentation is vital, and forms for release of information facilitate communication among treating clinicians.[29]

The Primary Care Clinician's Role

Family dynamics are complicated, and patterns of interaction can become quite ingrained. However, support for families can have a profound, positive, and enduring effect for children and those in their lives. For the PCC, attention to family functioning is inextricably linked to practice,[5,6,30] providing many opportunities for supporting the development of healthy families as well as for addressing problems as they may arise.

Indeed, the PCC-family relationship provides a unique opportunity for positive influence. Families are built on relationships, and the PCC supports the family by first developing a therapeutic alliance with the child and caregiver. In this important position, the clinician affirms intrinsic dignity and self-worth by modeling healthy, respectful interactions with each.

The preventive aspect of primary care integrates routine anticipatory guidance.[28] This helps parents understand their children, guides them through appropriate caregiving practices, and promotes healthy aspects of family development. Over time, the PCC gains understanding of differences in personalities, expectations, and the culture of parenting within the family. This allows further customization of care, with recognition of strengths and anticipation of needed support.

In addition to conducting office visits, most pediatric PCCs provide supplemental educational material (eg, *Connected Kids* [violence prevention handouts] available at https://patiented.solutions.aap.org) and refer families to parenting classes as available. Some clinicians incorporate group checkups or classes of their own to facilitate discussion, involve extended family members, and engender parent-to-parent support.[31] When family problems are apparent, the PCC may build on the above practices, remaining constructive and supportive.

The timing of child health supervision visits correlates with the transitional challenges of various developmental stages. Additional visits may be indicated for circumstances that challenge family members, such as the occurrence of night terrors or the experience of divorce. An up-to-date social history is invaluable.

The PCC who is sensitive to parental development may prevent problems that arise from misinterpretation ("My baby cries because she doesn't like me"), unrealistic expectations ("He should be toilet-trained by now"), parental self-doubt ("I feel so guilty going back to work"), discipline ("He just needs a good spanking"), and cultural issues ("My father thinks we spoil her").

The need for anticipatory guidance remains dynamic, even as the child matures and seems to be more self-sufficient. Each child is unique, and may challenge a parent in ways a sibling did not. A new parental influence or attitude may be introduced (such as through a remarriage/new partner, more contact with a grandparent, or a new child care or classroom setting). Misinterpretation by a caregiver may become quite problematic (even to the point of maltreatment) if a child is labeled "oppositional," "bossy," "mean," "moody," or "lazy," especially if there is little consideration of the factors that may overwhelm the child and keep him from successfully adapting to the demands of his daily tasks. What seems to be "nothing" to an adult may mean much more to a child.

Many factors that influence parenting behavior may not be readily apparent, even to the parents themselves. A particular age or situation may present a special challenge to a parent who similarly struggled (eg, a mother who was assaulted, a father who became overdependent on athletic competition for a sense of self-worth).

Typically, family roles are learned in the family of origin.[8,9] However, rapid cultural changes may result in much different family structures, needs, dynamics, and practices. Commonly, struggles within the family of origin resurface when the now grown child begins a family of her own. Even in the best of circumstances, there is some degree of differing opinion in regard to parental practices. Clearly, the PCC who monitors family development and provides appropriate intervention provides a tremendous support to parental efficacy, child development and sense of self-worth, and overall family health.

For any clinical encounter, the interpersonal interaction is of great importance. However, it is even more so for a family that is struggling. The PCC may be among the few consistent supports for the family. Although families typically place trust in the PCCs who care for their children, this should not be taken for granted. In fact, there are many cultural stereotypes (eg, industry influence, overuse of medications) that may cause a family to be wary of their PCC or treatment recommendations. One should always listen carefully to what the family is truly communicating and confirm shared understanding of the purpose of the visit.

Even if the child is the family member considered to need help, parents may be quite frustrated or ashamed of their perceived failure, and subsequently quite sensitive to any implied criticism. The clinician should remain nonjudgmental, acknowledging the parents' care for their child and expressing the desire to problem-solve with them. The clinician can both model respectful interactions and constructively guide interactions between family members during the office presentation.

Typically, several techniques are used.[32–36] Emotional effect is acknowledged. ("That must have been quite upsetting.") Expectations are clarified. ("We won't use that type of language.") Communication is fostered. ("I feel that we pay attention to each other better if the cell phone is put away.") Positive actions are encouraged. ("I like the way that you followed through with the consequences.") Education is provided.

It is important to have the appropriate family members present and to ensure that each has a chance to be heard. Even if the clinician disagrees with a statement or considers an emotion to be unwarranted, it is important to acknowledge an understanding of the perspective being communicated. Disagreement between any participants should be made transparent, with the goal of seeking a common point of agreement upon which to proceed. Problem-solving should be as concrete, achievable, and action centered as possible. The "next steps" should be agreed upon and documented as specifically as possible ("We will turn off the computer an hour before bedtime"). It is important to acknowledge family strengths, efforts, and successes.

Primary care clinician–family interaction may range from a longer, prescheduled, and defined "family meeting" to a few minutes of conversation during a child health supervision or an acute care visit.[37,38] If the allotted time does not seem to be sufficient to the task, this should be acknowledged, with agreement on the acute priority of the day. In this fashion, the PCC can accommodate a variety of methods to work with families while still working within the schedule constraints of a clinical practice. By the end of a particular encounter, however, one should always try to understand the situation as clearly as is feasible, ensure safety, have an agreed-upon plan for the next steps, and have scheduled follow-up.

Pediatric PCCs vary a great deal in regard to personality, style of practice, experience, training, abilities, and motivation to work with families. This is especially true when working in challenging situations. Many PCCs already feel overtaxed by time constraints, documentation, and other work-related demands. Subsequently, it can be quite daunting to address additional levels of complexity when working with patients and their families. However, techniques can be customized across a variety of practice settings, presenting patients, and professional skill levels.

It is critical for the PCC to understand, define, and communicate his or her own role. Caregivers by nature, PCCs may have varied emotional responses to the patients and families in their care. Although families can be a source of joy, they may also engender sadness or other emotions that may not be as transparent. Clinicians may feel frustrated with families who do not facilitate care or who challenge their skill level. They may feel anxious in sensitive or disagreeable situations, or feel dislike or anger toward certain patients or family members. They may be even more vulnerable to distress or countertransference in circumstances that resonate with their own life experiences. Often, the needs of the family seem insurmountable or can be met only with resources far outside the PCC's scope of practice. Subsequently, the effective pediatric PCC needs a certain degree of self-reflection to provide insight into her own emotions and behaviors, and must acknowledge tendencies for minimization or avoidance, maintain appropriate boundaries, develop reasonable expectations for her work, and determine the need for additional resources and support.

As adult learners, pediatric PCCs monitor their own "practice gaps" and seek information accordingly. A variety of resources is available to enhance the knowledge and skills that facilitate working with families.[10,14,15,22,23,28,37–48] In addition to the traditional written resources, organizational toolkits, workshops, and mentoring opportunities support the incorporation of knowledge and skills into clinical practice.

Pediatric PCCs will be most effective if they also use educational and community resources for both the children and the adults. There are many books, support groups, and Internet resources for common problems (eg, divorce, bereavement, alcohol use disorder, violence). Families with significant and chronic dysfunction will typically benefit from the specific ongoing guidance of family therapy, and the PCC should be aware of local mental health resources. When referral to additional providers is warranted, personal attention to family engagement will greatly facilitate follow-through with the recommendation.[34,49]

The AAP Task Force on Mental Health has recommended that PCCs develop "common factors" communication skills to elicit an accurate understanding, identify and address any barriers to the care and follow-up of identified problems, and build a therapeutic alliance with the child and family. These skills are described in Chapter 5, Effective Communication Methods: Common Factors Skills, and represented by the HELP mnemonic, described in Appendix 5. Such skills have been shown to be readily acquired by experienced clinicians and effective across a wide range of psychosocial problems commonly encountered in the primary care setting.[22,39,50]

Conclusion

Family dynamics are complex and vulnerable to a variety of influences. Pediatric practice, however, provides a unique and powerful opportunity to guide not only the development of healthy children but the development of healthy families as well. By understanding both adaptive patterns and maladaptive patterns of behavior, the PCC can prevent problems, detect issues as they emerge, and intervene at early stages. By honing communication skills, using professional resources, and identifying community services, the PCC can offer support, provide appropriate materials, and coordinate referrals for more specialized care. This results in profound benefits for children and their families, with the potential to affect generations to come.

AAP Policy

Garner AS, Shonkoff JP; American Academy of Pediatrics Committee on Psychosocial Aspects of Child and Family Health; Committee on Early Childhood, Adoption, and Dependent Care; and Section on Developmental and Behavioral Pediatrics. Early childhood adversity, toxic stress, and the role of the pediatrician: translating developmental science into lifelong health. *Pediatrics.* 2012;129(1):e224–e231. Reaffirmed July 2016 (pediatrics.aappublications.org/content/129/1/e224)

References

1. Garner AS, Shonkoff JP; American Academy of Pediatrics Committee on Psychosocial Aspects of Child and Family Health; Committee on Early Childhood, Adoption, and Dependent Care; and Section on Developmental and Behavioral Pediatrics. Early childhood adversity, toxic stress, and the role of the pediatrician: translating developmental science into lifelong health. *Pediatrics.* 2012;129(1):e224–e231

2. Felitti VJ. Adverse childhood experiences and adult health. *Acad Pediatr.* 2009; 9(3):131–132

3. Anda RF, Felitti VJ, Bremner JD, et al. The enduring effects of abuse and related adverse experiences in childhood. A convergence of evidence from neurobiology and epidemiology. *Eur Arch Psychiatry Clin Neurosci.* 2006;256(3):174–186

4. Felitti VJ, Anda RF, Nordenberg D, et al. Relationship of childhood abuse and household dysfunction to many of the leading causes of death in adults. The Adverse Childhood Experiences (ACE) Study. *Am J Prev Med.* 1998;14(4):245–258

5. Schor EL; American Academy of Pediatrics Task Force on the Family. Family pediatrics: report of the Task Force on the Family. *Pediatrics.* 2003;111(6, pt 2): 1541–1571

6. American Academy of Pediatrics Committee on Early Childhood, Adoption, and Dependent Care. The pediatrician's role in family support and family support programs. *Pediatrics.* 2011;128(6):e1680–e1684

7. Family medicine, definition of. American Academy of Family Physicians Web site. http://www.aafp.org/online/en/home/policy/policies/f/familydefinitionof.html. Published 1984. Accessed February 8, 2018

8. Nichols MP, Schwartz RC. *Family Therapy: Concepts and Methods.* 6th ed. Boston, MA: Pearson; 2004

9. Berk LE. *Child Development.* 7th ed. Boston, MA: Pearson Education Inc; 2006

10. The Resilience Project. American Academy of Pediatrics Web site. https://www.aap.org/theresilienceproject. Accessed February 8, 2018

11. Belsky J. The determinants of parenting: a process model. *Child Dev.* 1984;55(1):83–96

12. Glascoe FP, Leew S. Parenting behaviors, perceptions, and psychosocial risk: impacts on young children's development. *Pediatrics.* 2010;125(2):313–319

13. Widom CS, Maxfield M. An update on the "cycle of violence." *National Institute of Justice Research Brief.* Washington, DC: National Institute of Justice; 2001:1–8

14. National Center for Injury Prevention and Control. Strategic direction for child maltreatment prevention: preventing child maltreatment through the promotion of safe, stable, and nurturing relationships between children and caregivers. Centers for Disease Control and Prevention Web site. https://www.cdc.gov/violenceprevention/pdf/cm_strategic_direction--long-a.pdf. Accessed February 8, 2018

15. Merrick MT, ed. Interrupting child maltreatment across generations through safe, stable, nurturing relationships. *J Adolesc Health.* 2013;53(4):A1–A4, S1–S44

16. Shepherd S, Owen D, Fitch TJ, Marshall JL. Locus of control and academic achievement in high school students. *Psychol Rep.* 2006;98(2):318–322

17. Ainsworth MD. Patterns of infant-mother attachments: antecedents and effects on development. *Bull N Y Acad Med.* 1985;61(9):771–791

18. Bowlby J. Developmental psychiatry comes of age. *Am J Psychiatry.* 1988;145(1):1–10

19. Chapman DP, Whitfield CL, Felitti VJ, et al. Adverse childhood experiences and the risk of depressive disorders in adulthood. *J Affect Disord.* 2004;82(2):217–225

20. Wickrama KA, Conger RD, Lorenz FO, Jung T. Family antecedents and consequences of trajectories of depressive symptoms from adolescence to young adulthood: a life course investigation. *J Health Soc Behav.* 2008;49(4):468–483

21. Kahn RS, Brandt D, Whitaker RC. Combined effect of mothers' and fathers' mental health symptoms on children's behavioral and emotional well-being. *Arch Pediatr Adolesc Med.* 2004;158(8):721–729

22. Foy JM; American Academy of Pediatrics Task Force on Mental Health. Enhancing pediatric mental health care: report from the American Academy of Pediatrics Task Force on Mental Health. Introduction. *Pediatrics.* 2010;125(suppl 3):S69–S74

23. Preventing child maltreatment: a guide to taking action and generating evidence. World Health Organization Web site. http://www.who.int/violence_injury_prevention/publications/violence/child_maltreatment/en. Published 2006. Accessed February 8, 2018

24. Rush AJ, First MB, Blacker D. *Handbook of Psychiatric Measures.* Arlington, VA: American Psychiatric Publishing Inc; 2008

25. Kemper KJ, Kelleher KJ. Family psychosocial screening instruments and techniques. *Ambul Child Health.* 1996;1:325–339

26. National Center for Medical Home Implementation Web site. http://www.medicalhomeinfo.org. Accessed February 8, 2018

27. Cluster guidance. In: *Addressing Mental Health Concerns in Primary Care: A Clinician's Toolkit.* Elk Grove Village, IL: American Academy of Pediatrics; 2010

28. Hagan JF Jr, Shaw JS, Duncan PM, eds. *Bright Futures: Guidelines for Health Supervision of Infants, Children, and Adolescents.* 4th ed. Elk Grove Village, IL: American Academy of Pediatrics; 2017

29. US Department of Health and Human Services. HIPAA guidance materials. HHS Web site. https://www.hhs.gov/hipaa/for-professionals/privacy/guidance/index.html. Accessed February 8, 2018

30. Rushton FE. *Family Support in Community Pediatrics.* Westport, CT: Praeger; 1998

31. Barlow J, Stewart-Brown S. Behavior problems and group-based parent education programs. *J Dev Behav Pediatr.* 2000;21(5):356–370

32. Providing culturally effective, family-centered care. In: *Addressing Mental Health Concerns in Primary Care: A Clinician's Toolkit.* Elk Grove Village, IL: American Academy of Pediatrics; 2010

33. Generic or common factors interventions: HELP. In: *Addressing Mental Health Concerns in Primary Care: A Clinician's Toolkit.* Elk Grove Village, IL: American Academy of Pediatrics; 2010

34. Engaging children and parents using patient activation techniques. In: *Addressing Mental Health Concerns in Primary Care: A Clinician's Toolkit.* Elk Grove Village, IL: American Academy of Pediatrics; 2010

35. Brief supportive interviewing technique. In: *Addressing Mental Health Concerns in Primary Care: A Clinician's Toolkit.* Elk Grove Village, IL: American Academy of Pediatrics; 2010

36. Motivational counseling. In: *Addressing Mental Health Concerns in Primary Care: A Clinician's Toolkit.* Elk Grove Village, IL: American Academy of Pediatrics; 2010

37. Coleman WL. *Family-Focused Pediatrics: Interviewing Techniques and Other Strategies to Help Families Resolve Their Interactive and Emotional Problems.* 2nd ed. Elk Grove Village, IL: American Academy of Pediatrics; 2011

38. Allmond BW Jr, Tanner JL, Gofman HF. *The Family Is the Patient: Using Family Interviews in Children's Medical Care.* 2nd ed. Baltimore, MD: Williams & Wilkins; 1999

39. American Academy of Pediatrics. *Addressing Mental Health Concerns in Primary Care: A Clinician's Toolkit.* Elk Grove Village, IL: American Academy of Pediatrics; 2010

40. Spivak H, Sege R, Flanigan E, Licenziato V. *Connected Kids: Safe, Strong, Secure Clinical Guide.* Elk Grove Village, IL: American Academy of Pediatrics; 2006

41. Langford J, Wolf KG. *Guidelines for Family Support Practice.* 2nd ed. Chicago, IL: Family Resource Coalition; 2001

42. Cheng MK. New approaches for creating the therapeutic alliance: solution-focused interviewing, motivational interviewing, and the medication interest model. *Psychiatr Clin North Am.* 2007;30(2):157–166

43. Gleason MM, Shah P, Boris N. Assessment and interviewing. In: Kliegman RM, Behrman RE, Jenson HB, Stanton B, eds. *Nelson Textbook of Pediatrics.* 18th ed. Philadelphia, PA: WB Saunders; 2008

44. Shah P. Interviewing and counseling children and families. In: Voigt RG, Macias MM, Meyers SM, eds. *Developmental and Behavioral Pediatrics.* Elk Grove Village, IL: American Academy of Pediatrics; 2011

45. Sommers-Flanagan J, Sommers-Flanagan R. Our favorite tips for interviewing couples and families. *Psychiatr Clin North Am.* 2007;30(2):275–281

46. Stuart MR, Lieberman JA. *The Fifteen-Minute Hour: Applied Psychotherapy for the Primary Care Physician.* Westport, CT: Praeger; 2008

47. Whitaker T, Fiore DJ. *Dealing With Difficult Parents and With Parents in Difficult Situations.* Larchmont, NY: Eye On Education; 2001

48. Ginsburg KR; American Academy of Pediatrics Committee on Communications and Committee on Psychosocial Aspects of Child and Family Health. The importance of play in promoting healthy child development and maintaining strong parent-child bonds. *Pediatrics.* 2007;119(1):182–191

49. McKay MM, Hibbert R, Hoagwood K, et al. Integrating evidence-based engagement interventions into "real world" child mental health settings. *Brief Treat Crisis Interven.* 2004;4(2):177–186

50. Wissow LS, Gadomski A, Roter D, et al. Improving child and parent mental health in primary care: a cluster-randomized trial of communication skills training. *Pediatrics.* 2008;121(2):266–275

CHAPTER 19

Gender Expression and Identity

Robert J. Bidwell, MD

> *"The goal of care in working with gender variant children and transgender youths is to promote optimal physical, developmental, psychological, and social well-being. The challenge faced by clinicians is to achieve this goal within a context of nonacceptance and stigmatization by many people in society."*

Introduction

Definitions

Gender is a complex concept that is still not well understood. Researchers and theorists have attempted to study and explain various aspects of gender to improve their understanding of this important part of being human. *Gender role* represents a set of behaviors, attitudes, and interests that a society or culture believes are typically female or male. A child internalizes these cultural gender role expectations by the age of 3 to 5 years. *Gender expression* refers to how a person signifies gender in dress, speech, interests, and other outward signs. When a child displays behaviors, attitudes, or interests outside the cultural norm for the child's biological (genetic or anatomic) sex, it is referred to as *gender nonconforming* expression or *gender variant* expression. More recent terms include *gender creative* expression and *gender expansive* expression. For example, a boy with gender variant behavior may prefer playing house to playing football, may enjoy dressing up in his mother's clothes or trying on her makeup, may prefer long hair, and may be more stereotypically feminine in his mannerisms and speech, as determined by a particular culture. A girl with gender variant behavior may avoid wearing clothes that are culturally more associated with girls, may enjoy more physically aggressive play with boys, may prefer short hair, and may be more stereotypically masculine in her mannerisms.

In contrast, *gender identity* refers to a person's deepest inner sense of being female or male (or even something other than female or male) and is often established early in childhood. For most people, gender identity is congruent with biological sex or birth-assigned gender. For some, it is not. Although their bodies seem to tell them and the world around them that they are female or male, they have an inner identity that is of either the opposite gender or a sense of gender separate from female or male. These individuals are referred to as *transgender.*

Gender identity is distinct from *sexual orientation,* which refers to a person's affectional, romantic, or sexual attraction to others of the same sex (homosexual), the opposite sex (heterosexual), or both sexes (bisexual).

Transgender is also used sometimes as a broader umbrella term encompassing those who do not conform to cultural norms of being female or male. This group includes individuals whose gender identities are incongruent with their biological sexes and who may seek to change their bodies to make them more consistent with an inner sense of gender. These individuals are sometimes referred to as *transsexual* but are more commonly referred to as *transgender* in the narrower sense of the term, as described previously. Transgender in its broader sense has recently been referred to as the *trans* spectrum.* In addition to including those who experience an incongruence between their bodies and their inner gender identities, the trans* spectrum also includes those who cross-culturally defined gender boundaries, including cross-dressers (transvestites), drag kings and queens, and people who perceive themselves to be of both genders (bigender), to be of all genders (pangender), to be of no gender (agender), or as transcending the typical binary male-female conception of gender (gender nonbinary). It also includes those who may refer to themselves as *gender fluid* or *genderqueer* and those who are routinely gender variant in their attitudes, interests, and behaviors. In addition to being applied to adolescents, the term *transgender* is increasingly applied to prepubertal children who are persistent, insistent, and consistent in asserting a cross-gender identity.

In this chapter, *transgender* is used in its narrower sense, referring to gender identity. Transgender individuals often refer to themselves as *trans, trans*, TG,* or *T.* Many transgender people, but not all, experience significant *gender dysphoria,* a persistent discomfort with the gender assigned to them at birth and the societal gender role expectations that accompany it. These dysphoric feelings often begin in early childhood and increase with the appearance of unwanted physical changes at puberty. Many transgender individuals gradually move beyond the need to conform to societal expectations attached to a birth-assigned gender and increasingly present themselves to the world in a manner consistent with their gender identities. This process is known as *transition*. The transition process may be facilitated medically by pubertal suppression, cross-gender hormone therapy, or gender-affirmation surgery (also referred to as *sex-reassignment surgery*, or SRS), or varying combinations thereof. However, it not only is a physical process but also takes place on psychological, social, and spiritual levels. The terms *male-to-female* (MTF) transgender and *female-to-male* (FTM) transgender are used to describe the direction of transition from biological sex to actual gender identity. An FTM transgender person is often referred to as a *trans-man* and an MTF person as a *trans-woman*.

Prevalence

Most gender variant children and *youths* (defined in this chapter as children older than 6 years of age and adolescents, collectively) do not experience gender dysphoria, nor do they have gender identities that differ from their birth-assigned genders. The prevalence of gender variance in children and youths is uncertain, although studies have shown that gender variant behavior is common.[1-3] Persistent gender variant behavior and expressed wishes to be another gender are less common.[4-6] In a 2011 population-based survey of middle school students in San Francisco, when given a choice of identifying themselves as male, female, or transgender, 1.3% chose the last response. The World Professional Association for Transgender Health (WPATH) estimates that the prevalence of MTF transgender identity is 1 in 11,900 to 1 in 45,000 people and of FTM transgender identity is 1 in 30,400 to 1 in 200,000.[7] Some believe that these estimations are low because they are based on individuals seeking hormonal and surgical transition services: some transgender individuals do not have access to or do not want sex-reassignment services and so are not represented in the data. A recent meta-analysis of population-based surveys of US adults conducted between 2006 and 2016 suggested that transgender adults may represent 390 per 100,000 population.[8]

Gender Dysphoria

One of the most controversial issues related to gender expression and gender identity during childhood and adolescence is whether gender variance and transgenderism are causes for concern.[9-13] Do they represent a pathological abnormality, or are they simply part of the continuum of normal human expression and identity? Similar debates occurred around homosexuality until it was officially removed from the American Psychiatric Association (APA) list of mental disorders in 1973. Although controversial, until 2013 transgenderism (in the narrower sense) and transsexualism were represented in the fourth edition of the *Diagnostic and Statistical Manual of Mental Disorders* under the diagnostic category of *gender identity disorder* (GID).[14] Based on the work of the Workgroup on Sexual and Gender Identity Disorders, the APA fifth edition of the *Diagnostic and Statistical Manual of Mental Disorders* (*DSM-5*) introduced several important changes in terminology and diagnostic criteria related to gender identity, with separate criteria for children and for adolescents and adults.[15] The diagnostic category of GID was replaced by the less stigmatizing designation *gender dysphoria.* The controversy surrounding these diagnoses is well-documented.[16,17] The diagnostic criteria for childhood and for adolescent and adult gender dysphoria require a marked difference between a person's experienced or expressed gender and the gender assigned at birth. For a diagnosis of gender dysphoria to be made, this gender incongruence must have persisted for at least 6 months and resulted in significant distress or impairment in social, school, occupational, or other important areas of functioning.

At a basic level, the move from GID to gender dysphoria emphasizes that cross-gender *identity* is no longer considered disordered. Instead, it is the distress related to having a cross-gender identity, which is often caused in significant measure by growing up and living in a nonaccepting, often aggressively hostile, societal environment. Much of the controversy arising from the creation of both GID and gender dysphoria as *Diagnostic and Statistical Manual of Mental Disorders* diagnostic categories is the observation that any gender variant child or youth raised in a society that enforces a binary view of gender will predictably experience some degree of discomfort or distress related to gender expression and identity. Given the overt discrimination and violence that has occurred against transgender individuals in the United States, distress or impairment in social and other areas of functioning is not surprising. Evidence suggests that transgender individuals growing up in more-accepting societies experience less discomfort and distress related to their gender identities and gender expressions.[18]

Several developmental trajectories have been described for children with GID, which are presumably relevant for those now diagnosed as having gender dysphoria.[19] The diagnostic rubric of gender dysphoria is too recent to be reflected in a substantial body of literature. The studies on which these proposed trajectories are based are small and inconclusive. Taken as a whole, however, they suggest that many children diagnosed as having GID (and, more recently, gender dysphoria) eventually self-identify as gay or bisexual as adolescents or adults and no longer experience gender dysphoria. A smaller percentage later self-identify as heterosexual and also experience no gender dysphoria. A smaller but significant percentage, particularly children who are most consistent and insistent in asserting a cross-gender identity, continue to experience discomfort with their biological sexes into adolescence and adulthood, and they eventually self-identify as transgender.[20]

Care of Gender Variant Children and Transgender Youths

The American Academy of Pediatrics, the American Academy of Child and Adolescent Psychiatry, and the Society for Adolescent Health and Medicine have each issued official guidelines related to providing supportive care to children and youths facing issues of gender identity and gender expression.[19,21,22] In addition, several resources are available to pediatric clinicians (ie, primary care pediatricians, pediatric subspecialists, family physicians, internists, nurse practitioners, and family physicians who provide health care to children and adolescents) on providing culturally sensitive and relevant care to gender variant children and transgender youths and adults.[23–25]

Evaluation

History

Gender variant children and transgender youths may come to a pediatric clinician's office because of parental concerns or through school or child welfare agency referral. Transgender youths may also seek care themselves, often to discuss issues of safety and acceptance at home or school or concerns about sexually transmitted infections (STIs), or to request hormone therapy. However, many transgender patients see their pediatric clinicians not through referrals or acute care visits but rather in the context of routine adolescent health supervision evaluations. Many transgender patients hide any evidence of an inner gender identity; others are presumed, perhaps even by themselves, to be lesbian or gay. Clinicians should initiate discussion of sexuality and gender with all youths at each health supervision visit. Although many pediatric clinicians routinely discuss sexual activity and safer-sex practices, fewer discuss sexual orientation, and almost none of them address gender identity. However, as noted earlier, most transgender youths face significant confusion and distress related to their gender identities and face major risks from growing up in an often nonaccepting world. Pediatric clinicians must be willing to open the door to discussion of gender to reduce the turmoil and dangers that these youths face.

The clinician can begin to approach the issue of gender identity in the broader context of performing a HEADSSS mnemonic (home/environment, education and employment, activities, drugs, sexuality, suicide/depression, and safety) interview.[26] This approach will provide a sense of how things are going in various aspects of a youth's life, recognizing that many transgender youths face serious issues in each of these areas. Throughout this conversation, it is essential that the clinician use non-heterosexist, gender-neutral language, reflecting that no assumptions are being made about a youth's sexual orientation or gender identity or about those of family members or friends. To address gender identity within a broader sexual history, the clinician might say, "Sexuality and sexual feelings can be confusing sometimes. During puberty, bodies change in lots of different ways. Sexual feelings are changing as well. Some of my patients are not sure whether they are attracted to boys or girls or maybe both, and some of my patients even wonder whether they're more like a girl or a boy inside. All of this is completely normal but can be really confusing. So, I'm wondering what it's been like for you." After asking about attractions (sexual orientation), the clinician can simply ask, "And how about inside? Do you feel more like a girl or a boy or maybe something else?" For the patient who is not dealing with gender identity issues, these questions may seem odd. This discomfort can be addressed by a simple statement such as "These are questions I ask all my patients, and for some they're really important." For transgender youths, the questions may be lifesaving. Even if they decide not to acknowledge their gender identity concerns at the current visit, they have learned that someone is available with whom they can talk when the time is right. If youths acknowledge cross-gender feelings, the clinician can ask whether they have defined themselves by gender. Some may refer to themselves as transgender, while others may self-define as pansexual, pangender, bigender, gender fluid, genderqueer, or another designation. Some may refer to themselves as gay or lesbian. It is appropriate to ask each youth what the youth's particular self-designation means to the youth. This question demonstrates respect on the part of the clinician and can foster a sense of empowerment in the youth.

If youths acknowledge a transgender, a pangender, or another-gendered identity, the clinician should thank them for their trust in sharing this important and personal part of who they are. As a demonstration of understanding and respect, the clinician should then ask about preferred name and pronouns and use these through the remainder of the interview and subsequent visits. Patients should be reassured that the discussion of gender identity will remain confidential unless they give permission to share it with others or unless a risk of danger to someone exists. It is essential to ask, at an appropriate time in the interview, "Do you have any periods of feeling very sad? How long do they last? Have you ever had feelings of wanting to hurt yourself or kill yourself? Have you ever actually tried to do this?" If the clinician is uncomfortable with the depth of interviewing suggested in the following paragraphs, the clinician has a responsibility to refer the youth to someone else who can have this conversation.

The subsequent history may then focus on the youth's path to recognizing the youth's transgender identity: "When were you first aware of feeling more like a girl, a boy, or another gender? What was this experience like? How comfortable are you with your transgender identity now? What do you know about gender identity and what it means to be transgender? What are your hopes and dreams for the future? Do you see your future as enhanced or limited by being transgender?" The history may focus on the youth in the context of the world around the youth: "Have you told others (family, peers, teachers, or counselors) about your inner feelings of gender? Have these people responded in a supportive or negative way? Have you been bullied, harassed, scolded, ridiculed, or teased because of your gender identity? With whom do you spend time, and what kinds of things do you do together? Have you met other transgender adolescents or adults? Have you been in relationships, and have these relationships been healthy ones?

Have you been sexually active, and do you use safer-sex practices? How have you met your sexual and romantic partners? Have you ever been pregnant, impregnated anyone, or had an STI? How many different sexual partners have you had, and what have been their genders? Have you ever been touched sexually or forced to have sex without your permission?"

Understanding that transgender youths are often subjected to harassment and rejection at home and school, the clinician should ask about how they are treated in these settings and whether they have ever run away from home or dropped out of school. Have they needed to sell their bodies, deal drugs, or engage in other illegal activities to survive on the streets? Have they been involved with the child welfare or juvenile justice system, and how have they been treated within it? Have they ever used drugs or contemplated suicide? How do they believe their physical health has been, and do they have any health needs they believe are not being addressed? What do they know about gender transitions, and is that process something they have thought about? Have they actually begun the transition process? Have they begun to cross-dress? Have they begun puberty blockers or cross-gender hormone therapy, and, if so, where have they obtained this treatment? Have they injected silicone? Have they thought about gender-affirmation surgery or other transition-related procedures in the future?

Other questions to consider include "What have you found on the Internet or in various forms of media about transgender people?" "Do you know any transgender or lesbian, gay, or bisexual (LGB) people?" and "Whom do you have as supports?" Because eating disorders are common among sexual minorities and especially among transgender populations in which malnutrition can suppress pubertal progression, it is also important to ask, "Do you restrict your diet, binge and purge, or use laxatives or make yourself vomit?"

Not all these questions need to be addressed at the first visit. Follow-up visits should be made to address these issues on an ongoing basis. The clinician should be aware that the history, beyond providing specific information about the experience and needs of a transgender youth, is an opportunity for the clinician to interact with the patient in a comfortable, respectful, and caring manner that validates who the youth is as a human being. Many transgender youths have never experienced such acceptance before, and providing it is among the most fundamentally important things a clinician can do.

Physical Examination

The physical examination of children with gender variant behaviors or who express the desire to be other than their anatomic sexes should be guided by a comprehensive and accurate health history, including sexual and other risk behaviors. The content of the physical examination does not differ significantly from that of other youths. A complete examination, including the genitalia, should be a routine part of every child health supervision visit. On occasion, the clinician may observe a child wearing clothes or exhibiting behaviors or interests that are more typical of another gender. These behaviors or interests may or may not relate to the child's gender identity.

The clinician should remember that transgender youths may be heterosexually, homosexually, or bisexually active or not sexually active at all. Many transgender youths hide all public expressions of their gender identities. Some may have already begun the transition process and come to clinic displaying dress, hairstyles, makeup, and mannerisms usually associated with another gender but consistent with their gender identities. Occasionally, transgender patients may wear non–gender-defining street clothes but underwear appropriate for their gender identities. If patients have begun pubertal suppression, they will generally remain at Tanner stage 2 or 3 and, depending on the duration of suppression, may eventually show delay in pubertal development relative to their peers. If patients have already begun transition hormone therapy, they may show evidence of breast development (MTF), appearance of facial hair (FTM), and other expected changes of estrogen or testosterone treatment.

Clinicians should understand and respect the significant distress that many transgender youths experience related to their biologically determined pubertal changes, such as development of facial hair, deepening of the voice, breast development, and menstrual periods, which feel alien to them because of their gender identities. Some MTF-transgender youths may tuck their genitalia, placing their penis and testes between their legs so they are less visible. Some FTM-transgender youths may wear chest binders or baggy tops to make their breasts less visible. Some may also wear a "packer," which is padding or a phallic-shaped object worn in the front of the underwear or pants to give the appearance of having a penis.

In preparing for the examination, the clinician should discuss the rationale for suggesting the parts of the examination that might be particularly uncomfortable for a transgender youth, especially the breast and genital examinations. Clinicians should explain that their intention is to make the examination as comfortable as possible for the patient and to elicit the patient's guidance in how best to accomplish this task. Patients should be informed that they have a right to refuse any part of the examination. The clinician should ask transgender patients what words they would like used in referring to various body parts, for example, *genitalia* instead of *penis* or *vagina*. An FTM-transgender patient may prefer the term *chest* rather than *breast*. An MTF-transgender patient should be treated the same as other female patients and an FTM-transgender patient like other male patients in conducting the examination. Conducting all comprehensive physical examinations of MTF- and FTM-transgender patients with the patient in a gown and draped appropriately, to minimize exposure, is best. At the same time, acknowledging that the patient's anatomic features may suggest sex-specific evaluation, such as breast, testicular, or pelvic examination, is appropriate. For example, suggesting a pelvic examination for an FTM adolescent with unexplained vaginal discharge or bleeding might be appropriate. Most transgender patients will agree to the suggested examination if the medical rationale is presented in a factual and respectful manner, inviting the patient's questions and input on how to make the examination as comfortable as possible. All aspects of the physical examination should be for the purpose of medical necessity, not to satisfy clinician curiosity about possible genital or breast changes related to hormone or surgical transition therapy. As for all youths, a chaperone should be present during a breast examination, a genital examination, or an anorectal examination. The gender of the chaperone should be based on patient preference.

Promoting Resilience and Health

The goal of care in working with gender variant children and transgender youths is to promote optimal physical, developmental, psychological, and social well-being. The challenge faced by clinicians is to achieve this goal within a context of nonacceptance and stigmatization by many people in society. In this sense, gender variant children and transgender youths have life experiences and needs that are like those of LGB youths.

Another challenge faced by clinicians is how to advise and support families of gender variant and gender dysphoric children and youths when there has been a considerable lack of professional consensus on appropriate treatment approaches and goals in these age-groups. Because there has been insufficient research in these and related areas, treatment approaches and goals rely in large part on "expert opinion and experience" rather than scientific data. This insufficiency has led to the proposal of several different treatment approaches, particularly for preadolescents, based on differing philosophical foundations but very little science. This lack of evidence-based best-practice standards can present a dilemma for clinicians and families in trying to decide which of the varying approaches best meets the needs of a particular child. Fortunately, a 2012 issue of the *Journal of Homosexuality* is dedicated to assisting clinicians and parents by offering a comprehensive review of what is known and what has yet to be learned about gender variance and gender dysphoria in childhood, as well as various treatment approaches and their specified goals.[27] It also provides detailed descriptions of a number of well-established clinical programs and identified areas of consensus and disagreement among them.[28-30] Ethical implications of the various approaches are also discussed.[31] Because most pediatric clinicians work in communities without specialized child and youth gender clinics and may be the major source of information and support for gender variant and transgender patients and their families, it is imperative that clinicians become familiar with these issues, understand where they themselves stand philosophically on the continuum of treatment approaches, remain abreast of recent research findings, and be willing to reach out to experts at nationally recognized child and youth gender centers for consultation as the need arises.[32-34]

Although relatively little is known about gender variance, cross-gender identity, and gender dysphoria in childhood, the area that may be best understood is the likely developmental trajectories of prepubertal children with gender dysphoria. It appears that the dysphoria of many younger children with gender dysphoria does not persist into adolescence.[12] These children have been referred to as *desisters,* and their dysphoria usually disappears in later childhood, at about age 7 to 9 years. Research suggests that most desisters will go on to self-identify as lesbian or gay during adolescence, and a smaller percentage will identify as heterosexual. Children who insistently and consistently assert a cross-gender identity into adolescence have been referred to as *persisters,* and most eventually identify in adolescence and adulthood as transgender. An area of controversy has been whether treatment aimed at promoting a child's desistance is effective or, more important, ethical. This is among the most disputed aspects related to the treatment of gender variant expression, cross-gender identity, and gender dysphoria in preadolescence. While there is some controversy related to the treatment of transgender adolescents in timing and length of various transition treatments, most clinical experts support medical transition treatments in adolescence and adulthood, such as pubertal suppression, hormone therapy, and eventual gender-affirmation surgery. This is because research has shown that most transgender adolescents have a gender identity that will persist into adulthood. Furthermore, there is a robust body of evidence demonstrating that transition treatments are safe and lead to significant improvements in physical and emotional well-being.[35-39] There has been no similar body of research definitively supporting a single treatment approach over another in addressing gender dysphoria and gender variance in preadolescents. This has led to the confusing and sometimes contradictory choices facing clinicians and the parents and children they are trying their best to support.

Despite controversy, several shared themes can be found across most treatment programs for gender dysphoric and gender variant preadolescents.[31] Because many gender dysphoric children will be desisters and no longer gender dysphoric as they move into adolescence, it is generally agreed that the appropriate approach is to provide support and counseling to parents and children but not to provide medical transition treatment in childhood. Until recently, there has been a widely held view that social transition into living full-time as a child of another gender or use of a name and pronouns consistent with inner gender identity should probably be deferred until adolescence. However, a recent research study examined the experience of prepubertal children who identify as the gender opposite than assigned at birth and who are supported in living openly as that gender. While previous studies of children with GID often show significantly increased levels of depression and anxiety, children in this study showed no elevations in depression and only a slight elevation in anxiety compared to a general peer population. Although further research is needed to define the factors underlying their emotional well-being, this study suggests, at the very least, that supporting these children in their social transitions seems to do no harm and may, in fact, have a positive effect on their psychological well-being. This understanding has led to an increased willingness of clinicians to support the social transition of prepubertal children who clearly and consistently assert a cross-gender identity.

Another area of general agreement is that, ideally, support and counseling should be provided to gender dysphoric children and their families by a multidisciplinary team consisting of a primary care clinician (PCC), a psychiatrist or another mental health professional, and a social worker. These professionals can be valuable additions to the treatment plan in exploring a child's or youth's sense of gender identity, social and academic functioning, family relationships, cultural expectations, and self-esteem. They can help assess and support parents through the process of acceptance and, it is hoped, eventual celebration of their child. They can also address parental fears, concerns, and misconceptions, which will likely change in nature as a child grows older and moves into adolescence. Most treatment programs emphasize that their goal is not to prevent homosexuality or cross-gender identity. Instead, the stated goal for most is to prevent or ameliorate gender dysphoria, recognizing that not all children with cross-gender identity are gender dysphoric.

Despite these common themes among most programs, there are also significant and often controversial differences regarding what support and counseling actually mean among varying programs. These differences often reflect underlying philosophical differences and varying understandings of gender variance and gender identity, their etiologies, and the degree to which they are felt to reflect possible underlying pathology or simply another way of "being" in the world. At one end of the spectrum are programs that are prepared to focus on perceived psychopathology in a child, in a parent, or in family dynamics that either causes gender variant expression or cross-gender identity and dysphoria or allows them to persist.[28] Treatment often involves trying to help a child work through a cross-gender identity with the goal of decreasing gender dysphoria, even if it means engaging in efforts to decrease a child's desire to be another gender. Parents are asked to put limits on their child's cross-gender behaviors and to create more opportunities for their child to have interactions with temperamentally compatible same-sex peers, feeling that these kinds of interactions help solidify a child's "appropriate" sense of gender, consistent with natal sex, and perhaps counteract pathological influences that contribute to the creation or persistence of cross-gender identity. At the other end of the spectrum are professionals who believe the appropriate approach is to validate and celebrate the unique gender identity of each child,[40] respecting children's right to express their genders as they wish, while keeping them safe in an often nonaccepting and hostile world. Most programs working with gender variant and gender dysphoric children fall somewhere in the middle of the spectrum.[29,30,41] They tend not to focus on looking for sources of psychopathology as factors that contribute to a child's gender identity or gender dysphoria. Most feel that a good measure of the dysphoria experienced by children and youths comes from the negative responses of family, peers, and community to a child's cross-gender identity and expression. Therefore, a significant part of providing support to a child is to determine how safe and supportive that child's environment is and to work with extended families, schools, places of worship, and other settings to ensure that the child is safe and validated in all areas of the child's life. Parents are provided information about gender dysphoria and its possible developmental trajectories, as well as the understanding, skills, and resources to support their child effectively, no matter what their child's gender identity or sexual orientation might eventually be. Most pediatric clinicians take a watchful-waiting approach toward these children, allowing these children to express their genders, although sometimes suggesting certain limits (eg, being allowed to cross-dress at home but not when they go to school). As a child approaches adolescence, pediatric clinicians are especially watchful for evidence that the child's gender dysphoria, if present, may persist or desist. If it looks as if it may persist, discussions with parents and child about possible future choices related to transition take place (eg, the initiation of pubertal suppression early in puberty). If it seems that the child's gender dysphoria may desist, other discussions are to be had, including considering the possibility that the child may later recognize an LGB identity and providing family and child supportive resources in preparation for this possibility.

When faced with such a diverse and often contentious array of opinion and practice, what is a clinician to do when a family arrives in the clinic expressing concerns about their young child's gender variant behaviors, expressed cross-gender identity, or gender dysphoria? First, it is important to be familiar with the areas of consensus and controversy outlined in the previous paragraphs. Second, it is important to keep in mind the replacement of the GID diagnosis with gender dysphoria in the *DSM-5*. This replacement means that gender variant expression and cross-gender identity per se are now considered part of the normal spectrum of human diversity. Discomfort and distress over gender should be the focus of concern, and the goal of treatment is to prevent or ameliorate that distress, whether its origins are within a person's psyche, within a person's environment, or perhaps within both. It is important to remember that the goal of treatment is not to prevent homosexuality, and most clinicians would agree that it is also not to change a child's expressed gender identity. Clinicians should be aware of and willing to access local and national resources that can support them in the provision of informed care to these children and youths and their families. See Box 19-1. If possible, it is very helpful to bring together a multidisciplinary team as described earlier, to support the patient and the patient's family over time, from childhood through adolescence and possibly into adulthood.

Box 19-1. Resources for Clinicians Who Care for Gender Variant Children and Transgender Youths

- Brill S, Kenney L. *The Transgender Teen: A Handbook for Parents and Professionals Supporting Transgender and Non-binary Teens.* San Francisco, CA: Cleis Press Inc; 2016

- Brill S, Pepper R. *The Transgender Child: A Handbook for Families and Professionals.* San Francisco, CA: Cleis Press Inc; 2008

- Centers for Disease Control and Prevention. Transgender persons. Centers for Disease Control and Prevention Web site. https://www.cdc.gov/lgbthealth/transgender.htm. Updated May 18, 2017. Accessed February 20, 2018

- *Guidelines for Care of Lesbian, Gay, Bisexual, and Transgender Patients.* San Francisco, CA: Gay and Lesbian Medical Association; 2006. http://glma.org/_data/n_0001/resources/live/GLMA%20guidelines%202006%20FINAL.pdf. Accessed February 20, 2018

- Makadon HJ, Mayer KH, Potter J, Goldhammer H, eds. *The Fenway Guide to Lesbian, Gay, Bisexual and Transgender Health.* Philadelphia, PA: American College of Physicians; 2008

- Mallon GP, DeCrescenzo T. Transgender children and youth: a child welfare practice perspective. *Child Welfare.* 2006;85(2):215–241

- Ryan C. *Helping Families Support Their Lesbian, Gay, Bisexual, and Transgender (LGBT) Children.* Washington, DC: National Center for Cultural Competence, Georgetown University Center for Child and Human Development; 2009

- World Professional Association for Transgender Health. Standards of care for the health of transsexual, transgender, and gender nonconforming people. *Int J Transgend.* 2012;13(4):165–232.

It is important to be open with parents about the varying approaches to working with gender variant and gender dysphoric children and about the parents' underlying assumptions and goals. It is also important for clinicians to let parents know where they are on the spectrum of professional opinion about the appropriate treatment approach to these children and their families. Clinicians or other team members should open the opportunity for a discussion of parental concerns, fears, and degree of comfort related to their child's gender identity and expression. They should also be asked what their hopes and expectations around treatment might be. Parents should be informed clearly that the goals of treatment are to prevent or diminish a child's distress around gender but not to change a child's gender identity or sexual orientation. Often parents fear that their child might someday be lesbian or gay, and they may not have thought about the possibility of their child being transgender. The clinician should gently remind parents that any child might be gay, lesbian, bisexual, or transgender and should let them know of the medical profession's position that all these possibilities are considered normal developmental outcomes, while recognizing that not all segments of society yet agree. The clinician should also share, in lay terms, what is known about the developmental trajectories of children experiencing gender dysphoria, that is, that in adolescence many come to realize a lesbian or gay identity, while a smaller number are transgender. Over time, as a child gets older, this issue should be revisited, offering parents an opportunity to share their thoughts or concerns and allowing the clinician to correct misconceptions and connect parents, children, and youths to supportive resources.

Above all, clinicians should remind parents of the importance of expressing their unconditional love for their child and refraining from comments or actions that demonstrate disapproval of their child's gender expression or identity. The Family Acceptance Project at San Francisco University has conducted research demonstrating the important role that parents play in keeping their lesbian, gay, bisexual, or transgender (LGBT) children healthy and safe through the provision of acceptance and love.[42] The clinician should share this understanding with all families and provide them the skills and resources to accept and support their children no matter what a gender identity or sexual orientation might be.

The following sections continue the discussion by focusing on how clinicians can recognize and address the needs of gender variant children and transgender youths.

Physical Well-being

Gender variant children and transgender youths face the same health issues as other young people. The health care they receive should be based on a comprehensive history, physical examination, and evaluative studies, not on a gender expression or identity. Nevertheless, the clinician should recognize that these children and youths often grow up in hostile environments that may have a negative effect on their physical well-being. Among these negative effects are the physical sequelae of substance use, poor nutrition caused by homelessness or disordered eating, unprotected sexual behaviors, self-harm, injuries caused by physical and sexual victimization, and hormone or surgical transition treatments accessed outside of health care settings.

Developmental, Social, and Emotional Well-being

In most ways, children with gender variant expression and transgender youths are the same as their peers. They have the same needs for protection, nurturance, and love and the same hopes and dreams for the future. They grow up in the same families and communities and attend the same schools and places of worship. Like other children, they face the fundamental task of achieving a sense of identity that integrates all aspects of who they are, including their sexual orientations and gender identities. This integration of sexual orientation and gender identity, accompanied by a growing sense of comfort with that orientation and identity, is essential for the optimal health and well-being of each child and youth.

However, the experience of growing up as a child with gender variant expression or as a transgender youth is different in several important ways.[9,43,44] Unlike their peers, these young people face an often lonely and sometimes frightening journey of self-discovery, attempting to understand 2 of the most fundamental aspects of who they are as human beings: their gender identities and their sexual orientations. Some of these children will recognize, often at a young age, that the inner sense of being female, male, or another gender they feel differs from the gender that was assigned to them at birth. Some children and youths accommodate themselves to this growing awareness. Most, however, experience significant confusion and distress, wondering what their feelings mean and uncertain of who they are. Growing up in a society that believes that a person is either male or female and that gender expression and identity must strictly reflect biological sex undoubtedly intensifies a sense that something inside them has gone wrong. Many of these individuals become filled with an overwhelming mix of confusion, shame, anger, self-hatred, and despair. It is important to remember that many gender dysphoric children eventually self-identify as LGB and no longer experience gender dysphoria as adolescents. Being LGB in an often disapproving society may bring its own distinct set of developmental challenges.

The pediatric clinician's role as educator and counselor is as important as that of medical provider in caring for gender variant children, transgender youths, and their families. The clinician should avoid assumptions based on stereotypes and listen carefully to understand each patient's unique experience and needs. In general, the counseling of gender variant children and transgender youths will address 6 areas: self-acceptance and validation of gender expression and identity; safety; connectedness to supportive others; self-disclosure, or coming out; healthy relationships and sexual decision-making; and optimism for the future. Addressing each of these areas is essential in ensuring the healthy development of these patients. These areas should be addressed over time and not all at an initial presentation or single visit.

Self-acceptance and Validation

The clinician can play an important role in countering the effects of disapproval and the pathologizing of gender variant expression and identity. For the gender variant child, the clinician should state that although being different in this society can be painful, the child's gender variant behavior can be healthy for that child. For transgender youths, the clinician should acknowledge the controversy around the use of gender dysphoria as a diagnostic category. Clinicians should present being transgender as part of the tapestry of normal human identity and clarify that the primary issue of concern is distress that can often come from having a transgender identity in a society that is unaccepting. This validating reassurance of healthiness and normalcy is perhaps the most powerful statement a clinician can make to gender variant children and transgender youths and their families.

More and more older gender variant children and transgender youths know a significant amount about gender, gender identity, and gender expression. Many have done extensive research on the Internet, accessing YouTube videos and Web sites that are easily searchable or connecting with other gender variant children and transgender youths on social media. Others, however, continue to be very isolated and know little or nothing about the nature and meaning of any emerging sense of identity. Therefore, the clinician should conduct an initial inquiry into what the child or youth knows and has seen or read and focus on correcting misconceptions, providing validation, and supporting empowerment. Gender variant children can be reassured that many ways exist of being a boy or a girl and that their way is one of these many ways. They can also be told that some children feel more like a girl inside and some more like a boy, or perhaps another gender, and that however they feel in gender identity is all right. Transgender youths should be provided information on sexual orientation, gender identity, and what it means to be transgender. Some of these youths may go through a period of confusion, not knowing whether they are gay, lesbian, bisexual, straight, transgender, or a combination of these. The clinician should inform the youth that such uncertainty is normal and that over time the youth will have a clearer understanding of who the youth is. The clinician may also provide brochures to youths who are facing issues of gender identity or refer them to supportive Web sites.[45] See Box 19-2.

Youths of an ethnic minority or another minority who are transgender may have an especially difficult time. The clinician should discuss these issues with their patients openly and connect them to appropriate supportive resources within their communities and online.

Box 19-2. Resources for Gender Variant Children and Transgender Youths

- Advocates for Youth. I think I might be transgender, now what do I do? Advocates for Youth Web site. http://www.advocatesforyouth.org/component/content/article/731-i-think-i-might-be-transgender-now-what-do-i-do. Accessed February 20, 2018

- Gender spectrum. Resources: teens. Gender Spectrum Web site. https://www.genderspectrum.org/resources/teens-2. Accessed February 20, 2018

- Get support. PFLAG Web site. https://www.pflag.org. Accessed February 20, 2018

- Harbor Camps, Inc. Camp Aranu'tiq Web site. https://www.camparanutiq.org. Accessed February 20, 2018

- The Trevor Project Web site. https://www.thetrevorproject.org. Accessed February 20, 2018

Safety

Because gender variant children and transgender youths endure higher rates of physical and sexual assault, harassment, discrimination, and social rejection, clinicians should ask gender variant children and transgender youths about their safety in their homes, schools, places of worship, and broader community. If harassment or other harmful treatment is acknowledged, the clinician should work with the child or youth and the family to identify and implement appropriate strategies to end the violence. Many of these children and youths feel shame and are afraid to advocate for their own safety. They may think they deserve the harm inflicted on them, or they may simply accept that this is the way the world is. The clinician should tell children and youths that they do not deserve such treatment and that they should expect and demand safety and respect from everyone in their lives and in all settings. Because gender variant children and transgender youths have so few advocates, the clinician should offer to join with them in approaching every venue in which they experience violence, including the home and school, to work out a plan to end violence immediately and completely.

Isolation

Because gender variant children and transgender youths experience profound isolation and loneliness, their physical and emotional health may be compromised. Pediatric clinicians should address the issue of isolation by giving accurate information about gender expression and gender identity. They should provide supportive and reassuring counseling, or they should refer the child or youth to colleagues who have the time, comfort, and expertise to provide the child or youth accepting and supportive care and counseling. Clinicians should connect these children and youths to local community resources such as support groups and other youth programs. Children, youths, and families who do not have access to local programs should be informed about national organizations and Web sites created specifically for gender nonconforming children, transgender youths, and their families. Boxes 19-2 and 19-3 contain examples of these resources.

Clinicians can also point out positive gender variant and transgender role models in the community or nationally. In certain circumstances, it is appropriate for transgender clinicians to present themselves as role models to transgender youths and their families.

Self-disclosure, or Coming Out

Transgender youths often reach a point in their development at which they feel a strong urge to disclose their gender identities to others. Transgender youths often have a history of gender variant expression as children. Therefore, others may have already assumed or sensed that these youths may be transgender or lesbian or gay. Some transgender youths, however, successfully conceal their gender identities, either by adapting their gender expressions to fit societal expectations consistent with their biological sexes or by labeling themselves or allowing others to perceive them as gay or lesbian. The process of disclosure to family and friends is often emotional and traumatic. Transgender youths who disclose their gender identities (come out) risk condemnation and rejection by family and peers. Therefore, coming out should be considered carefully, weighing the risks and benefits. It is sometimes suggested that if a youth expects a negative response from parents, the youth should wait to disclose until legally and financially independent. However, many youths think that continuing to live a lie is intolerable and harmful to one's self-esteem, and they come out earlier. A clinician should never reveal a youth's gender identity to parents without permission unless imminent risk of harm exists. A clinician can play an important role in the process of disclosure by helping youths decide whether they are ready to come out to family or friends and helping them choose an appropriate time, place, and approach for disclosure. Clinicians who feel they do not have the skills to provide such counseling effectively should refer to or collaborate with a therapist who can guide the youth and support the family through the coming-out process.

Relationships and Sexual Decision-making

Most transgender youths have difficulty in meeting other transgender youths to establish friendships and share mutual support. Clinicians should help connect transgender youths to local LGBT teen support groups and LGBT-supportive programs in the community, if they exist. This task can be accomplished ethically without parental notification. Clinicians can suggest national telephone hotlines or Web sites from which transgender youths can receive accurate information and supportive counseling and can communicate with other transgender youths. See Box 19-2. If these options are unavailable, the clinician can serve as a supportive and reassuring lifeline until the youth is old enough to become independent and possibly move away to attend school or work in a community that is more accepting of transgender people.

Transgender youths may be heterosexual, homosexual, or bisexual in their attractions and behaviors. Given the prevailing societal disapproval of transgender individuals, however, many transgender youths are afraid to reveal their gender identities to those with whom they might be interested in establishing a relationship. Therefore, some transgender youths find that their only options for exploring emotional and physical intimacy are through anonymous sexual encounters on the streets, in parks, or through Internet hookups. In addition to being potentially dangerous, these encounters are often accompanied by feelings of shame and degradation, which are harmful to a youth's sense of identity and self-worth. That many transgender youths are eager to engage in the typical courting practices of adolescence, which normally take place in safer and more affirming circumstances, is evidenced in the great popularity of LGBT youth proms and other social gatherings in more and more communities across the United States.

Transgender youths who are in relationships face many of the same questions as their nontransgender peers: "Am I in love?" "What do I want from a relationship?" "Do I really want to be in this relationship?" "How do I know if this is a good relationship?" "How do I get out of this relationship?" In addition, transgender youths face the exceedingly difficult questions of how and when to tell a potential boyfriend or girlfriend about one's gender identity. A transgender-supportive clinician or therapist can help youths reflect on and find answers to these questions.

As with other youths, many transgender youths know little about sexuality and how to make healthy sexual choices. Abstinence is always the appropriate option for youths who do not feel ready for a sexual relationship. Transgender youths should understand that when they are ready for a sexual relationship, they can expect to lead healthy and fulfilling sexual lives. All youths who have decided they are ready for a sexual relationship should be advised to limit their number of sexual partners and avoid mixing sex and alcohol or drugs so as to reduce their risk for infection, trauma, and sexual assault. Transgender youths, like other youths and depending on the sexual behaviors they engage in, are at risk for unplanned pregnancy and should be counseled on contraception. Pregnancy not only could lead to medical risks but can often be extremely psychologically traumatizing to a gender variant or transgender youth. Safer-sex practices related to oral, vaginal, and anal sex should be reviewed in detail. Transgender youths should also be aware that *no* always means *no* in negotiating sex, and any forced or coerced sexual experience represents sexual assault.

Optimism for the Future

Clinicians should not only focus on the risks that transgender youths face but also identify specific strengths that have allowed them to survive and sometimes thrive in the face of an often hostile environment. They should also challenge the belief of many transgender youths that their futures will be significantly limited by their gender identities. Although some communities are more accepting of transgender people than others are, many transgender adults lead happy, healthy, and productive lives. Although growing up transgender is often challenging, the future should be seen as hopeful and exciting.

Care of Transitioning Youths

Transition represents the emotional, psychological, social, physical, and legal processes transgender people experience to assume a body and gender role consistent with a gender identity. The transition process often begins in childhood and continues through adolescence into adulthood. Pubertal suppression, hormone therapy, and surgery are often the final medical steps in this process. Clinicians play an essential role in facilitating the patient's transition from female to male, from male to female, or perhaps to another gender. Primary care clinicians have often known their gender variant and gender dysphoric patients since early childhood. As puberty approaches and it seems that gender dysphoria may persist into adolescence, PCCs are in an advantageous position to provide patient and parents with detailed and accurate information about the nature and timing of transition, its limitations and benefits, and the choices that lie ahead. It is also important to share with families that, just as there is a degree of controversy around the understanding and management of gender dysphoria and gender variance in childhood, there is also controversy around certain aspects of the provision of medical transition care from early puberty through adolescence. This understanding is essential for patients and parents to give informed consent to treatment. At the same time, it is imperative for the clinician to be clear about where the clinician stands within the spectrum of opinion on the medical management of transition, including pubertal suppression, hormone therapy, and gender-affirmation surgery.

Whether or not the pediatric clinician will be the one prescribing hormone therapy, the clinician has an important role in helping patients and families identify possible natural transition points for initiating hormone therapy, such as when a patient is changing schools (eg, from middle school to high school) and when a family is planning to move to a new home and neighborhood. Once such transition points are identified, it is important that the clinician work with school personnel before transition begins, educating them about what it means to be transgender and the social and psychological benefits of transition. The potential risk of harassment by other students or by school staff should also be addressed. To ensure both respectful treatment and safety in the school setting, the clinician should advocate for the development of an Individualized Education Program or another formal assurance that the transgender student's preferred name and pronouns will be used in all school settings, both inside the classroom and outside the classroom and regardless of whether the student is present, and that appropriate restrooms and changing rooms are identified and accessible. The clinician should understand that obtaining a legal name change and a change of gender designation on a birth certificate is an important aspect of social transition for many transgender children and youths and is directly relevant to the patient's safety and well-being in school and other settings. Clinicians should also become familiar with state laws regarding these issues and be ready to help facilitate the process of achieving these changes, as guided by both patient and parents.

In addition to facilitating and monitoring social and psychological aspects of transition, pediatric clinicians are playing an increasingly central role in the initiation and management of physical transition, including both pubertal suppression and hormone therapy. Many clinicians still feel they do not have the training, experience, or time to do so effectively. Therefore, they refer their patients with significant gender variance or gender dysphoria to gender specialists and other colleagues whom they feel have greater expertise in assessing gender issues and providing transgender care. At the same time, they retain their role as PCC and provider of a medical home. Many larger communities have endocrinologists and adolescent medicine, family practice, and internal medicine physicians, as well as mental health specialists, who are experienced in providing medical care and counseling to gender dysphoric youths considering transition. Such clinicians can often be located through local LGBT community centers or national organizations such as GLMA. Many pediatric clinicians, however, practice in smaller communities with few or no physicians who have such expertise. Primary care clinicians in these settings should reach out to regional or other gender experts, through telemedicine and other means, to request their guidance in the evaluation and treatment of children and youths experiencing significant gender variance or gender dysphoria. Thus, through necessity, many pediatric clinicians have become experts on transgender care. They recognize that for most gender dysphoric youths entering puberty, the provision of transition-related treatments, such as pubertal suppression and hormone therapy (outlined in the Pubertal Suppression and Hormone Therapy sections of this chapter), is not elective but instead represents the standard of care, with the early institution of treatment predicting optimal improvement in both physical well-being and psychological well-being.[19,36,38,39]

Guidelines are available to help clinicians facilitate the transition process. WPATH in 2011 published the seventh edition of *Standards of Care for the Health of Transsexual, Transgender, and Gender Nonconforming People,* which is considered to be among the most authoritative guides to providing medical and mental health transition counseling, treatment, and support.[7] The Endocrine Society has also developed detailed clinical practice guidelines on hormone transition therapy for transgender adolescents and adults.[37] In addition, several health centers experienced in providing comprehensive transgender health care have developed their own clinical guidelines.[32,33] These latter guidelines often approach transgender care on the basis of an informed-consent model, which is premised on a belief in the ability of patients (and if a minor, their parents as well) to determine their own transition paths if provided complete and unbiased information about transition choices and their benefits and limitations. This model differs markedly from the traditional approaches to transition care, including those represented in earlier versions of the WPATH standards of care, which presented a very prescriptive and linear path to transition. Under these earlier standards, transition was presided over by medical and mental health gatekeepers who could decide who was eligible for transition treatments, as well as the nature, sequence, and timing of those treatments. The latest edition of the WPATH standards of care differs significantly from previous versions. It is much more patient centered and allows for a flexible approach in which recommendations related to transition care may be modified case by case to address a patient's specific needs and circumstances. The ultimate goal of the current WPATH standards of care is to reduce symptoms of gender dysphoria and maximize physical and psychological well-being. It explicitly emphasizes that efforts to change an individual's gender identity or expression are considered unethical.

Regarding physical interventions for youths considering transition, WPATH suggests an approach consisting of 3 stages: fully reversible interventions, using gonadotropin-releasing hormone (GnRH) analogs in early puberty to suppress estrogen and testosterone production, thereby delaying the progression of puberty; partially reversible interventions, consisting of hormone therapy to masculinize or feminize the body; and irreversible interventions such as gender-affirmation surgery, generally occurring in adulthood. WPATH advocates a staged approach to allow the youth and parents time to adjust to one stage before moving on to the next. The involvement of a multidisciplinary team to support the youth and family through the significant changes of physical, psychological, and social transitions is highly recommended, with the understanding that the role of each team member is to facilitate the process of timely transition and not to stand as a gatekeeper obstructing the path to receiving appropriate care, as has occurred in the past.

Despite WPATH's staged model of transition care, it is important to recognize that the path of transition is not the same for everyone. Some individuals are satisfied to live their lives consistent with their gender identities in a social sense but have no urge to initiate hormone therapy or undergo surgery. Others seek hormone therapy but feel that surgical alteration of their bodies is unnecessary. Still others may choose partial surgical gender reassignment; for example, many FTM transgender individuals choose mastectomy but not genital reconstruction. In addition, the transition process is not necessarily a linear one. Some individuals move back and forth between feelings of being more feminine or masculine and may present themselves differently to the world at different times in gender role and expression. This fluidity of identity and expression should be expected and supported by the clinician.

Pubertal Suppression

Pubertal suppression has become the standard of care for children entering puberty with persistent gender dysphoria, and it is advocated by both WPATH and the Endocrine Society. Puberty is suppressed through the administration of GnRH analogs, very similar to the treatment of precocious puberty in younger children. Pubertal suppression as treatment for gender dysphoria represents an off-label use of this medication. The GnRH analogs suppress the secretion of luteinizing hormone from the pituitary gland, resulting in suppressed levels of testosterone and estrogen, thereby postponing the development of secondary sexual characteristics. One proposed benefit of pubertal suppression is that it allows a youth additional time to better understand the youth's gender identity and, with increasing maturity, be able to make more informed decisions about whether to proceed with gender transition. A second benefit is that pubertal suppression can prevent or postpone the emotional trauma that can accompany the development of secondary sexual characteristics reflecting natal sex for most transgender youths, resulting in decreased symptoms of gender dysphoria. A third benefit is that pubertal suppression prevents the development of secondary sexual characteristics that often make later physical transition much more difficult. Hormone therapy is much more effective in bringing about desired physical changes if the undesired pubertal changes that reflect natal sex have not taken place. Suppression of unwanted pubertal changes may also decrease the need for more-invasive interventions later, such as breast surgery, electrolysis, and tracheal shaving.

For a child experiencing persistent or emerging gender dysphoria, pubertal suppression treatment should be offered when the first signs of puberty appear (which may occur as early as age 9 years).[37] Suppression should continue until the youth is able to confidently specify a gender identity. If a youth decides that a gender identity is consistent with natal sex, pubertal suppression is ended, and puberty allowed to proceed. The hormonal influences of suppression are completely reversible with no compromise to subsequent pubertal development. If a youth confirms a transgender identity, pubertal suppression is ended, and cross-gender hormone therapy is begun.

During pubertal suppression, the involvement of a supportive pediatric endocrinologist is recommended. Research on the use of GnRH analogs suggests the possibility of decreased bone mineral density in some patients during suppression treatment. However, current research suggests that children who have been on suppressive therapy catch up on bone growth once they progress through puberty or are started on cross-gender hormone therapy. Suppression therapy may also lead to irregular menses in biological females, particularly if started later in pubertal development. An endocrinologist can help address these issues and can monitor attainment of gender-appropriate height, making appropriate adjustments to treatment as necessary. The few potential risks of suppression treatment must be weighed against the growing body of research that documents the positive outcomes on physical and psychological well-being resulting from the use of pubertal suppression in the treatment of gender dysphoric youths in early puberty and adolescence.

Gender dysphoric youths whose natal sex is male should be informed, along with their parents, that pubertal suppression could result in insufficient penile tissue if later penile-inversion vaginoplasty is desired. However, skin grafts and colonic tissue may be used instead. Clinicians should also have detailed discussions with patients and their parents about the effects of both pubertal suppression and cross-gender hormone therapy on future fertility. Youths who receive only pubertal suppression treatment should progress to full fertility once pubertal suppression is discontinued and pubertal development resumes. Those who move from pubertal suppression directly to cross-gender hormone therapy will likely experience some degree of impaired fertility. Some patients may choose to have a hormone-free interval between pubertal suppression and the initiation of cross-hormone therapy to permit collection of sperm and oocytes for cryopreservation. Others have interrupted cross-gender hormone therapy later in life for the same purpose. The important thing is that this essential conversation takes place and that patients and their families are made aware of fertility experts who they may turn to for further consultation. Finally, families should be informed that pubertal suppression treatment is expensive and may not be covered by some insurance plans, although this coverage will likely change as such treatment is increasingly recognized as a standard of care. Clinicians should be ready to act as advocates on patients' behalves with insurance companies that refuse to cover pubertal suppression treatment. They should emphasize that pubertal suppression represents the standard of care for gender dysphoric children and that denial of this care can result in significant psychological and physical harm.

The primary controversy related to pubertal suppression therapy relates to when it should be started. Gender specialists agree that for children who have long-standing or emerging intense gender dysphoria at the onset of puberty, pubertal suppression should be initiated early. While earlier guidelines suggest beginning therapy at Tanner stage 2 or 3, most now advocate beginning treatment with the first physical or hormonal evidence of puberty, early in Tanner stage 2. For many children, this stage would mean with the first appearance of pubic hair.

Hormone Therapy

Offering hormone therapy, like offering pubertal suppression, represents the standard of care for youths persisting in gender dysphoria and committed to transition. Several protocols are available that address the evaluation and hormone therapy of transgender youths. There is uniform agreement across protocols on the appropriateness of hormone therapy for transgender youths, supported by research that shows the significant benefits of hormonal transition in both physical well-being and psychological well-being. Certain aspects of these protocols, however, continue to be controversial. The most significant among these controversies reflects a debate among clinicians about the appropriate age for initiating hormone therapy. Historically, the age of 16 years was most often cited, accompanied by a belief that a 16-year-old would be better able than a younger youth to make informed, mature decisions around treatment that could lead to irreversible physical changes. In fact, age 16 was initially recommended solely because the age of majority in the Netherlands, where most early treatment protocols were developed, was age 16, and it represented the age at which youths in that country could consent to their own care. The latest edition of WPATH's standards of care as well as the recommendations of others who are working in the field of transgender health allow for flexibility in determining the age of hormone therapy initiation, advising that such decisions should be made case by case, with age 16 set only as a guideline and with allowances made for earlier initiation.[7,38,46] In fact, many families and youths seek care much earlier than age 16, and many centers initiate hormone therapy much earlier than age 16 years and sometimes as young as age 12 years. Staff of these centers see no reason to delay treatment unnecessarily, because the trauma of experiencing puberty that reflects natal sex or being told to wait for years in a suspended peripubertal state as peers continue to develop is significant and may even be life-threatening.

Clinicians should discuss these issues openly with families and youths, considering the questions "For this particular youth, what is the rationale for suppressing puberty for 3 to 5 years? Does this youth in fact display uncertainty regarding this youth's gender identity that dictates waiting this long to end suppressive treatment or initiate hormone therapy?"

While many centers operate under a belief that mental health support is an essential component of transition, it should not delay or become a barrier to accessing appropriate and timely treatment. The WPATH's standards of care state directly that "refusing timely medical interventions for adolescents might prolong gender dysphoria and contribute to an appearance that could provoke abuse and stigmatization. As the level of gender-related abuse is strongly associated with the degree of psychiatric distress during adolescence…, withholding puberty suppression and subsequent feminizing and masculinizing hormone therapy is not a neutral option for adolescents."

Male-to-Female Hormone Therapy

Estrogen is the mainstay of MTF-transgender hormone therapy. For adolescents, most clinicians prescribe estrogen sublingually or transdermally, to prevent first-pass metabolism. Protocols also cite oral and injectable forms as options. For transgender individuals, many of the side effects of estrogen therapy are in fact desirable effects. Expected changes include breast development, softening of skin, increase in subcutaneous fat and its redistribution to the thighs and buttocks, diminished body hair, fewer erections, and testicular atrophy. Patients may also experience decreased libido, weight gain, and emotional changes. Some of these changes may be irreversible, continuing even after possible discontinuation of treatment. Fertility will be impaired while on estrogen therapy and possibly even if estrogen therapy is discontinued. This impairment should be discussed openly with patients and their parents, as should the option of cryopreservation of sperm if desired. Estrogen therapy is generally safe in adolescents.[47] Although clinicians should be aware of the precautions generally noted for estrogen therapy, including the possibility of blood clots in high-risk populations such as smokers, medical contraindications to estrogen therapy in adolescents are rare.

Antiandrogens, such as spironolactone, finasteride, and GnRH analogs, are routinely added to the regimen to suppress the action of endogenous testosterone, augment breast development, and soften facial and body hair. Gonadectomy serves a similar purpose, although it is generally not considered until age 18 years or older as part of gender-affirmation surgery.

Female-to-Male Hormone Therapy

The FTM transition is facilitated through the use of testosterone administered through injection, patch, or topical gel. Testosterone treatment is generally safe in adolescents. Among the potentially desirable side effects of testosterone treatment for these patients are increased facial and body hair, clitoral enlargement, vagina atrophy, cessation of menses, male pattern baldness, deepening of voice, decreased fat mass, increased muscle mass and strength, a more masculine body shape, increased weight, more-prominent veins, coarser skin, and mild breast atrophy. Patients may also notice increased acne, mood changes, and increased libido. Some of these changes may be irreversible. Fertility will likely be impaired during testosterone treatment, although it may return if treatment is interrupted. Clinicians should discuss this impairment openly with patients and their families and should also discuss options for cryopreservation of oocytes before treatment is begun.

Other Treatments

Some transgender individuals will seek other treatments to facilitate physical and psychosocial transitions to their appropriate genders. Often these treatments will occur after the adolescent years, partly because these procedures are expensive and not yet covered by many insurance plans. Because many of these treatments involve irreversible changes, most protocols recommend deferring them until at least age 18 years, especially those that represent gender-affirmation surgery. Male-to-female– transgender individuals may seek plastic surgery, including penectomy, orchiectomy, vaginoplasty, clitoroplasty, vulvoplasty, breast and gluteal augmentation, tracheal shaving, and facial reconstruction. Electrolysis or other hair-removal procedures may be sought. Silicone injections may also be sought to obtain a more feminine body contour. Female-to-male– transgender individuals may seek chest plastic surgery, hysterectomy, oophorectomy, phalloplasty, and other genital reconstructions. Both MTF individuals and FTM individuals may seek voice therapy and professional guidance in how to present themselves as male, female, or another gender through body language, facial expression, gait, posture, and mannerisms.

Although these surgical, cosmetic, and other procedures often take place after adolescence, discussing these options and their benefits and limitations and making appropriate referrals should be part of the clinician's anticipatory guidance of transgender youths.

Parents

Parents who come to recognize their child's gender variant behavior or transgender identity may experience a variety of emotions: confusion, fear, sadness, concern, embarrassment, guilt, anger, or disgust, but also acceptance and celebration. These feelings should be discussed openly and with compassion. Many parents fear for their child's safety and happiness. Many of them fear that their child may eventually self-identify as lesbian or gay. In many instances, these concerns and fears are not raised on visits to the clinician or are referred to only indirectly ("My son is a sensitive child" or "My daughter is definitely a tomboy"). The clinician should be sensitive to any cues of parental worry about gender variance and ask parents simply, "Do you have any concerns about your child's behaviors?" or, even better, "Have you had any concerns that your son's [daughter's] behaviors or interests are more feminine [masculine] than other children's his [her] age?" Most concerned parents, although perhaps embarrassed, are relieved to have such a discussion. The clinician's primary role in working with parents is to help them understand and celebrate their gender variant child and support them in their efforts to keep their child happy, healthy, and safe.

Parents should be referred to Web sites, books, brochures, and media resources geared to parents of gender nonconforming children and youths. See Box 19-3.

Parents should be assured that with love, validation, and support their children should grow up to be happy, healthy, and productive adults, no matter what a child's gender expression, gender identity, or sexual orientation might be. The Children's National Medical Center has developed guidelines to help parents in their provision of support for their children (Box 19-4), and Box 19-5 lists pitfalls parents should try to avoid.

> **Box 19-3. Resources for Parents of Gender Variant Children and Transgender Youths**
>
> ▪ Brill S, Kenney L. *The Transgender Teen: A Handbook for Parents and Professionals Supporting Transgender and Non-binary Teens.* San Francisco, CA: Cleis Press Inc; 2016
>
> ▪ Brill S, Pepper R. *The Transgender Child: A Handbook for Families and Professionals.* San Francisco, CA: Cleis Press Inc; 2008
>
> ▪ Gender Spectrum. Resources: parenting and family. Gender Spectrum Web site. https://www.genderspectrum.org/resources/parenting-and-family-2. Accessed February 20, 2018
>
> ▪ Marian Wright Edelman Institute, San Francisco State University. Family Acceptance Project Web site. http://familyproject.sfsu.edu. Accessed February 20, 2018

When to Refer

Refer to a child behavioral, adolescent, or gender specialist whenever a child or youth

▶ Shows significant gender variant behaviors, particularly if they are concerning to parents or have resulted in rejection or mistreatment by family members, peers, or others. Ideally, referral will be made before possible dysphoria arises.

▶ Shows signs or symptoms of gender dysphoria, including expression of dissatisfaction or distress related to a birth-assigned gender or insistence that one is of another gender.

Refer to a child and adolescent psychiatrist or another mental health professional whenever a child or youth

▶ Experiences persistent or recurrent depressed or anxious mood that interferes with function

▶ Has acute or recurrent suicidal ideation or self-injury

▶ Evidences isolation from peers or family members

▶ Engages in substance use or other high-risk behaviors

It should be noted that referrals for therapy to change a gender identity or expression of a child or youth are considered unethical.[7]

Box 19-4. Children's National Medical Center Outreach Program Guidelines for Parents of Gender Variant Children and Transgender Youths

- Love your child for who your child is. Love, acceptance, understanding, and support are especially important when peers and society are often intolerant of difference.

- Question traditional assumptions about gender roles and sexual orientation. Do not allow societal expectations to come between you and your child.

- Create a safe space for your child, allowing your child to always be who the child is, especially in the child's own home.

- Seek out socially accepted activities (eg, sports, arts, hobbies) that respect your child's interests while helping your child fit in socially.

- Validate your child and your child's interests, supporting the idea that more than one way exists to be a girl or a boy. Speak openly and calmly about gender variance with your child. Talk about these subjects in positive terms, and listen as your child expresses feelings of being different.

- Seek out supportive resources (eg, books, videos, Web sites, support groups) for parents, families, and children.

- Talk about gender variance with other significant people in your child's life, including siblings, extended family members, babysitters, and family friends.

- Prepare your child to deal with bullying. Let your child know that a child does not deserve to be hurt. Be aware of behaviors that suggest bullying and may be occurring, such as school refusal, crying excessively, and reporting aches and pains.

- Be your child's advocate. Expect and insist on acceptance, respect, and safety wherever your child is. Parents may need to educate school staff and others about the special experience and needs of gender variant children.

Box 19-5. Children's National Medical Center Pitfalls to Avoid as Parents of Gender Variant Children and Transgender Youths

- Avoid finding fault. No blame exists. Your child's gender variance came from within, not from you as parents. Blame will get in the way of enjoying your child.

- Do not pressure your child to change, because doing so will cause much pain and harm.

- Do not blame your child. Do not accept bullying as *just the way things are*. No one has the right to torment or criticize others because they are different.

AAP Policy

American Academy of Pediatrics Committee on Adolescence. Office-based care for lesbian, gay, bisexual, transgender, and questioning youth. *Pediatrics.* 2013;132(1): 198–203 (pediatrics.aappublications.org/content/132/1/198)

References

1. Achenbach TM. *Manual for Child Behavior Check List/4-18 and 1991 Profile.* Burlington, VT: University of Vermont Dept of Psychiatry; 1991

2. Sandberg DE, Meyer-Bahlburg HF, Ehrhardt AA, Yager TJ. The prevalence of gender-atypical behavior in elementary school children. *J Am Acad Child Adolesc Psychiatry.* 1993;32(2):306–314

3. Steensma TD, van der Ende J, Verhulst FC, Cohen-Kettenis PT. Gender variance in childhood and sexual orientation in adulthood: a prospective study. *J Sex Med.* 2013;10(11):2723–2733

4. Achenbach TM, Edelbrock C. *Manual for the Youth Self-report and Profile.* Burlington, VT: University of Vermont Dept of Psychiatry; 1987

5. Meyer WJ III. Gender identity disorder: an emerging problem for pediatricians. *Pediatrics.* 2012;129(3):571–573

6. van Beijsterveldt CEM, Hudziak JJ, Boomsma DI. Genetic and environmental influences on cross-gender behavior and relation to behavior problems: a study of Dutch twins at ages 7 and 10 years. *Arch Sex Behav.* 2006;35(6):647–658

7. World Professional Association for Transgender Health. Standards of care for the health of transsexual, transgender, and gender-nonconforming people. *Int J Transgend.* 2012;13(4):165–232

8. Meerwijk EL, Sevelius JM. Transgender population size in the United States: a meta-regression of population-based probability samples. *Am J Public Health.* 2017;107(2):e1–e8

9. Mallon GP, DeCrescenzo T. Transgender children and youth: a child welfare practice perspective. *Child Welfare.* 2006;85(2):215–241

10. Richardson J. Response: finding the disorder in gender identity disorder. *Harvard Rev Psychiatry.* 1999;7(1):43–50

11. Zucker KJ, Spitzer RL. Was the gender identity disorder of childhood diagnosis introduced into *DSM-III* as a backdoor maneuver to replace homosexuality? A historical note. *J Sex Marital Ther.* 2005;31(1):31–42

12. Zucker KJ. Gender identity development and issues. *Child Adolesc Psychiatr Clin North Am.* 2004;13(3):551–568

13. Pleak RR. Ethical issues in diagnosing and treating gender-dysphoric children and adolescents. In: Rottnek M, ed. *Sissies and Tomboys: Gender Nonconformity and Homosexual Childhood.* New York, NY: New York University Press; 1999:34–51

14. American Psychiatric Association. *Diagnostic and Statistical Manual of Mental Disorders.* 4th ed. Arlington, VA: American Psychiatric Association; 2000

15. American Psychiatric Association. *Diagnostic and Statistical Manual of Mental Disorders.* 5th ed. Arlington, VA: American Psychiatric Association Publishing; 2013

16. Drescher J. Controversies in gender diagnoses. *LGBT Health.* 2014;1(1):10–14
17. Zucker KJ, Cohen-Kettenis PT, Drescher J, Meyer-Bahlburg HF, Pfäfflin F, Womack WM. Memo outlining evidence for change for gender identity disorder in the *DSM-5. Arch Sex Behav.* 2013;42(5):901–914
18. Vasey PL, Bartlett NH. What can the Samoan "Fa'afafine" teach us about the Western concept of gender identity disorder in childhood? *Perspect Biol Med.* 2007;50(4):481–490
19. Adelson SL; American Academy of Child and Adolescent Psychiatry Committee on Quality Issues. Practice parameter on gay, lesbian, or bisexual sexual orientation, gender nonconformity, and gender discordance in children and adolescents. *J Am Acad Child Adolesc Psychiatry.* 2012;51(9):957–974
20. Green R. *The "Sissy Boy Syndrome" and the Development of Homosexuality.* New Haven, CT: Yale University Press; 1987
21. American Academy of Pediatrics Committee on Adolescence. Office-based care for lesbian, gay, bisexual, transgender, and questioning youth. *Pediatrics.* 2013;132(1):198–203
22. Society for Adolescent Health and Medicine. Recommendations for promoting the health and well-being of lesbian, gay, bisexual, and transgender adolescents: a position paper of the Society for Adolescent Health and Medicine. *J Adolesc Health.* 2013;52(4):506–510
23. *Guidelines for Care of Lesbian, Gay, Bisexual, and Transgender Patients.* San Francisco, CA: Gay and Lesbian Medical Association; 2006. GLMA Web site. http://glma.org/_data/n_0001/resources/live/GLMA%20guidelines%202006%20FINAL.pdf. Accessed February 20, 2018
24. Kaiser Permanente National Diversity Council, Kaiser Permanente National Diversity Department. *A Provider's Handbook on Culturally Competent Care: Lesbian, Gay, Bisexual, and Transgendered Population.* 2nd ed. Oakland, CA: Kaiser Permanente; 2004
25. Centers for Disease Control and Prevention. Transgender persons. Centers for Disease Control and Prevention Web site. https://www.cdc.gov/lgbthealth/transgender.htm. Updated May 18, 2017. Accessed February 20, 2018
26. Goldenring JM, Rosen DS. Getting into adolescents' heads: an essential update. *Contemp Pediatr.* 2004;21(1):64–90
27. Drescher J, Byne W. Gender dysphoric/gender variant (GD/GV) children and adolescents: summarizing what we know and what we have yet to learn. *J Homosex.* 2012;59(3):501–510
28. Zucker KJ, Wood H, Singh D, Bradley SJ. A developmental, biopsychosocial model for the treatment of children with gender identity disorder. *J Homosex.* 2012;59(3):369–397
29. Menvielle E. A comprehensive program for children with gender variant behaviors and gender identity disorders. *J Homosex.* 2012;59(3):357–368
30. de Vries AL, Cohen-Kettenis PT. Clinical management of gender dysphoria in children and adolescents: the Dutch approach. *J Homosex.* 2012;59(3):301–320

31. Stein E. Commentary on the treatment of gender variant and gender dysphoric children and adolescents: common themes and ethical reflections. *J Homosex.* 2012;59(3):480–500

32. Tom Waddell Health Center. *Protocols for Hormonal Reassignment of Gender.* San Francisco, CA: Tom Waddell Health Center; 2013. San Francisco Department of Public Health Web site. https://www.sfdph.org/dph/comupg/oservices/medSvs/hlthCtrs/TransGendprotocols122006.pdf. Accessed February 20, 2018

33. Center of Excellence for Transgender Health, University of California, San Francisco. Guidelines for the primary and gender-affirming care of transgender and gender nonbinary people. Center of Excellence for Transgender Health Web site. http://transhealth.ucsf.edu/tcoe?page=protocol-00-00. Accessed February 20, 2018

34. Hsieh S, Leininger J. Resource list: clinical care programs for gender-nonconforming children and adolescents. *Pediatr Ann.* 2014;43(6):238–244

35. Connolly MD, Zervos MJ, Barone CJ II, Johnson CC, Joseph CL. The mental health of transgender youth: advances in understanding. *J Adolesc Health.* 2016;59(5):489–495

36. Gorin-Lazard A, Baumstarck K, Boyer L, et al. Hormonal therapy is associated with better self-esteem, mood, and quality of life in transsexuals. *J Nerv Ment Dis.* 2013;201(11):996–1000

37. Hembree WC, Cohen-Kettenis P, Delemarre-van de Waal HA, et al. Endocrine treatment of transsexual persons: an Endocrine Society clinical practice guideline. *J Clin Endocrinol Metab.* 2009;94(9):3132–3154

38. Spack NP, Edwards-Leeper L, Feldman HA, et al. Children and adolescents with gender identity disorder referred to a pediatric medical center. *Pediatrics.* 2012;129(3):418–425

39. de Vries AL, McGuire JK, Steensma TD, Wagenaar EC, Doreleijers TA, Cohen-Kettenis PT. Young adult psychological outcome after puberty suppression and gender reassignment. *Pediatrics.* 2014;134(4):696–704

40. Ehrensaft D. From gender identity disorder to gender identity creativity: true gender self child therapy. *J Homosex.* 2012;59(3):337–356

41. Edwards-Leeper L, Spack NP. Psychological evaluation and medical treatment of transgender youth in an interdisciplinary "Gender Management Service" (GeMS) in a major pediatric center. *J Homosex.* 2012;59(3):321–336

42. Ryan C, Huebner D, Diaz RM, Sanchez J. Family rejection as a predictor of negative health outcomes in white and Latino lesbian, gay, and bisexual young adults. *Pediatrics.* 2009;123(1):346–352

43. DeCrescenzo T, Mallon GP. *Serving Transgender Youth: The Role of Child Welfare Systems.* Arlington, VA: Child Welfare League of America; 2002

44. Woronoff R, Estrada R, Sommer S; Child Welfare League of America, Lambda Legal Defense and Education Fund. *Out of the Margins: A Report on Regional Listening Forums Highlighting the Experience of Lesbian, Gay, Bisexual, Transgender, and Questioning Youth in Care.* New York, NY: Lambda Legal Defense and Education Fund; 2006

45. Advocates for Youth. I think I might be transgender, now what do I do? Advocates for Youth Web site. http://www.advocatesforyouth.org/component/content/article/731-i-think-i-might-be-transgender-now-what-do-i-do. Accessed February 20, 2018

46. Olson J, Forbes C, Belzer M. Management of the transgender adolescent. *Arch Pediatr Adolesc Med.* 2011;165(2):171–176

47. van Kesteren PJ, Asscheman H, Megens JA, Gooren LJ. Mortality and morbidity in transsexual subjects treated with cross-sex hormones. *Clin Endocrinol (Oxf).* 1997;47(3):337–342

Inattention and Impulsivity

Lawrence S. Wissow, MD, MPH

> "The care of a child experiencing symptoms of inattention and impulsivity can begin in the primary care setting from the time symptoms are recognized, even if the child's symptoms do not rise to the level of a disorder and regardless of whether referral to a mental health specialist is ultimately part of the care plan."

Introduction

Symptoms of inattention and impulsivity affect many children, including a large number whose symptoms do not rise to the level of a disorder. Attention-deficit/hyperactivity disorder (ADHD) occurs in about 8% of children and youths,[1] who experience significant impairment in their functioning because of their symptoms. As part of their condition, individuals with ADHD often have deficits in social skills, impairing their abilities to function well in school and social settings.[2] Attention-deficit/hyperactivity disorder is frequently comorbid with learning difficulties, and the 2 conditions can mimic each other in school or during cognitive tasks outside of school (including time devoted to doing homework). Thus, ADHD can result in significant adverse consequences. Follow-up studies have found that children with ADHD, particularly those untreated, are at greater risk for school failure, underemployment, difficulty with legal authorities, substance use, and morbidity from risky behaviors, including motor vehicle crashes and sexually transmitted infections.[3]

The guidance in this chapter applies to the care of children and *youths* (defined here as children and adolescents aged 6–18 years), collectively called *children* unless otherwise specified, presenting with undifferentiated symptoms of inattention and impulsivity in pediatric clinical settings. Its intended audience is pediatric primary care clinicians (PCCs): pediatricians, family physicians, internists, nurse practitioners, and physician assistants who provide frontline, longitudinal health care to children.

This chapter is based on the work of the World Health Organization, whose recommendations may be updated annually. The most up-to-date information can be found at www.who.int/mental_health/publications/mhGAP_intervention_guide/en.

Findings Suggesting Inattention and Impulsivity

Inattention and impulsivity occur commonly during childhood. When these symptoms occur more persistently and to a greater degree than is seen in a child's peers, there may be cause for concern. Often, the child's teacher is the first to observe the symptoms or to encourage medical attention for the child. A summary of the symptoms and clinical findings that suggest inattention and impulsivity can be found in Box 20-1. These symptoms may be elicited from parents, teachers, or children. Because observers often disagree about behavioral and emotional symptoms, collecting information from all 3 sources can be helpful, and the process of reconciling differences can itself be therapeutic.

Tools to Assist With Identification

Because many children do not spontaneously disclose their symptoms, standardized wide-range psychosocial screening instruments may be used to identify children with emotional and behavioral difficulties that may include symptoms of inattention and impulsivity. Diagnostic criteria for ADHD require presence of symptoms in more than one setting; therefore,

---

Box 20-1. Indications of Inattention and Impulsivity in History From Patient or Parent

- Excitability, impatience, angry outbursts (more than is seen in peers)
- Wandering attention (greater than is seen in peers)
- Difficulties with behavior at home and in the classroom
- Academic difficulties
- Parents and teachers presuming diagnosis of ADHD or seeking diagnosis of ADHD

Abbreviation: ADHD, attention-deficit/hyperactivity disorder.

collateral reports from the school or child care center, as well as the parent or parents, are critical elements in the identification process. Several instruments have versions to collect information from the child, parents, and teachers. Table 20-1 provides an overview of general psychosocial screening tools available in the public domain, along with results raising concerns in the areas of inattention and impulsivity. Use of additional instruments, such as the NICHQ Vanderbilt ADHD assessment scales, can then help confirm findings of the initial screening, corroborate a concern raised by a teacher or parent, and serve as a benchmark to track treatment progress. However, it is important to remember that the symptoms of ADHD are nonspecific; positive scores on an ADHD assessment scale confirm that the child has a problem but do not necessarily say which problem or combination of problems may underlie the symptoms. Use of a functional assessment tool such as the Impact Supplement of the Strengths and Difficulties Questionnaires (SDQ) or the Columbia Impairment Scale

Table 20-1. General Psychosocial Screening/Results Suggesting Inattention and Impulsivity

Screening Instrument	Score
PSC-35	• Total score ≥24 for children aged ≤5 y. • ≥28 for those 6–16 y. • ≥30 for those aged ≥17 y. *and* • Further discussion of items related to attention and impulse control confirms a concern in that area.
PSC-17	• Attention subscale is ≥7. *and* • Further discussion of items related to attention and impulse control confirms a concern in that area.
SDQ	• Total symptom score of >19. • Hyperactivity scale score of 7–10 (see instructions at www.sdqinfo.com). • Impact scale (back of form) score of 1 (medium impairment) or ≥2 (high impairment). *and* • Further discussion of items related to attention and impulse control confirms a concern in that area.

Abbreviations: PSC, Pediatric Symptom Checklist; SDQ, Strengths and Difficulties Questionnaires.

will assist in determining whether the child is significantly impaired by the symptoms. Use of a tool to assess the effect of the child's problem on other members of the family may also be helpful; the CGSQ (Caregiver Strain Questionnaire) is an example of such a tool. Appendix 2, Mental Health Tools for Pediatrics, provides more information about these and other screening instruments.

Assessment

Assessment begins by differentiating the child's symptoms from normal behavior. All children may be inattentive or impulsive at times, but for some children inattention and impulsivity limit their adaptability to normal peer and family situations and interfere with learning. Inattention and impulsivity are typical characteristics of preschool-aged children, but extremes of these behaviors warrant further evaluation (eg, concern that the behavior is harming family or peer relationships, interfering with learning, putting the child at risk for expulsion from child care or school because of behavior). Boisterousness or dreaminess can be normal behavior patterns in older children. Children with limited social experiences and those whose environment is relatively less structured may seem impulsive and inattentive compared with their peers, especially when entering highly structured situations such as a classroom or organized group activities.

Table 20-2 provides a summary of conditions, such as hearing or vision problems, receptive and expressive language problems, learning disorders, and sleep deprivation, that may mimic or co-occur with inattention and impulsivity problems.

Table 20-2. Conditions That May Mimic or Co-occur With Inattention and Impulsivity	
Condition	**Rationale**
Hearing or vision problems	All children who seem inattentive should be screened for sensory deficits.
Sleep deprivation	Sleep problems can cause inattention and irritability. ADHD may contribute to difficulty sleeping.

Table 20-2. Conditions That May Mimic or Co-occur With Inattention and Impulsivity (*continued*)

Condition	Rationale
ADHD	Diagnosis requires that a child have symptoms for at least 6 months, appearing before age 12 and present in at least 2 settings (eg, home and school); involving a persistent pattern of inattention (eg, careless with detail, seems not to listen, poorly organized, distractible, forgetful, does not finish tasks, loses things, avoids tasks that require sustained attention) or hyperactivity-impulsivity (eg, fidgety, noisy, talkative, can't wait turn, difficulty staying in seat, interrupts, high level of motor activity) or both; interfering with functioning or development; and not better explained by some other condition or situation in which the child finds himself or herself.[a]
Learning problems or disabilities	If symptoms of inattention and impulsivity are associated with problems of school performance, the child may be experiencing learning difficulties. See Chapter 21, Learning Difficulty, to explore this possibility.
Developmental problems	Children with overall intellectual or social limitations may seem less able than their age-mates to control their impulses and to focus and maintain their attention.
Language impairment or disorder	Children with receptive or expressive language impairment may be frustrated and inattentive at least in part because of difficulty understanding what others say or being able to express themselves. Similar problems can arise when children are learning a new language and cannot yet fully function at the level of their peers or teachers.
Depression	May co-occur with ADHD. Marked sleep disturbance, disturbed appetite, low mood, or tearfulness could indicate that depression is a factor contributing to attention difficulties. See Chapter 22, Low Mood.
Exposure to ACEs	Children who have experienced or witnessed trauma, violence, a natural disaster, separation from a parent, parental divorce or separation, parental substance use, neglect, or physical, emotional, or sexual abuse are at high risk of developing symptoms suggesting inattention and impulsivity. These symptoms may mask or be expressions of emotional difficulties such as adjustment disorder or PTSD. Some symptoms of PTSD may resemble symptoms of ADHD (eg, hypervigilance may mimic hyperactivity, dissociation may mimic inattention). These children may also manifest other forms of anxiety. Inquiring about previous trauma in a confidential setting is important. See Chapter 14, Anxiety and Trauma-Related Distress.

Table 20-2. Conditions That May Mimic or Co-occur With Inattention and Impulsivity (*continued*)	
Condition	Rationale
Anxiety	Anxious children may experience difficulty concentrating. See Chapter 14, Anxiety and Trauma-Related Distress.
Bereavement	Most children will experience the death of a family member or friend sometime in childhood. Other losses may also trigger grief responses, for example, separation or divorce of parents, relocation, change of school, deployment of a parent in military service, breakup with a girlfriend or boyfriend, or remarriage of parent. Such losses are traumatic. They may result in such symptoms as sadness, anxiety, difficulty concentrating, poor impulse control, or academic decline immediately following the loss and, in some instances, more persistently. See also Chapter 22, Low Mood, and the discussion of PTSD in Chapter 14, Anxiety and Trauma-Related Distress.
Physical illness	Medical issues that can mimic or provoke symptoms of inattention and impulsivity include thyroid disease, hypoglycemia, hyperglycemia, unwanted side effects of medications (eg, bronchodilators), and endocrine tumors (eg, rarely pheochromocytoma).
Substance use	Children with symptoms of inattention and impulsivity may self-medicate with alcohol, nicotine, or other drugs. Conversely, children using substances may manifest inattention, impulsivity, and deteriorating school performance.
Conduct or oppositional defiant disorders	See Chapter 15, Disruptive Behavior and Aggression, to differentiate these symptoms from problems of inattention and impulsivity and ADHD.
Tourette syndrome	Children with repetitive movements (tics) should be identified. In children with Tourette syndrome, ADHD symptoms may precede onset of tics. Stimulant medication may worsen tics. It is important to tailor treatment to the child's most pressing symptoms before deciding the risks and benefits of using stimulants in children with both problems.

Abbreviations: ACE, adverse childhood experience; ADHD, attention-deficit/hyperactivity disorder; PTSD, post-traumatic stress disorder.

[a] For specific criteria, refer to the *Diagnostic and Statistical Manual of Mental Disorders*.

Plan of Care for Children With Inattention and Impulsivity

The care of a child experiencing symptoms of inattention and impulsivity can begin in the primary care setting from the time symptoms are recognized, even if the child's symptoms do not rise to the level of a disorder and regardless of whether referral to a mental health specialist is ultimately part of the care plan.

Engaging Child and Family in Care

Without engagement, most families will not seek or persist in care. The process may require multiple primary care visits.[4]

Reinforce strengths of the child and family (eg, good relationships with at least one parent or important adult, prosocial peers, concerned or caring family, help seeking, connection to positive organizations) as a method of engagement, and identify any barriers to addressing the problem (eg, stigma, family conflict, resistance to treatment). Use "common factors" techniques,[5] represented by the HELP mnemonic in Box 20-2 and discussed in-depth in Chapter 5, Effective Communication Methods: Common Factors Skills, to build trust and optimism, reach agreement on incremental next steps, develop a plan of care, and collaboratively determine the role of the PCC. A key step is to reach agreement that there is a reason to consider intervention and, ideally, that there are concrete problems that the family would like to see addressed. Regardless of other roles, PCCs can encourage a positive view of treatment on the part of the child and family.

Box 20-2. Common Factors Mnemonic: HELP Build a Therapeutic Alliance

H = Hope

E = Empathy

L^2 = Language, Loyalty

P^3 = Permission, Partnership, Plan

Adapted with permission from American Academy of Pediatrics. *Addressing Mental Health Concerns in Primary Care: A Clinician's Toolkit*. Elk Grove Village, IL: American Academy of Pediatrics; 2010. For the fully annotated mnemonic, please refer to Appendix 5.

Offering Psychoeducation About ADHD, the Differential Diagnosis, and the Process of Arriving at a Diagnosis

Parents have likely heard about ADHD from other sources; their knowledge and concerns about the conditions may vary widely. Parents may have worries about being coerced into labeling their child with the condition by demands from the PCC or schools. The PCC can ask about what they know and what questions they may have. She can explain the process of making a provisional diagnosis and investigating alternatives, including language and learning problems, anxiety, and normal variation in development and temperament. Perhaps most important, the PCC can assure parents that she will not be jumping to a diagnosis; rather, she will work with them to collect relevant information, make a plan of treatment, and then reevaluate the situation as time goes on. At some point, parents will also want to know more about the natural history of the condition and the implications it may have for their child's future. It is reasonable to say that these sorts of problems are common and highly amenable to treatment of various kinds and, while sometimes persistent, tend to be more easily managed as the child gets older.

Encouraging Healthy Habits

Regular exercise and outdoor play are beneficial to all children and may be particularly helpful to inattentive and impulsive children. These children may also benefit from participation in structured sports activities, which offer exercise as well as the opportunity to build social skills such as taking turns, following rules, and handling success and disappointment. Also important are regular sleep habits, special time with parents, praise for good behavior, and reinforcement of the child's strengths. Limiting media exposure may be particularly important for these children. Television (TV) programs, movies, and computer games can be overstimulating; long hours in these activities can produce irritability. Unrestricted access to a TV or computer, especially in the child's bedroom, can contribute to loss of sleep, failure to do homework, and the risk of seeing programming that contributes to increased activity.

Reducing Stress

Consider the child's social environment (eg, family social history, parental depression screening, results of any family assessment tools administered, reports from child care or school). Symptoms of inattention and hyperactivity will generally worsen in stressful settings. The PCC can guide parents in providing a safe, structured environment and coach parents in working constructively with the child's school. The PCC can also address stresses on family members; for example, if family members have problems with mood or irritability, they will have more difficulty adapting to and moderating the child's behavior.

Offering Initial Interventions

The strategies described in the following text are common elements of evidence-based and evidence-informed psychosocial interventions for management of children's behavior. They are applicable to the care of children with mild or emerging symptoms of inattention and impulsivity and to those with impairing symptoms that do not rise to the level of a disorder. They can also be used along with other specific interventions for ADHD.

Guide parents in managing the child's behavior. Good practices include

▶ **Tangible rewards:** Rewards or privileges contingent on performance of routine tasks (eg, TV or computer time contingent on attaining a realistic goal). These rewards are most effective when coupled with a system for helping the child be aware of his or her own level of functioning, including charts that monitor events such as completion of homework without a reminder, staying on task in school for a prearranged time before taking a break, and carrying out chores at home before being asked.

▶ **Parent praise:** Conscious effort by parent to identify and comment on positive aspects of child's behavior (eg, compliment child, especially when desired action is spontaneous).

▶ **Parent monitoring:** Use of some systematic means to rate the child's burden of specific ADHD symptoms and overall social, emotional, and academic function (eg, weekly use of NICHQ Vanderbilt ADHD assessment scales or a customized checklist, often with simultaneous teacher ratings). Monitoring helps the parent advocate for the child and can help take pressure off the child by giving short-term, objective measures of progress.

▶ **Time-out:** Avoiding reinforcement of undesired behavior through arguing or allowing the behavior to continue (eg, child is required to sit without attention or activity for a brief period as a consequence for an undesired behavior).

▶ **Commands and limit setting:** Use of clear, simple commands that ideally give the child a warning of impending expected behavior, an opportunity to perform it, a warning of consequences for nonperformance, and a consistent consequence (eg, "You can do 1 more puzzle and then we have to go…now it's time to go…if you don't put the puzzle away now, you can't choose the music we listen to in the car.").

If there are battles over homework, offer guidelines. Box 20-3 provides suggestions for parents to consider in addressing homework issues.

If child meets diagnostic criteria for ADHD, consider specific therapy. The course of treatment depends on the child's age and should be noted in the overall care plan. For preschool-aged children (4–5 years of age), evidence-based, parent-administered behavioral therapy or evidence-based,

---

Box 20-3. Strategies for Working Constructively With a Child's School

- Obtain consent for the clinician to exchange information with the child's teacher.
- Establish constructive 3-way (parent, teacher, and pediatrician) communication with the school.
- Ask if testing has been requested and taken place to detect special educational needs.
- Monitor academic progress, helping to reinforce successes and identify particular subjects or educational settings in which more support is needed.
- Advocate for appropriate classroom strategies.
  - Have the child sit at the front of the class.
  - If possible, engage the child in active learning (eg, have the child go to the blackboard to write answers to questions).
  - Give extra time to stay organized (eg, write down assignments, make sure that all needed materials are taken home or gathered for a project, have the child repeat back what he or she is to do).
  - Break longer assignments into shorter pieces (also helpful for homework).
  - Coordinate reports of behavior with home; for example, consider a daily report card of behavior and subsequent rewards or consequences.

teacher-administered behavioral therapy (or both) is considered the first line of treatment. Use of medications may be considered, ideally with specialist consultation, if behavioral treatment does not provide sufficient improvement or if evidence-based treatment is not available.

For elementary school–aged children (6–11 years of age), either US Food and Drug Administration (FDA)–approved medications for ADHD or evidence-based behavioral therapy administered by a parent or a teacher (or both) are considered first-line treatment of ADHD; both medication and therapy are preferred. The evidence is particularly strong for stimulant medications and sufficient but less strong for atomoxetine, extended-release guanfacine, and extended-release clonidine (in that order). Use of stimulant medication requires careful monitoring of growth parameters. See Chapter 11, Psychotropic Medications in Primary Care, for further guidance on the selection and monitoring of these medications.

For preadolescents and adolescents (12–18 years of age), FDA-approved medications for ADHD (with the assent of the patient) along with behavioral therapy are considered treatment of ADHD.[6]

Providing Resources

Families may find support and resources from organizations such as Children and Adults with Attention-Deficit/Hyperactivity Disorder (www.chadd.org). Examples of helpful publications include *ADHD: What Every Parent Needs to Know,* by Michael I. Reiff, and *Addressing ADD Naturally,* by Kathi J. Kemper. Provide the family with contact numbers and resources in case of emergency.

Monitoring the Child's Progress Toward Therapeutic Goals

Child care, preschool, or school reports can be helpful in monitoring progress. The NICHQ Vanderbilt ADHD assessment scales (parent and teacher), SDQ (parent and teacher), and Pediatric Symptom Checklist (commonly known as PSC) can be helpful in monitoring progress with symptoms and functioning. (See Appendix 2.) Both medications and behavioral treatments need careful titration to achieve their desired positive effects without the development of harmful, unintended, or undesired side effects. The need for higher-than-recommended doses of medication could be a sign of difficulties with adherence, a need to switch to a different medication, or a need to reconsider the primary or secondary diagnosis. Behavioral treatments can be difficult to implement and maintain. Primary care clinicians can work with families to adapt behavioral suggestions to family circumstances and to explore barriers to other aspects of treatment, including effective engagement with schools.

It is important for the clinician to help the family understand that it is not uncommon for treatment to be successful for a period and then seem to lose effectiveness. This situation can happen when there are new stresses or demands or when, after a period of success, there has been a letup on treatment. If modifying existing treatment and exploring ways of dealing with new stresses do not help get function back to baseline, then new treatments, or new diagnoses, need to be considered. In particular, as school demands increase, learning issues may need to be considered, even if they were not seen as contributing problems in the past.

Involving Specialists

Involve one or more specialists if the child does not respond to initial interventions or if the following clinical circumstances exist:

▶ Child has severe functional impairment.

▶ Child has severely disruptive behavior or aggression.

▶ Child has comorbid depression or post-traumatic stress disorder, or child has problems with mood, behavior, and development that seem more prominent than difficulties with attention or impulsivity.

▶ Symptoms are threatening school performance or the achievement of other developmentally important goals (eg, developing and sustaining friendships).

▶ The child or parent is very distressed by the symptom or symptoms.

▶ There are co-occurring behavioral problems. (The combination of shyness, anxiety, and behavioral problems is thought to be particularly risky for future behavioral problems of a more serious nature.)

▶ The child's symptoms were preceded by serious trauma.

▶ The child has ADHD and contraindications to stimulants or marked side effects with stimulants.

▶ The child's problems are occurring in the context of other family emotional or behavioral problems that have not been alleviated with primary care interventions.

When specialty care is needed, ensure that it is evidence informed and assist the family in accessing it. Pharmacological interventions and a number of evidence-based and evidence-informed psychosocial interventions are available for the treatment of ADHD in children and adolescents. Ideally, those referred for care in the mental health specialty system would have access to the safest and most effective treatments. Box 20-4 provides a summary of these interventions. Children referred for mental health specialty care complete the referral process only 61% of the time, and a significantly smaller number persist in care.[7]

Note that not all evidence-based interventions may be available in every community. If a particular intervention is not available, this lack of intervention becomes an opportunity to collaborate with others in the community to advocate on behalf of children. Increasingly, states offer both telepsychiatry services and consultation and referral support "warmlines" that help PCCs provide initial treatment and locate resources. The availability of the latter form of help is tracked at the National Network of Child Psychiatry Access Programs (www.nncpap.org).

Reach agreement on respective roles in the child's care. If the child is referred to mental health specialty care, the PCC may be responsible for initiating medication or adjusting doses, monitoring response to treatment, monitoring adverse effects, engaging and encouraging the child's and family's positive views of treatment, and coordinating care provided by parents, school, medical home, and specialists. In fact, the child may improve just knowing that the PCC is involved and interested. Resources to help clinicians in these roles include Appendixes 4, 6, and 7 and Chapter 11, Psychotropic Medications in Primary Care. Additionally, the American Academy of Pediatrics publishes *ADHD: Caring for Children With ADHD; A Resource Toolkit for Clinicians,* which is available at https://shop.aap.org.

Box 20-4. American Academy of Pediatrics Recommendations for Treatment of Attention-deficit/Hyperactivity Disorder

- Recommendations for treatment of children and adolescents with ADHD vary depending on the patient's age.
  - For *preschool-aged children (4–5 years of age),* the PCC should prescribe evidence-based, parent-administered behavioral therapy or evidence-based, teacher-administered behavioral therapy (or both) as the first line of treatment (quality of evidence A/strong recommendation) and may prescribe methylphenidate if the behavioral interventions do not provide significant improvement and there is moderate-to-severe continuing disturbance in the child's function. In areas in which evidence-based behavioral treatments are not available, the clinician needs to weigh the risks of starting medication at an early age against the harm of delaying diagnosis and treatment (quality of evidence B/recommendation).
  - For *elementary school–aged children (6–11 years of age),* the PCC should prescribe either FDA-approved medications for ADHD (quality of evidence A/strong recommendation) or evidence-based behavioral therapy administered by a parent or a teacher (or both) as treatment of ADHD; both medication and therapy are preferred (quality of evidence B/strong recommendation). The evidence is particularly strong for stimulant medications and sufficient but less strong for atomoxetine, extended-release guanfacine, and extended-release clonidine (quality of evidence A/strong recommendation). The school environment, program, or placement is a part of any treatment plan.
  - For *preadolescents and adolescents (12–18 years of age),* the PCC should prescribe FDA-approved medications for ADHD with the assent of the patient (quality of evidence A/strong recommendation) and may prescribe behavioral therapy as treatment of ADHD (quality of evidence C/recommendation); both medication and therapy are preferred.
- PCCs should titrate doses of medication for ADHD to achieve maximum benefit with minimum adverse effects (quality of evidence B/strong recommendation).

For more information, see American Academy of Pediatrics Subcommittee on Attention-deficit/Hyperactivity Disorder and Steering Committee on Quality Improvement. ADHD: clinical practice guideline for the diagnosis, evaluation, and treatment of attention-deficit/hyperactivity disorder in children and adolescents. *Pediatrics.* 2011;128(5):1007–1022 (pediatrics.aappublications.org/content/128/5/1007).

Abbreviations: ADHD, attention-deficit/hyperactivity disorder; PCC, primary care clinician; FDA, US Food and Drug Administration.

See also Chapter 11, Psychotropic Medications in Primary Care, for guidance on primary care prescribing.

Adapted with permission from American Academy of Pediatrics Subcommittee on Attention-deficit/Hyperactivity Disorder and Steering Committee on Quality Improvement. ADHD: clinical practice guideline for the diagnosis, evaluation, and treatment of attention-deficit/hyperactivity disorder in children and adolescents. *Pediatrics.* 2011;128(5):1007–1022.

Acknowledgments: The author and editor wish to acknowledge the contributions of Linda Paul, MPH, manager of the American Academy of Pediatrics Mental Health Leadership Work Group.

AAP Policy

American Academy of Pediatrics Subcommittee on Attention-deficit/Hyperactivity Disorder and Steering Committee on Quality Improvement and Management. ADHD: clinical practice guideline for the diagnosis, evaluation, and treatment of attention-deficit/hyperactivity disorder in children and adolescents. *Pediatrics.* 2011;128(5):1007–1022 (pediatrics.aappublications.org/content/128/5/1007)

References

1. Visser SN, Lesesne CA, Perou R. National estimates and factors associated with medication treatment for childhood attention-deficit/hyperactivity disorder. *Pediatrics.* 2007;119(suppl 1):S99–S106

2. McQuade JD, Hoza B. Peer problems in attention deficit hyperactivity disorder: current status and future directions. *Dev Disabil Res Rev.* 2008;14(4):320–324

3. Wolraich ML, Wibbelsman CJ, Brown TE, et al. Attention-deficit/hyperactivity disorder among adolescents: a review of the diagnosis, treatment, and clinical implications. *Pediatrics.* 2005;115(6):1734–1746

4. Foy JM; American Academy of Pediatrics Task Force on Mental Health. Enhancing pediatric mental health care: algorithms for primary care. *Pediatrics.* 2010; 125(suppl 3):S109–S125

5. Wissow LS, Gadomski A, Roter D, et al. A cluster-randomized trial of mental health communication skills for pediatric generalists. *Pediatrics.* 2008;121(2): 266–275

6. American Academy of Pediatrics Subcommittee on Attention-deficit/Hyperactivity Disorder and Steering Committee on Quality Improvement and Management. ADHD: clinical practice guideline for the diagnosis, evaluation, and treatment of attention-deficit/hyperactivity disorder in children and adolescents. *Pediatrics.* 2011;128(5):1007–1022

7. Rushton J, Bruckman D, Kelleher K. Primary care referral of children with psychosocial problems. *Arch Pediatr Adolesc Med.* 2002;156(6):592–598

CHAPTER 21

Learning Difficulty

Barbara L. Frankowski, MD, MPH

"The care of a child experiencing learning difficulties can begin in the primary care setting from the time symptoms are recognized, even if the child's problems do not rise to the level of a disorder and regardless of whether referral to the school or to a mental health specialist is ultimately part of the care plan."

Background and Significance

Learning difficulties can occur at any age and for a variety of reasons. They invariably cause frustration for the child or adolescent, which can lead to or compound behavioral problems and emotional distress. The effects of learning difficulties, whatever their causes, can be profound, with economic and emotional consequences far into adult life. Children and adolescents (collectively called *children* in this chapter) who do not receive timely intervention are at risk not only for academic failure but also for the psychosocial morbidities that accompany limited academic achievement, such as substance use and juvenile delinquency.[1] Some children with learning difficulties are among the 7%[2] of US 15- through 24-year-olds who drop out of school, leading to chronic unemployment, poverty, and higher risk of health problems throughout adulthood. The drop-out rate is higher among minority populations of black non-Hispanics (8%) and Hispanics (22.5%) than white children.[2] Clearly, learning difficulties are an important concern for primary care clinicians (PCCs)—that is, pediatricians, family physicians, internists, nurse practitioners, and physician assistant who provide frontline, longitudinal health care to children.

Primary Care Clinician's Role

It is the PCC's role to recognize that a child is experiencing difficulty in learning, to help the family sort out the cause of the child's learning difficulties, to identify referral sources for psychological and educational assessment, to ensure that the child receives the educational resources he or she needs and is entitled to, to address any medical or mental health problems that may be associated with the child's learning difficulties, and to guide the family in advocating and providing a supportive environment for the child.

Recognition of Children With Learning Difficulties

The PCC has opportunities at routine health supervision visits to elicit parental concerns, to monitor children's developmental progresses and functioning, and to screen for developmental delays and symptoms of social-emotional problems. The PCC may also receive referrals from child care or school personnel who have observed that the child has difficulty learning compared with his or her peers or is experiencing behavioral problems in the classroom. There may be a family history of learning problems, compounding concerns about the child's progress in learning. See Box 21-1 and Table 21-1 for signs and symptoms that a child is experiencing learning difficulties.

Box 21-1. Symptoms and Clinical Findings Suggesting Learning Difficulties

Indications From Child's or Parent's History

- Child has experienced a delay in language development or has difficulty understanding language despite normal hearing and vision.
- Child has difficulty following directions.
- Child has difficulty learning letters, numbers, and colors.
- Child has struggled to read, grasp math concepts, or write in comparison with her peers.
- Letter reversals (*b/d*), inversions (*m/w*), transpositions (*felt/left*), substitutions (*house/home*), or confusion of arithmetic signs persist past peers.
- Child avoids reading aloud, writing, or homework.
- Child or parent is frustrated with the child's academic performance.
- Parent perceives child is "lazy" in school.
- Child is perceived as an "underachiever."
- Classroom behavior or inattention has become a problem.
- Other family members have experienced learning difficulties or did not complete high school.

Table 21-1. Findings Suggesting Learning Difficulty

Measurement	Score
End-of-grade test scores or achievement test scores	Percentiles are low (≤15%) or markedly scattered, or the child is performing considerably less well than would be expected for his or her intelligence.
Report cards	Grades are low or markedly scattered.
Intelligence tests	Percentiles are within the reference range or significantly higher than measures of academic achievement.

Causes of Learning Difficulties

Lack of School Readiness

Some young children experience difficulties in learning because they are not yet ready for the school experience, socially, emotionally, or physically; because they do not have language and literacy skills comparable with their peers; or because their family or culture does not value their education. Box 21-2 outlines the specific traits a child should ideally possess in order to be ready for school, and Box 21-3 identifies key family and community supports for preparing a child for school.

Box 21-2. Traits for School Readiness

- Physical well-being and motor development: good health status and alertness; any physical disabilities identified and accommodated

- Social-emotional development: turn-taking, cooperation, empathy, and the ability to express his or her own emotions

- Approaches to learning: enthusiasm, curiosity, family and cultural values supportive of learning

- Language development: skills in understanding and speaking the language spoken in the classroom; adequate vocabulary and other literacy skills, including print awareness, story sense, and writing and drawing processes

- General knowledge and cognition: sound-letter association, awareness of spatial relations, and number concepts

---

Box 21-3. Preparing the Child for School: Key Elements

- At least a high school education or equivalent for parents
- High-quality prenatal health care for the mother
- Optimal nutrition for mother and child
- Comprehensive health care for the child
- Daily physical activity
- Daily time with parent in learning activities (eg, reading, conversation, family meals)
- Access to high-quality preschool for children in impoverished environments
- Access to programs for children and parents who speak English as a second language

---

Finally, many schools are not prepared to educate children with the full range of abilities and disabilities. Measurement of children's readiness for kindergarten should be used to assess the effectiveness of community-based programs and to prepare schools to meet the child's ongoing needs, rather than to exclude or delay children from their formal educational experiences.[3] Box 21-4 highlights key elements of schools that are ready for children.

Medical, Mental Health, and Developmental Problems

Learning difficulties may also be caused by cognitive limitations; a language or learning disorder; vision or hearing impairment; behavioral and emotional problems; a chronic disease that affects the child's concentration, interpersonal relationships, or school attendance; sleep deprivation; or medication affecting concentration or alertness. See Table 21-2 for a listing of problems that can cause or co-occur with learning difficulties.

Box 21-4. Preparing the School for the Child: Key Elements

- High-quality preschools for children in impoverished environments
- Programs and teacher training for children of all ability levels
- Preschool screening of children aimed at measuring the outcome of their preschool programs and at identifying and addressing students' needs (not at excluding children or delaying their school entry)

Table 21-2. Conditions That May Cause Poor School Performance or Co-occur With Learning Difficulties

Condition	Rationale
Hearing or vision problems	All children who are experiencing learning difficulties should be screened for sensory deficits.
Sleep deprivation	Sleep problems can cause inattention and irritability and contribute to poor school performance; conversely, poor school performance and homework struggles may contribute to difficulty sleeping. See Chapter 28, Sleep Disturbances.
Developmental problems	Children with overall intellectual or social limitations will learn more slowly than their age-mates. Children with low achievement and low intellectual levels often have the same problems as children with learning disabilities.
ADHD	Children who are inattentive or impulsive may manifest poor academic performance. They may have problems with getting the work completed and turned in, rather than skill deficits. Conversely, children experiencing academic difficulties may seem restless and inattentive. See Chapter 20, Inattention and Impulsivity.
Exposure to ACEs	Children who have experienced or witnessed trauma, violence, a natural disaster, separation from a parent, parental divorce or separation, parental substance use, neglect, or physical, emotional, or sexual abuse are at high risk of developing emotional difficulties such as adjustment disorder or PTSD. Children with PTSD can manifest poor concentration, memory problems, school refusal, and academic decline. These children may also manifest other forms of anxiety. Physicians may want to consider speaking separately and confidentially with the child and parents to explore this possibility. Parents are often unaware of exposures that children may have had at school or in the community. There may be major traumas in the family (eg, serious illness in a parent, maltreatment of the child, death or incarceration of a loved one) that are similarly not discussed or disclosed. The 3 hallmark symptom clusters of PTSD are reexperiencing, avoidance of memories or situations that recall the trauma, and hypervigilance (ie, increased worry about safety, startling or anxiousness at unexpected sounds or events). See also Chapter 14, Anxiety and Trauma-Related Distress.

Table 21-2. Conditions That May Cause Poor School Performance or Co-occur With Learning Difficulties (*continued*)

Condition	Rationale
Anxiety	Anxious children may experience difficulty concentrating and perform poorly on tests. See Chapter 14, Anxiety and Trauma-Related Distress.
Bereavement	Most children will experience the death of a family member or friend sometime in their childhoods. Other losses may also trigger grief responses—separation or divorce of parents, relocation, change of school, deployment of a parent in military service, breakup with a girlfriend or boyfriend, or remarriage of parent. Such losses are traumatic. They may result in such symptoms as sadness, anxiety, difficulty concentrating, poor impulse control, or academic decline immediately following the loss and in some instances, more persistently. See also Chapter 22, Low Mood, and the discussion of PTSD in Chapter 14, Anxiety and Trauma-Related Distress.
Depression	Depression may cause a decline in school performance, result from poor school performance, or simply coexist with learning disabilities. Marked sleep disturbance, disturbed appetite, low mood, or tearfulness could indicate that a child (or more commonly, an adolescent) is depressed. See Chapter 22, Low Mood.
Physical illness	Medical issues that may have an effect on school performance include all illnesses that may interfere with the child's attendance. Some illnesses (or symptoms caused by the illnesses) can affect attention in the classroom (eg, hypothyroidism or hyperthyroidism, neurological disorders, post-traumatic brain injury, undiagnosed diabetes), as can adverse effects of medications such as bronchodilators or anticonvulsants.
Substance use	Children frustrated with their school performances may use substances such as alcohol, nicotine, or other drugs to alleviate their frustrations, or self-medicate with caffeine or cocaine. Conversely, children using substances may manifest inattention, impulsivity, and deteriorating school performance. See Chapter 31, Substance Use 2: Use of Other Substances.
Conduct or oppositional defiant disorders	These disorders may cause poor academic performance, and frustration with poor academic performance can exacerbate conduct or oppositional problems. See Chapter 15, Disruptive Behavior and Aggression.

Table 21-2. Conditions That May Cause Poor School Performance or Co-occur With Learning Difficulties (*continued*)	
Condition	**Rationale**
Autism spectrum disorder, including high-functioning autism spectrum disorder, which was formerly known as pervasive development disorder, and Asperger syndrome	Children who have these difficulties also have problems with social relatedness (eg, poor eye contact, preference for solitary activities, language [often stilted], and range of interests [persistent and intense interest in a particular activity or subject]). They often will have very rigid expectations for routine and become anxious or angry if these expectations are not met. As such, these children may manifest difficulties in the classroom and many of the symptoms associated with learning disorders.

Abbreviations: ACE, adverse childhood experience; ADHD, attention-deficit/hyperactivity disorder; PTSD, post-traumatic stress disorder.

Learning Disabilities

Rarely diagnosed before a child enters school, learning disabilities (LDs) represent a broad array of specific learning challenges that significantly impede a child's ability to perform at the expected grade level. They generally occur in the context of normal sensory functioning and otherwise normal cognitive capabilities and, by definition, are not the result of a primary emotional disorder or lack of opportunity (although frustration and low self-esteem associated with LDs may contribute to development of problems such as anxiety, depression, or oppositional attitudes). Learning disabilities are clearly familial, with genetics contributing substantially to a child's risk.[4] It is estimated that between 5.0% and 17.5% of individuals meet diagnostic criteria for LDs and approximately 2 million US school children aged 6 to 11 years are affected.[5] Eighty percent of those identified have dyslexia or a reading disorder.

Assessment of Children With Learning Difficulties

Assessment begins by differentiating the child's symptoms from normal behavior. Children learn at different rates. Typically developing children younger than 7 years may reverse and transpose letters and experience some frustration with new learning tasks, particularly if the child has had limited preschool experience or other children in the classroom have had more exposure to formal school experiences. Many children will have one or more of the symptoms in Box 21-1 from time to time. Children who have missed school for an illness, changed schools, or experienced a significant loss may experience transient problems with school functioning. Some parents have unrealistic expectations, based on their own learning experiences or that of older siblings or children of friends.

It is important to explore sources of stress in the family, school, or community, as any of these can cause inattentiveness and distraction in the child.

A full physical and psychosocial assessment of the child will serve to identify conditions that can cause or co-occur with learning difficulties (see Table 21-2).

Two categories of medical risk deserve special attention: prematurity and cyanotic congenital heart disease. Preterm infants are at significantly higher risk for global developmental delays and for LDs.[6] In particular, children born at less than 32 weeks' gestation or who experience perinatal and postnatal complications such as prolonged ventilation, intracranial hemorrhage, sepsis, seizures, prolonged acidosis, or hypoglycemia are at higher risk for neurodevelopmental sequelae. Similarly, children surviving severe congenital cardiac anomalies are at high risk for LDs.[7] Several genetic disorders have been linked to risk for various forms of LD. In particular, children with Klinefelter syndrome, Turner syndrome, velocardiofacial syndrome, and spina bifida with shunted hydrocephalus have all been shown to be at significant risk for LDs.[8] When one of these risk factors is identified, the PCC should have a low threshold to refer for psychological and educational assessment.

Adolescents who present with learning difficulties are a particular challenge for the PCC. An adolescent who has been progressing normally with academics may suddenly develop learning difficulties. It is possible that the adolescent may have a mild LD for which he or she has compensated in lower grades, but which is now causing difficulty in meeting the more rigorous demands of middle or high school. The adolescent may have mild attentional problems, together or separately, that have not required any special intervention up until this point. However, it is also possible that the adolescent has other problems causing or contributing to learning difficulties, such as inadequate amounts of sleep, poor nutrition, inadequate physical activity, anxiety, depression, or substance use. The adolescent could also, or alternatively, be struggling with issues of sexual orientation or bullying that cause stress in the school environment. It is important to consider all these possibilities when assessing an adolescent with learning difficulties.

To further the assessment of any child or adolescent with learning difficulties, the PCC can communicate with school personnel (eg, guidance counselor, classroom teacher, school psychologist) to request data and observations such as

▶ **Intelligence testing:** School personnel may be willing to administer a cognitive screening test or, if there are apparent discrepancies between intelligence and academic achievement, a full battery of psychological tests.

▶ **Achievement testing:** School personnel can provide a screening test or reports of achievement or end-of-grade tests.

▶ **Full psychoeducational evaluation:** School psychologist or community psychologist may provide, by referral.

▶ **School placement and special services.**

▶ **Individualized Educational Program (IEP) or 504 plan,** if in place.

▶ **History of academic progress, behavior and discipline, and peer interactions.**

Use of additional screening instruments such as the NICHQ Vanderbilt ADHD assessment scales and general psychosocial screenings (Pediatric Symptom Checklist [PSC]-35, PSC-17, and Strengths and Difficulties Questionnaires [SDQ]) can be used to identify children who may have psychosocial problems contributing to their learning difficulties. See Appendix 2, Mental Health Tools for Pediatrics, for further information about these tools.

Plan of Care for Children With Learning Difficulties

The care of a child experiencing learning difficulties can begin in the primary care setting from the time symptoms are recognized, even if the child's problems do not rise to the level of a disorder and regardless of whether referral to the school or to a mental health specialist is ultimately part of the care plan.

Engaging Child and Family in Care

Without engagement, most families will not seek or persist in care. The process may require multiple primary care visits.

Reinforce strengths of the youth (defined in this chapter as children aged 6–18 years) and family as a method of engagement and identify any barriers to addressing the problem (eg, stigma, family conflict, resistance to academic testing or special education). Use "common factors" techniques,[9] represented by the HELP mnemonic in Box 21-5, to build trust and optimism, reach agreement on incremental next steps, develop a plan of care, and collaboratively determine the role of the PCC. Regardless of other roles, the PCC can encourage a positive view of treatment on the part of the youth and family.

Encouraging Healthy Habits

Encourage exercise, outdoor play, balanced and consistent diet, sleep (critically important to mental health), avoidance of exposure to frightening or violent media, limitation of screen time to less than 1 to 2 hours per day, special time with parents, acknowledgment of child's strengths, and special efforts to support the child and help him or her to feel competent, special, positive, and appreciated.

Reducing Stress

Consider the child's social environment (eg, family social history, parental depression screening, results of any family assessment tools administered, reports from child care or school). Questions to raise might include

---

Box 21-5. Common Factors Mnemonic: HELP Build a Therapeutic Alliance

H = Hope

E = Empathy

L^2 = Language, Loyalty

P^3 = Permission, Partnership, Plan

Adapted from American Academy of Pediatrics. *Addressing Mental Health Concerns in Primary Care: A Clinician's Toolkit.* Elk Grove Village, IL: American Academy of Pediatrics; 2010. For the fully annotated mnemonic, please refer to Appendix 5.

Is the parent punitive or critical? If parents' psychosocial problems are affecting their relationship with the child, explore their readiness to address these problems as part of helping their child. Encourage praise for their child's efforts. Urge parents to avoid comparisons with siblings or peers and to keep up the child's self-esteem. Urge parents to nurture the child's nonacademic gifts, such as art or music, and encourage participation in extracurricular activities that provide social experiences uncomplicated by academic performance and competition (eg, scouts, faith-based youth group, boys' or girls' club).

Are there battles over homework? Advise parents that the child is not lazy. Provide guidance about helping with homework (and requesting modified assignments, as appropriate). See Box 21-6 on guidelines to prevent homework battles.

Box 21-6. Guidelines for Parents: Preventing Homework Battles

- Establish a routine (not waiting until evening to get started).
- Identify another student your child can call to clarify homework assignments.
- Limit distractions (eg, TV, computer, phone).
- Assist child in dividing assignments into small, manageable segments (especially important for long-range assignments and large projects).
- Assist child in getting started (eg, read directions together, watch child complete first items).
- Monitor without taking over.
- Praise good effort and completion of tasks.
- Do not insist on perfection.
- Offer incentives ("When you've finished, we can…").
- Help child study for tests.
- Do not force child to spend excessive time on homework; write a note to the teacher if the child put forth good effort but was not able to complete it.
- If child fails to turn in completed work, develop a system with the teacher to collect it on arrival.
- If unable to provide homework supervision and assistance, or if homework battles are adversely affecting the parent-child relationship, ask the teacher for help finding a tutor.

Abbreviation: TV, television.

Is the child exposed to criticism or teasing at school? Is the child's teacher supportive and patient? Provide strategies for communication between school personnel and home; coach them to praise progress and effort, not just outcomes, and to address teasing or bullying.

Are school authorities proceeding with assessment in accordance with the child's rights? Inform parents about the child's rights under the Individuals with Disabilities Education Act (IDEA) and Section 504 of the Rehabilitation Act. It is important to obtain information about how these 2 acts are specifically implemented in your state and school districts. If a child has an LD, he or she qualifies for specialized educational services, and IDEA requires that the school develop an IEP. The IEP documents the child's current level of functioning, establishes goals, and delineates the services needed to meet those goals in the least restrictive environment possible. The parent is entitled to meet with school personnel to review and approve the IEP. If the child does not qualify for specialized educational services but has minor challenges that can be helped by minor classroom modifications (eg, preferential seating, homework modifications), the school may develop a 504 plan for the child. If the parent is dissatisfied with the school's response to the child's needs, there is an appeal process within the school system.

If the school is not adequately addressing the child's needs, the PCC may offer referral to a community mental health specialist such as a psychologist or developmental-behavioral pediatrician, or an educational tutor. Results of this assessment may provide support for the parent's advocacy efforts in the school system or may guide the family in developing tutorial assistance for the child.

Whatever interventions are planned, it is important to acknowledge and reinforce protective factors (eg, good relationships with at least one parent or important adult, prosocial peers, concerned or caring family, help seeking, and connection to positive organization[s]).

Offering Initial Interventions

The strategies described herein are applicable to the care of children with mild or emerging learning difficulties, as well as diagnosed learning disorders. They can also be used as initial primary care treatment of children with learning difficulties while readying children for further assessment or educational services or while awaiting access to evaluation and treatment. In addition, PCCs can address any comorbid conditions and, if there are battles over homework, offer parents guidelines to prevent them. (See Box 21-6.)

Providing Resources

Families may find the National Center for Learning Disabilities (www. ncld.org) a helpful source for information and support. Parents with questions about special education law may wish to consult a dedicated resource like Wrightslaw (www.wrightslaw.com). The American Academy of Pediatrics has developed a number of helpful handouts, publications, and Web sites, including *Individualized Education Program (IEP) Meeting Checklist* (www.brightfutures.org/mentalhealth/pdf/families/mc/ iep.pdf), "Learning Disabilities: What Parents Need to Know" (www. healthychildren.org/English/healthissues/conditions/learning-disabilities/ Pages/Learning-Disabilities-What-Parents-Need-To-Know.aspx), *Reading for Children: Grades 1–6* (www.brightfutures.org/mentalhealth/pdf/ families/mc/grades.pdf), and *Your Child's Mental Health: When to Seek Help and Where to Get Help* (https://patiented.solutions.aap.org).

Monitoring the Child's Progress Toward Educational Goals

School reports can be helpful in monitoring progress. Screening instruments that gather information from multiple reporters (youth, parent, teacher), such as the SDQ, can be helpful in monitoring progress with symptoms and functioning.

Involving Specialist(s)

Involve education or mental health specialist(s) if child does not respond to initial interventions or if indicated by the following clinical circumstances:

▶ The child or parent is very distressed by the symptom(s).

▶ There are co-occurring behavioral problems not responsive to primary care management.

▶ School evaluation is incomplete or untimely.

▶ Parent's relationship with school is adversarial.

▶ Child and family have conflicts not responsive to primary care management.

▶ Parent is very negative toward child or unresponsive to primary care guidance.

Consider seeing a geneticist for a diagnostic genetic workup if there are persistent concerns that interventions are not producing results.

Reach agreement on respective roles in the child's care. The PCC may be responsible for advising the family about the child's rights under IDEA, reducing stresses on the child while awaiting further assessment and treatment, engaging and encouraging the child's positive view of his or her evaluation and specialized instruction, monitoring academic progress, observing for and addressing any comorbidities, and coordinating care provided by parents, school, medical home, and specialists. Resources available to help PCCs in this role include The LD Navigator from the National Center for Learning Disabilities (http://ldnavigator.ncld.org) and *Practice Parameters* from the American Academy of Child and Adolescent Psychiatry (www.aacap.org/cs/root/member_information/practice_information/practice_parameters/practice_parameters). The PCC may also review with the family whether the child's school interventions are evidence-based ones, or refer to a developmental-behavioral pediatrician who is more knowledgeable in this area.

AAP Policy

Adams RC, Tapia C; American Academy of Pediatrics Council on Children With Disabilities. Early intervention, IDEA Part C services, and the medical home: collaboration for best practice and best outcomes. *Pediatrics.* 2013;132(4):e1073–e1088. Reaffirmed May 2017 (pediatrics.aappublications.org/content/132/4/e1073)

American Academy of Pediatrics Council on Children With Disabilities. Provision of educationally related services for children and adolescents with chronic diseases and disabling conditions. *Pediatrics.* 2007;119(6):1218–1223. Reaffirmed November 2014 (pediatrics.aappublications.org/content/119/6/1218)

American Academy of Pediatrics Council on Children With Disabilities and Medical Home Implementation Project Advisory Committee. Patient- and family-centered care coordination: a framework for integrating care for children and youth across multiple systems. *Pediatrics.* 2014;133(5):e1451–e1460 (pediatrics.aappublications.org/content/133/5/e1451)

American Academy of Pediatrics Section on Ophthalmology and Council on Children With Disabilities, American Academy of Ophthalmology, American Association for Pediatric Ophthalmology and Strabismus, American Association of Certified Orthoptists. Learning disabilities, dyslexia, and vision. *Pediatrics.* 2009;124(2):837–844. Reaffirmed July 2014 (pediatrics.aappublications.org/content/124/2/837)

Moeschler JB, Shevell M; American Academy of Pediatrics Committee on Genetics. Comprehensive evaluation of the child with intellectual disability or global developmental delays. *Pediatrics.* 2014;134(3):e903–e918 (pediatrics.aappublications.org/content/134/3/e903)

References

1. Esser G, Schmidt MH. Children with specific reading retardation—early determinants and long-term outcome. *Acta Paedopsychiatr.* 1994;56(3):229–237
2. Shin HB. *School Enrollment—Social and Economic Characteristic of Students: October 2003.* Washington, DC: US Census Bureau; 2005. https://www.census.gov/prod/2005pubs/p20-554.pdf. Accessed February 8, 2018
3. High PC; American Academy of Pediatrics Committee on Early Childhood, Adoption, and Dependent Care and Council on School Health. School readiness. *Pediatrics.* 2008;121(4):e1008–e1015
4. Pennington BF. Genetics of learning disabilities. *J Child Neurol.* 1995;10(suppl 1):S69–S77
5. American Academy of Pediatrics Section on Ophthalmology and Council on Children with Disabilities, American Academy of Ophthalmology, American Association for Pediatric Ophthalmology and Strabismus, American Association of Certified Orthoptists. Learning disabilities, dyslexia, and vision. *Pediatrics.* 2009;124(2):837–844
6. Rais-Bahrami K, Short BL. Premature and small-for-dates infants. In: Batshaw ML, Pellegrino L, Roizen NJ, eds. *Children With Disabilities.* 6th ed. Baltimore, MD: Paul H. Brookes Publishing; 2007:107–122
7. Bellinger DC, Wypij D, duPlessis AJ, et al. Neurodevelopmental status at eight years in children with dextro-transposition of the great arteries: the Boston Circulatory Arrest Trial. *J Thorac Cardiovasc Surg.* 2003;126(5):1385–1396
8. Rourke BP, Ahmad SA, Collins DW, Hayman-Abello BA, Hayman-Abello SE, Warriner EM. Child clinical/pediatric neuropsychology: some recent advances. *Annu Rev Psychol.* 2002;53:309–339
9. Kemper KJ, Wissow L, Foy JM, Shore SE. *Core Communication Skills for Primary Clinicians.* Winston-Salem, NC: Wake Forest School of Medicine. http://nwahec.org/45737. Accessed February 8, 2018

CHAPTER 22

Low Mood

Lawrence S. Wissow, MD, MPH

> *"One can 'prescribe pleasure' by telling youths and families that caring for oneself, including engaging in activities that were previously pleasurable, is not weakness but rather an important part of self-care, just as athletes need to rest or stretch in addition to testing their limits in workouts."*

The term *low mood* encompasses a variety of symptoms and feelings that can have a range of impact on a child's or an adolescent's functioning. Symptoms can include withdrawal from usual activities and changes to sleep or eating; feelings can include sadness, low self-worth, and hopelessness; and impact on the individual can range from a noticeable but minor impact on energy and optimism to actively pursuing self-harm. In adults, much of this range can be summed up as various degrees of low mood. However, in children and adolescents, symptoms may also include irritability, aggression, and even recklessness. In this chapter, we use the term *depression* (with a small *d*) to refer to the entire range of issues that can be associated with low mood in children and adolescents and may mask the core feelings of sadness and hopelessness.

Symptoms of depression affect many children and adolescents, including a large number whose symptoms do not rise to the level of a disorder but who nonetheless experience considerable morbidity.[1] It is estimated that at any given time in the United States up to 3% of children younger than 13 years and up to 6% of adolescents experience depression. Larger numbers of symptoms and feelings and greater functional impact may reach a threshold for diagnosis of major depressive disorder (MDD). Estimates of lifetime prevalence of MDD are significantly higher, at up to 20%.[2]

Depression may remit on its own or after treatment but recur spontaneously at times of developmental transitions or with new stressors (both positive and negative). Depression is among the mental health problems associated with suicidal ideation, suicide attempts, and completed suicide. Other associated problems include negative effects on school performance, early pregnancy, and impairment of function in the work, social, and family environments.[3] Risk factors for the development of depression among children and adolescents include family history (heritability is approximately 40%), adverse childhood experiences, temperament, and the existence of a major non–mood disorder or a chronic or disabling medical condition.[4] Children and adolescents who seem depressed may have relatives who have also experienced depression or other mental disorders. Finding such a history may reinforce the need to thoroughly evaluate concerns about the patient, especially if there is a family history of suicide. Knowing that other family members have experienced the same problems can increase empathy for the patient's problems and may well provide role models for successful treatment.

There is some evidence that both initial onset and recurrence of depression may be preventable.[5] Nurturing care during the critical first years after birth, warm and confiding family relationships, learning active coping strategies for predictable stressors, promoting a sense of self-efficacy through learning to work through problems, and trying to maintain regular patterns of sleep and exercise may all be protective. If parents have mental health problems (especially depression), helping their children understand and cope with changing parental mood and behavior may help prevent the children themselves from becoming depressed. If a child or an adolescent has received treatment for depression, continuing treatment beyond the early stages of recovery is associated with a reduced risk of relapse or recurrence.

The guidance in this chapter applies primarily to the care of youths (children and adolescents aged 6–18 years) presenting with undifferentiated depression in pediatric clinical settings. (For guidance in the care of younger children, see Chapter 17, Emotional or Behavioral Disturbance in Children Younger Than 5 Years.) This chapter's primary audience is primary care clinicians (PCCs): pediatricians, family physicians, internists, nurse practitioners, and physician assistants who provide longitudinal, frontline health care to children and adolescents. It is based on the work of the World Health Organization, whose recommendations may be updated annually. The most up-to-date information can be found at www.who.int/mental_health/publications/mhGAP_intervention_guide/en.

Findings Suggesting Depression

Although depression may come on without an apparent trigger, even among those who seem highly successful and privileged, it can often develop after one or more stresses or losses or in conjunction with prolonged anxiety. Most children and adolescents will experience an event that induces low mood or sadness, such as breakup with a friend, the death of a loved one or pet, or other losses resulting from life changes such as a move, a family member's military deployment, or parents' separation. A sadness experience of greater intensity or duration than is typical for the child's or adolescent's peers is a cause for concern and may indicate depression.

Symptoms of depression vary. A summary of the symptoms and clinical findings that suggest depression in youths can be found in Box 22-1. For those familiar with the symptoms of depression in adults, it is important

---

Box 22-1. Symptoms and Clinical Findings Suggesting Depression in Youths (Children and Adolescents Aged 6–18 Years)

Indications From History From Youth or Parent

- Low or sad mood present most days
- Loss of interest in school or other activities present most days
- Loss of pleasure in activities formerly enjoyed (When is last time he/you had fun?)
- Suicidal thoughts or acts
- Irritability
- Academic difficulties
- Withdrawal from friends and family
- Physical symptoms such as headaches, abdominal pain, trouble sleeping, fatigue, or poor control of a chronic illness
- Hopelessness
- Poor concentration
- Poor or excessive sleep for developmental stage
- Weight loss (or failure to gain weight normally) or excessive weight gain
- Low self-esteem
- Loss of energy
- Agitation or slowing of movement or speech

Box 22-1. Symptoms and Clinical Findings Suggesting Depression in Youths (Children and Adolescents Aged 6–18 Years) (*continued*)

Risk Factors for Increased Susceptibility to Depression in Youths

- ACEs (eg, mother who experienced postpartum depression)
- Prior trauma or bereavement
- Family breakdown
- Shy personality
- Peer relationship problems
- Breakup of a relationship; setback or disappointment

Abbreviation: ACE, adverse childhood experience.

to remember that, among youths, irritability may be a more prominent symptom than sadness is. In some cases, withdrawal from usual activities or decreased interaction with friends and family may be the only obvious sign, possibly coupled with a change in appetite, sleep, or level of energy.

Symptoms may be elicited from parents or youths but ideally from both parent and youth. Youths may be better able to report on feelings that do not result in behavior change that is obvious to others; on the other hand, youths may not be aware of how their appearances or behaviors have changed in ways that are apparent to others.

Tools to Assist With Identification

Because many youths do not spontaneously disclose their symptoms, standardized psychosocial screening instruments may be used to identify those with symptoms of depression. The American Academy of Pediatrics and Bright Futures recommend annual screening of adolescents for depression beginning at 12 years of age using a validated tool. Several instruments have versions to collect information from youths, parents, and teachers. Table 22-1 provides examples of general psychosocial screening results suggesting that a child may be depressed. Additional instruments such as the Patient Health Questionnaire for Adolescents (PHQ-A) or PHQ-A Depression Screen, Beck Depression Inventory-Primary Care (also known as Fast Screen), or the Modified Patient Health Questionnaire-9 (commonly known as PHQ-9) can also be used to screen adolescents for

Table 22-1. General Psychosocial Screening/Results Suggesting Depression in Children and Youths

Screening Instrument	Score Suggesting Depression
PSC-35	• Total score ≥24 for children aged ≤5 y. • ≥28 for those 6–16 y. • ≥30 for those aged ≥17 y. *and* • Further discussion of items related to depressive symptoms confirms a concern in that area.
PSC-17	• Internalizing subscale is ≥5. *and* • Further discussion of items related to depressive symptoms confirms a concern in that area.
SDQ	• Total symptom score of >19. • Emotional symptom score of 7–10 (see instructions at www.sdqinfo.com). • Impact scale (back of form) score of 1 (medium impairment) or ≥2 (high impairment). *and* • Further discussion of items related to depression confirms a concern in that area.

Abbreviations: PSC, Pediatric Symptom Checklist; SDQ, Strengths and Difficulties Questionnaires.

depression or to help confirm findings of a general psychosocial screening. See Appendix 2, Mental Health Tools for Pediatrics, for more information about these and other instruments.

It is important to differentiate the use of these tools as screening instruments at routine visits vs their use to refine concerns that have already been raised. When used as screening tools, they tend to have relatively low sensitivity and positive predictive value. That is, positive results need further discussion to understand the meaning of the result, and negative results may not be reassuring if the parent or youth is truly concerned. When used to follow up on existing concerns, results still need discussion with families but are more likely be a fair indicator of the nature and severity of the child's problems. The use of a functional assessment tool such as the Strengths and Difficulties Questionnaires (SDQ) or Columbia Impairment Scale (commonly known as CIS) will assist the PCC in determining whether the child's functioning is significantly impaired by the symptoms. Use of a tool to assess the impact of the child's problem on other members of the family may also be helpful; the CGSQ (Caregiver Strain Questionnaire) is one example. See Appendix 2, Mental Health Tools for Pediatrics.

Assessment

Assessment begins by differentiating the child's symptoms from normal behavior. All children may be sad or irritable at times, but for some children these symptoms limit adaptability to normal peer and family situations, interfere with learning, or precipitate suicidal thoughts. Of particular concern is MDD; fifth edition of *Diagnostic Manual of Mental Disorders* (commonly known as *DSM-5*) criteria for MDD are shown in Box 22-2. There are also some conditions that may mimic or co-occur with depression. Table 22-2 provides a summary of these conditions.

For a child with symptoms of depression, the psychosocial assessment process always includes determination of suicide risk, as described in Box 22-3.

Box 22-2. Criteria for Major Depressive Episode (*DSM-5*)

A. Five (or more) of the following symptoms have been present during the same 2-week period and represent a change from previous functioning; at least 1 of the symptoms is either depressed mood or loss of interest or pleasure. **Note:** Do not include symptoms that are clearly attributable to another medical condition.

1. Depressed mood most of the day, nearly every day, as indicated by either subjective report (eg, feels sad, empty, hopeless) or observation made by others (eg, seems tearful). **Note:** In children and adolescents, can be irritable mood.

2. Markedly diminished interest or pleasure in all, or almost all, activities most of the day, nearly every day (as indicated by either subjective account or observation).

3. Significant weight loss when not dieting or weight gain (eg, a change of more than 5% of body weight in a month), or decrease or increase in appetite nearly every day. **Note:** In children, consider failure to make expected weight gain.

4. Insomnia or hypersomnia nearly every day.

Box 22-2. Criteria for Major Depressive Episode (*DSM-5*) (*continued*)

⑤ Psychomotor agitation or retardation nearly every day (observable by others, not merely subjective feelings of restlessness or being slowed down).

⑥ Fatigue or loss of energy nearly every day.

⑦ Feelings of worthlessness or excessive or inappropriate guilt (which may be delusional) nearly every day (not merely self-reproach or guilt about being sick).

⑧ Diminished ability to think or concentrate, or indecisiveness, nearly every day (either by subjective account or as observed by others).

⑨ Recurrent thoughts of death (not just fear of dying), recurrent suicidal ideation without a specific plan, or a suicide attempt or a specific plan for committing suicide.

B. The symptoms cause clinically significant distress or impairment in social, occupational, or other important areas of functioning.

C. The episode is not attributable to the physiologic effects of a substance or to another medical condition. **Note:** Criteria A–C represent a major depressive episode.

Note: Responses to a significant loss (eg, bereavement, financial ruin, losses from a natural disaster, a serious medical illness or disability) may include the feelings of intense sadness, rumination about the loss, insomnia, poor appetite and weight loss as noted in Criterion A, which may resemble a depressive episode. Although such symptoms may be understandable or considered appropriate to the loss, the presence of a major depressive episode in addition to the normal response to a significant loss should also be carefully considered. This decision inevitably requires the exercise of clinical judgment based on the individual's history and the cultural norms for the expression of distress in the context of loss.

D. The occurrence of the major depressive episode is not better explained by schizoaffective disorder, schizophrenia, schizophreniform disorder, delusional disorder, or other specified and unspecified schizophrenia spectrum and other psychotic disorders.

E. There has never been a manic episode or a hypomanic episode. **Note:** This exclusion does not apply if all of the manic-like or hypomanic-like episodes are substance-induced or are attributable to the psychological effects of another medical condition.

From American Psychiatric Association. *Diagnostic and Statistical Manual of Mental Disorders.* 5th ed. Washington, DC: American Psychiatric Association Publishing; 2013, with permission.

Table 22-2. Conditions That May Mimic or Co-occur With Depression

Condition	Rationale
Sleep deprivation	Sleep problems can cause irritability and labile mood; conversely, depression may contribute to difficulty sleeping. See Chapter 28, Sleep Disturbances.
Somatic concerns	Depressed children may present with a variety of somatic concerns (eg, GI symptoms, headaches, chest pain). Conversely, acute or chronic medical conditions or pain syndromes may cause depression.
Learning problems or disabilities	If symptoms of depression are associated with problems of school performance, the child may be experiencing learning difficulties. See Chapter 21, Learning Difficulty, to explore this possibility.
Exposure to ACEs	Children who have experienced or witnessed trauma, violence, a natural disaster, separation from a parent, parental divorce or separation, parental substance use, neglect, or physical, emotional, or sexual abuse are at high risk of developing emotional difficulties such as adjustment disorder, PTSD, and depression. Denial of trauma symptoms does not mean trauma did not occur; questions about ACEs should be repeated as a trusting relationship is established. See also Chapter 14, Anxiety and Trauma-Related Distress.
Maltreatment	Children who have experienced neglect or physical, emotional, or sexual abuse are at high risk of developing emotional difficulties such as depression; this possibility should always be considered.
Anxiety	Depression often co-occurs with anxiety. See Chapter 14, Anxiety and Trauma-Related Distress.
Bereavement	Most children will experience the death of a family member or friend sometime in childhood. Other losses may also trigger grief responses, for example, separation or divorce of parents, relocation, change of school, deployment of a parent in military service, breakup with a girlfriend or boyfriend, or remarriage of parent. Such losses are traumatic. They may result in feelings of sadness, despair, insecurity, or anxiety immediately following the loss and, in some instances, more persistent anxiety or mood symptoms or disorders. Furthermore, they may make the child more susceptible to impaired functioning at the time of subsequent losses. See also the discussion of PTSD in Chapter 14, Anxiety and Trauma-Related Distress.

Table 22-2. Conditions That May Mimic or Co-occur With Depression (*continued*)	
Condition	**Rationale**
Physical illness and harmful medication side effects	Medical issues that can mimic or provoke symptoms of depression include hypothyroidism, lupus, chronic fatigue syndrome, diabetes, and anemia. Children with any chronic medical condition are more likely to experience depression than their peers are (and depression may contribute to poor management of the condition). Medications commonly used in adolescence can be associated with depression (eg, acne preparations, oral contraceptives, interferon, corticosteroids).
Substance use	Children with symptoms of depression may self-medicate with alcohol, nicotine, or other drugs. Conversely, children using substances may manifest depression and deteriorating school performance. See Chapter 31, Substance Use 2: Use of Other Substances.
Conduct or oppositional defiant disorders	Oppositional children may manifest depressive symptoms. Children with conduct problems are at higher risk for suicide. See Chapter 15, Disruptive Behavior and Aggression.
Psychosis	Depression can be complicated by problems with thinking that go beyond the distortions or hopelessness of low mood. These problems include delusions (ie, strongly held and usually odd false beliefs about others, one's body, or one's self), paranoia (ie, strongly felt and unjustified concerns that others are following or intend harm), or hallucinations (ie, seeing or hearing things that others don't hear or see). Individuals often don't volunteer that they are having these sorts of thoughts; asking is important if the person's interactions seem unusual. (Do you ever feel your eyes or ears play tricks on you?)
Bipolar disorders	Adults and older adolescents with bipolar disorder may have markedly varying low mood (depression) or high mood (mania), cycling over weeks or months. Diagnosis of bipolar disorder in children remains controversial. It may be considered in children who cycle through low and high moods very rapidly and in children with explosive or destructive tantrums, dangerous or hypersexual behavior, aggression, irritability, bossiness with adults, driven creativity (sometimes depicting graphic violence), excessive talking, separation anxiety, chronic depression, sleep disturbance, delusions, hallucinations, psychosis, and talk of homicide or suicide. See also Chapter 20, Inattention and Impulsivity; Chapter 15, Disruptive Behavior and Aggression; and Chapter 14, Anxiety and Trauma-Related Distress.

Abbreviations: ACE, adverse childhood experience; GI gastrointestinal; PTSD, post-traumatic stress disorder.

Box 22-3. Determining Suicide Risk

"Are there others in the family (present or past generations) who have had depression or a bipolar disorder or who have attempted suicide?" Youths and parents may need opportunities to answer these questions confidentially because this information is not always shared among family members. Positive responses, especially a family history of suicide, increase concern. Other risk factors include substance use, a model among peers or famous individuals known to the youth, or a recent traumatic or shameful episode. A past attempt by the youth is the single strongest risk factor for future attempts and may warrant mental health referral for the current episode if the youth is not in ongoing care.

The severity of suicidal thoughts can be assessed with several questions and tools. See Appendix 2, Mental Health Tools for Pediatrics. Examples include the following questions:

- *"Have you ever felt bad enough that you wished you were dead?"*
- *"Have you had any thoughts about wanting to kill yourself?"*
- *"Have you ever tried to hurt or kill yourself or come close to hurting or killing yourself?"*
- *"Do you have a plan?"*
- *"Do you have a way to carry out your plan?"*

One way of approaching suicidality is to think of your inquiry as a staged process. A significant minority of adolescents have transient suicidal thoughts or what psychiatrists call "passive death wishes," that is, thoughts that perhaps death would be a way out of problems or stresses but without thinking of a way to harm themselves. Absent the risk factors discussed previously, these youths likely need exploration of stressors and assessment for depression or other mental health problems. A smaller group will have thought about ways of harming themselves but without a concrete plan or making any preparations. Again, absent past attempts, ongoing stressors, a model in the media or among peers, or substance use, these youths need support and further evaluation but are not at high risk of harming themselves. Youths with plans for harming themselves (no matter what the likelihood of success) or who have gathered or identified the means (ropes, medications, knives, or other weapons) are at high risk of harming themselves. They require both a short-term plan for safety and an urgent mental health evaluation.

PCCs frequently encounter youths who superficially harm themselves with sharp objects or by rubbing their skin, usually on the arms or thighs in places that are readily covered by clothing. Collectively referred to as *cutting,* these behaviors are often described by young people as helping them relieve tension or worry, and they often stop when other means of relief are made available. Cutting in the context of persistent low mood, or a stated desire to harm oneself, suggests a need for urgent evaluation.

For more information, see Chapter 27, Self-injury.

Abbreviation: PCC, primary care clinician.

Plan of Care for Youths With Depression

Suicidal intent is an emergency requiring immediate treatment and close supervision of the youth at all times. The care of a youth experiencing depression can begin in the primary care setting from the time symptoms are recognized, even if the youth's symptoms do not rise to the level of a disorder and regardless of whether referral to a mental health specialist is ultimately part of the care plan.

Engaging Youth and Family in Care

Without engagement, most families will not seek or persist in care. The process may require multiple primary care visits.[6] Even when they are evaluated in emergency facilities, youths not admitted may not receive follow-up mental health care.[7] Tracking by PCCs may help reconnect youths with care or reinforce the need to continue seeing a mental health specialist.

Reinforce strengths of the youth and family (eg, good relationships with at least one parent or important adult, prosocial peers, concerned or caring family, help seeking, connection to positive organizations) as a method of engagement and identify any barriers to addressing the problem (eg, stigma, family conflict, resistance to treatment). Use "common factors" techniques,[8] represented by the HELP mnemonic (Box 22-4), to build trust and optimism, reach agreement on incremental next steps, develop a plan of care, and collaboratively determine the role of the PCC. Regardless of other roles, the PCC can encourage a positive view of treatment on the part of the youth and family.

Box 22-4. Common Factors Mnemonic: HELP Build a Therapeutic Alliance

H = Hope

E = Empathy

L^2 = Language, Loyalty

P^3 = Permission, Partnership, Plan

Adapted with permission from American Academy of Pediatrics. *Addressing Mental Health Concerns in Primary Care: A Clinician's Toolkit.* Elk Grove Village, IL: American Academy of Pediatrics; 2010. For the fully annotated mnemonic, please refer to Appendix 5.

Providing Psychoeducation

Depression is very common and not the result of lack of coping ability or personal strength. Often, the family has a history of the condition; talking about this history may reduce stigma and increase empathy and a willingness to seek care, but doing so may also be met with resistance. To assist family members in understanding the disorder, additional points to highlight include that the youth is not making the symptoms up, what looks like laziness or crossness can be symptoms of depression, and the hopelessness of depression is a symptom, not an accurate reflection of reality. However, this negative view of the world and of future possibilities can be hard to penetrate. In addition, the clinician can emphasize that treatment works, although it can take several weeks for improvement, and the affected individual is often the last person to recognize that it has taken place.

Families should be encouraged to address risk factors for maintenance of depression and for the risk of suicidal acts. Weapons should ideally be removed from the home or secured, and a careful survey should be made for potentially lethal medications or household chemicals, including pesticides. Suicidal and depressive thoughts can be spread through social networks and, increasingly, through social media. Not all close, confiding relationships are supportive: teens, in particular, are prone to seek out friends who validate their glum view of the world. Electronic communication has been found, paradoxically, to promote isolation at the same time as it seems to be increasing connectedness. Although doing so is not often easy, parents can be helped to both monitor and limit the use of e-mail, texts, and social media posts until the youth has recovered.

The clinician may also, at this point, talk about how there are many types of treatment for depression, including various forms of psychosocial care, and, for teens, medications. It may be useful to ask about what the teen and family have thought of or heard about treatment; in that way, the clinician can discover if they are anxious that the discussion is leading to a suggestion they would not be willing to accept.

Encouraging Healthy Habits

Encourage exercise, outdoor play, healthy diet, sleep, one-on-one time with parents, praise for positive behavior, and acknowledgment of the youth's strengths. Limit screen time and agree to monitoring of social media. Caring for oneself can be presented honestly as therapeutic. One can "prescribe pleasure" by telling youths and families that caring for oneself, including engaging in activities that were previously pleasurable, is not weakness but rather an important part of self-care, just as athletes need to rest or stretch in addition to testing their limits in workouts.

Reducing Stress

Consider the youth's social environment (eg, family social history, parental depression screening, results of any family assessment tools administered, reports from child care or school). Questions to raise might include

▶ **Is the youth or are other family members experiencing grief and loss issues?** Grief and loss are virtually universal childhood experiences. Youths vary widely in their reactions to these events, depending on their developmental levels, temperaments, prior states of mental health, coping mechanisms, parental responses, and support systems. Also helpful can be supportive counseling, explaining to youths what they might reasonably expect, inviting them to participate in funerals or other ceremonies to the level they feel comfortable, active listening while allowing the youth to express his or her grief, providing guidance about the grief process, and identifying and addressing feelings of guilt. When a parent is also grieving, youths may need time alone with the clinician because they may be reluctant to increase parental sadness. Providing follow-up to see how the family is coping with a loss can help the youth and provide opportunities to assess for more serious reactions, such as complicated bereavement, depression, or post-traumatic stress disorder. Providing referral to community resources may also be helpful. Increasingly, involvement of hospice and palliative care services at the end of life includes support for bereaved family members and specific programs for surviving children. The effects of profound losses, such as the death of a sibling or parent during childhood or removal from parents, last a lifetime. The clinician will need to view all future physical and mental health issues in the family through the prism of this loss. Overlooking such experiences and failing to follow up on the child and family's progress after a traumatic event are lost opportunities to connect with the child and family around important mental health issues.

▶ **Is the youth or family experiencing unusual stress?** The family can work to try to reduce stresses and increase support for the youth. This effort may involve reasonable and short-term changes in demands and responsibilities, including negotiating extensions for assignments or other ways of reducing stress at school; it can also include seeking help for others in the family who are distressed. If a parent is grieving a loss or manifesting symptoms of depression, it is particularly important that the parent address his or her own needs and find additional support for the youth and other family members.

▶ **Does the house have weapons or medications in it?** Guns should be removed from the home; other weapons, medications (including over-the-counter preparations and acetaminophen), and alcohol should be removed from the home, destroyed, or secured. In farm communities, there may be toxic products (such as insecticides or fertilizers) that may need to be secured. Depressed individuals should be dissuaded from operating dangerous machinery or engaging in other activities that require care and normal risk aversion to avoid injury.

Offering Initial Interventions to Address the Depressive Symptoms

The strategies described in the following text are common elements of evidence-based psychosocial interventions for depression in youths. They are applicable to the care of youths with mild or emerging depressive symptoms and to those with impairing symptoms that do not rise to the level of a disorder. They can also be used as initial treatment of youths with a depressive disorder while readying them for or awaiting access to specialty care.

Help the youth develop cognitive and coping skills. Find agreement with the youth and family on a description of the problem. Many negative thoughts can be empathetically challenged and looked at from another perspective. Helpful metaphors include "Long journeys start with a single step" and "The glass is half full, not half empty." Relaxation techniques and visualization (eg, practicing relaxation cued by a pleasant memory, imagining being in a pleasant place) can be helpful for sleep and for anxiety-provoking situations. The clinician can also ask the youth what he or she does to feel better or relax and, if appropriate, prescribe more of that (*behavioral activation*). If the young person has withdrawn from social contacts or activities, the clinician can help plan a return. Young people often cite irritation with others as the cause of their withdrawal; clinicians can empathize with this irritation, point out that it may be partly caused by the young person's depression, and suggest some tactics for tolerating it until things improve. Encourage a focus on strengths rather than weaknesses and doing more of what the youth is good at. Distraction is also good therapy: if the youth is ruminating on a particular stressor, give permission to think about or engage with something else. Many young people will suggest that particular music helps them feel better.

Help the youth develop problem-solving skills. Determine what small achievable act would help the youth feel that he is on the way to overcoming his problems. Suggest that the youth list difficulties, prioritize them, and concentrate efforts on one issue at a time. Avoid downplaying social crises that are important to the young person, even if, from an adult perspective, they seem trivial. Instead, offer to help the young person evaluate the options as he sees them, seeking, if there is an opening, permission to offer alternatives that may not have been raised.

Rehearse behavior and social skills. Reactions to particular situations or people often seem to trigger or maintain low mood. If these triggers can be identified, assist the youth in developing and practicing means of avoidance or alternative responses. Practice doing things and thinking thoughts that improve mood.

Create a safety and emergency plan. Developed in partnership with the family, a treatment plan includes a listing of telephone numbers to call in the event of a sudden increase in distress. This listing should be specific to the youth's community and circumstances (eg, the number for a suicide or depression hotline, on-call telephone number for the practice, area mental health crisis response team contact information). The family should also be instructed to proactively remove lethal means and monitor for suicide risk factors such as increased agitation, stressors, loss of rational thinking, expressed wishes to die, previous attempts, and comorbid conduct disorder or aggressive outbursts.

Providing Resources

The American Academy of Pediatrics has created a number of helpful tools for families: "Childhood Depression: What Parents Can Do to Help" (www.healthychildren.org/English/health-issues/conditions/emotional-problems/Pages/Childhood-Depression-What-Parents-Can-Do-To-Help.aspx); "Help Stop Teenage Suicide" (www.healthychildren.org/English/

health-issues/conditions/emotional-problems/Pages/Help-Stop-Teen-Suicide.aspx); *Teen Suicide, Mood Disorder, and Depression* (https://patiented.solutions.aap.org); and "Ten Things Parents Can Do to Prevent Suicide" (www.healthychildren.org/English/health-issues/conditions/emotional-problems/Pages/Ten-Things-Parents-Can-Do-to-Prevent-Suicide.aspx). Provide the family with contact numbers and resources in case of emergency.

Monitoring the Youth's Progress Toward Therapeutic Goals

Child care, preschool, or school reports can be helpful in monitoring progress. Screening instruments that gather information from multiple reporters (eg, youth, parent, teacher), such as the SDQ and PSC, can be helpful in monitoring progress with symptoms and functioning.

It is important for the clinician to work with the family to understand that it is not uncommon for treatment to be successful for a period and then seem to lose effectiveness. This setback can happen when there are new stresses or demands or when, after a period of success, there has been a letup on treatment. If troubleshooting existing treatment and ways of dealing with new stresses does not help get function back to baseline, new treatments, or new diagnoses, need to be considered. In particular, as school demands increase, learning issues may need to be considered, even if they were not seen as contributing problems in the past.

Involving Specialists

Involve specialists if the youth does not respond to initial interventions or if indicated by the following clinical circumstances:

► A preadolescent child manifests depression or suicidal ideation.

► An adolescent with depressive symptoms has made a prior suicide attempt, developed a plan (especially with means available), or known a friend or acquaintance who has committed suicide.

► An adolescent's functioning is significantly impaired.

► Symptoms are threatening the achievement of developmentally important goals (eg, attending school, spending time with friends).

► The adolescent has mental health comorbidities such as substance use or odd behavior suggestive of an emerging psychotic disorder.

▶ The adolescent also has symptoms of a bipolar disorder, that is, elevated (often more driven rather than positive) mood and energy associated with irritability and behavior that seems audacious for her age (grandiosity).

▶ Depressive symptoms were preceded by serious trauma.

For youths with a diagnosis of moderate to severe MDD, data indicate superior efficacy of a combination of cognitive behavioral therapy (CBT) and a selective serotonin reuptake inhibitor (SSRI) compared with either CBT alone (which may not be sufficiently helpful for these more severe cases) or an SSRI alone.[9] Thus, youths with MDD would ideally receive treatment from a licensed therapist with training in CBT (see following text).

When specialty care is needed, ensure that it is evidence informed and assist the family in accessing it. A variety of evidence-based and evidence-informed psychosocial interventions, and some pharmacological interventions, are available for the treatment of depressive disorders in children and adolescents. Ideally, those referred for care in the mental health specialty system would have access to the safest and most effective treatments. Table 22-3 provides a summary of these interventions. Box 22-5 summarizes psychopharmacological interventions approved at the time of this book's publication by the US Food and Drug Administration for treatment of MDD in children and adolescents. Youths referred for mental health specialty care complete the referral process only 61% of the time, and a significantly smaller number persist in care.[10,11] Approaches to improving the referral process include making sure that the family is ready for this step in care, that they have some idea of what the specialty care will involve, and that they understand what the PCC's ongoing role may be. If the specialty appointment is not likely to occur shortly, the PCC can work with the patient and family on a plan to manage the problem as well as possible in the meantime.

Reach agreement on respective roles in the youth's care. If the youth is referred to mental health specialty care for a depressive disorder, his or her PCC may be responsible for initiating medication or adjusting doses, monitoring response to treatment, monitoring adverse effects, engaging and encouraging the youth's and family's positive views of treatment, and

Table 22-3. Psychosocial and Psychopharmacological Therapies for Depression: Evidence Base as of April 2018

Problem Area	Level 1 – Best Support	Level 2 – Good Support	Level 3 – Moderate Support	Level 4 – Minimal Support	Level 5 – No Support
Depressive or Withdrawn Behaviors	CBT, CBT and Medication, CBT with Parents, Client Centered Therapy, Family Therapy	Attention Training, Cognitive Behavioral Psychoeducation, Expression, Interpersonal Therapy, MI/Engagement and CBT, Physical Exercise, Problem Solving, Relaxation	None	Self Control Training, Self Modeling, Social Skills	CBT and Anger Control, CBT and Behavioral Sleep Intervention, CBT and PMT, Goal Setting, Life Skills, Mindfulness, Play Therapy, PMT, PMT and Emotion Regulation, Psychodynamic Therapy, Psychoeducation
Suicidality	None	Attachment Therapy, CBT with Parents, Counselors Care, Counselors Care and Support Training, Interpersonal Therapy, Multisystemic Therapy, Parent Coping/Stress Management, Psychodynamic Therapy, Social Support	None	None	Accelerated Hospitalization, Case Management, CBT, Communication Skills, Counselors Care and Anger Management

Abbreviations: CBT, Cognitive Behavior Therapy; MI, Motivational Interviewing; PMT, Parent Management Training; Level 5 refers to treatments whose tests were unsupportive or inconclusive. This report updates and replaces the "Blue Menu" originally distributed by the Hawaii Department of Health, Child and Adolescent Mental Health Division, Evidence-Based Services Committee from 2002–2009.

Excerpted from PracticeWise Evidence-Based Child and Adolescent Psychosocial Interventions, created for the period October 2017–April 2018, using the PracticeWise Evidence-Based Services Database, available at www.practicewise.com. See Appendix 6 for the full table and details on background and evidence. For biannual updates go to www.aap.org/en-us/documents/crpsychosocialinterventions.pdf.

Box 22-5. US Food and Drug Administration–Approved Psychopharmacological Interventions for Children and Adolescents (as of March 12, 2018)[a,b]	
Diagnostic Area	**Psychopharmacological Intervention**
MDD	SSRIs (fluoxetine [starting at age 8 y] and escitalopram [starting at age 13 y]) are currently the only drugs approved by the FDA for treating MDD among youths. Some data indicate superior efficacy of combination CBT and SSRI vs CBT or SSRI alone.

Abbreviations: CBT, cognitive behavioral therapy; FDA, US Food and Drug Administration; MDD, major depressive disorder; SSRI, selective serotonin reuptake inhibitor.

[a] For up-to-date information about FDA-approved interventions, go to www.fda.gov/ScienceResearch/SpecialTopics/PediatricTherapeuticsResearch/default.htm.

[b] See also Chapter 11, Psychotropic Medications in Primary Care, for guidance in primary care prescribing.

coordinating care provided by parents, school, medical home, and specialists. In fact, the youth may improve just knowing that the PCC is involved and interested.

Primary care clinicians frequently lament that it is difficult to obtain follow-up information from mental health specialists. There are many potential barriers, including misinterpretations of confidentiality rules by primary care or mental health providers and their differing work schedules. Documenting each family's permission for the exchange of information between the PCC and mental health specialists, both at the time of referral and on an ongoing basis, is one way to avoid delays in treatment. Resources available to help PCCs in this role and related roles include the *Guidelines for Adolescent Depression-Primary Care (GLAD-PC) Toolkit* at www.glad-pc.org.

Note that not all evidence-based interventions may be available in every community. If a particular intervention is not available, this lack of intervention becomes an opportunity to collaborate with others in the community to advocate on behalf of children. Increasingly, states offer both telepsychiatry services and consultation and referral support "warmlines" that help PCCs provide initial treatment and locate resources. The availability of the latter form of help is tracked at www.nncpap.org.

Acknowledgments: The author and editor wish to acknowledge the contributions of Linda Paul, MPH, manager of the American Academy of Pediatrics Mental Health Leadership Work Group.

AAP Policy

American Academy of Pediatrics Committee on Practice and Ambulatory Medicine and Bright Futures Periodicity Schedule Workgroup. 2017 recommendations for preventive pediatric health care. *Pediatrics.* 2017;139(4):e20170254 (pediatrics. aappublications.org/content/139/4/e20170254)

References

1. Carrellas NW, Biederman J, Uchida M. How prevalent and morbid are subthreshold manifestations of major depression in adolescents? A literature review. *J Affect Disord.* 2017;210:166–173

2. Williams SB, O'Connor EA, Eder M, Whitlock EP. Screening for child and adolescent depression in primary care settings: a systematic evidence review for the US Preventive Services Task Force. *Pediatrics.* 2009;123(4):e716–e735

3. Fergusson DM, Woodward LJ. Mental health, educational, and social role outcomes of adolescents with depression. *Arch Gen Psychiatry.* 2002;59(3):225–231

4. American Psychiatric Association. *Diagnostic and Statistical Manual of Mental Disorders.* 5th ed. Washington, DC: American Psychiatric Association Publishing; 2013

5. Brown CH, Brincks A, Huang S, et al. Two-year impact of prevention programs on adolescent depression: an integrative data analysis approach. *Prev Sci.* 2016. doi: 10.1007/s11121-016-0737-1

6. Foy JM; American Academy of Pediatrics Task Force on Mental Health. Enhancing pediatric mental health care: algorithms for primary care. *Pediatrics.* 2010;125(suppl 3):S109–S125

7. Asarnow JR, Baraff LJ, Berk M. An emergency department intervention for linking pediatric suicidal patients to follow-up mental health treatment. *Psychiatr Serv.* 2011;62(11):1303–1309

8. Kemper KJ, Wissow L, Foy JM, Shore SE. *Core Communication Skills for Primary Clinicians.* Winston-Salem, NC: Wake Forest School of Medicine. http://nwahec. org/45737. Accessed February 8, 2018

9. Hodes M, Garralda E. NICE guidelines on depression in children and young people: not always following the evidence. *BJPsych Bull.* 2007;31(10):361–362

10. Manfredi C, Lacey L, Warnecke R. Results of an intervention to improve compliance with referrals for evaluation of suspected malignancies at neighborhood public health centers. *Am J Public Health.* 1990;80(1):85–87

11. Friman PC, Finney JW, Rapoff MA, Christophersen ER. Improving pediatric appointment keeping with reminders and reduced response requirement. *J Appl Behav Anal.* 1985;18(4):315–321

CHAPTER 23

Maternal Depression

Marian Earls, MD

"The non-stigmatizing, longitudinal pediatric relationship lends itself to identifying maternal depression and supporting maternal and child health."

Perinatal depression is a pertinent issue for the primary care clinician (PCC) because of the significant associated risks to the health and well-being of the infant and family. Perinatal depression is an example of an adverse childhood experience (ACE) that has potential long-term adverse health complications for the mother, the father, the infant, and the mother-infant dyad. Postpartum depression may adversely affect the child's early brain development and lead to increased costs of medical care, inappropriate medical care, child abuse and neglect, discontinuation of breastfeeding, and family dysfunction. Pediatric practices, as medical homes, can establish a system to implement postpartum depression screening and to identify and use community resources for the treatment and referral of the mother with depression and support for the mother-infant (dyad) relationship.[1] This chapter specifically offers guidance to the PCC who is providing care for the infant of a depressed mother.

Background

Up to 12% of all women may experience depression in a given year. Socioeconomic status is a compounding factor, and if a woman has low income, the prevalence of depression is doubled to 25%. Forty percent to 60% of mothers who have low income report depressive symptoms (but do not necessarily meet criteria for a depressive disorder).[2] Specifically, depression occurs in 8.5% to 11% of women during pregnancy and in 6.5% to 12.9% of women during the postpartum period. Major depression, as a subset of those statistics, occurs in 3.1% to 4.9% and 1% to 6.8%, respectively. The peak for minor depression occurs at 2 to 3 months' postpartum; the peak for major depression, at 6 weeks' postpartum.[3] Another peak occurs at 6 months' postpartum.

The spectrum of postpartum depression encompasses "postpartum blues" to postpartum mood disorders (PPMDs), which include postpartum depression and postpartum psychosis. Fifty percent to 80% of all mothers experience postpartum blues after birth. These symptoms are transient (beginning a few days after birth and lasting up to 2 weeks), but they do not impair function. Symptoms include crying, depressed mood, irritability, anxiety, and confusion.

Postpartum depression meets fifth edition of the *Diagnostic and Statistical Manual of Mental Disorders*[4] criteria as a minor or major depressive disorder. If a woman experiences PPMD, she is likely to experience it again with subsequent pregnancies. However, PPMD can affect mothers even without a previous history after earlier births. A mother is at increased risk for depression if her infant has difficult temperament, was born preterm, or has a chronic health condition. If a mother has difficulty reading her infant's cues, bonding may be difficult and interaction impaired.

Postpartum psychosis is a relatively rare event. Only 1% to 3% of women experience postpartum psychosis. Occurring in the first 4 weeks after birth, impairment is serious and may include paranoia, mood shifts, hallucinations or delusions, and suicidal or homicidal thoughts. Postpartum psychosis requires immediate medical attention.

Effects of Maternal Depression

The Infant

Depression may cause the mother to disengage emotionally, making it difficult for her to read her baby's cues, causing the infant to withdraw from daily activities, impairing interaction between mother and baby, and compromising bonding. Research on early brain development, toxic stress, epigenetics, and ACEs has revealed the physiologic impact of the infant's environment on health, development, and learning in the short and long term.[5]

An infant in the environment of significant maternal depression is at risk for toxic stress and its consequences. Toxic stress is an unhealthy prolonged activation of the stress response, unbuffered by a caregiver. Physiologic responses to stress in the infant's environment affect the infant's social-emotional development. The activation of the physiologic stress response system results in increased levels of stress hormones. Persistent elevation of cortisol level can disrupt the developing brain's architecture in the areas of the amygdala, hippocampus, and prefrontal cortex and therefore ultimately affect learning, memory, and behavioral and emotional adaptation. When an infant lives in an environment of neglect, magnetic resonance imaging may reveal visible changes in the frontal lobes.[6,7] The infant, therefore, is at risk for impaired social interaction, delays in language and cognitive development, failure to thrive, and reactive attachment disorder of infancy.[8]

Early signs and symptoms in the infant include poor orientation skills and tracking, lower activity level, and negative temperament. The developing infant may appear sad, lethargic, and withdrawn. The infant may have little interest in exploration. There may be feeding or sleeping problems. The infant may cry a lot and have difficulty with both self-comforting and being soothed. As early as 2 months of age, the infant looks at the depressed mother less frequently and may demonstrate poor state regulation, less interaction with objects, and lower activity level. The infant is likely to exhibit no caregiver preference and to go to anyone. The infant may resist touch or be clingy. Infants are at risk for insecure attachment. Children with insecure attachment are more likely to develop behavioral problems and conduct disorder. Higher cortisol levels in preschoolers are linked with anxiety, social wariness, and withdrawal.[9] Attachment disorders, behavioral problems, and depression can occur in childhood and adolescence. When mothers experience depression, the children, as they age, often have poor self-control, poor peer relationships, school problems, aggression, special education needs, grade retention, and early school exit.

The Mother

Maternal depression impairs parenting skills. The mother's perception of the infant's behavior is less positive than that of her nondepressed peers. Her interaction is less attuned to the infant's cues and may be more controlling. On the other hand, she may have apathy toward the baby and indifference to caregiving. She is likely to have impaired attention and judgment for health and safety. Furthermore, there is an adverse effect on breastfeeding. The Agency for Healthcare Research and Quality evidence report *Breastfeeding and Maternal and Infant Health Outcomes in Developed Countries* reviewed 6 prospective cohort studies regarding postpartum depression and breastfeeding. It revealed an association between not breastfeeding, or early cessation of breast-feeding, and postpartum depression.[10]

Early response is urgent. If the mother continues to experience depression with no intervention for the dyad, the child's developmental issues are likely to persist and be less responsive to intervention over time.[11]

Role of the Primary Care Clinician

Postpartum depression leads to adverse effects on infant brain develop-ment, cessation of breastfeeding, family dysfunction, inappropriate medi-cal treatment of the infant, and increased costs of care. To have a positive effect on the health of the child and family, medical homes can be timely and proactive by implementing screening, supporting the mother-child relationship, and identifying and using community resources for referral and treatment. Primary care clinicians who care for children need to promote awareness of the need for screening in the obstetric and pediatric periodicity of care schedules, use evidence-based interventions focused on healthy attachment and parent-child relationships, and promote training for professionals who care for very young children (0–5 years of age).

The American Academy of Pediatrics policy statement "The Future of Pediatrics: Mental Health Competencies for Pediatric Primary Care" recognized the unique advantage of the primary care physician for surveillance, screening, and working with families to improve mental health outcomes.[12] "The primary care advantage" derives from the follow-ing characteristics:

▶ Longitudinal, trusting relationship with the family

▶ Family centeredness

▶ Unique opportunities for prevention and anticipatory guidance

▶ Understanding of common social-emotional and learning issues in the context of development

▶ Experience in coordinating with specialists in the care of CYSHCN (children and youths with special health care needs)

▶ Familiarity with chronic care principles and practice improvement

Bright Futures: Guidance for Health Supervision of Infants, Children, and Adolescents, 4th Edition, health promotion themes include Lifelong Health for Families and Communities, Family Support, Healthy Development, and Mental Health. Bright Futures includes surveillance for family social-emotional well-being by recommending that PCCs elicit parental strengths and protective factors and ask about social determinants of health. Specifically, *Bright Futures,* 4th Edition, recommends using a strength-based approach (ie, eliciting and reinforcing strengths and protective factors) to perform a history at every contact beginning with the prenatal visit.[13] Beginning with the newborn visit, *Bright Futures,* 4th Edition, recommends psychosocial and behavioral assessment at every visit (described as "family centered and [possibly including] an assessment of child social-emotional health, caregiver depression, and social determinants of health"); formal maternal depression screening at intervals during infancy); developmental screening at 9 months, 18 months, and 2½ years; and developmental surveillance at regular intervals throughout childhood and adolescence.[14] When history, psychosocial and behavioral assessment, surveillance, or screening is positive for depression, a PCC can use a "common factors" approach (see Chapter 5, Effective Communication Methods: Common Factors Skills) to engage families, build a therapeutic alliance, and address any barriers to help seeking for mental health and social problems.

Screening for Postpartum Depression

On the basis of peak times for the occurrence of the spectrum of PPMD, the 1-, 2-, 4-, and 6-month infant health supervision visits are appropriate times to screen for maternal depression. Screening tools are simple and include the Edinburgh Postnatal Depression Scale (EPDS) or the Patient Health Questionnaire-2 (PHQ-2) or Patient Health Questionnaire-9 (PHQ-9), both of which are endorsed by the US Preventive Services Task Force.[15] These questionnaires are also in the public domain. The EPDS has 10 multiple choice questions and is completed by the mother. It is also embedded in the Survey of Well-being of Young Children (SWYC). A score of 10 or greater indicates possible depression. The EPDS also contains 2 questions regarding anxiety, which is a common component of postpartum depression. The screening is available in English and Spanish and can be accessed online. The PHQ-2, followed by the PHQ-9 when the PHQ-2 is positive for depression, has only 2 questions and is not specific to the postpartum period. It can be used during pregnancy, for surveillance, and to indicate risk for depression in adults in general.[15] See Appendix 2, Mental Health Tools for Pediatrics, for descriptions of these tools.

When Screening Shows a Concern

When a maternal depression screening is positive, management will vary according to the degree of concern and need. At the very least, the finding will require support and demystification and notation of it on the child's record to prompt heightened surveillance of the child and follow-up of the mother. Management includes

► Triage for psychiatric or social emergency

► Communication

► Demystification

► Support resources (family and community)

► Referrals

 – For the mother

  ■ Evidence-based therapy by a licensed mental health specialist and, if pharmacotherapy is indicated, by a prescribing clinician

  ■ For the breastfeeding mother, lactation support from an experienced provider

 – For the dyad

  ■ If attachment issues are identified, evidence-based therapy by a pediatric mental health specialist regarding attachment and bonding

 – For the child

  ■ Early intervention (EI) (for targeted promotion of social-emotional development)

  ■ Follow-up social-emotional screening in the primary care practice

Discussion of each of these elements of management follows.

Emergency

Immediate action is necessary if the EPDS score is 20 or greater, if question 10 on the EPDS is positive, if question 9 on the PHQ-9 is positive, if the mother expresses concern about her or her baby's safety, or if the PCC suspects that the mother is suicidal, homicidal, severely depressed, manic, or psychotic. Referral to emergency mental health services (most communities have mental health crisis teams or services) is needed and the mother should leave with a support person (not alone) and with a safety plan.

Communication and Demystification

Demystification is directed at removing the mystery about maternal depression, that is, emphasizing that postpartum depression happens with many women, that the mother is not at fault or a bad mother, that depression is treatable, and that the PCC is a resource and other help is available. She can be reassured that having a baby is a time of transition that can be difficult when there are other stressors but can be eased when there are other supports. A brief intervention, framed by common factors principles, could include

▶ Promote the strength of the mother-infant relationship.

▶ Encourage and reassure the mother regarding any concerns about breastfeeding.

▶ Encourage the mother's understanding and response to the baby's cues.

▶ Encourage the mother to read and talk to the infant.

▶ Encourage routines for predictability and security.

▶ Encourage focus on the mother's wellness: sleep, diet, exercise, and stress relief.

▶ Promote the mother's realistic expectations and prioritization of important things.

▶ Encourage the mother's social connections.

Support and Referral Resources for Mother

Depending on her needs, intervention for the mother may include support, therapy, medication, emergency mental health services, and hospitalization. Referrals for the mother could be to her own PCC or her obstetrician (either of whom may have an integrated mental health specialist [MHS] linked with his or her practice), or to a MHS for individual or couple's therapy. Note, however, that mild depression does not generally require medication. If a mother is referred, a key component is follow-up with the mother to be certain that she is receiving treatment and support and, if so, that depressive symptoms are decreased.

Follow-up and Referral for the Infant and Dyad

When maternal depression screening is positive, follow-up before the next routine visit should occur. To follow up on depression concerns and the effect on the mother-infant relationship, use of a screening for infant social-emotional development and interaction is appropriate. The Ages & Stages Questionnaires: Social-Emotional, Second Edition (commonly known as ASQ:SE-2) is one such tool. It is parent completed and has a single cutoff score. It provides information about infant caregiver interaction and screens affect, self-regulation, adaptive functioning, autonomy, compliance, and communication. Another infant social-emotional screening instrument in the public domain is the Baby Pediatric Symptom Checklist (also embedded in the SWYC). It assesses irritability, inflexibility, and difficulty with routines and is to be used for babies and children younger than 18 months.[16]

Intervention for the infant and dyad includes the follow-up social-emotional screening (described in the previous section of this chapter) and, if attachment issues are indicated, therapy with a pediatric MHS regarding attachment and bonding. It also includes referral to Part C (EI services for 0- to 3-year-olds).

Referrals for the dyad should be to a professional who has expertise in the treatment of very young children (0–5 years of age). Evidence-based treatments include Circle of Security, Parent-Child Interactive Therapy, Child-Parent Psychotherapy, and Attachment and Biobehavioral Catch-up.[17,18] Part C services can provide modeling and support for interaction and play with the infant to promote healthy development.

Support for the Family

The father may also have depression, and the incidence may be higher if the mother is depressed. A father who is not depressed may be a protective factor for the mother.

If the practice has an integrated mental health provider, such as a licensed clinical social worker or counselor, that provider can provide immediate triage for a positive screening, administer secondary screenings, offer support and follow-up, facilitate referrals, and coordinate follow-up with the PCC.

Other community resources for the family include

- ▶ Public health nurses

- ▶ Lactation specialists

- ▶ Parent educators

- ▶ Family support groups

- ▶ Parent-child groups

- ▶ Mother's morning out

- ▶ Early Head Start

- ▶ Mentoring and home visitation such as Parents as Teachers, Healthy Families America, Nurse-Family Partnership, and faith-based or other volunteers

Practical Issues Regarding Implementation

Introduction of Screening Into a Primary Care Practice

Planning to begin postpartum depression screening includes the essential component of simultaneously planning the process for linking the mother, infant, and family to appropriate support and intervention resources. Implementation of these screening and referral processes requires a quality improvement approach to office process. Ideally, the quality team at the practice would include front office, nursing, and clinical staff and family advisors. Outreach to referral sources to discuss referral planning facilitates referral relationships. For these processes, outreach to identify MHSs who provide infant and early childhood services is particularly important.

Integration of a Mental Health Specialist Into Primary Care

In an integrated model, the MHS is located within the primary care practice and is part of the medical home team, practicing in the clinic alongside the PCC, allowing shared visits, warm handoffs (in-person introduction and transfer of trust), and brief interventions. The MHS may also provide some traditional behavioral health services but will accommodate interruptions to participate flexibly in primary care visits. In the instance that there is a positive screening for maternal depression, the PCC can do a warm handoff to that clinician in real time. In a brief visit, the MHS can provide triage, support, and facilitation of a referral if indicated. Follow-up (by phone or in person) with the mother and serving as a liaison with a community MHS providing dyadic therapy is also a function of the MHS. Finally, the MHS can provide follow-up social-emotional screening for the infant.

Summary

Early brain development research highlights the importance of a healthy mother-infant relationship. Unrecognized and untreated, postpartum depression places this relationship and the infant at risk. The non-stigmatizing, longitudinal pediatric relationship lends itself to identifying maternal depression and supporting maternal and child health. Universal early, routine, structured psychosocial screening opens the door to broader communication with families and the medical home about mental health–related concerns. The PCC-family relationship provides the primary care advantage to facilitate promotion and prevention for healthy attachment and social-emotional development for the infant.

AAP Policy

American Academy of Pediatrics Committee on Psychosocial Aspects of Child and Family Health and Task Force on Mental Health. The future of pediatrics: mental health competencies for pediatric primary care. *Pediatrics*. 2009;124(1):410–421. Reaffirmed August 2013 (pediatrics.aappublications.org/content/124/1/410)

Cohen GJ; American Academy of Pediatrics Committee on Psychosocial Aspects of Child and Family Health. The prenatal visit. *Pediatrics*. 2009;124(4):1227–1232. Reaffirmed May 2014 (pediatrics.aappublications.org/content/124/4/1227)

Earls MF; American Academy of Pediatrics Committee on the Psychosocial Aspects of Child and Family Health. Incorporating recognition and management of perinatal and postpartum depression into pediatric practice. *Pediatrics*. 2010;126(5):1032–1039. Reaffirmed December 2014 (pediatrics.aappublications.org/content/126/5/1032)

References

1. Earls MF; American Academy of Pediatrics Committee on the Psychosocial Aspects of Child and Family Health. Incorporating recognition and management of perinatal and postpartum depression into pediatric practice. *Pediatrics*. 2010; 126(5):1032–1039

2. Isaacs M. *Community Care Networks for Depression in Low-Income Communities and Communities of Color: A Review of the Literature*. Washington, DC: Howard University School of Social Work and National Alliance of Multiethnic Behavioral Health Associations; 2004

3. Kahn RS, Wise PH, Wilson K. Maternal smoking, drinking and depression: a generational link between socioeconomic status and child behavior problems [abstract]. *Pediatr Res*. 2002;51(pt 2):191A

4. American Psychiatric Association. *Diagnostic and Statistical Manual of Mental Disorders*. 5th ed. Washington, DC: American Psychiatric Association; 2013

5. American Academy of Pediatrics Committee on Psychosocial Aspects of Child and Family Health; Committee on Early Childhood, Adoption, and Dependent Care; and Section on Developmental and Behavioral Pediatrics. Early childhood adversity, toxic stress, and the role of the pediatrician: translating developmental science into lifelong health. *Pediatrics*. 2012;129(1):e224–e231

6. De Bellis MD, Thomas LA. Biologic findings of post-traumatic stress disorder and child maltreatment. *Curr Psychiatry Rep*. 2003;5(2):108–117

7. Hagele DM. The impact of maltreatment on the developing child. *N C Med J*. 2005;66(5):356–339

8. Zero to Three. *Diagnostic Classification of Mental Health and Developmental Disorders of Infancy and Early Childhood*. Washington, DC: Zero to Three; 2016

9. Essex MJ, Klein MH, Cho E, Kalin NH. Maternal stress beginning in infancy may sensitize children to later stress exposure: effects on cortisol and behavior. *Biol Psychiatry*. 2002;52(8):776–784

10. Agency for Healthcare Research and Quality. *Breastfeeding and Maternal and Infant Health Outcomes in Developed Countries*. Rockville, MD: Agency for Healthcare Research and Quality; 2007:130–131. AHRQ publication 07-E007

11. Riley AW, Brotman M. *The Effects of Maternal Depression on the School Readiness of Low-Income Children*. Baltimore, MD: Annie E. Casey Foundation, Johns Hopkins Bloomberg School of Public Health; 2003

12. American Academy of Pediatrics Committee on Psychosocial Aspects of Child and Family Health and Task Force on Mental Health. The future of pediatrics: mental health competencies for pediatric primary care. *Pediatrics*. 2009;124(1):410–421

13. Cohen GJ; American Academy of Pediatrics Committee on Psychosocial Aspects of Child and Family Health. The prenatal visit. *Pediatrics*. 2009;124(4):1227–1232

14. Hagan JF Jr, Shaw JS, Duncan PM, eds. *Bright Futures: Guidelines for Health Supervision of Infants, Children, and Adolescents*. 4th ed. Elk Grove Village, IL: American Academy of Pediatrics; 2017

15. Siu AL; US Preventive Services Task Force. Screening for depression in adults. *JAMA*. 2016;315(4):380–387

16. Sheldrick RC, Henson BS, Neger EN, Merchant S, Murphy JM, Perrin EC. The baby pediatric symptom checklist: development and initial validation of a new social/emotional screening instrument for very young children. *Acad Pediatr.* 2013;13(1):72–80

17. Appleyard K, Berlin L. *Supporting Healthy Relationships Between Young Children and Their Parents: Lessons From Attachment Theory and Research* [brief]. Durham, NC: Duke University Center for Child and Family Policy; 2007

18. Berlin LJ, Zeanah CH, Lieberman AF. Prevention and intervention programs for supporting early attachment security. In: Cassidy J, Shaver PR, eds. *Handbook of Attachment: Theory, Research, and Clinical Applications.* 2nd ed. New York, NY: Guilford Press; 2008:745–761

CHAPTER 24

Medically Unexplained Symptoms

Rebecca Baum, MD, and John Campo, MD

> "Rather than focusing on false dichotomies between physical
> and psychological health, it is preferable to recognize
> the connection between psychology and physiology:
> the term somatization is used to reflect the experience of
> the individual, including his subjective experience, distress,
> and desire to seek medical care, in the setting of medically
> unexplained symptoms."

Background

Medically unexplained symptoms (MUSs) can present significant challenges and frustrations to the children and adolescents affected by them and their families, and to the primary care clinicians (PCCs)—pediatricians, family physicians, internists, nurse practitioners, and physician assistants—and pediatric subspecialists involved in their care. While medically unexplained physical symptoms are often associated with mental health issues, children and adolescents with MUSs often present in primary care and general medical settings rather than the mental health setting. Patients with MUSs often experience increased utilization of health care services,[1] with multiple visits in the primary care, pediatric subspecialist, and/or emergency department settings, and are at risk for potentially dangerous and unnecessary evaluations, laboratory tests, and procedures.[2] Patients and families may be frustrated and confused by clinicians' communicating that "nothing is wrong" despite continued pain and impairment. Medically unexplained symptoms are thus an important entity for PCCs and pediatric subspecialists (collectively encompassed by the term *pediatric clinicians* in this chapter) to recognize to help facilitate accurate assessment and intervention.

Historically, physicians have been trained in the biomedical model that explains the presence of physical symptoms with a diagnosis based on the presence of pathology consistent with a specific disease.[3] In this model, unexplained symptoms may not be presumed to be real, or they may be considered representative of a mental disorder. This dichotomous approach, termed *dualism,* distinguishes between physical and mental disorders by virtue of whether there is evidence of a biomedical explanation. It is increasingly being recognized that such dualistic thinking is inadequate to address the entity of MUSs. Using this model, pediatric clinicians may complicate care, or they may even put patients at risk, in an attempt to prevent "missing" explanatory physical disease. Families and patients may feel stigmatized, misunderstood, and lacking in an explanation for their symptoms.

Our current understanding of pain suggests that it is an unpleasant sensory and emotional experience representative of physiologic changes and tissue damage. This approach suggests that pain is a derivative of demonstrable tissue pathology, yet pain can also be experienced subjectively in the absence of demonstrable pathology. Similarly, the level of pain experienced in association with a given degree of tissue damage may also vary. Rather than focusing on false dichotomies between physical and psychological health, it is preferable to recognize the connection between psychology and physiology.[4] The term *somatization* is used to reflect the experience of the individual, including his subjective experience, distress, and desire to seek medical care, in the setting of MUSs.[5]

Epidemiology

Medically unexplained symptoms are often encountered across childhood and adolescence, with pain and fatigue being especially common in all age-groups. It is also important to remember that the presence of one type of MUS typically predicts the presence of other MUSs. In preschool children, abdominal pain is a common manifestation.[6] Among children and adolescents, headache and abdominal pain are the most prevalent symptoms,[7,8] although other types of pain, such as limb and chest pain, are often reported.[9] Fatigue is a particularly common concern in teens.[10] Other symptoms include urinary, cardiovascular, rheumatologic, and gastrointestinal concerns. Medically unexplained symptoms suggesting neurological or sensory impairment, often referred to as *conversion symptoms,* are relatively unusual in community settings yet more common in specialty settings. A study of teens in the Ontario Child Health Study suggested a prevalence of recurrent somatic symptoms in the primary care setting of 4% for boys and 11% for girls.[11] Other studies report that between 2% and 20% of children in primary care settings present with MUS.[9] Boys and girls may have different clinical presentations, with some studies suggesting that girls report more somatic symptoms than boys do and more frequently report symptoms of headache or abdominal pain than boys do, particularly with increasing age into adolescence.[10–12] All types of MUSs can be associated with significant impairment for patients and their families. Impairment may include missed school days, increased health care use, patient and family distress, limitation of activities, impaired peer interactions, and significant effect on family functioning.[13] Pediatric MUSs are also well-known risk markers for current and future anxiety and depressive disorders,[14] and they may predict suicide attempts and completion later in life.[15]

The precise etiology of MUSs is unknown. Certain associations and risk factors have been identified (Box 24-1). In general, children with emotional and behavioral problems are more likely to experience MUSs than are otherwise healthy children. In a primary care sample, children

---

Box 24-1. Risk Factors for the Development of Medically Unexplained Symptoms

- Genetics
- Modeling
- Physical illness
- School stressors
- Family stressors
- High-achieving families
- Parental overprotection
- Secondary gain[a]
- Impaired or limited coping mechanisms
- Difficulty identifying/expressing feelings
- Difficulty with transitions
- Psychiatric comorbidity
- Trauma

---

[a] *Secondary gain* refers to the social and familial reinforcement of the symptom.

Derived from Ibeziako P, Bujoreanu S. Approach to psychosomatic illness in adolescents. *Curr Opin Pediatr.* 2011;23(4):384–389.

identified as somatizers had a higher frequency of emotional and behavioral problems, including internalizing symptoms such as worrying, fear of new situations, and problems with separation.[13] Children and adolescents with diagnosed mental disorders such as anxiety, depression, and disruptive behavioral disorders have also been found to exhibit more somatic symptoms, including headache, abdominal pain, and musculoskeletal pain.[10,12]

Classification

Definitions for conditions characterized by chronic pain and physical distress are detailed in the fifth edition of the *Diagnostic and Statistical Manual of Mental Disorders* (*DSM-5*), under the category of "Somatic Symptom and Related Disorders." This category replaces that of "Somatoform Disorders" in the fourth edition of the *Diagnostic and Statistical Manual of Mental Disorders* (*DSM-IV*). These disorders are characterized by pain or other somatic symptoms in association with impairment in functioning and significant individual distress. Somatic symptom disorder (SSD) is the diagnosis applied in the presence of distressing or impairing somatic symptoms along with excessive, maladaptive, or disproportionate thoughts or feelings about the physical symptoms. See Table 24-1 for additional disorders in this category, including illness anxiety disorder, which replaces hypochondriasis; conversion disorder, and psychological factors affecting medical condition. Factitious disorder, defined by the intentional falsification of symptoms with the apparent goal of achieving behavioral and social benefits associated with the sick role, is now included in this category as well. Historically, these disorders were considered when a medical explanation could not be found, although, in many cases, it can be difficult and counterproductive to fully exclude an exhaustive list of potential medical conditions. In the *DSM-5*, the key component of these disorders is the presence of somatic symptoms *and* the way they are interpreted by the patient, rather than solely by the lack of medical explanation. Children and adolescents (both encompassed by the terms *child* and *children* in this chapter unless otherwise specified) with these disorders experience significant impairment across one or several domains, including relationships with peers or parents, school functioning, and participation in extracurricular activities. Table 24-1 describes the categories of somatic

Table 24-1. Classification of Somatic Symptom and Related Disorders

Disorder	Description
SSD	• Presence of ≥1 somatic symptoms that are distressing or result in significant disruption of daily life. • Excessive thoughts, feelings, or behaviors related to the somatic symptoms. • Symptoms must be persistent (usually >6 mo).
Illness anxiety disorder	• Preoccupation with having a serious illness (≥6 mo). • If a medical condition or strong family history is present, worry is out of proportion to the likelihood of severe illness; somatic symptoms, if present, are mild. • High degree of anxiety about one's health. • Excessive engagement in health-related behavior or avoidance of necessary health care.
Conversion disorder	• Presence of ≥1 symptoms of altered voluntary motor or sensory function that result in significant distress or impairment. • Evaluation suggests that symptoms are incompatible with recognized medical conditions.
Psychological factors affecting other medical conditions	• Presence of psychological or behavioral factors that result in delayed recovery or added health risk, interfere with treatment, or escalate the need for medical treatment. • An underlying medical condition must be present.
Factitious disorder (imposed on self or imposed on another)	• Intentional falsification of physical or psychological signs or symptoms or infliction of injury. • Deceptive behavior is present.
Other specified somatic symptom and related disorder	• Presence of somatic symptoms that cause significant distress or impairment but do not meet full criteria for another category of somatic symptom and related disorders • May be used when symptoms are brief (eg, 6 mo) or just below the diagnostic criteria
Unspecified somatic symptom and related disorder	• Presence of somatic symptoms that cause significant distress or impairment but do not meet full criteria for another category of somatic symptom and related disorders • Used only in unusual situations when there is insufficient information to make a more specific diagnosis

Abbreviation: SSD, somatic symptom disorder.
Derived from American Psychiatric Association. *Diagnostic and Statistical Manual of Mental Disorders.* 5th ed. Arlington, VA: American Psychiatric Association; 2013.

symptom and related disorders according to the *DSM-5,* with the same criteria applied to both adults and children.

When considering the presence of an SSD, it is important to assess for physical disorders that may be causing or contributing to the child's symptoms. However, the pediatric clinician is cautioned to avoid unnecessary testing once it can be reasonably assumed that a general medical disorder has been excluded.[16] It is recommended that SSDs be included in the differential diagnosis rather than relegated to a diagnosis of exclusion. Other conditions to include in the differential diagnosis of MUSs include *psychological factors affecting other medical conditions,* which describes the presence of psychological factors and symptoms associated with an underlying medical condition. Conditions such as anxiety and depression may also result in pain and fatigue and should thus be considered the primary diagnosis in those circumstances.

Assessment

An empathetic and collaborative approach is recommended when considering MUSs. Children affected by MUSs and their families may be frustrated by frequent office visits, multiple laboratory tests, and being told that "nothing is wrong" despite patient distress. While the approach to each child should be individualized, general principles can help guide successful assessment. Important aspects to consider during the assessment process are presented in Box 24-2. Medically unexplained symptoms should be approached just as any other symptom in the pediatric history, with a review of symptom characteristics, including duration, frequency, intensity, and moderating factors. Special attention should be paid to environmental stressors, opportunities for secondary gain, and emotional factors such as anxiety, depression, or other psychological symptoms.

In addition to a careful history, standardized tools can be helpful in the assessment process. The Children's Somatization Inventory (commonly known as CSI) can be used to assess for the presence of multiple somatic symptoms. It has been revised to a 24-item questionnaire that includes parent and child (aged ≥7 years) versions and is available in the public domain.[17] The Functional Disability Inventory is a 15-item questionnaire with parent and child (aged ≥8 years) versions that can be used to assess health status across multiple domains.[18] General screening tools for

> **Box 24-2. Important Principles in the Assessment of Children With Medically Unexplained Symptoms**
>
> - Acknowledge symptoms, patient experience, and family concerns.
> - Review past evaluations and treatment.
> - Investigate fears related to symptoms.
> - Remain alert to unrecognized medical diagnosis.
> - Avoid unnecessary tests.
> - Avoid diagnosis by exclusion.
> - Understand symptom timing, context, and characteristics.
>
> Derived from Campo JV, Fritz G. A management model for pediatric somatization. *Psychosomatics.* 2001;42(6):467–476.

emotional and behavioral concerns in the public domain, such as the Pediatric Symptom Checklist and the Strengths and Difficulties Questionnaires, can also be helpful in identifying children at risk for mental health problems. See Appendix 2, Mental Health Tools for Pediatrics, for more information about these screening instruments.

Management

Collaborative care in the management of MUSs requires communicating diagnostic impressions to the family in a clear and honest manner.[19] Families may benefit from a discussion of the interplay between physiologic and emotional factors, with reassurance that the absence of diagnosable medical disease does not minimize the child's distress or negate the reality of the problem. Pediatric clinicians should be mindful of the stigma associated with mental health conditions and avoid the mind-body dualism that may characterize MUSs as being "all in your head."[16] The use of placebo and other forms of deception in attempts to achieve diagnosis or reduce symptoms is discouraged.[16]

Once diagnostic impressions are communicated and questions are discussed, the clinician must attempt to shift the family's focus from the cause of symptoms to improving the child's functioning and reducing distress.[20] The clinician should facilitate the development of a treatment plan that addresses physical pain, stress reduction, and reduction of stigma while fostering hope that the child will improve. Parents and caregivers must understand that rehabilitative expectations in the face of the child's real distress are not cruel, and clinicians should communicate that the child is fundamentally strong, competent, and capable of overcoming the distress and challenge presented by the illness. Goals should be developed collaboratively and should be meaningful to the child and family. In many cases, treatment will involve an interprofessional approach involving medical, mental health, and allied health disciplines. Clear communication across disciplines is essential.

Several interventions have been proposed for the treatment of SSDs and thus MUSs (Table 24-2). Treatments may be delivered independently or in combination, although the use of medication alone without supportive therapies is discouraged.

Patients with MUSs are often successfully treated in primary care settings, particularly when symptoms are less intense or impairing, but a substantial portion of treatment for some patients may occur outside the realm of primary care, often in pediatric subspecialty settings. In these circumstances, an important role for the PCC is one of care coordination, hope, and support. Primary care clinicians may be especially helpful in conveying information about previous clinical observations and diagnostic evaluation, educating the patient and family, and making timely referrals to mental health specialists as indicated. Primary care clinicians play a key role in supporting families through the assessment and treatment process, which includes conveying an understanding that their concerns will be taken seriously and addressing parental anxiety, if present. Primary care clinicians in underserved areas may find themselves providing more direct care, given challenges related to mental health and specialty care access. The psychiatric literature contains excellent resources for clinicians who are interested in the assessment and initial management of MUSs. In addition, a number of states are offering clinicians psychiatric consultation resources that can provide guidance, education, and, in some cases, facilitated referrals provided by Child and Adolescent Psychiatry.[21,22] More information about these programs can be accessed through the National Network of Child Psychiatry Access Programs.[23] Somatic symptom disorders may present significant challenges in the primary care and pediatric subspecialty settings. Seeking advice and support from colleagues and specialists can be helpful in alleviating the frustration that can sometimes accompany the care of patients with MUSs.

Table 24-2. Interventions for Children With Somatic Symptoms and Related Disorders

Intervention	Characteristics
CBT	May involve a combination of • Cognitive restructuring (eg, "I realize I have some pain today, but I can still go for a walk with my friends.") • Relaxation • Graded exposure to unpleasant experiences
Rehabilitative approach	Focus on coping and improving health status
Behavioral intervention	Approaches include • Reinforcement of healthy behaviors • Minimization of secondary gain
Self-management	Possible techniques include mindfulness, hypnosis, guided imagery, and relaxation.
Family intervention	Involves work with the family system that may inadvertently reinforce the sick role
Maximal treatment of psychiatric comorbidities	Important to consider given the high prevalence of mental health conditions in children with MUSs
Medication management	Should be considered for • The treatment of underlying mental health conditions • Somatic symptoms that accompany mental health conditions

Abbreviations: CBT, cognitive behavioral therapy; MUS, medically unexplained symptom.
Derived from Dell ML, Campo JV. Somatoform disorders in children and adolescents. *Psychiatr Clin North Am.* 2011;34(3):643–660.

Prognosis

In general, the prognosis for children presenting with MUSs is favorable, but proper symptom recognition and intervention are essential.[4] An association has been documented between MUSs in children and subsequent anxiety or depression in adulthood, as well as between anxiety and depression in childhood and subsequent impairing somatic symptoms in adulthood.[14,24] Further studies will be needed to determine whether identification and intervention in childhood can mitigate the development of lifelong symptoms. Meanwhile, it is clear that PCCs play a key role in the initial treatment of the child with MUSs, as well as in family support and care coordination. Pediatric subspecialists are encouraged to consider MUSs in their differential diagnosis, when appropriate, and to approach the possibility with empathy and collaboration. These strategies can reduce child and family frustration, lead to improved outcomes, and be a rewarding experience for the clinician who is able to help guide families through this complex process.

References

1. Barsky AJ, Orav EJ, Bates DW. Somatization increases medical utilization and costs independent of psychiatric and medical comorbidity. *Arch Gen Psychiatry.* 2005;62(8):903–910

2. Sumathipala A, Siribaddana S, Hewege S, Sumathipala K, Prince M, Mann A. Understanding the explanatory model of the patient on their medically unexplained symptoms and its implication on treatment development research: a Sri Lanka study. *BMC Psychiatry.* 2008;8:54

3. Chambers TL. Semeiology—a well established and challenging paediatric speciality. *Arch Dis Child.* 2003;88(4):281–282

4. Ibeziako P, Bujoreanu S. Approach to psychosomatic illness in adolescents. *Curr Opin Pediatr.* 2011;23(4):384–389

5. Lipowski ZJ. Somatization: the concept and its clinical application. *Am J Psychiatry.* 1988;145(11):1358–1368

6. Domènech-Llaberia E, Jané C, Canals J, Ballespí S, Esparó G, Garralda E. Parental reports of somatic symptoms in preschool children: prevalence and associations in a Spanish sample. *J Am Acad Child Adolesc Psychiatry.* 2004;43(5):598–604

7. Egger HL, Angold A, Costello EJ. Headaches and psychopathology in children and adolescents. *J Am Acad Child Adolesc Psychiatry.* 1998;37(9):951–958

8. Hyams JS, Burke G, Davis PM, Rzepski B, Andrulonis PA. Abdominal pain and irritable bowel syndrome in adolescents: a community-based study. *J Pediatr.* 1996;129(2):220–226

9. Goodman JE, McGrath PJ. The epidemiology of pain in children and adolescents: a review. *Pain.* 1991;46(3):247–264

10. Larsson BS. Somatic complaints and their relationship to depressive symptoms in Swedish adolescents. *J Child Psychol Psychiatry.* 1991;32(5):821–832

11. Offord DR, Boyle MH, Szatmari P, et al. Ontario Child Health Study. II. Six-month prevalence of disorder and rates of service utilization. *Arch Gen Psychiatry.* 1987; 44(9):832–836

12. Egger HL, Costello EJ, Erkanli A, Angold A. Somatic complaints and psychopathology in children and adolescents: stomach aches, musculoskeletal pains, and headaches. *J Am Acad Child Adolesc Psychiatry.* 1999;38(7):852–860

13. Campo JV, Jansen-McWilliams L, Comer DM, Kelleher KJ. Somatization in pediatric primary care: association with psychopathology, functional impairment, and use of services. *J Am Acad Child Adolesc Psychiatry.* 1999;38(9):1093–1101

14. Shanahan L, Zucker N, Copeland WE, et al. Childhood somatic complaints predict generalized anxiety and depressive disorders during young adulthood in a community sample. *Psychol Med.* 2015;45(8):1721–1730

15. Luntamo T, Sourander A, Gyllenberg D, et al. Do headache and abdominal pain in childhood predict suicides and severe suicide attempts? Finnish nationwide 1981 birth cohort study. *Child Psychiatry Hum Dev.* 2014;45(1):110–118

16. Campo JV, Fritz G. A management model for pediatric somatization. *Psychosomatics.* 2001;42(6):467–476

17. Walker LS, Beck JE, Garber J, Lambert W. Children's Somatization Inventory: psychometric properties of the revised form (CSI-24). *J Pediatr Psychol.* 2009; 34(4):430–440

18. Claar RL, Walker LS. Functional assessment of pediatric pain patients: psychometric properties of the functional disability inventory. *Pain.* 2006; 121(1–2):77–84

19. Dell ML, Campo JV. Somatoform disorders in children and adolescents. *Psychiatr Clin North Am.* 2011;34(3):643–660

20. Griffin A, Christie D. Taking the psycho out of psychosomatic: using systemic approaches in a paediatric setting for the treatment of adolescents with unexplained physical symptoms. *Clin Child Psychol Psychiatry.* 2008;13(4):531–542

21. Sarvet B, Gold J, Bostic JQ, et al. Improving access to mental health care for children: the Massachusetts Child Psychiatry Access Project. *Pediatrics.* 2010; 126(6):1191–1200

22. Pediatric Psychiatry Network Web site. http://ppn.mh.ohio.gov/default.aspx. Accessed February 9, 2018

23. National Network of Child Psychiatry Access Programs Web site. http://www. nncpap.org. Accessed February 9, 2018

24. Campo JV. Annual research review: functional somatic symptoms and associated anxiety and depression—developmental psychopathology in pediatric practice. *J Child Psychol Psychiatry.* 2012;53(5):575–592

CHAPTER 25

Nonadherence to Medical Treatment

Robin S. Everhart, PhD, and Barbara H. Fiese, PhD

> "*Adherence rates tend to be higher when patients have access to a consistent primary care clinician, particularly one whom the family views as empathetic and with whom they have established rapport.*"

In cases of pediatric chronic illnesses, adherence is defined as the extent to which a child's health-related behaviors coincide with agreed recommendations from a healthcare professional.[1] Adherence refers to not only taking medications as prescribed but also adhering to other aspects of health care recommendations, such as wearing a seat belt, exercise, nutrition, and sleep. Because many underlying factors contribute to a family's ability to effectively manage child conditions, adherence in pediatrics is complex. Behaviors, as well as mental health, of both the parent and the child or adolescent (called simply *child* or *children* in this chapter unless otherwise specified), must be considered. Nonadherence may result from delayed or forgotten doses, child oppositional behaviors, child anxiety, difficulty with pill swallowing, lack of knowledge, family conflict, and parents feeling overwhelmed or stressed. Parent mental health and child mental health have been recognized as important components of adherence. In particular, when parents of younger pediatric patients are experiencing symptoms of depression or anxiety, they may be less likely to maintain set routines around treatment adherence behaviors or prioritize daily adherence. Similarly, children with chronic conditions who are experiencing mental health difficulties may lack the motivation, concentration, or desire to adhere to treatment regimens.[2] The association between mental health and adherence behaviors is likely bidirectional: when children are less adherent to their treatment, they may experience an exacerbation of symptoms, which, in turn, can influence both child mental health and parent mental health. This chapter focuses primarily on adherence with medication use to illustrate the extent and consequences of nonadherence in pediatrics; factors associated with nonadherence, especially mental health within families; and strategies to improve adherence within a pediatric population. The primary intended audience for this chapter is pediatric primary care clinicians (hereafter referred to as PCCs): pediatricians, family physicians, internists, nurse practitioners, and physician assistants who provide health care to children. Pediatric subspecialists and other pediatric health care professionals, particularly those involved in longitudinal relationships with children and families, may also find it useful. The term *pediatric clinicians* is used when referring to PCCs and pediatric subspecialists.

Rates of Adherence

Adherence rates among pediatric populations are estimated to be about 50%.[3] Rates of adherence, however, vary across pediatric conditions, with adherence to short-term treatments, which show immediate effects, typically higher than adherence to long-term treatments. For example, rates of adherence to airway clearance and diet recommendations for children with cystic fibrosis (CF) are often between 20% and 40%.[4] Rates of nonadherence to dietary aspects of HIV treatment regimens have been reported at more than 90%.[5] Rates of medication nonadherence for transplant recipients are estimated at 43%.[6] In cases of pediatric asthma, rates of adherence to daily controller medications have been reported to range from 34%[7] to 71%.[8] Rates of adherence vary within conditions for a variety of reasons, including measurement of adherence and which component of the treatment regimen is being reported (eg, diet, medication). Self-reported measures of adherence, although cost-effective and easy to administer, often lead to higher estimates of adherence because of social desirability bias.[3] Thus, rates of adherence reported to pediatric clinicians by children and parents may actually be lower than reported.[9] Reports of adherence are often more accurate when patients are asked to recall the last 24 hours (eg, cued recall) or when electronic monitoring devices (eg, metered-dose inhalers) are used.[9]

Consequences of Poor Adherence

Depending on the pediatric condition, the consequences of poor adherence to a medical treatment may include disease complications, disease progression, increased symptoms, higher rates of health care use, and even mortality. For instance, in both cases of CF and cases of asthma, increased health care use has been associated with lower rates of adherence.[7,10] In fact, estimates of the cost to the health care system are close to $300 billion.[11] For infectious diseases, problems with nonadherence may cause relapses of infections or the emergence of resistant microbial strains.[12]

Nonadherence can also compromise the efficacy of the medical regimen. Certain children who have diabetes mellitus are hospitalized repeatedly for ketoacidosis and demonstrate highly elevated hemoglobin A_{1C} levels related to nonadherence to the prescribed regimen for insulin therapy.[13] Furthermore, nonadherence can adversely affect medical decisions and evaluation of treatment efficacy, leading to inappropriate increases in dose, changes in the scheduling regimen, or additional medical tests or procedures. Although poor adherence affects current and future disease-related outcomes, poor adherence can also affect other areas of the child's daily life, including school attendance and overall quality of life.[14]

Factors Contributing to Adherence

Adherence among pediatric populations is complex and determined by multiple factors, including child and caregiver mental health, other child and caregiver characteristics (eg, patient desire for autonomy), and family factors (eg, family conflict, cultural beliefs). Although communication with PCCs, health literacy, and factors specific to the disease and its treatment are also components of adherence, in this chapter we have focused on those components most central to child mental health and caregiver mental health. It should also be noted that rates of adherence have been found to decline in adolescence.[3] A description of several central factors that may affect pediatric adherence and that may serve as discussion points for clinicians working with pediatric patients is presented in Table 25-1.

Child Mental Health and Caregiver Mental Health

Because pediatric conditions are typically managed by the child's parent or caregiver (and more so by children as they enter adolescence), emotional difficulties in either caregiver or child can contribute to lower rates of adherence.[15,16] For instance, in cases of pediatric asthma, maternal depressive symptoms have been associated with incorrect use of inhalers and forgetting doses.[17] Depressive symptoms in children with asthma can also lead to nonadherence or chronic lung inflammation or both, which

Table 25-1. Risk Factors for Lower Rates of Pediatric Adherence	
Level	**Factor**
Child/caregiver mental health and other factors	Emotional difficulties (eg, depressive or anxious symptoms)
	Oppositional child behaviors
	Limited disease-related knowledge or skills
	Adolescence (eg, denial, autonomy seeking, peer influence)
	Insufficient parental monitoring
Family	Disorganized family environment
	Conflict, disengagement, criticism
	Difficulty integrating adherence into routines
	Cultural beliefs related to medication necessity
PCC communication	Mistrust from family
	Unclear communication about therapies
	Short-term relationship with PCC
Disease related	Chronic therapies
	Complicated regimens with several components
	Unpleasant-tasting medications
	Uncomfortable treatments (eg, airway clearance)

Abbreviation: PCC, primary care clinician.

may result in poor asthma control and jeopardize future emotional and physical functioning.[18] Children and preadolescents (aged 1–13 years) with CF of parents with symptoms of depression had lower rates of pancreatic enzyme therapy adherence than children and preadolescents of parents without depressive symptoms. In fact, parental depression had an indirect effect on child and adolescent weight via pancreatic enzyme therapy adherence.[19]

Per the adolescent diabetes literature, higher levels of depressive symptoms have been associated with poor adherence to diabetes management, including less frequent blood glucose concentration monitoring.[20] A more recent study showed that among adolescents with higher levels of depressive symptoms, the relationship between parent and adolescent was disrupted such that parents were less involved in their adolescent's diabetes management.[21] This decrease in involvement is especially problematic given that adolescents whose parents are involved in their diabetes care tend to experience improved glycemic control.[22]

Other Child and Caregiver Factors

Oppositional child behaviors, such as tantrums, can also make it difficult for caregivers to administer child medications and adhere to nutritional components of the treatment regimen.[4,23] Caregiver and child knowledge and disease-related skills can also affect adherence. Poor aerosol delivery or misunderstandings about the use of preventive medications have been linked to lower rates of adherence.[24,25] Caregivers may also have difficulty with instructions involving medication dosing and mistakenly choose the incorrect dosing device for liquid medications.[26]

As children mature into adolescents, their adherence rates often decline as they struggle for independence and autonomy in their medical care. When parents cannot directly monitor treatment behaviors, adherence declines.[27] A strategy may be to include children early on in disease management behaviors so that the transition to independence in management behaviors is easier when children reach adolescence. Denial and rebelliousness among adolescents with chronic conditions further complicate adherence.[28] For instance, teenagers with CF may smoke or impose weight-loss regimens, which contradict medical advice. Negative attitudes about PCCs, reluctance to adhere to treatments in front of peers, and denial of the consequences of nonadherence can also contribute to lower adherence rates in adolescence.[29,30]

Family Factors

A cohesive family climate (ie, a family that works together well) and supportive family interactions have been found to promote adherence in cases of pediatric conditions such as diabetes and CF.[31,32] Family conflict, disengagement, criticism, and high levels of stress can hinder adherence.[33,34] Families that have clear daily management practices that allow them to effectively incorporate a child's treatment regimen into existing family routines will likely have greater success in adhering to treatments.[35] Child cooperation, parental presence, and positive attention have all been related to higher respiratory adherence among children with CF.[36]

The family's perception of the illness and treatment and its sense of control over the illness influence its adherence to a therapeutic regimen.

Among parents of children with asthma, fears and misconceptions about preventive medications can negatively affect patient adherence.[37] Cultural beliefs related to medication necessity have been found to predict adherence[38]; lower rates of adherence have also been linked to the use of complementary and integrative medications.[39] In line with the Health Belief Model, caregivers who show concern about their child's illness, perceive the illness as a threat, and believe in the accuracy of the diagnosis and the benefits of treatment are more likely to adhere to a therapeutic regimen.[40]

Communication With the Primary Care Clinician

Effective communication between a child's family and PCC can enhance patient adherence significantly.[41] Parents and PCCs have been found to disagree on up to 17% of the medications prescribed.[4] Adherence rates tend to be higher when patients have access to a consistent PCC, particularly one whom the family views as empathetic and with whom they have established rapport.[41,42] Improved patient-PCC communication has also been found to decrease health care use and missed school days for children with asthma.[43] For adolescents, it is important that the PCC also establish rapport directly with the patient and spend time speaking with the patient individually without parents present.[44] Prior to such discussions, the PCC should ask for assent in the treatment from children and adolescents. Other factors that can improve adherence in patient-PCC communication include treatment plans that are discussed verbally and sent home in written form.[45]

Disease-Related Factors

Lower rates of adherence are associated with treatments that require long-term medications, multiple medications and components of the regimen, and frequent medication administration.[46,47] Other important issues include the ease and comfort of administration, volume of medication, and palatability.

Strategies for Improving Adherence

Pediatric clinicians may find it useful to frame their recommendations regarding treatment adherence within the context of the child and family. This framework may require that the PCC tailor recommendations according to how the family can succeed at adherence. Some families may be able to handle multiple components of the treatment regimen reasonably well, whereas others may need considerable encouragement and support to succeed at one aspect of the pediatric treatment regimen. Strategies for improving adherence to pediatric health care recommendations are provided in Box 25-1.

Because pediatric clinicians have limited time with each patient and family, they may find it useful to begin the conversation by asking about nonadherence. The clinician might ask, "What has gotten in the way of helping your child take all his medications this week?" or "What has been the area of your child's treatment regimen that you've had the hardest

---

Box 25-1. Strategies for Improving Adherence

Child, Caregiver, and Family Focused

- Assess and provide appropriate referrals for oppositional behaviors, risk-taking behaviors, and psychological difficulties.
- Focus on how the family can succeed: What can they accomplish that will build efficacy related to adherence?
- Ask about family beliefs, fears, and misconceptions about disease and treatment.
- Assess how well the family is balancing adolescent autonomy and parental supervision over adherence.
- Provide written information that addresses family concerns.
- Enlist other family members as support.
- Focus on incorporating adherence into daily family routines.

Primary Care Clinician Communication and Treatment

- Establish rapport early by normalizing nonadherence and asking what makes adherence difficult.
- Spend time speaking with adolescents without parents present.
- Practice techniques with the child and caregiver in the clinic.
- Be aware of palatability of different medications and possibility of prescribing generic medications.
- Increase continuity of care.
- Keep treatments as simple as possible.
- Provide written treatment plans.

time with this week?" By doing so, the clinician is normalizing adherence, building rapport with the family, and diving right into issues that the caregiver might be hesitant to bring up. The PCC should then follow up on that area with concrete, written strategies folded into daily routines that the family can take with them, refer to, and work to improve.

Primary care clinicians should also be prepared to address family beliefs, fears, and misconceptions concerning the child's disease and treatment. They can ask specific questions about medication concerns and worries, including adverse effects, dependency, and long-term use. Some families may benefit from individualized, written information that is focused on the family's understanding of disease, medication and other needs, and the importance of treatments. Other strategies might include providing additional sources of information or enlisting support from other family members with sensitivity toward their cultural beliefs. For some caregivers, practicing techniques (eg, aerosol delivery) in the office with the PCC or nursing staff may improve their confidence and ability to use the device, which may improve adherence at home.

Screening for Mental Health Difficulties

Another strategy to improve adherence is recognizing depressive symptoms, oppositional child behaviors, adolescent risk-taking behaviors, and families that may not be supportive of each other. Primary care clinicians should incorporate a brief discussion of parent mental health and child mental health into each clinic session. This discussion may include a series of questions such as "How are you doing?" "How have you been able to find time for yourself this week?" or "How would you describe your mood today?" These questions can be asked of both the parent and the child. A short discussion on the link between mental health and nonadherence may also be useful, with an emphasis on why it is important for parents to remember to take care of their physical and mental health as well.

In fact, given the recently documented prevalence of both anxiety and depression in patients with CF and their parent caregivers,[48] the Cystic Fibrosis Foundation and the European Cystic Fibrosis Society developed new guidelines for the screening and treatment of depression and anxiety in CF patients ($\geq$12 years) and their caregivers. These guidelines include using tools such as the Patient Health Questionnaire-9 (commonly known as PHQ-9) to screen for depression and the Generalized Anxiety

Disorder (7-item) Scale to screen for anxiety by someone on the care team trained in mental health.[49] Appendix 2, Mental Health Tools for Pediatrics, provides more information about these and other screening instruments. We suggest that pediatric care teams of other chronic diseases consider using a similar model that highlights the importance of mental health in pediatric patients with chronic conditions.

On the basis of routine screenings or other discussions around mental health, PCCs may need to provide referrals for adult or child psychological services, as well as family-focused therapy. They may also want to focus on the family structure and how the family has integrated treatment behaviors into its daily routine. Is there a set time for treatments every day? If not, how can the family go about altering a daily routine to include medical adherence? Primary care clinicians may find it necessary to consult a caseworker or psychologist for families that "seem" extremely overwhelmed by the child's treatment regimen. The PCC should also consider how the family is balancing an adolescent's desire for independence with parental monitoring of adherence behaviors. Some adolescents will require little monitoring and will easily assume responsibility for treatment behaviors; for others, it will be a gradual process that slowly allows the parent to assume less of the day-to-day responsibilities.[50] Patient-PCC interactions can be improved by increasing continuity of care and clinician awareness of family concerns. Treatment goals should be set in collaboration with the child and family, using motivational interviewing (MI) and other "common factors" techniques to address barriers such as resistance, discouragement, or conflict. (See Chapter 5, Effective Communication Methods: Common Factors Skills.) The PCC should explain likely adverse effects and suggest ways that these effects can be minimized. Routine supervision with adherence monitoring may be necessary to ensure continuation of therapies for chronic disease. This monitoring may involve follow-up appointments, telephone calls, home visits, blood level monitoring, or counting unused pills. In fact, recent reports have shown that text message reminders can increase medication adherence, including among children with inflammatory bowel disease,[51] adolescents with asthma,[52] and youths with sickle cell anemia.[53] Moreover, other members of the health care team, including nurses and social workers, can help provide support for families to improve adherence, monitor mental health symptoms, and assist with written instructions, referrals, and education.

Finally, a treatment should be as simple as possible to maximize the likelihood of patient adherence. Here again, MI and other common factors techniques can be applied to a problem-solving session with the patient and family, aiming to reach agreement on the best path forward. Medications can be prescribed by using the shortest regimen that is reasonable, and dosing can be tailored to the patient's daily routine. Furthermore, being aware of the palatability of different medications when there is a choice in medication can also be helpful in improving adherence. In some cases, generic drugs may be preferable to reduce the cost of the treatment. Issues of access to prescribed therapies should be addressed beginning with the original encounter; the PCC should prescribe the medication entailing the least out-of-pocket expense for the patient whenever possible.

Summary

Nonadherence is a common challenge that pediatric PCCs and other child health professionals face in treating pediatric patients. Increased rates of nonadherence can contribute to a range of consequences, including increased symptoms, disease progression, the emergence of resistant microbial strains, and even mortality. Nonadherence can also adversely affect medical decisions and the evaluation of treatment efficacy. Barriers at the child, caregiver, and family level, including mental health difficulties, clinician level, and the disease itself, can contribute to lower rates of adherence. Mental health screening and psychosocial therapy for symptoms in the child and family have gained attention with certain pediatric conditions, such as CF. Future research and treatment approaches should continue to bring awareness to the consistent link between mental health of patients and mental health of parents and treatment adherence behaviors. Moreover, the role of patients, in partnership with families and their PCCs, is important to emphasize and cultivate to increase adherence. Primary care clinicians who recognize barriers specific to an individual family and work with the family to address those barriers through a tailored approach may have greater success at promoting adherence. Adherence is a complicated issue requiring a multifactorial approach that includes providing accurate, concise, and easy-to-understand information to families; understanding health-related beliefs and barriers to adherence; improving communication between clinicians and families; and simplifying and individualizing the treatment. Ideally, patients will receive adherence monitoring, with consistent follow-up and support from the health care team. Barriers to adherence should be identified early in therapy to allow for timely intervention and to minimize negative consequences.

Acknowledgments: The authors would like to acknowledge the contributions of Jill S. Halterman, MD, MPH, and colleagues in the original chapter, Adherence to Pediatric Health Care Recommendations.

References

1. Modi AC, Pai AL, Hommel KA, et al. Pediatric self-management: a framework for research, practice, and policy. *Pediatrics.* 2012;129(2):e473–e485
2. Bitsko M, Everhart RS, Rubin BK. The adolescent with asthma. *Paediatr Respir Rev.* 2013;15(2):146–153
3. Rapoff MA. *Adherence to Pediatric Medical Regimens.* New York, NY: Kluwer Academic/Plenum Publishers; 1999
4. Modi AC, Quittner AL. Barriers to treatment adherence for children with cystic fibrosis and asthma: what gets in the way? *J Pediatr Psychol.* 2006;31(8):846–858
5. Marhefka SL, Tepper VJ, Farley JJ, Sleasman JW, Mellins CA. Brief report: assessing adherence to pediatric antiretroviral regimens using the 24-hour recall interview. *J Pediatr Psychol.* 2006;31(9):989–994
6. Dobbels F, Ruppar T, De Geest S, Decorte A, Van Damme-Lombaerts V, Fine RN. Adherence to immunosuppressive regimen in pediatric kidney transplant recipients: a systematic review. *Pediatr Transplant.* 2010;14(5):603–613
7. McNally KA, Rohan J, Schluchter M, et al. Adherence to combined montelukast and fluticasone treatment in economically disadvantaged African American youth with asthma. *J Asthma.* 2009;46(9):921–927
8. Burgess SW, Sly PD, Morawska A, Devadason SG. Assessing adherence and factors associated with adherence in young children with asthma. *Respirology.* 2008;13(4):559–563
9. Quittner AL, Modi AC, Lemanek KL, Ievers-Landis CE, Rapoff MA. Evidence-based assessment of adherence to medical treatments in pediatric psychology. *J Pediatr Psychol.* 2008;33(9):916–936
10. Quittner AL, Zhang J, Marynchenko M, et al. Pulmonary medication adherence and health-care use in cystic fibrosis. *Chest.* 2014;146(1):142–151
11. DiMatteo MR. Variations in patients' adherence to medical recommendations: a quantitative review of 50 years of research. *Med Care.* 2004;42(3):200–209
12. Wainberg M, Friedland G. Public health implications of antiretroviral therapy and HIV drug resistance. *JAMA.* 1998;279(24):1977–1983
13. Morris AD, Boyle DI, McMahon AD, Greene SA, MacDonald TM, Newton RW. Adherence to insulin treatment, glycaemic control, and ketoacidosis in insulin-dependent diabetes mellitus. *Lancet.* 1997;350(9090):1505–1510
14. Bender B, Milgrom H, Rand C, Ackerson L. Psychological factors associated with medication nonadherence in asthmatic children. *J Asthma.* 1998;35(4):347–353

15. Smith BA, Wood BL. Psychological factors affecting disease activity in children and adolescents with cystic fibrosis: medical adherence as a mediator. *Curr Opin Pediatr.* 2007;19(5):553–558

16. Kovacs M, Goldston D, Obrosky DS, Iyengar S. Prevalence and predictors of pervasive noncompliance with medical treatment among youths with insulin-dependent diabetes mellitus. *J Am Acad Child Adolesc Psychiatry.* 1992;31(6):1112–1119

17. Bartlett SJ, Krishnan JA, Riekert KA, Butz AM, Malveaux FJ, Rand CS. Maternal depressive symptoms and adherence to therapy in inner-city children with asthma. *Pediatrics.* 2004;113(2):229–237

18. Bender BG. Risk taking, depression, adherence, and symptom control in adolescents and young adults with asthma. *Am J Respir Crit Care Med.* 2006; 173(9):953–957

19. Barker D, Quittner AL. Parental depression and pancreatic enzymes in children with cystic fibrosis. *Pediatrics.* 2016;137(2):e20152296

20. McGrady ME, Laffel L, Drotar D, Repaske D, Hood KK. Depressive symptoms and glycemic control in adolescents with type 1 diabetes: mediational role of blood glucose monitoring. *Diabetes Care.* 2009;32(5):804–806

21. Wu YP, Hilliard ME, Rausch J, Dolan LM, Hood KK. Family involvement with the diabetes regimen in young people: the role of adolescent depressive symptoms. *Diabet Med.* 2013;30(5):596–602

22. Vesco AT, Anderson BJ, Laffel LM, Dolan LM, Ingerski LM, Hood K. Responsibility sharing between adolescents with type 1 diabetes and their caregivers: importance of adolescent perceptions on diabetes management and control. *J Pediatr Psychol.* 2010;35(10):1168–1177

23. Spieth L, Stark LJ, Mitchell M, et al. Observational assessment of family functioning at mealtime in preschool children with cystic fibrosis. *J Pediatr Psychol.* 2001;26(4):215–224

24. Farber HJ, Capra AM, Finkelstein JA, et al. Misunderstanding of asthma controller medications: association with nonadherence. *J Asthma.* 2003;40(1):17–25

25. Everard ML. Aerosol delivery to children. *Pediatr Ann.* 2006;35(9):630–636

26. Madlon-Kay DJ, Mosch FS. Liquid medication dosing errors. *J Fam Pract.* 2000;49(8):741–744

27. Zindani GN, Streetman DD, Streetman DS, Nasr SZ. Adherence to treatment in children and adolescent patients with cystic fibrosis. *J Adolesc Health.* 2006;38(1):13–17

28. Suris JC, Michaud PA, Akre C, Sawyer SM. Health risk behaviors in adolescents with chronic conditions. *Pediatrics.* 2008;122(5):e1113–e1118

29. Cohen R, Franco K, Motlow F, Reznik M, Ozuah PO. Perceptions and attitudes of adolescents with asthma. *J Asthma.* 2003;40(2):207–211

30. Rhee H, Wenzel J, Steeves RH. Adolescents' psychosocial experiences living with asthma: a focus group study. *J Pediatr Health Care.* 2007;21(2):99–107

31. Cohen DM, Lumley MA, Naar-King S, Partridge T, Cakan N. Child behavior problems and family functioning as predictors of adherence and glycemic control in economically disadvantaged children with type 1 diabetes: a prospective study. *J Pediatr Psychol.* 2004;29(3):171–184

32. DeLambo KE, Ievers-Landis CE, Drotar D, Quittner AL. Association of observed family relationship quality and problem-solving skills with treatment adherence in older children and adolescents with cystic fibrosis. *J Pediatr Psychol.* 2004;29(5): 343–353

33. Lewandowski A, Drotar D. The relationship between parent-reported social support and adherence to medical treatment in families of adolescents with type I diabetes. *J Pediatr Psychol.* 2007;32(4):427–436

34. Fiese BH, Everhart RS. Medical adherence and childhood chronic illness: family daily management skills and emotional climate as emerging contributors. *Curr Opin Pediatr.* 2006;18(5):551–557

35. Lewin AB, Heidgerken AD, Geffken GR, et al. The relation between family factors and metabolic control: the role of diabetes adherence. *J Pediatr Psychol.* 2006; 31(2):174–183

36. Butcher JL, Nasr SZ. Direct observation of respiratory treatments in cystic fibrosis: parent-child interactions relate to medical regimen adherence. *J Pediatr Psychol.* 2015;40:8–17

37. Conn KM, Halterman JS, Fisher SG, Yoos HL, Chin NP, Szilagyi PG. Parental beliefs about medications and medication adherence among urban children with asthma. *Ambul Pediatr.* 2005;5(5):306–310

38. McQuaid EL, Everhart RS, Seifer R, et al. Medication adherence among Latino and non-Latino white children with asthma. *Pediatrics.* 2012;129(6):e1404–e1410

39. Koinis-Mitchell D, McQuaid EL, Friedman D, et al. Latino caregivers' beliefs about asthma: causes, symptoms, and practices. *J Asthma.* 2008;45(3):205–210

40. Janz NK, Becker MH. The Health Belief Model: a decade later. *Health Educ Q.* 1984;11(1):1–47

41. De Civita M, Dobkin PL. Pediatric adherence as a multidimensional and dynamic construct, involving a triadic partnership. *J Pediatr Psychol.* 2004;29(3):157–169

42. Litt IF, Cuskey WR. Compliance with medical regimens during adolescence. *Pediatr Clin North Am.* 1980;27(1):3–15

43. Carpenter DM, Ayala GX, Williams DM, Yeatts KB, Davis S, Sleath B. The relationship between patient-provider communication and quality of life for children with asthma and their caregivers. *J Asthma.* 2013;50(7):791–798

44. Brand PL. The clinician's guide on monitoring children with asthma. *Paediatr Respir Rev.* 2013;14(2):119–125

45. Bratton DL, Price M, Gavin L, et al. Impact of a multidisciplinary day program on disease and healthcare costs in children and adolescents with severe asthma: a two-year follow-up study. *Pediatr Pulmonol.* 2001;31(3):177–189

46. Lemanek KL, Kamps J, Chung NB. Empirically supported treatments in pediatric psychology: regimen adherence. *J Pediatr Psychol.* 2001;26(5):253–257

47. Naar-King S, Podolski CL, Ellis DA, Frey MA, Templin T. Social ecological model of illness management in high-risk youths with type I diabetes. *J Consult Clin Psychol.* 2006;74(4):785–789

48. Quittner AL, Goldbeck L, Abbott J, et al. Prevalence of depression and anxiety in patients with cystic fibrosis and parent caregivers: results of The International Depression Epidemiological Study across nine countries. *Thorax.* 2014;69(12):1090–1097

49. Quittner AL, Abbott J, Georgiopoulos AM, et al. International Committee on Mental Health in Cystic Fibrosis: Cystic Fibrosis Foundation and European Cystic Fibrosis Society consensus statements for screening and treating depression and anxiety. *Thorax.* 2016;71(1):26–34

50. Duncan CL, Hogan MB, Tien KJ, et al. Efficacy of a parent-youth teamwork intervention to promote adherence in pediatric asthma. *J Pediatr Psychol.* 2013;38(6):617–628

51. Miloh T, Shub M, Montes R, Ingebo K, Silber G, Pasternak B. Text messaging effect on adherence in children with inflammatory bowel disease. *J Pediatr Gastroenterol Nutr.* 2017;64(6):939–942

52. Johnson KB, Patterson BL, Ho YX, et al. The feasibility of text reminders to improve medication adherence in adolescents with asthma. *J Am Med Inform Assoc.* 2016;23(3):449–455

53. Estepp JH, Winter B, Johnson M, Smeltzer MP, Howard SC, Hankins JS. Improved hydroxyurea effect with the use of text messaging in children with sickle cell anemia. *Pediatr Blood Cancer.* 2014;61(11):2031–2036

CHAPTER 26

School Absenteeism and School Refusal

Ronald V. Marino, DO, MPH

> "...the variability in absenteeism among children who have the same medical condition suggests that individual and family responses to a physical condition are more important than the actual condition in determining attendance."

A major developmental task of childhood is separating from the family and accepting the functional demands of society. One of the most obvious indicators that this process may not be proceeding normally is lack of attendance at school. Assessing a child's school attendance and functioning in the context of biopsychosocial health supervision is the responsibility of pediatric primary care clinicians (PCCs): pediatricians, family physicians, internists, nurse practitioners, and physician assistants who provide frontline, longitudinal care to children and adolescents (collectively called simply *children* in this chapter unless otherwise specified).

Nonattendance may be the consequence of a variety of underlying causes. *Absenteeism* is generally considered to be parentally sanctioned nonattendance, most commonly attributed to medical illness. *Truancy* is nonattendance without parental consent, in which the time allegedly spent at school is often spent engaging in antisocial behaviors or rebelling against authority. *School refusal* is characterized by inappropriate fear about leaving home, inappropriate fear of school, or both.

When confronted with nonattendance, PCCs must carefully consider not only physical maladies but also the mental and social functioning of the child and family.

Absenteeism

Excessive absenteeism is important to PCCs because it is an excellent marker for physical and mental health problems (Box 26-1). It also is negatively correlated with social adjustment and academic performance. In fact, excessive absenteeism and failure to read at the appropriate level in the

Box 26-1. Chronic School Absence: Differential Diagnosis

- School refusal
- Parental overresponse to minor illnesses
- Chronic physical disease with poor adaptation
- Learning disability with poor adaptation
- Untreated mental health issues (eg, anxiety, depression)
- Bullying
- Truancy
- Substance use disorder
- Psychosis
- Teenage pregnancy
- Family dysfunction (including violence and abuse)

third grade are the 2 strongest predictors of subsequent dropping out of school. According to the National Center for Education Statistics, in 2005 19% of fourth graders and 20% of eighth graders missed at least 3 days of school in the past month. More specifically, 7% of fourth graders and 7% of eighth graders missed at least 5 days of school in the past month. National surveys indicate that healthy children average 4 or 5 absences a school year, whereas children who have a chronic disease are typically absent at least twice as often.[1,2] Educators think that missing more than 10 days in a 90-day semester results in difficulty staying at grade level.[3]

Acute physical health problems are given as the reason for nonattendance 75% of the time. However, the variability in absenteeism among children who have the same medical condition suggests that individual and family responses to a physical condition are more important than the actual condition in determining attendance.[3] The decision not to attend school reflects subtle and complex relationships among the physical, social, and psychological states of the student, family, and community. Individual rates of absenteeism tend to be stable for a given child and for a given school district.

The health conditions most commonly associated with nonattendance include upper respiratory tract infections, headaches, abdominal distress, menstrual cramps, and sleep disorders.[3,4] Parental characteristics associated with excessive absenteeism include lower socioeconomic class, cigarette smoking, chronic parental illness (including mental illness), lower educational expectations, and vulnerable child syndrome.[5-7] A plethora of nonmedical conditions, including transportation difficulties, illness of other family members, religious holidays, family vacations, inclement weather, and professional appointments, are also reasons children miss school. Chronically ill children typically miss more school than their healthy peers do. This tendency may result from a wide variety of causes, including acute exacerbations of the underlying condition, health care visits, adverse effects of medications, and parental misconceptions about the child's ability to attend school. Healthy adjustment by the child and family to the chronic condition minimizes the potential effect of the increase in school days missed. A significant increase in absenteeism over baseline is always a warning sign. Exploring the reasons why a child seeks to avoid school is the PCC's responsibility. Sudden changes in school attendance may be the first concrete symptom of family dysfunction, mental illness, physical deterioration of the student or a family member, alcohol or drug use disorder, or school refusal.

School Refusal

Difficulties attending school despite caregivers' support have been a problem for children, families, schools, and health care professionals since the early 20th century. Initial views of school refusal focused on truancy and its link to delinquency. In 1932, Broadwin focused attention on the frequent role of anxiety in attendance difficulties, and, in 1939, Partridge[8] labeled this clinical condition *psychoneurotic truancy*. Johnson et al[9] introduced the term *school phobia* in 1941, stressing that the child's anxiety about separating from mother was displaced to fear of attending school. This view was strengthened further in the 1950s, when Estes et al[10] concluded that school phobia was a variant of separation anxiety.

This view and nomenclature persisted until the late 1970s, when the term *school refusal* was introduced. The term has descriptive merits that recognize the heterogeneity of the underlying disorders. These disorders include, but are not limited to, major depression, simple and social phobia, and separation anxiety disorder. Criteria for making this diagnosis include severe difficulty in attending school or refusal to attend school, severe emotional upset when attempting to go to school, absence of significant antisocial disorders, and staying at home with the parent's knowledge.

A variety of physical symptoms often accompany the child's request to not attend school. Symptoms can be quite impressive to parents and may emulate organic medical problems.

Prevalence

The prevalence of school refusal varies widely and has been estimated to be between 0.4% and 18.0%.[11,12] The incidence of school refusal has 2 peaks; the first is associated with entering primary school (4–6 years), and the second is at the age of 11 to 12 years, a time of change from elementary to intermediate school, as well as the onset of early adolescence. The American Academy of Pediatrics estimates that 5% of elementary school children and 2% of junior high students experience school refusal. The symptoms of school refusal are associated with several psychiatric disorders. In an outpatient sample of referred children, 22% had separation anxiety disorder, 11% had generalized anxiety disorder, 8% had oppositional defiant disorder, and 5% had major depressive disorder. Twenty percent to 30% of school-refusing children do not qualify for any specific psychiatric diagnosis.[11,13]

Child-Related Factors

Children who have school refusal usually have at least average intelligence and academic achievement. Cultural norms encourage girls to admit fear and discourage boys from doing the same. The actual incidence of school refusal is nearly identical between the sexes. Younger children report more fear of being scolded or of performing before a group, whereas older children seem to be more intimidated by tests and the possibility of failure. Vague somatic symptoms, typically offered as a rationale for nonattendance, may belie the underlying anxiety that is frequently present. Symptoms may amplify in response to parental pressure to attend or to excel (or to do both) in school. Overdependence or concern about the well-being of a parent is also a common underlying dynamic. Serious or chronic illness in the parent may lead to school refusal. Depression has often been noted, as have panic disorder and agoraphobia. Because there are reports of suicide among school refusers, any reference to this possibility must be addressed seriously.

Family Factors

The family context is always a major factor in understanding a child's health. Marital conflict or constricted communication patterns are often found in families with school refusers. The child's presence at home caused by physical illness may provide a cohesive force to an otherwise unstable marital relationship. Families of youths with school refusal behavior are often marked by poverty, poor cohesion and considerable conflict, enmeshment, isolation, and detachment.[14,15]

Common patterns of communication in families in which school refusal occurs have been described[16]: both parents are overly concerned and solicitous of the child's medical problem; one parent, typically the mother, is overprotective and concerned, whereas the other overtly disagrees; and one parent, typically the mother, is overinvolved in caring for the child's every need, whereas the other parent is emotionally absent. Because children are reared in many diverse family situations, PCCs must remain open and attentive to family structure and dynamics to develop an effective treatment plan.[17]

School Environment Factors

The role of the school environment in school refusal has received little attention. Institutional factors such as changing classrooms or lack of privacy in the school bathroom have been associated with fear of school. The physical environment may include uncomfortable temperatures, mold, or allergens, which predispose to illness or student discomfort. Humiliation caused by an insensitive teacher may also be a precipitating stressor in the onset of clinical symptoms. Temperamental mismatch among teacher, student, and parents may serve a maintaining role.

Bullying and social humiliation are increasing in frequency, and students who are bullied often develop somatic symptoms as a coping mechanism.[18] The increased use of social media has created a new and potentially dangerous phenomenon in cyberbullying. *Cyberbullying* is defined as willful and repeated harm inflicted through computers, cell phones, and other electronic devices. More than 20% of 4,400 randomly selected 11- to 18-year-olds indicated they had been subjected to cyberbullying at some point in their lives.[19] In 2005, 24% of students aged 12 to 18 years reported gangs at their schools; this report was more common among urban (36%) than suburban (21%) or rural (16%)

schools. In addition, 28% of students aged 12 to 18 years were reportedly bullied at school in the past 6 months. Most said bullying occurred 1 to 2 times in 6 months, but 25% were bullied 1 to 2 times per month, 11% were bullied 1 to 2 times per week, and 8% were reportedly bullied almost daily.[20] Both traditional bullying and cyberbullying have been implicated as sources of severe emotional distress among students who are bullied, even leading to suicide. Violence in secondary schools provides children a seemingly appropriate reason for refusing to attend school. Twenty-six percent of junior and senior high school students have been assaulted on school grounds, 20% of students admitted bringing a knife or gun to school, and 10% admitted not going to school because of fear of violence.[12,21] Media attention to school violence may further accelerate a child's anxiety and school refusal. Clearly, school-associated stressors are emerging as a concern in understanding and treating school refusal.

Associated Stressors

While exploring factors related to the child, parent, family, and school environment, the PCC must also search for a precipitating event or stress that may have tipped the balance in causing a child to refuse to attend school. Illness or injury of a family member or of the child may be the initial reason for nonattendance. Similarly, the death of a relative or close friend may precipitate the refusal. Moving to a new home, community, or school may also contribute to refusal. The longer a child has been out of school, the more difficult and stressful returning can become.

Clinical Management

In 1958, Eisenberg[22] stated, "[I]t is essential that the paralyzing force of the school phobia on the child's whole life be recognized. The symptom itself serves to isolate him from normal experience and makes further psychological growth almost impossible. If we do no more than check this central symptom, we have nonetheless done a great deal." The foundations of any clinical treatment plan are rapport, trust, and respect. The initial interview should serve not only as a means of gathering data but also as the start of a therapeutic alliance. Primary care clinicians should use a sensitive, holistic approach to data gathering, because the history-taking technique provides the first opportunity for creating a healing rapport. Factors related to the child, parents, family, and school environment must be investigated when exploring school maladaptation. An open mind that recognizes the unique and complex interactions of temperament, stressful life events, family systems function, learning style, parental medical or psychiatric conditions, and school system variables will be helpful in solving this problem. The child must understand that involving a PCC in treatment reflects the seriousness of the symptoms and marks a turning point in changing the avoidant behavior.

Organic disease should be ruled out through a thorough history and physical examination, coupled with judicious laboratory evaluation. Chapter 24, Medically Unexplained Symptoms, provides clear guidance on recognizing and treating somatic symptoms and related disorders. Briefly, time spent in conducting a thorough medical examination communicates the PCC's sincere acceptance of the child's symptoms as being real. Parents are better able to confront the lack of organic disease when a clinician who is completely familiar with the child's history and physical examination discusses the subject with them. A biopsychosocial approach from the outset also aids family acceptance of psychiatric concerns. The laboratory should be used in a symptom-specific, noninvasive, cost-effective manner consistent with ruling out possible organic disease. Additionally, addressing the potential contributions of parental disorders or specific environmental problems will be helpful in formulating a treatment plan. Readers are directed to the chapter on medically unexplained symptoms for a more in-depth discussion of these conditions.

The parents, PCC, and school personnel must all agree that returning to school as quickly as possible is the immediate goal of treatment. Allowing the child to stay home while awaiting laboratory data results or using home tutors only delays the inevitable and makes the return to school more difficult. A specific plan must be developed to respond to clinical symptoms. Objective criteria for school absence, such as a measured fever, should be consistently used in modifying performance expectations, both at home and in school. Parents in doubt should seek the guidance of the child's PCC regarding the significance of acute symptoms before keeping the child home. In addition, the significant attachment figures in the child's life must make it clear they will adhere to the therapeutic program consistently and persistently. In most cases of school refusal, especially in the elementary years, the aforementioned program, carried out under the guidance of the PCC, is curative. Other treatment modalities, typically used by a mental health specialist, include desensitization, psychotherapy, hypnotherapy, cognitive restructuring, and behavior modification. A variety of psychopharmacological agents have been used to manage anxiety- or depression-based school refusal. Selective serotonin reuptake inhibitors (SSRIs) predominate the scant literature and have been found to be useful in some individuals.[12] Concerns about a possible relationship between SSRIs and risk of suicide in children and adolescents have reduced the number of primary care physicians willing to prescribe these medications. Children who are recalcitrant to behavioral interventions may require referral to a mental health specialist. Suggested criteria for mental health referral are listed in Box 26-2.

Mental health specialists typically use cognitive behavioral therapy with or without SSRIs.[23-25] Severe cases may require inpatient treatment.[26]

Prognosis

Most children who refuse to attend school quickly overcome the difficulty with appropriate clinical management. Intermittent relapses associated with stress or new separation experiences, such as camp or sleepovers, occur in approximately 5% of children. Children who require psychiatric management do not fare as well.[21] Most published series in the psychiatric literature reveal significant cohorts of patients requiring ongoing therapy and having persistent difficulties in emancipating themselves from their families.[22,27] Phobias, depression, and anxiety are more common in adults who have a history of childhood school refusal.[28] Table 26-1 lists long-term sequelae in children with school refusal.[29]

Box 26-2. Criteria for Mental Health Referral

- Unresponsive to management
- Out of school for 2 mo
- Onset in adolescence
- Psychosis
- Depression
- Panic reactions
- Parental inability to cooperate with treatment plan

Table 26-1. Long-term Sequelae in Children With School Refusal	
Outcome	**Prevalence**
Interrupted compulsory school	18%
Did not complete high school	45%
Adult psychiatric outpatient care	43%
Adult psychiatric inpatient care	6%
Criminal offense	6%
Still living with parents after 20-year follow-up	14%
Married at 20-year follow-up	41%

Information from Bernstein GA, Hektner JM, Borchardt CM, McMillan MH. Treatment of school refusal: one-year follow-up. *J Am Acad Child Adolesc Psychiatry*. 2001;40(2):206–213 and Flakierska-Praquin N, Lindström M, Gillberg C. School phobia with separation anxiety disorder: a comparative 20- to 29-year follow-up study of 35 school refusers. *Compr Psychiatry*. 1997;38(1):17–22. From Fremont WD. School refusal in children and adolescents. *Am Fam Physician*. 2003;68(8):1555–1560. Reproduced with permission.

Prevention

Anticipatory guidance is an excellent means of primary prevention, and it allows the PCC to advise parents on developmentally appropriate separation guidelines. For example, by the time an infant is 6 months of age, the parents should be able to spend some evenings out alone. By the time a toddler is 1 year of age, peer contact should be encouraged. Toddlers should experience babysitters while awake. By age 3 years, the child should experience being away from home without a parent, such as in a playgroup or at a neighbor's home. Age 4 years is a good time to consider preschool for the child. Such guidance can be shared in the context of routine health supervision. Parents should also be discouraged from keeping children home because of minor illness, and PCCs must avoid unnecessary medical restrictions.

Preventing vulnerable child syndrome is also important when caring for ill children. This disorder arises when parents think that their child's life has been threatened significantly, and it may result in separation difficulties, overprotection, bodily concerns, and underachievement in school.[7] Parents need to be informed about the true significance and prognosis of any medical difficulty the child has experienced. Primary care clinicians have a responsibility to avoid creating iatrogenic misconceptions about a child's health. They can accomplish this task by using everyday language as much as possible, rather than medical jargon, and by demystifying anxiety associated with insignificant findings, such as a functional murmur. Parents need to be reassured that children who have recovered fully from an acute illness are at no increased risk for future illness. By inquiring about children's school attendance and promoting healthy parenting styles, PCCs can help prevent school refusal.

Truancy and Dropping Out

Truancy is a good predictor of dropping out at a later date. Many schools in inner cities report daily absence rates above 20%, with most of these rates thought to be the result of truancy; an equal or greater percentage of inner-city school children never finish high school. Truancy is a serious social problem that can have lifelong consequences. Unemployment or underemployment, criminal behavior, marital problems, and chronic social maladjustment are often seen in children with truancy or children who drop out. These same long-term outcomes have been identified in groups of children who have learning disabilities. One risk factor for truancy is learning disability and its associated school failure.

Truancy has also been noted among children who have a history of having been sexually abused. Other risk factors are low socioeconomic status, conduct disorder, gang membership, substance use disorder, cigarette smoking, and family discord. Early recognition of children at risk should prompt immediate intervention to promote optimal adjustment. Mobilization of resources in the school, community, and family is critical to help prevent progression from truancy to dropping out. Creative programs to foster school attendance and success have been conducted with variable results. An emerging new truancy variant is the child who goes to school or its immediate environment but does not attend class. This child is participating in the social aspects of the school community but is shunning the academics. Primary care clinicians can assume an advocacy role in guiding and supporting therapeutic interventions in the educational and social welfare arenas.

Conclusion

Absenteeism is a symptom that has multiple causes. Because success in school is often the foundation for continuing success in life, PCCs must devote thoughtful attention to understanding and treating absentees. Using a biopsychosocial model and mobilizing multidisciplinary resources are the keys to clinical success.

AAP Policy

American Academy of Pediatrics Council on School Health. Out-of-school suspension and expulsion. *Pediatrics.* 2013;131(3):e1000–e1007 (pediatrics.aappublications.org/content/131/3/e1000)

Christian CW; American Academy of Pediatrics Committee on Child Abuse and Neglect. The evaluation of suspected child physical abuse. *Pediatrics.* 2015;135(5): e1337–e1354 (pediatrics.aappublications.org/content/135/5/e1337)

Jenny C, Crawford-Jakubiak JE; American Academy of Pediatrics Committee on Child Abuse and Neglect. The evaluation of children in the primary care setting when sexual abuse is suspected. *Pediatrics.* 2013;132(2):e558–e567 (pediatrics. aappublications.org/content/132/2/e558)

Thackeray JD, Hibbard R, Dowd MD; American Academy of Pediatrics Committee on Child Abuse and Neglect and Committee on Injury, Violence, and Poison Prevention. Intimate partner violence: the role of the pediatrician. *Pediatrics.* 2010;125(5): 1094–1100. Reaffirmed January 2014 (pediatrics.aappublications.org/content/125/5/1094)

References

1. Fowler MG, Johnson MP, Atkinson SS. School achievement and absence in children with chronic health conditions. *J Pediatr.* 1985;106(4):683–687
2. Klerman LV. School absence—a health perspective. *Pediatr Clin North Am.* 1988;35(6):1253–1269
3. Weitzman M, Klerman LV, Alpert JJ, Lamb GA, Kayne H, Rose L. Factors associated with excessive school absence. *Pediatrician.* 1986;13(2–3):74–80
4. Bernstein GA, Massie ED, Thuras PD, Perwien AR, Borchardt CM, Crosby RD. Somatic symptoms in anxious-depressed school refusers. *J Am Acad Child Adolesc Psychiatry.* 1997;36(5):661–668
5. Charlton A, Blair V. Absence from school related to children's and parental smoking habits. *BMJ.* 1989;298(6666):90–92
6. Cassino C, Auerbach M, Kammerman S, et al. Effect of maternal asthma on performance of parenting tasks and children's school attendance. *J Asthma.* 1997;34(6):499–507
7. Green M, Solnit AJ. Reactions to the threatened loss of a child: a vulnerable child syndrome. Pediatric management of the dying child, part III. *Pediatrics.* 1964;34:58–66

8. Partridge JM. Truancy. *J Mental Sci.* 1939;85:45–81
9. Johnson AM, Falstein EI, Szurek SA, et al. School phobia. *Am J Orthopsychiatry.* 1941;11(4):702–711
10. Estes HR, Haylett CH, Johnson M. Separation anxiety. *Am J Psychother.* 1956; 10(4):682–695
11. Granell de Aldaz E, Vivas E, Gelfand DM, Feldman L. Estimating the prevalence of school refusal and school-related fears. A Venezuelan sample. *J Nerv Mental Dis.* 1984;172(12):722–729
12. Kearney CA. School absenteeism and school refusal behavior in youth: a contemporary review. *Clin Psychol Rev.* 2008;28(3):451–471
13. Hella B, Bernstein GA. Panic disorder and school refusal. *Child Adolesc Psychiatr Clin N Am.* 2012;21(3):593–606
14. Berg I. Absence from school and mental health. *Br J Psychiatry.* 1992;161:154–166
15. Hansen C, Sanders SL, Massaro S, Last CG. Predictors of severity of absenteeism in children with anxiety-based school refusal. *J Clin Child Psychol.* 1998;27(3):246–254
16. Nader PR, Bullock D, Caldwell B. School phobia. *Pediatr Clin North Am.* 1975; 22(3):605–617
17. Hersov L. School refusal. *Br Med J.* 1972;3(5818):102–104
18. Torrens Armstrong AM, McCormack Brown KR, Brindley R, Coreil J, McDermott RJ. Frequent fliers, school phobias, and the sick student: school health personnel's perceptions of students who refuse school. *J Sch Health.* 2011;81(9):552–559
19. Cyberbullying Research Center. 2010 cyberbullying data. Cyberbullying Research Center Web site. http://www.cyberbullying.us/2010-data. Accessed February 9, 2018
20. National Center for Education Statistics. *Student Reports of Bullying and Cyberbullying: Results From the 2011 School Crime Supplement to the National Crime Victimization Survey.* Washington, DC: National Center for Education Statistics; 2013. https://nces.ed.gov/pubs2013/2013329.pdf. Accessed February 9, 2018
21. Associated Press. Study: 1 in 5 NY students were armed. *Newsday.* February 14, 1994:19
22. Eisenberg L. School phobia: a study in the communication of anxiety. *Am J Psychiatry.* 1958;114(8):712–718
23. Last CG, Hansen C, Franco N. Cognitive-behavioral treatment of school phobia. *J Am Acad Child Adolesc Psychiatry.* 1998;37(4):404–411
24. Bernstein GA, Borchardt CM, Perwien AR, et al. Imipramine plus cognitive-behavioral therapy in the treatment of school refusal. *J Am Acad Child Adolesc Psychiatry.* 2000;39(3):276–283
25. Walkup JT, Albano AM, Piacentini J, et al. Cognitive behavioral therapy, sertraline, or a combination in childhood anxiety. *N Engl J Med.* 2008;359(26):2753–2766
26. Walter D, Hautmann C, Rizk S, et al. Short term effects of inpatient cognitive behavioral treatment of adolescents with anxious-depressed school absenteeism: an observational study. *Eur Child Adolesc Psychiatry.* 2010;19(11):835–844
27. Flakierska-Praquin N, Lindström M, Gillberg C. School phobia with separation anxiety disorder: a comparative 20- to 29-year follow-up study of 35 school refusers. *Compr Psychiatry.* 1997;38(1):17–22
28. Bernstein GA, Hektner JM, Borchardt CM, McMillan MH. Treatment of school refusal: one-year follow-up. *J Am Acad Child Adolesc Psychiatry.* 2001;40(2):206–213
29. Fremont WP. School refusal in children and adolescents. *Am Fam Physician.* 2003;68(8):1555–1560

CHAPTER 27

Self-injury

Nancy Heath, PhD; Jessica R. Toste, PhD;
Timothy R. Moore, PhD, LP, BCBA-D; and Frank Symons, PhD

> " *...self-injury is generally understood to be a completely different phenomenon in typically vs atypically developing children and adolescents. While there are many differences in presentation and treatment approaches, these behaviors can be understood as possibly serving either an automatic or a social function in both populations.* "

Foundations of Self-injury

Self-injury in children and adolescents may be grouped into 2 classifications: self-injury with intent to die (suicidal behaviors) and self-injury without intent to die (nonsuicidal self-injurious behaviors [SIBs]). Two of the best-known behaviors within the nonsuicidal classification are *nonsuicidal self-injury* (NSSI), occurring in typically developing children and adolescents, and *self-injurious behavior*, most common among children and adolescents with intellectual and developmental disabilities (IDDs). Over the past decade, it has become increasingly apparent that NSSI is a widespread and significant mental health concern among adolescents. However, although SIB is encountered less frequently in clinical practice, it is generally the more severe behavior. Thus, both forms of self-injury pose significant challenges to pediatric primary care clinicians (PCCs): pediatricians, family physicians, internists, nurse practitioners, and physician assistants who provide frontline care to children and adolescents (collectively referred to as simply *children* in this chapter unless otherwise specified). This chapter describes the independent and converging characteristics and features of each of these presentations of self-injury.

Definition and Types of Self-injury

Nonsuicidal self-injury refers to the deliberate destruction of one's own body tissue, occurring without suicidal intent and for purposes not socially sanctioned. Thus, NSSI excludes piercings and tattoos. Most commonly, NSSI includes superficial to moderate self-cutting, burning, scratching, and bruising. Nonsuicidal self-injury occurs among typically developing children and adolescents. This behavior is often engaged in repetitively over long periods of time, with increasing severity, and, although distinct from suicidal behaviors, NSSI has been found to be a significant risk factor for future suicidal behaviors.[1] Furthermore, these self-inflicted injuries can result in medical complications, infection, or permanent scarring. Historically, this behavior has also been referred to as *self-mutilation, self-harm,* and *parasuicide.* The definition of NSSI excludes extreme forms of body mutilation (eg, amputation, enucleation) seen in patients with psychosis, as well as stereotypical self-injury seen among individuals with IDDs.

Self-injurious behavior among children and adolescents with IDDs shares a similar definition with NSSI. *Self-injurious behavior* is defined as physical acts directed to one's own body that result in or produce tissue damage or that have the possibility of producing tissue damage if left unchecked. However, the most common forms of SIB are different from those of NSSI, and they may include head banging, biting, scratching, pinching, and rubbing. Chronic SIB poses tremendous challenges for affected individuals and their families. Indeed, SIB is among the most disturbing and serious of all behaviors exhibited by children with IDDs, because it has profound implications for a child's health and quality of life. Self-injurious behavior often leads to increased risk for institutionalization and social stigmatization and to decreased opportunities to learn.

Epidemiology

The onset of NSSI most commonly occurs in late preadolescence and early adolescence (12–14 years), although it is increasingly common for this behavior to occur among prepubertal children.[2] Research has found that between 14% and 20% of adolescents in community samples report having engaged in NSSI at least once during their lifetimes, with approximately one-quarter indicating they have engaged in it repetitively. Studies of mental health issues in college students have reported comparable lifetime prevalence estimates, suggesting that rates of NSSI are similar from adolescence to young adulthood. Furthermore, recent research suggests that approximately 4% to 7% of children aged 8 to 12 years report some form of NSSI.[2] In contrast to studies conducted with adolescents in community samples, lifetime prevalence estimates of NSSI among adolescents in clinical samples are substantially higher, with rates ranging from 60% to 80%.[3]

Interestingly, while research has found NSSI rates to be much higher among females in clinical settings,[4] the same pattern is not consistently found among females in community samples. Some studies have found a female predominance in the behavior,[5,6] while others conclude that there may be little or no gender difference in occurrence of NSSI.[7-10] In a review of the literature of NSSI among adolescents, Heath and colleagues[11] found that studies reporting gender differences have included overdose and medication misuse or have focused exclusively on cutting, both of which have been found to be largely female behaviors. It has been found that females are more likely to cut, whereas males are more prone to self-hitting.[5] Thus, it is important to avoid the assumption that NSSI is a predominantly female behavior in community practice, even though girls are more likely to be seen in clinical settings.

Findings regarding age of onset and gender patterns for SIB are notably different from those for NSSI. Self-injurious behavior occurs at all levels of IDDs across the life span, with greater frequency typically reported among children with more severe intellectual impairments. The specific age of onset is typically unknown, but reports documenting SIB have included children as young as 18 months.[12] Epidemiological estimates vary depending on study design, sampling frame, and participant characteristics, but a reasonable lifetime prevalence estimate would be that approximately 20% of individuals with IDDs will exhibit some form of self-injury.[13] Unlike with NSSI, there are clear gender differences in occurrence of SIB, with males overrepresented by a ratio of approximately 4:1. There have been no studies directly addressing ethnic differences in the prevalence of NSSI or SIB among children with IDDs.

Etiology and Function

For many years, self-injury occurring outside the IDD population was believed to be indicative of severe psychiatric disorders, particularly borderline personality disorder (BPD).[14,15] However, research has shown that NSSI is not limited to individuals with BPD. Research has revealed that this behavior serves a number of different functions.[16-18] These functions may be understood as falling into 2 broad categories: functions that serve an internal or automatic purpose (eg, to elicit a calm feeling or eliminate tension) or functions that serve an external or social purpose (eg, as a form of communication or to elicit a response). For most individuals who engage in NSSI, emotion regulation difficulties are at the root of this behavior.[16,19-22] These adolescents and young adults experience their intense negative emotions as intolerable and use NSSI to gain relief.

Although use of NSSI to regulate internal states or emotions has received the most support in the literature, for some adolescents and young adults it seems that social factors may also play a role in this behavior.[11,23] It has been suggested that in these cases NSSI serves as a form of communication to parents and peers when alternative forms of communication are perceived as being ineffective.[17] Thus, for typically developing adolescents, the primary function of the behavior is to obtain relief from an internal state or experience. In contrast, as discussed below, SIB among children and adolescents with IDDs is most often found to serve an environmental or a social function (eg, to gain attention from others or to escape from task demands); however, it is recognized that an automatic function may also be involved in many cases (eg, to attain relief from pain caused by an underlying medical condition).

Advances in behavioral assessment technology have led to remarkable progress in identifying environmental[24-26] and biological[27,28] variables underlying SIB. While the etiology of SIB may be related to an undiagnosed painful medical condition in some cases,[29] the specific etiology of SIB is unknown in most cases. Little is known about the behavioral or biological mechanisms influencing the early development of SIB in young children with IDDs.[30] Communication impairment associated with IDDs is a primary risk factor, as is the overall severity of the intellectual impairment.

Co-occurring Disorders

Research on co-occurrence is crucial for knowing how to assess and treat adolescents and young adults who engage in different forms of self-injury. For example, because the underlying functions of NSSI are similar to those of other mental health issues, it is necessary to be aware of which conditions tend to occur with NSSI and how to effectively assess and monitor them. Some of the most commonly co-occurring disorders include mood disorders, anxiety disorders, impulse control or conduct problems, uncontrolled anger, BPD, alcohol or substance use disorder, eating disorders, and suicidality.[31]

Similarly, a number of IDD-related syndromes tend to occur with SIB. The most common of these include Lesch-Nyhan syndrome, fragile X syndrome, de Lange syndrome, Prader-Willi syndrome, and Rett syndrome.[32,33] Whether there are mechanisms specific to any single genetic disorder and the expression of SIB is unclear but unlikely.

Evaluation

Diagnostic and treatment approaches to NSSI and SIB differ substantially. Nonsuicidal self-injury is largely hidden and may range in severity or treatment needs; therefore, much of the focus for the PCC is on early risk assessment and referral to appropriate treatment. In contrast, SIB necessitates an initial ruling out of a possible underlying medical condition followed by the need for a full behavioral evaluation by a behavior analyst certified by the Behavior Analyst Certification Board (https://bacb.com). Interestingly, despite the obvious differences between the diagnostic approaches to NSSI and SIB, both share the difficulty of preconceived notions regarding the behavior (based on common misconceptions) and the lack of consideration of both internal functions and external functions. For clarity, the following section is divided into separate, brief reviews of NSSI and SIB.

Nonsuicidal Self-injury

Signs and Symptoms

A particularly challenging aspect of NSSI among children is that it is a largely hidden behavior. Most adolescents engaging in the behavior make great efforts to keep the behavior secret, perhaps revealing only to friends or peers in online communities.[34] Despite the child's reluctance to reveal the behavior, physical examination of the child will reveal fresh injuries, scars, burns, or unexplained bruises that are clearly indicative of NSSI. Some individuals will limit themselves to pin or razor blade scratching that they may explain as "cat scratches." Awareness of NSSI in typically developing adolescents ensures that PCCs are cautious in their interpretation of signs of injury (eg, bruising, burning, cutting) as signs of physical abuse (intentional harm by another).

One of the most significant obstacles to identification of NSSI by PCCs is a lack of awareness of this behavior. It is widely thought that self-injury is largely a female behavior and limited to self-cutting; thus, NSSI is often overlooked in boys or when other methods of injury are involved. Rather than understanding the underlying emotion regulation or "coping" function, PCCs who encounter cases of NSSI often misidentify it as a suicide attempt or physical abuse, or they assume that there are underlying disorders (eg, BPD, eating disorders). Additionally, PCCs must recognize the high rate of occurrence for NSSI in adolescents and young adults and that the behavior is not limited to specific social cliques (eg, "emos" or "goths").

Diagnostic Approach

Of particular importance is the need to distinguish between NSSI and suicidal behaviors. In the past, researchers have often failed to distinguish between self-injury with and without suicidal intent.[11] However, suicide attempts and NSSI are distinct behaviors and should be understood, managed, and treated differently. Suicide attempts are behaviors that may or may not result in injury, for which there is intent to die. In contrast, NSSI is a behavior in which immediate tissue damage is present, but for which there is no intent to die. In essence, suicidal behaviors express a wish to stop living, whereas NSSI is reported by the adolescent or young adult as an attempt to feel better without any conscious desire to die. Nevertheless, these behaviors are not mutually exclusive, and some adolescents and young adults engage in both, albeit at different times and with different intents. Therefore, it is important to evaluate for both suicidal self-injury and NSSI.

Risk Assessment and Effective Referral

A key role of the PCC is to complete a risk assessment to determine the current risk level and make appropriate referrals. Assessment includes evaluation of risk for suicide, physical injury, and the presence of other co-occurring risk factors. In determining risk-level status, the clinician must recognize that there is no simple formula for determining whether a patient is at high or low risk. Nevertheless, if there is increased risk for suicide or physical injury, or if there are significant mental health concerns, the risk-level status of the patient increases. Despite the extensive list of factors contributing to risk stratification, many patients who self-injure remain in the low-risk category. These patients may have mild, nonclinical levels of depression, anxiety, negative body image, or self-derogation and may seem to be functioning extremely well academically, socially, and within their home environments. Despite this apparent positive presentation, research has found that engaging in NSSI (even if only a few times) indicates problematic emotional regulation and a need for intervention to develop more adaptive coping strategies.[35] Furthermore, it is known that risk level for suicide by individuals who engage in NSSI is substantial and subject to change over time; thus, regular reassessment is essential.

Self-injurious Behavior

Signs and Symptoms

The PCC should be aware that SIB injuries can have pattern-mark appearances and can be mistaken for physical abuse. Children with developmental disabilities, however, may be at higher risk for abuse or neglect. Careful history, risk assessment, and physical examination are warranted.

Presence of SIB often includes biting of the hands, arms, or lips; banging the head on solid surfaces; hitting the head or face with a closed fist or an open palm; eye poking; or scratching, picking, pinching, or rubbing skin.[36] Mild, moderate, or permanent tissue damage and disfigurement, possibly life-threatening, can occur if SIB is left untreated.[37]

Diagnostic Approach

Behavioral evaluation of SIB is predicated on 3 empirically based assumptions: SIB is functional, learned behavior (ie, a function, in part, of its circumstances and consequences); the momentary likelihood of SIB is influenced by antecedent stimulus conditions (ie, it occurs more often in the presence of certain people, places, materials, demand contexts, and biological states than in others); and intervention linked to function (ie, related to antecedents and consequences) rather than form alone will result in superior, clinically significant outcomes.[38-40] Behavioral evaluations require effort, time, and trained staff to administer and interpret, but they lead to effective interventions more quickly than alternatives not based on behavioral function.

Functional Assessment and Analysis of Behavior

Primary care clinicians who eliminate the possibility of underlying medical conditions and determine that SIB warrants evaluation should refer the patient to a board-certified behavior analyst (BCBA). State-by-state and provincial listings of BCBAs are available. Two broad categories of clinical evaluation procedures are available: functional assessment[41-44] and functional analysis.[24,45] Both types of evaluations are designed to generate information about environmental antecedents to, and contingent consequences of, behavior that can be directly linked to interventions. Functional assessments generate descriptive accounts of contextual and antecedent precursors to behavior as well as outcomes produced by behavior. The functional assessment interview[42] is typically administered face-to-face, and it can be completed in approximately 1 hour (shorter or longer depending on the complexity of the behavior and level of information desired). The Questions About Behavioral Function,[43] Functional Analysis Screening Tool,[41] and Motivation Assessment Scale[44] are more time-efficient survey forms that can be completed by caregivers at home or school. It is best practice to corroborate any interview and survey information with observations of the behavior, because these screening instruments have been found to generate hypotheses about the function of SIB different from observational accounts, such as experimental functional analysis.[46,47] Nevertheless, strong hypotheses of the function of SIB can be generated by these types of descriptive functional assessments and effective interventions can be developed based on those hypotheses.

Experimental functional analysis involves systematic manipulation of the antecedents to, and consequences for, SIB, and it involves direct observation of the effects of these consequences.[24] Typically, children are evaluated in clinical settings and the occurrence of SIB is compared across test and control conditions to determine whether SIB is sensitive to social consequences. The usual consequences evaluated are possible positive and negative reinforcers in the form of attention from others, escape from task demands, access to tangible items, or other preferred situations. When the presentations of antecedent and consequence stimuli are arranged systematically in a single-subject experimental design, causal claims between SIB and its consequences can be made. Experimental functional analysis requires highly trained professionals to administer and interpret its findings (and is therefore costlier), but the trade-off is confirmation of the environment-behavior relationship responsible for the maintenance of SIB, resulting in prompter implementation of the proper intervention.

Management and Treatment

Effective treatment of NSSI begins with appropriate assessment. This assessment includes a full history of the behavior, including age of onset; incidence over time; and specific aspects of the behavior over time, including the history of method (or methods), frequency, location (or locations), number of injuries per episode, and medical severity of injuries. These variables may change with time, indicating an overall profile of increasing severity or a pattern of waxing and waning reflective of periods of stress.[35] Currently, the only treatment approach for NSSI that has some empirical support (including randomized controlled trials) is dialectical behavioral therapy (DBT),[48] which has been found to be effective both with adults and with adolescents.[49] However, none of these studies used community samples of adolescents engaging only in NSSI; rather, this approach has been found to be effective with individuals with severe NSSI and co-occurring suicidal behaviors. Dialectical behavioral therapy focuses on specific treatment goals arranged in a hierarchy of importance as follows: decreasing life-threatening and NSSI behaviors; eliminating behaviors that interfere with therapy; decreasing behaviors that interfere with quality of life (eg, substance use, high-risk sex); and skills training in mindfulness, distress tolerance, emotion regulation, and interpersonal effectiveness to help manage psychological distress.[50,51] This approach is intensive and demanding of resources, requiring a therapist trained in DBT. Although DBT has been referred to as the "gold standard" of treatment, less intensive treatment approaches that incorporate the key elements of mindfulness, distress tolerance, emotion regulation, and interpersonal skills to some degree may be effective with community samples of adolescents who engage in NSSI.[52,53] Regardless, at a minimum the PCC working with the young person must be aware of the elements of DBT.

A child with an IDD presenting with SIB should be evaluated for any possible illness or the likelihood of an acute or chronic condition that may be painful. Treating the underlying medical condition may lead to reduced SIB. For behavioral assessment, referral to a qualified specialist (eg, BCBA) is recommended. The evidence for SIB treatment based on behavioral evaluation is large and growing.[54,55] Best practice calls for linking behavioral evaluation results directly to intervention strategies. These interventions include modifications to the antecedent environment, to limit the presence of variables known to be associated with the onset of self-injury,[56] and approaches to decreasing self-injury that emphasize reinforcement of desired behavior (including reinforcement of new or underused communication strategies that serve the same behavioral function as SIB)[57-59] and that de-emphasize the use of punishment.[54] Specifics of any treatment regimen should be individualized with respect to the patient's preferences, strengths, needs, and scope of SIB, as well as with consideration of the caregivers' preferences, strengths, capacities, and available family and community supports.[60,61] Studies of neurobiological factors associated with SIB have identified a role for opioidergic, dopaminergic, and serotonergic systems in the pathophysiology of SIB. These findings are in line with the results of a growing body of controlled psychopharmacological studies demonstrating that SIB can be reduced to different degrees by agents that have actions in these neurochemical systems. One main difficulty to date is that it is not clear who will respond to what medication under what circumstances.[33]

Ongoing Care

The main consideration in the ongoing care of patients who have engaged in NSSI is the need for regular follow-up and suicide risk assessment. Although many individuals will stop and not resume the behavior (exact numbers are unclear at this time), some adolescents will relapse and show a sharp escalation in severity following a stressor. While the prognosis is excellent for most adolescents who engage in NSSI at a low or moderate severity level, as a group they remain at significantly greater risk for suicide. Similarly, while tremendous advances have been made in the past 3 decades in our understanding and treatment of SIB, there is little evidence that the scientific community has effectively reduced the long-term burden of SIB on families and society. Prevalence estimates continue to suggest approximately 20% of people with IDDs exhibit SIB,[62] suggesting an ongoing need for intensive intervention with an emphasis on sustainability by incumbent supports.

Self-injury Similarities and Differences

In summary, self-injury is generally understood to be a completely different phenomenon in typically vs atypically developing children and adolescents. While there are many differences in presentation and treatment approaches, these behaviors can be understood as possibly serving either an automatic or a social function in both populations. Furthermore, it is essential in both instances to evaluate for the underlying functions to understand the reinforcers of these behaviors. Treatment for NSSI and SIB requires a detailed analysis and understanding of what is reinforcing the behavior and ultimately trying to interrupt this reinforcement chain.

Effectively disrupting the response-reinforcer contingency depends, in part, on recognizing that self-injury elicits reactions from individuals in the patient's or individual's environment, which can create a complex situation (ie, it is a natural response on the part of a clinician to want to react and stop an individual from harming himself or herself). Documentation and clear communication to share information about any planned intervention is essential to effective outcomes. Resources are available to assist both families and clinicians: for example, the Self-injury Outreach and Support Web site (http://sioutreach.org) and the Self-Injury and Recovery Research and Resources Web site (www.selfinjury.bctr.cornell.edu).

References

1. Guan K, Fox KR, Prinstein MJ. Nonsuicidal self-injury as a time-invariant predictor of adolescent suicide ideation and attempts in a diverse community sample. *J Consult Clin Psychol.* 2012;80(5):842–849
2. Barrocas AL, Hankin BL, Young JF, Abela JR. Rates of nonsuicidal self-injury in youth: age, sex, and behavioral methods in a community sample. *Pediatrics.* 2012;130(1):39–45
3. Heath NL, Schaub K, Holly S, Nixon MK. Self-injury today: review of population and clinical studies in adolescents. In: Nixon MK, Heath NL, eds. *Self-injury in Youth: The Essential Guide to Assessment and Intervention.* New York, NY: Routledge Press/Taylor & Francis Group; 2009
4. Claes L, Vanderycken W, Vertommen H. Eating-disordered patients with and without self-injurious behaviors: a comparison of psychopathological features. *Eur Eat Disord Rev.* 2003;11(5):379–396
5. Sornberger MJ, Heath NL, Toste JR, McLouth R. Nonsuicidal self-injury and gender: patterns of prevalence, methods, and locations among adolescents. *Suicide Life Threat Behav.* 2012;42(3):266–278
6. Nixon MK, Cloutier P, Jansson SM. Nonsuicidal self-harm in youth: a population-based survey. *CMAJ.* 2008;178(3):306–312
7. Lloyd-Richardson EE, Perrine N, Dierker L, Kelley ML. Characteristics and functions of non-suicidal self-injury in a community sample of adolescents. *Psychol Med.* 2007;37(8):1183–1192
8. Muehlenkamp JJ, Gutierrez PM. Risk for suicide attempts among adolescents who engage in nonsuicidal self-injury. *Arch Suicide Res.* 2007;11(1):69–82
9. Muehlenkamp JJ, Gutierrez PM. An investigation of differences between self-injurious behavior and suicide attempts in a sample of adolescents. *Suicide Life Threat Behav.* 2004;34(1):12–23
10. Izutsu T, Shimotsu S, Matsumoto T, et al. Deliberate self-harm and childhood hyperactivity in junior high school students. *Eur Child Adolesc Psychiatry.* 2006; 15(3):172–176
11. Heath NL, Ross S, Toste JR, Charlebois A, Nedecheva T. Retrospective analysis of social factors and nonsuicidal self-injury among young adults. *Can J Behav Sci.* 2009;41(3):180–186

12. Moore TR, Gilles E, McComas JJ, Symons FJ. Functional analysis and treatment of self-injurious behaviour in a young child with traumatic brain injury. *Brain Inj.* 2010;24(12):1511–1518

13. MacLean WE, Dornbush K. Self-injury in a statewide sample of young children with developmental disabilities. *J Ment Health Res Intellect Disabil.* 2012;5(3–4): 236–245

14. Gerson J, Stanley B. Suicidal and self-injurious behavior in personality disorder: controversies and treatment directions. *Curr Psychiatry Rep.* 2002;4(1):30–38

15. Paris J. Understanding self-mutilation in borderline personality disorder. *Harv Rev Psychiatry.* 2005;13(3):179–185

16. Klonsky ED. The functions of deliberate self-injury: a review of the evidence. *Clin Psychol Rev.* 2007;27(2):226–239

17. Nock MK. Actions speak louder than words: an elaborated theoretical model of the social functions of self-injury and other harmful behaviors. *Appl Prev Psychol.* 2008;12(4):159–168

18. Nock MK, Prinstein MJ. A functional approach to the assessment of self-mutilative behavior. *J Consult Clin Psychol.* 2004;72(5):885–890

19. Chapman AL, Gratz KL, Brown MZ. Solving the puzzle of deliberate self-harm: the experiential avoidance model. *Behav Res Ther.* 2006;44(3):371–394

20. Heath NL, Toste JR, Nedecheva T, Charlebois A. An examination of non-suicidal self-injury in college students. *J Ment Health Couns.* 2008;30(2):137–156

21. Klonsky ED. The functions of self-injury in young adults who cut themselves: clarifying the evidence for affect-regulation. *Psychiatry Res.* 2009;166(2–3): 260–268

22. Nock MK, Prinstein MJ. Contextual features and behavioral functions of self-mutilation among adolescents. *J Abnorm Psychol.* 2005;114(1):140–146

23. Hilt LM, Nock MK, Lloyd-Richardson EE, Prinstein MJ. Longitudinal study of nonsuicidal self-injury among young adolescents. *J Early Adolesc.* 2008;28(3): 455–469

24. Iwata BA, Dorsey MF, Slifer KJ, Bauman KE, Richman GS. Toward a functional analysis of self-injury. *J Appl Behav Anal.* 1994;27(2):197–209

25. Sprague JR, Horner RH. Functional assessment and intervention in community settings. *Ment Retard Dev Disabil Res Rev.* 1995;1(2):89–93

26. Wacker DP, Berg WK, Harding JW, et al. Evaluation and long-term treatment of aberrant behavior displayed by young children with disabilities. *J Dev Behav Pediatr.* 1998;19(4):260–266

27. Carr EG, Smith CE. Biological setting events for self-injury. *Ment Retard Dev Disabil Res Rev.* 1995;1(2):94–98

28. Sandman CA, Hetrick W, Taylor DV, Chicz-DeMet A. Dissociation of POMC peptides after self-injury predicts responses to centrally acting opiate blockers. *Am J Ment Retard.* 1997;102(2):182–199

29. Bosch J, Van Dyke C, Smith SM, Poulton S. Role of medical conditions in the exacerbation of self-injurious behavior: an exploratory study. *Ment Retard.* 1997;35(2):124–130

30. Richman DM. Annotation: early intervention and prevention of self-injurious behaviour exhibited by young children with developmental disabilities. *J Intellect Disabil Res.* 2008;52(pt 1):3–17

31. Lofthouse N, Muehlenkamp JJ, Adler R. Nonsuicidal self-injury and co-occurrence. In: Nixon MK, Heath NL, eds. *Self-injury in Youth: The Essential Guide to Assessment and Intervention.* New York, NY: Routledge Press/Taylor & Francis Group; 2009

32. MacLean WE, Symons F. Self-injurious behavior in infancy and young childhood. *Infants Young Child.* 2002;14(4):31–41

33. Schroeder S, Thompson T, Oster-Granite ML. *Self-injurious Behavior: Genes, Brain, and Behavior.* Washington, DC: American Psychological Association; 2002

34. Adler PA, Adler P. The demedicalization of self-injury: from psychopathology to sociological deviance. *J Contemp Ethnog.* 2007;36(5):537–550

35. Heath NL, Nixon MK. Assessment of nonsuicidal self-injury in youth. In: Nixon MK, Heath NL, eds. *Self-injury in Youth: The Essential Guide to Assessment and Intervention.* New York, NY: Routledge Press/Taylor & Francis Group; 2009

36. Symons FJ, Thompson T. Self-injurious behaviour and body site preference. *J Intellect Disabil Res.* 1997;41(pt 6):456–468

37. Luiselli JK, Matson JL, Singh NN, eds. *Self-injurious Behavior: Analysis, Assessment, and Treatment.* New York, NY: Springer; 1992

38. Carr EG, Durand VM. Reducing behavior problems through functional communication training. *J Appl Behav Anal.* 1985;18(2):111–126

39. Day HM, Horner RH, O'Neill RE. Multiple functions of problem behaviors: assessment and intervention. *J Appl Behav Anal.* 1994;27(2):279–289

40. Repp AC, Felce D, Barton LE. Basing the treatment of stereotypic and self-injurious behaviors on hypotheses of their causes. *J Appl Behav Anal.* 1988; 21(3):281–289

41. Iwata BA, Deleon IG, Roscoe EM. Reliability and validity of the functional analysis screening tool. *J Appl Behav Anal.* 2013;46(1):271–284

42. O'Neill RE, Albin RW, Storey K, Horner RH, Sprague JR. *Functional Assessment and Program Development for Problem Behavior: A Practical Handbook.* Stamford, CT: Cengage Learning; 2015

43. Paclawskyj TR, Matson JL, Rush KS, Smalls Y, Vollmer TR. Questions About Behavioral Function (QABF): a behavioral checklist for functional assessment of aberrant behavior. *Res Dev Disabil.* 2000;21(3):223–239

44. Durand VM, Crimmins DB. Identifying the variables maintaining self-injurious behavior. *J Autism Dev Dis.* 1988;18(1):99–117

45. Northup J, Wacker D, Sasso G, et al. A brief functional analysis of aggressive and alternative behavior in an outclinic setting. *J Appl Behav Anal.* 1991;24(3):509–522

46. Hall SS. Comparing descriptive, experimental and informant-based assessments of problem behaviors. *Res Dev Disabil.* 2005;26(6):514–526

47. Paclawskyj TR, Matson JL, Rush KS, Smalls Y, Vollmer TR. Assessment of the convergent validity of the Questions About Behavioral Function scale with analogue functional analysis and the Motivation Assessment Scale. *J Intellect Disabil Res.* 2001;45(pt 6):484–494

48. Lynch TR, Cozza C. Behavior therapy for nonsuicidal self-injury. In: Nock MK, ed. *Understanding Nonsuicidal Self-injury: Origins, Assessment, and Treatment.* Washington, DC: American Psychological Association; 2009

49. Miller AL, Muehlenkamp JJ, Jacobson CM. Special issues in treating adolescent nonsuicidal self-injury. In: Nock MK, ed. *Understanding Nonsuicidal Self-injury: Origins, Assessment, and Treatment.* Washington, DC: American Psychological Association; 2009

50. Miller AL, Rathus JH. Dialectical behavior therapy: adaptations and new applications. Introduction. *Cogn Behav Pract.* 2000;7(4):420–425

51. Miller AL, Rathus JH, Linehan MM. *Dialectical Behavior Therapy With Suicidal Adolescents.* New York, NY: Guilford Press; 2006

52. Gratz KL, Chapman AL. *Freedom From Self-harm: Overcoming Self-injury With Skills From DBT and Other Treatments.* Oakland, CA: New Harbinger Publications Inc; 2009

53. Hollander M. *Helping Teens Who Cut: Understanding and Ending Self-injury.* New York, NY: Guilford Press; 2008

54. Kahng S, Iwata BA, Lewin AB. Behavioral treatment of self-injury, 1964 to 2000. *Am J Ment Retard.* 2002;107(3):212–221

55. Tiger JH, Hanley GP, Bruzek J. Functional communication training: a review and practical guide. *Behav Anal Pract.* 2008;1(1):16–23

56. Kern L, Clarke S. Antecedent and setting event interventions. In: Bambara LM, Kern L, eds. *Individualized Supports for Students With Problem Behaviors: Designing Positive Behavior Support Plans.* New York, NY: Guilford Press; 2005

57. Durand VM, Carr EG. Functional communication training to reduce challenging behavior: maintenance and application in new settings. *J Appl Behav Anal.* 1991; 24(2):251–264

58. Petscher ES, Rey C, Bailey JS. A review of empirical support for differential reinforcement of alternative behavior. *Res Dev Disabil.* 2009;30(3):409–425

59. Wacker DP, Berg WK, Harding JW, Barretto A, Rankin B, Ganzer J. Treatment effectiveness, stimulus generalization, and acceptability to parents of functional communication training. *Educ Psychol.* 2005;25(2–3):233–256

60. Lucyshyn JM, Albin RW, Nixon CD. Embedding comprehensive behavioral support in family ecology: an experimental, single-case analysis. *J Consult Clin Psychol.* 1997;65(2):241–251

61. Moes DR, Frea WD. Using family context to inform intervention planning for the treatment of a child with autism. *J Posit Behav Interv.* 2000;2(1):40–46

62. Lowe K, Allen D, Jones E, Brophy S, Moore K, James W. Challenging behaviours: prevalence and topographies. *J Intellect Disabil Res.* 2007;51(pt 8):625–636

CHAPTER 28

Sleep Disturbances

Anne May, MD, and Mark L. Splaingard, MD

> "*...maturational concerns need to be distinguished from sleep-related disorders, which have specific medical criteria with functional and health-related consequences.*"

Sleep questions and concerns are a frequent topic during pediatric visits. Parents are often concerned about normal sleep patterns and about ensuring adequate sleep for their child. Problems with a child's sleep frequently stress the entire family. The sleep deprivation that parents experience because of their child's sleep problems can affect parents' resilience and the consistency and quality of their parenting.

When evaluating concerns about a child's sleep, it is important for the primary care clinician (PCC)—that is, the pediatrician, family physician, internist, nurse practitioner, or physician assistant who provides the child's or adolescent's frontline, longitudinal health care—to determine the nature of the parent's concern. Sleep patterns vary widely among children and adolescents (collectively called *children* in the remainder of this chapter unless otherwise specified), and often it is a normal variation in sleep development that causes concern for parents. These maturational concerns need to be distinguished from sleep-related disorders, which have specific medical criteria with functional and health-related consequences. A true sleep disorder consistently affects daytime functioning. Sleep problems may be associated with a psychiatric or behavioral disorder, a developmental disorder, or a medical problem. This chapter is designed to provide guidance for PCCs in determining the type of sleep concern that is present, so interventions can be tailored to each child and family's situation.

Determining the frequency of sleep disturbances in pediatric patients can be challenging, and estimates of prevalence of sleep disturbances in children vary widely. This determination is particularly challenging with maturational sleep problems as opposed to sleep-related disorders, such as obstructive sleep apnea (OSA), which have distinct criteria for diagnosis. In addition, cultural and ethnic variations, underreporting by parents, and underdiagnosis by PCCs have been issues in determining prevalence.[1] Sleep problems are conservatively estimated to occur in approximately 25% of healthy children younger than 5 years and in up to 80% of children with special needs. They are reported in greater than 70% of children with depression and, when present, are associated with more severe depression and a higher rate of suicide completion.[2,3] Sleep disturbances are also common in children with other mental disorders and contribute to the challenges of their care. Successful management of pediatric sleep problems often results in improved sleep and daytime functioning for all members of the household.[4]

Evaluation of Children for Inadequate Sleep

Children rarely report sleeping problems. The PCC may suspect poor sleep on the basis of findings during routine surveillance at child health supervision visits or signs and symptoms suggesting sleep deprivation (Box 28-1). Most commonly, a parent or another caregiver brings the problem to the PCC's attention. The most common concerns are the child's inability to fall asleep or remain asleep, daytime sleepiness, and abnormal behaviors during sleep (snoring, gasping, or yelling). In sorting out a concern about sleep, history is the major initial diagnostic tool.

Because parental perception of sleep problems varies widely,[5] the first step in a sleep evaluation is correctly identifying the concerns of the family. A strong subjective component can be found for many pediatric

---

Box 28-1. Symptoms and Signs of Inadequate Amount of Sleep

- EDS (rare in young children)
- Hyperactivity or impaired attention
- Poor school performance (eg, impaired concentration, vigilance)
- Behavior problems (eg, bad mood, irritability)
- Obesity (possibly linked to inadequate sleep)
- Failure to thrive

Abbreviation: EDS, excessive daytime sleepiness.

sleep problems, such as in the typical case of the toddler with night awakenings who wants to get into the parental bed:

► The parents in family A do not consider this desire to be a problem. Both parents are good sleepers and do not care if their child sleeps in their bed.

► The parents in family B believe strongly that their child does not belong in their bed and that their bedroom is the only place they have to themselves.

► The parents in family C have let their child into their bed in the past, but another child (newborn) is due in 3 months, and they would like their child to transition to spending the night in her own bed.

► The parents in family D do not consider letting their child into their bed to be a problem, but their child's restless sleep and snoring are keeping them (the parents) up at night.

These examples illustrate the variety of responses to a common sleep issue in the young child. All these families have caring parents and normally developing toddlers. Some of the parents regard the behavior as a sleep problem, whereas others do not. The parents in family B are more likely than the parents in family A to consult a pediatric PCC about their child's sleep.

Sleep evaluation should include a history of bedtime, wake time, duration of time until the child falls asleep, and the frequency of overnight awakenings. Inquiring about a bedtime routine, or lack thereof, may provide helpful information about the child's activity prior to attempting sleep. In addition, the PCC should try to get an idea of the environment where the child usually sleeps. This evaluation may include determining the location of the sleeping area (eg, own bedroom, parents' room, common spaces) as well as the temperature, light level, noise level, and electronic devices in the sleeping area. Questionnaires for general screening or for evaluating sleep concerns, such as the BEARS Sleep Screening Algorithm (see Appendix 2, Mental Health Tools for Pediatrics), may be helpful in gathering data in busy practices. It is important for the clinician to determine the level of parental concern, elicit maladaptive patterns, and help formulate a differential diagnosis. Table 28-1 lists sample questions to clarify sleep problems. Having the parents keep a sleep chart is helpful (Figure 28-1); it may demonstrate a consistent

Table 28-1. Questions to Clarify Sleep Problems

Questions	To Clarify
To the Parents	
When and how did the child's sleep problems start?	Secondary gain
Did other changes in the child's life occur around this time? • What methods have you tried to solve this problem? • What ideas have you had about solving this problem? • What have others told you about this problem?	Traumas or stress
What is the atmosphere in the room where the child sleeps with regard to temperature, darkness, noise, presence of siblings, and type of bed?	Environmental sleep disorder
When is the last time the child eats before falling asleep?	Inadequate sleep hygiene
	Sleep-onset association disorder
Does the child consume any caffeine or nicotine in the evening?	Insomnia caused by substance or drug effects
What is the child doing just before bedtime?	Inadequate sleep hygiene
	Limit-setting disorder
	Bedtime resistance
What routines do you use to put the child to bed?	Inadequate sleep hygiene
	Limit-setting disorder
	Bedtime resistance
What exactly do you do at bedtime?	Sleep-onset association disorder
How does the child act at bedtime?	Bedtime resistance
Where and with whom does the child sleep?	Sleep-onset association disorder
What does your spouse or partner think about this arrangement?	Family conflict
Who else has something to say about the child's sleeping?	Family conflict
Is the child already asleep when you put him or her into the crib or bed?	Sleep-onset association disorder

Table 28-1. Questions to Clarify Sleep Problems (*continued*)	
Questions	**To Clarify**
To the Parents	
What time is the child put into bed?	Limit-setting disorder
	Inadequate sleep hygiene
	Circadian rhythm sleep disorders
What time is the child asleep?	Limit-setting disorder
	Inadequate sleep hygiene
	Circadian rhythm sleep disorders
Does the child do anything unusual during sleep?	—
Snoring, gasping, apnea?	SDB
Leg kicking, thrashing?	Periodic limb movement disorder, restless legs syndrome
Bed-wetting?	Nocturnal enuresis
Shaking, screaming?	Nocturnal seizures
	Parasomnias
What times does the child wake up?	Night feeders
	Sleep-onset association disorder
How does the child appear, or what does he or she do after waking?	Parasomnias
	Developmental night waking
	Trained night feeders
	Seizures
What works to resettle the child?	Sleep-onset association disorder
	Trained night waking
	Trained night feeding
	Gastroesophageal reflux
How is that process for you?	Secondary gain
Does the child snore or seem to stop breathing during the night?	SDB
What time is the child up for the day?	Circadian rhythm sleep disorders
	Mood disorders
Is the schedule the same on weekends, or does the child sleep in?	Limit-setting disorder or sleep-phase delay

Table 28-1. Questions to Clarify Sleep Problems (*continued*)	
Questions	**To Clarify**
To the Parents	
How does the child wake up in the morning?	Circadian rhythm sleep disorder or sleep-phase delay
When you wake the child, does he or she seem rested and cheerful?	Circadian rhythm sleep disorder or sleep-phase delay
	Inadequate sleep
What time does the child eat in the morning?	Circadian rhythm sleep disorder or sleep-phase advance
	Limit-setting disorder
If age >3 y, does the child remember what happened during the night?	Parasomnia (not remembered)
	Nightmares (remembered)
	Panic attacks (remembered)
Does the child fall asleep during the day? If so, when, where, and for how long?	Circadian rhythm sleep disorders
	Idiopathic hypersomnia or narcolepsy
How is the child settled for naps?	Sleep-onset association disorder
	Limit-setting disorder
Does the child sleep differently at other people's houses? If so, how?	Sleep-onset association disorder
	Limit-setting disorder
Has the child ever been given any medications for sleep? What was the medication? How did it work?	Insomnia caused by a psychiatric or behavioral condition
Has anyone in the family ever had sleep problems? Did either of you have sleep problems as children?	Genetic factors (short or long sleeper)
To the Child	
What do you think about before you go to sleep?	Anxiety or mood disorder
	Limit-setting disorder
How do you feel when you wake up in the night?	Nightmares
	Disorders of arousal
	Anxiety or mood disorder
Do you still feel sleepy in the morning?	Inadequate sleep
	Circadian rhythm sleep disorder or sleep-phase delay

Questions	To Clarify
Table 28-1. Questions to Clarify Sleep Problems (*continued*)	
To the Child	
How do you feel about this sleeping problem?	Anxiety
	Secondary gain
What do you think your parents should do about this?	Secondary gain
How are your concentration and grades at school?	Sleep-related breathing disorder
	Sleep-phase delay
	Periodic limb movement disorder
	Narcolepsy
	Idiopathic hypersomnia

Abbreviation: SDB, sleep-disordered breathing.

pattern, which may improve with the use of sleep hygiene principles. Resources to assist parents include a handout from the American Academy of Pediatrics, *Sleep Problems in Children,* which is available online at https://patiented.solutions.aap.org. A general medical, developmental, and mental health history assessment should include any medications, any herbal products, and any drug, alcohol, or tobacco use. Given that many sleep disorders have a strong familial component, a history of parental sleep issues may be helpful.

In addition to focusing on the child's sleep habits, recognizing parental perceptions and differences of opinion about sleep often are critical in problem-solving efforts. Co-sleeping (one or both parents sharing a bed with one or more children) serves as a good example of this point. Co-sleeping is a common practice in many cultures and households. Bed sharing with newborns and infants remains controversial, and American Academy of Pediatrics policy about safe sleep practices advises against this because of an increase in rates of SIDS (sudden infant death syndrome).[6] When it is agreeable to both parents, co-sleeping outside of the newborn period and infancy is not associated with greater-than-average behavioral or emotional problems in the child. If, however, co-sleeping is a source of discord between parents or reflects a parent's

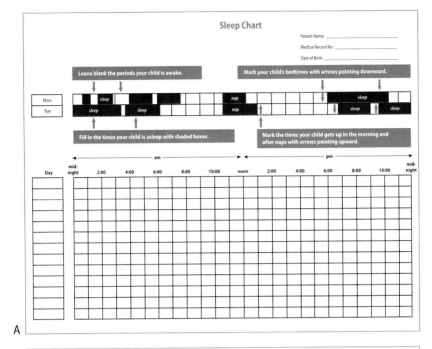

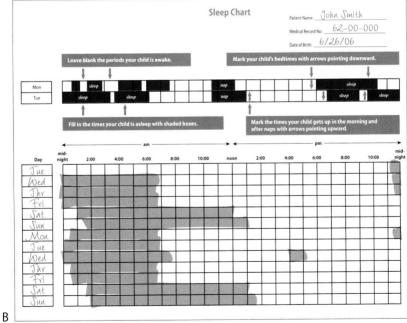

Figure 28-1. A, Sleep log. B, Sleep log showing sleep-phase delay.

inability to manage the child's behavioral bedtime problems, it should be addressed as a sleep problem.

Parental mental health needs to be screened in assessing sleep difficulties because the emotional stability of parents may affect both the perception of problems in children and the ability to carry out a treatment plan. Histories from babysitters or relatives who observe the child's sleep may be diagnostic, especially when problems seen at home are not seen in these settings. The family may provide audiotapes or videotapes that may be helpful.

The history itself is often diagnostic, but some patients need to undergo overnight polysomnography (PSG) for further assessment. While PSG is rarely helpful in diagnosing and treating insomnia or behavioral sleep concerns, a PSG provides clinically useful information about sleep stages, sleep disruption, respiratory status during various sleep stages, leg movements, and changes in cardiac rate and rhythm during sleep. The PSG also provides a picture of the relationship of sleep-related measurements. For instance, OSA may cause arousals, cardiac deceleration, and oxygen desaturation; these findings may be mild during non–rapid eye movement (NREM) sleep but profound during rapid eye movement (REM) sleep. Finally, the observations of the overnight sleep technologist provide valuable insight in making a diagnosis. These data are essential in diagnosing and treating OSA, narcolepsy, and periodic limb movement disorder.

Maturational Issues

Day-Night Reversals

The earliest parental concern about sleep is often day-night reversal, occurring around 2 weeks of age. This problem is predictable because consolidated nocturnal sleep has not yet developed. Parental concerns provide the pediatrician a valuable opportunity to assess parental coping skills and help parents understand the normal unfolding of the child's physiologic regulation. Day-night reversals can be shifted by establishing a general bedtime, keeping the lights off or low, and keeping handling and interaction to a minimum during nighttime feedings. In the morning, lights should be bright and social interaction encouraged. Lack of sleep at this age is unusual and should alert the clinician to medical problems, especially if associated with irritability.

Delayed Settling

Another common problem is a delay in the much desired milestone of sleeping through the night. One definition of settling or sleeping through the night is 5 hours of continuous sleep after midnight for 4 consecutive weeks. Unrealistic parental expectations for sleeping through the night are common. Anders observed that 44% of parents of 2-month-olds reported that their infant slept throughout the night when, in fact, recording on time-lapse videotape showed that only 15% slept throughout the night without awakening.[7]

The issue of sleeping through the night may have important ramifications for the breastfeeding newborn or infant. Despite the widely recognized and undisputed advantages of human milk for infants, the duration of lactation in the United States is still well below the recommended goal of 50% at 6 months in all ethnic groups.[8] The perceptions of normal maternal and infant sleep patterns may be an important factor in failure to sustain lactation. Although breastfed infants are typically assumed to feed more frequently and to have shorter meal intervals than bottle-fed infants do, widely disparate differences in sleep patterns, crying, fussiness, and colic behavior between breastfed infants and bottle-fed infants have been reported. The perception that breastfed infants typically *settle* at an older age than bottle-fed infants do, and awaken more frequently at night, is quoted in the popular press as an *advantage* of formula feeding. As a corollary, a mother's need for an uninterrupted night's sleep may inadvertently promote the early cessation of breastfeeding.

In fact, breastfeeding need not be associated with increased night wakening by 12 weeks of age; both breastfed infants and bottle-fed infants can respond to behavioral interventions aimed at increasing sleep time during the night.[9-11] Additional evidence is emerging that continuing lactation can actually increase maternal slow-wave (restorative) sleep because of increased circulating prolactin levels.[12] The circadian rhythm of tryptophan secretion in mother's milk may help promote nocturnal infant sleep and is being mimicked by investigators exploring varying amounts of tryptophan in day and night formulas.[13]

Infants who appear to have a low threshold of sensitivity by temperamental disposition also tend to settle later. Preterm infants tend to settle around the time expected for their gestational ages, although variability is greater than among term infants. Delays in central nervous system (CNS) maturation are often associated with delays in settling. Infants with frank neurological impairments may not only be delayed in settling but also have other medical issues that need to be addressed to allow settling to occur.

Awakenings From Sleep (Fragmentation) Associated With Development

Waking at night occurs in more than 80% of children and, of course, in infants who still need to feed. Night waking is problematic only when the child cannot return to sleep on his or her own. As many as 20% of 2-year-olds, 14% of 3-year-olds, and 6.5% of 5- to 12-year-olds have problematic night awakenings.[14]

Trained Night Feeding

In Western industrialized societies, between 60% and 70% of either breastfed infants or bottle-fed infants are reported to be settling or sleeping through the night by 12 weeks of age without any specific behavioral interventions.[10,15] Nonetheless, some infants older than 6 months who wake up during the night are immediately fed to encourage their return to sleep. Their sleep cycles may be changed by the introduction of food to produce an arousal—basically, learned hunger—and they will consume a full feeding during the night. Trained night feeding should generally not be diagnosed before 6 months' post-term because of the frequent need for a feeding during the night in younger or preterm infants. Infants who learned to sleep through the night and subsequently begin waking during the night and seeming genuinely hungry are probably ready for solid foods (if they are >4–6 months) or need increased volumes or number of feedings during the day and evening if they are formula fed. Breastfed infants may respond better to more frequent evening feedings (cluster feeding) of smaller but richer (higher lipid content) human milk.

Trained night feeding can be prevented by teaching parents ways to recognize when an infant is fussy because of hunger and when fussiness arises from other causes, such as boredom. Parents should not automatically feed a fussy infant unless the infant appears hungry. Parents who go to their infants older than 4 months at the first sound of stirring should also be encouraged to allow their infants the opportunity to return to sleep without intervention. Expectations of the appropriate need for a late (eg, 10:00 pm) feeding should be clarified. Daytime feeding intervals can be adjusted gradually and any sleep associations retrained simultaneously. If night feedings are an established pattern, the formula-fed infant can be fed 30 mL (1 fl oz) less each night. This tactic will usually help resolve trained night feeding in approximately 1 week.

Trained Night Waking

Waking at night without requiring a feeding in the infant between 4 and 8 months of age is called *trained night waking*. This pattern often begins when the infant is ill or subjected to travel or some other change in routine, but the pattern may persist because the infant gets a secondary reward from the parent's attention. One parent may believe that quieting the infant quickly is necessary to prevent disturbing other family members or neighbors. In some instances, parents who have little time to spend with the infant during the day enjoy this time with the infant and reinforce the night waking by playing with him or her. Trained night waking is also common in infants who have difficult temperaments.

Management of trained night waking that causes persistent family disruption requires management of the precipitant stress and, ideally, collaboration with the spouse or neighbors to tolerate some crying during the treatment. Bedtime routines need to be established, perhaps providing bedding or infant clothing with a maternal scent, and the infant should be put into bed awake. Daytime naps should be limited to 2 hours to consolidate the longest sleep period at night. When awakening during the night, the infant should be allowed 1 to 2 minutes of crying before being checked, but not fed, and then checked every 2 to 5 minutes in most circumstances. The infant may be touched but not picked up, rocked, or cuddled. For success, this approach may require the more involved parent to take a shower, turn up music, or find some other distraction.

Developmental Night Waking

Although most infants are sleeping through the night by 6 months of age, many begin awakening again around 8 to 10 months of age. This new behavior, called *developmental night waking,* corresponds to several coincident developmental processes, including increased mobility, fear reactions to strangers, and object permanence (ability to remember and seek something or someone, such as a parent, that is out of sight).

The best management is advising parents at the 6-month health supervision visit to expect a recurrence of night waking. Because of differences in cultures, not all parents will see this circumstance as a problem. For parents who do, they should be advised to wait a few minutes before going to the infant but to avoid feeding or other reinforcements. If waking is already established, the parents should have the contributing developmental forces explained and be advised to create a bedtime routine, including a transitional object and a dim night-light. When the infant awakens, he or she should be given at least 2 minutes to self-soothe, with some fussing tolerated as part of the process. If fussing continues, one parent can go to reassure the infant briefly, without touching or feeding, and settle down within sight to sleep the rest of the night without talking to the infant. The infant often becomes enraged instead of fearful, which is more tolerable to the parent, who can see that the infant is safe. Some parents are more comfortable than others with this plan. For children who are no longer constrained to a crib, the parent must prevent body contact with the child by giving him or her the alternative that the parent will leave the room, to prevent establishing a sleep association. Further interactions should be brief and minimally interactive. Eventually, the child will no longer require the parent's presence to return to sleep after nocturnal awakenings.[16]

Bedtime Fears

Preschool-aged and early school-aged children often have bedtime fears. These may be generated by stresses such as separation from parents, aggressive peers, sibling birth, or the death of a grandparent. Exposure to frightening movies or video games can also contribute to these fears. The child's fears should be acknowledged, and he or she should be reassured that the parents will keep him or her safe. Older children benefit from relaxation exercises accompanied by empowerment stories. A night-light may be helpful.

Behavioral Insomnia of Childhood

Behavioral insomnia of childhood is a frequent problem that arises as children transition from sleep in infancy and toddlerhood to later childhood. These issues occur when children have learned specific behavioral patterns to assist in falling asleep or in avoiding sleep. Treatment consists of teaching new behaviors and shifting the family dynamic so that old behaviors are no longer acceptable.

Sleep-Onset Associations

Infants and children develop habits of falling asleep in accustomed circumstances, such as in a bed, in a parent's arms, or while being fed. These sleep-onset associations may begin in the first 2 months of life and may be viewed as a problem by the family when an infant older than 6 months needs prolonged parental assistance to fall asleep at the beginning of the night and after each nocturnal arousal. This pattern is a conditioned response, and the infant is unable to fall asleep unless the conditions allowing sleep onset are recreated. Parents may report that their own sleep is severely disrupted because they need to help the infant resettle several times each night. Treatment is straightforward: the infant learns to make the transition from wake to sleep without expecting a parent's participation. Parents should be advised to place the infant while still awake into the crib for both nighttime sleeping and naps starting by 48 weeks' post-gestational age. A helpful tactic is for the infant's bedding to have the mother's scent for comfort. If a problematic sleep-onset association has already developed, parents may need to institute a graduated extinction program to help infants and children older than 6 months learn to fall asleep on their own over several weeks.[17]

Although graduated extinction is a very effective treatment, parental distress is a common issue during the initial portions of using an extinction strategy. Warning parents what to expect and addressing fears about harming or creating a sense of abandonment in the child may alleviate some parental concern. Successful treatment requires consistency, and it is important that all nighttime caregivers are able to implement the extinction technique. If the parents are uncertain that they will be able to consistently implement extinction strategy, it may be advisable to delay treatment until that is possible. Parents should be educated that the extinction process may take longer if the disruptive sleep pattern becomes more well-established as the child becomes older.[16]

Limit-Setting Issues

Bedtime routines should take 30 minutes or less. Consistently longer bedtime routines may reflect parental difficulty in setting limits. Prolonged bedtime routines are often associated with multiple "curtain calls" for stories, hugs, water, and trips to the toilet. Toddlers and preschool-aged children no longer sleeping in a crib may reappear after being put to bed, thus prolonging the routine. These curtain calls are unintentionally reinforced by the parental attention needed to return the child to bed, even if done with obvious displeasure.

The best management of prolonged bedtime routines is prevention through reasonable daily schedules, assurance of adequate special individual time with each parent every day, and careful limit setting. This approach reduces the child's separation anxiety as well as parental guilt. The bedtime routine should be limited to a defined set of activities or length of time. Parents may then either notify the child that they will not respond to further requests or say "only one more" and adhere to this declaration. Parents should be warned to avoid responding to the excuses that will likely ensue. Having the parent promise to check the child frequently can also be reassuring. Bedtime should occur when the child is tired to enhance his or her tendency to fall asleep. Naps should not occur close to bedtime.

Positive reinforcement may enhance limit setting. Children who stay in bed without calling out may be motivated by simple rewards with stickers in the morning or an extra story the following night. Parents may need coaching on limit setting or referral to a psychologist if discipline is a major problem.

Other Difficulties Falling or Staying Asleep

Dyssomnia, the term for insomnia that does not meet disorder criteria, occurs mainly in preschool-aged and older children.

This includes difficulties either falling asleep (sleep onset) or staying asleep (sleep maintenance) caused by environmental disruptions. A detailed history of sleep environment and bedtime behaviors is needed to explore these issues. Excessive noise or light, uncomfortable bedding, excessive room temperature, interference of pets, or outside noises are commonly found. By older patients, the use of personal electronics at bedtime and during overnight awakenings also contributes to these issues. Treatment is simply to eliminate or correct the environmental condition or distraction, if possible. This change may be particularly challenging in crowded households, in homes with individuals who work different schedules, or when multiple homes or multiple locations or both are used for sleep. In these circumstances, involving the family in creating suggestions that eliminate disruptions is important, to ensure that these environmental changes are achievable at home.

Therapies have been devised by many cultures to restore the essential health-giving function of sleep. Herbal remedies such as chamomile (*Matricaria chamomilla*) and other soothing teas are common. Any treatment that involves scheduled rest and mental preparation for sleep would be expected to result in improvement.

Sleep Concerns Associated With Psychiatric or Behavioral Disorders

Although sleep problems may occur in association with almost any mental disorder (Table 28-2), mood disorders are among the most common. It has become more appreciated that many children and adolescents referred to a sleep center for evaluation of insomnia exhibit clinical symptoms of an accompanying mood disorder.[18] It is debated whether insomnia and concomitant chronic sleep insufficiency are affecting psychopathology or are merely early symptoms of underlying or developing mood disorders.[19] Depression may cause sleep-onset insomnia, although this condition is less common in young children than in other age-groups. The early-morning waking of adults with depression is not usually seen before puberty and is only rarely seen among adolescents, for whom hypersomnia is a more common concern than insomnia is.[20] Studies suggest that children with depression accompanied by either insomnia or hypersomnia are more severely affected, having more depressive symptoms and comorbid anxiety disorders.[2] The sleep problems that are intrinsic to depression are complicated by intrusive thoughts or worries that may interfere with sleep maintenance. It is common to treat depression and insomnia concurrently.[21] This approach is supported by adult literature, which suggests that treatment of insomnia is necessary for remission of depressive symptoms.[22] Treatments of sleeping problems in children with depression may include cognitive behavioral therapy (CBT) and antidepressants.[23] Little is written about the treatment of depression-induced hypersomnia. In the presence of clinically impairing hypersomnia, common approaches may involve off-label trials of stimulants or stimulating antidepressants. However, in the patient with depression, this approach should be undertaken with

Table 28-2. Behavioral and Psychiatric Disorders Associated With Sleep Problems in Children and Adolescents

Diagnosis	Sleep Problems
Depression	Sleep-onset or maintenance insomnia seen in 50% of children with depression
	Early-morning awakenings
	EDS seen in 25% of children with depression
	Sleep concerns are prevalent symptoms of major depression in adolescents.
Bipolar disorder	Decreased need for sleep without fatigue
	Insomnia
Seasonal affective disorder	Prevalence of 3%–4% in children with EDS; fatigue in winter
Anxiety disorder	Increased night awakenings, nighttime fears
	Increased sleep-onset insomnia, bedtime problems
	Increased EDS
OCD	Decreased TST
ASD, pervasive developmental disorder	Sleep-onset insomnia, difficulty settling at night, prolonged and frequent nocturnal awakenings
	Shortened duration of sleep
	Irregular sleep-wake pattern
	Parasomnia (including RBD)
ADHD	Sleep-onset or maintenance insomnia
	Nocturnal wakening, OSA, excessive periodic limb movements

Abbreviations: ADHD, attention-deficit/hyperactivity disorder; ASD, autism spectrum disorder; EDS, excessive daytime sleepiness; OCD, obsessive-compulsive disorder; OSA, obstructive sleep apnea; RBD, REM sleep behavioral disorder; REM, rapid eye movement; total sleep time.
Derived from Ivanenko A, Crabtree VM, Gozal D. Sleep in children with psychiatric disorders. *Pediatr Clin North Am.* 2004;51(1):51–68.

the assistance of a psychiatrist, a sleep medicine specialist, or another provider familiar with the use of these medications.

In addition to depression, other mood disorders may affect sleep in children. Children with bipolar disorders may have a dramatically reduced need for sleep (<4 hours a day) during the manic phase. Anxiety and panic disorders may result in difficulties falling asleep because of specific or nonspecific fears. These patients may also have difficulties returning to sleep if aroused during the night.

Children who have been abused have frequent sleep problems, including nightmares, increased activity during sleep, and sleep-onset and sleep-maintenance insomnia.[24] Personality disorders in adolescence have been associated with sleep-onset insomnia. Psychoses may include troubling intrusive thoughts, especially at night, which also lead to insomnia.

Insomnia or hypersomnia caused by substance use or substance use disorder should be considered in older children and adolescents with sleep disorders. Alcohol can induce sleep, but it causes sleep fragmentation in the latter portion of the night. When alcohol is metabolized, sympathetic tone increases, leading to abrupt arousals and sleep-maintenance insomnia. Withdrawal from chronic alcohol use may cause severe insomnia. Stimulants such as cocaine and amphetamines can cause severe insomnia. Some antidepressants, such as fluoxetine, may cause insomnia, whereas others, such as tricyclic antidepressants, trazodone, or mirtazapine, may cause excessive daytime sleepiness (EDS). Antidepressants may eliminate REM atonia, thus precipitating REM sleep behavioral disorder (RBD), a condition during which an individual acts out the contents of one's dreams, potentially posing a risk to oneself or others. Atypical antipsychotics such as aripiprazole may cause stimulation, whereas others, such as olanzapine, cause sedation. Many medications for pain can cause daytime sedation. Timing of medications should be considered when evaluating patients for insomnia and hypersomnia.

Sleep Concerns Associated With Developmental Disorders

Learning disabilities are associated with increased rates of sleep disturbance, including night waking and trouble falling asleep. Half of these sleep difficulties persist for more than 3 years.[25] Systematic review of the literature suggests that children with attention-deficit/hyperactivity disorder (ADHD) have higher daytime sleepiness, more movements during sleep, and higher apnea-hypopnea indexes compared with control patients. Reported sleep problems also include trouble settling to sleep and multiple awakenings from sleep.[26] Medications used to treat ADHD may prolong sleep-onset latency. Clonidine at bedtime has been found to be effective in improving the sleep of 85% of these children when behavioral measures failed.[27]

Many children with autism spectrum disorder (ASD) have difficulties falling asleep, frequent nocturnal awakenings, and early-morning waking. Children with ASD frequently have insomnia that may benefit from behavioral interventions, melatonin therapy, or medications.[28] In addition, many children with ASD require less sleep than their peers do. This tendency may pose a safety risk for patients awake after the household has fallen asleep, or it may lead to challenges for parents and caregivers, when the child needs less sleep than the rest of the household. Asperger syndrome has been associated with insomnia and RBD. Children who have Tourette syndrome have increased risk of parasomnias.

Sleep Concerns Associated With Medical Problems

Sleep problems are seen in patients with a variety of medical conditions (Table 28-3). These sleep problems can be caused by circadian variations associated with some of these diseases, such as asthma. They can also occur because of the physiologic changes that accompany sleep and how those changes interact with these medical conditions.

Sleep-Related Asthma

Asthma episodes are increased during sleep, presumably because the neuroendocrine regulators of respiration are sensitive to circadian regulation. This sensitivity may lead to an increase in asthma symptoms overnight. In one study of children with asthma, 34% awakened at least once a week, and 5% awakened every night, from asthma symptoms. Daytime sequelae were common, with 59% reporting daytime sleepiness and 51% reporting difficulty with concentration. If nocturnal symptoms of asthma are poorly controlled, the recurrent awakenings may lead to fragmented and insufficient nocturnal sleep. Children who have sleep-related asthma may develop anxiety associated with breathing discomfort when they are in bed. This anxiety may lead to bedtime resistance. The relationship between underlying medical issues and quality of sleep is highlighted in asthma, as these concerns improve with successful asthma management.[29,30]

Table 28-3. Medical Disorders Associated With Sleep Problems in Childhood

Diagnosis	Sleep Problems
Asthma	Circadian variation in • PEF (nadir at 4:00 am) • Cutaneous immediate hypersensitivity to house dust allergen • Airway inflammation
	Sleep-related changes • Decrease in lung volumes and increased airway resistance • Increased airway resistance and decreased intrapulmonary blood volume • Decreased mucociliary clearance • Nocturnal gastroesophageal reflux
Cystic fibrosis	OSA can be common in children aged <7 y.
	Nocturnal oxygen desaturation in children aged >7 y • Hypoventilation, especially during REM sleep, caused by de-recruitment of ventilatory muscles • Ventilation-perfusion mismatch caused by decreased functional residual capacity • Occurs more frequently with forced expiratory volume of <65% or resting oxygen saturation while sitting of <94%
Craniofacial abnormalities (eg, Pierre Robin sequence, Goldenhar syndrome, Down syndrome, Treacher Collins syndrome, velocardiofacial syndrome, cleft lip and palate)	Upper airway obstruction
	Nocturnal hypoventilation
Gastroesophageal reflux	Increased night awakening and pain
	Delayed sleep onset
	May result in nocturnal stridor, cough, and wheezing
Down syndrome	Upper airway obstruction with OSA in 30%–60% of children with Down syndrome
	Decreased REM sleep associated with low IQ

Table 28-3. Medical Disorders Associated With Sleep Problems in Childhood (*continued*)

Diagnosis	Sleep Problems
Sickle cell disease	Episodic and continuous nocturnal hypoxemia in 40% of children with sickle cell disease and caused by either OSA or primary lung disease
Obesity	OSA • Obesity-hypoventilation syndrome: hypercapnia, hypoxemia, and daytime somnolence
Scoliosis or congenital neuromuscular disorder (eg, Duchenne muscular dystrophy, spinal muscular atrophy)	Nocturnal hypoventilation
	Nocturnal hypoxemia: EDS and morning headaches
	OSA
	Restless sleep
	Frequent awakenings
Traumatic brain injuries	Sleep-onset and sleep-maintenance insomnia
	EDS
	Dreaming disturbances
	Nocturnal hypoventilation
Spina bifida	Obstructive, central, or mixed apnea
	Nocturnal hypoventilation may cause severe EDS.

Abbreviations: EDS, excessive daytime sleepiness; OSA, obstructive sleep apnea; PEF, peak expiratory flow; REM, rapid eye movement.
Derived from Bandla H, Splaingard M. Sleep problems in children with common medical disorders. *Pediatr Clin North Am.* 2004;51(1):203–227.

Gastroesophageal Reflux Disease

Gastroesophageal reflux disease (GERD) may produce sleep problems in a variety of ways. The reflux can be painful, resulting in night waking and crying. Reflux has also been associated with both central sleep apnea (CSA) and OSA in infants and young children. The diagnosis of GERD may not always be obvious, owing to lack of usual signs, including excessive spitting up, re-swallowing motions, increased fussiness, refusal of feedings, and failure to thrive. Failure to be consoled while being held can be a clue that the child is experiencing pain. Holding a child with GERD upright reduces the amount of acid in the esophagus and may comfort the child. The use of a pH or impedance probe to detect gastroesophageal reflux, or esophagoscopy to assess for esophageal erosions, may be needed to determine the cause of nighttime pain.

Neurological Disorders

Any CNS impairment can result in dysregulation of the sleep cycle. As many as 85% of children who have major developmental disabilities may experience chronic sleep problems.[31] Behavioral sleep problems in these children can be improved by establishing a bedtime routine and putting the child to bed when sleep onset is likely to occur quickly. If the child has persistent difficulty falling asleep, it may be helpful to establish a new pattern by delaying the usual bedtime for 30 minutes and then removing the child from bed if sleep does not occur in 15 to 20 minutes. After removing the child from bed, the parent should keep him or her awake for 30 minutes. This procedure is repeated until the child falls asleep within 15 minutes of being put into bed. Wake-up time is kept constant, and daytime naps should not be allowed for children older than 4 years.

Other factors such as timing of medications, need for repositioning during the night, pain, nighttime feedings, and caregiver anxiety can contribute to sleep problems in the child with neurological impairment. Melatonin administered at bedtime has been shown to be helpful in some children who have CNS problems or blindness as the cause of their sleep disturbances. Melatonin should be used cautiously in children with seizure disorders.

Tumors of the third ventricle or posterior hypothalamus may also cause daytime sleepiness. Brainstem lesions or Chiari malformation type II, both of which are common in children with myelomeningoceles, can cause severe CSA or vocal cord paralysis. Vocal cord paralysis in turn, can cause OSA.

Sleep-Related Epilepsy

Approximately 20% of patients with epilepsy have seizures only during sleep, most often at the time of sleep-wake transitions. Seizures occurring during the night may disrupt sleep by causing multiple awakenings. Nocturnal seizures may manifest themselves as unusual behaviors at night. The possibility of a seizure disorder should be considered in adolescents with new-onset parasomnias. Atypical seizures may produce EDS.

Sleep-Related Headaches

Most headaches occurring during sleep occur during REM sleep. Cluster headaches are more frequent at night than in the daytime and often disrupt sleep. Headaches on awakening are unusual; the child should be evaluated carefully for the presence of increased intracranial pressure or hypercapnia caused by hypoventilation.

Degenerative Disorders

Degenerative brain disorders result in frequent awakenings, difficulty falling asleep, early-morning waking, sleep deprivation, and daytime sleepiness.

Other Medical Disorders

Any condition causing pain at night, such as juvenile idiopathic arthritis, can result in disrupted sleep.[32] Eczema that causes associated scratching results in frequent awakenings. Painful menstrual cramps may also disrupt sleep.

Common Sleep Disorders

Primary Insomnia

Insomnia is a condition that is characterized by difficulty falling or staying asleep and associated daytime dysfunction. It can be seen in children with normal development but is generally transient and resolves within a month. Chronic insomnia occurs when children have difficulty initiating or maintaining sleep, bedtime resistance, or early awakening at least 3 nights per week, for at least 3 months. In addition, daytime symptoms, such as behavioral problems, hyperactivity, inattention, or sleepiness must be present.

In most cases, pediatric insomnia should be managed with CBT interventions (Box 28-2). It is not uncommon for families to move bedtimes forward or provide methods of distraction while trying to fall asleep (such as the use of electronics or prolonged reading). Although the intention is to increase sleep, the long-term effect of these interventions is worsened insomnia. Cognitive behavioral therapy for sleep is designed to retrain many of these behaviors. Medication for primary insomnia

> ### Box 28-2. Key Points of Cognitive Behavioral Therapy for Insomnia
>
> - **Sleep hygiene:** Creating an environment that is conducive to good sleep.
>
> - **Sleep restriction:** Limiting the time spent in bed while awake. This therapy may involve having older children leave their bed/bedroom if they are unable to fall asleep within 20 min of "lights out."
>
> - **Stimulus control:** Using bed/bedroom for sleep only.
>
> - **Relaxation therapy:** Using guided imagery or progressive muscle relaxation to achieve a calm and relaxed state.
>
> - **Cognitive therapy:** Identifying and targeting cognitive distortions regarding the consequences of insomnia.
>
> ---
>
> Derived from Lofthouse N, Gilchrist R, Splaingard M. Mood-related sleep problems in children and adolescents. *Child Adolesc Psychiatr Clin N Am.* 2009;18(4):893–916.

in healthy children is controversial, but medications such as diphenhydramine, clonidine, and melatonin have been used in pediatric patients with insomnia. Indiscriminate medication use can mislead PCCs and families about the causes of insomnia and mask the behavioral management needed.[33]

Sleep-Disordered Breathing

The PCC is often confronted with the problem of what to do with the child who snores. Snoring is common; OSA is less common.

Young children with sleep-disordered breathing (SDB) may not have obesity, unlike typical adult patients. Some groups of children are at particularly high risk for SDB, including those with craniofacial anomalies, chromosomal syndromes, and neuromuscular disorders. Children with Down syndrome, Prader-Willi syndrome, cleft palate, achondroplasia, muscular dystrophy, cerebral palsy, and other underlying disorders should be routinely screened for sleep problems.[34] Although children with Down syndrome, for instance, typically have learning difficulties, treatment of SDB may result in improved daytime performance.[35]

While many children with obstructive SDB improve after adenotonsillectomy, 70% to 90% of patients may still have sleep apnea at repeat PSG.[36]

On occasion, nasal continuous positive airway pressure (commonly known as CPAP) or even tracheotomy may be required.

The question of whether all children should undergo sleep studies before undergoing adenotonsillectomy is controversial. Certain groups of children are clearly at higher risk for perioperative complications and may warrant PSG as part of a preoperative evaluation, especially if outpatient surgery is being contemplated. Children younger than 3 years, children with morbid obesity or chromosomal or craniofacial anomalies, children with underlying neuromuscular disorders, and those with other underlying medical conditions that make them higher-risk surgical patients should be considered for preoperative PSG.[36-38]

Central sleep apnea can also occur in children. This may be the result of underlying neurological, pulmonary, or cardiac disease. In some instances, magnetic resonance imaging (commonly known as MRI) of the brainstem may be indicated to assess for a Chiari malformation, or genetic testing to evaluate for congenital central hypoventilation may be warranted. Consultation with a sleep specialist is recommended to assist with evaluation and treatment of CSA when no apparent etiologic origin is known.

Circadian Rhythm Sleep Disorders

Because the natural circadian cycle is approximately 24.5 hours, some individuals are vulnerable to shifting sleep cycles. Circadian rhythm sleep disorders occur when a person's sleep is of normal duration but occurs at a time that does not allow adequate sleep in the context of the person's life. For example, an adolescent who is unable to fall asleep until 4:00 am and cannot wake before noon is said to have a circadian rhythm sleep disorder (sleep-phase delay) and is likely to have problems functioning in a usual school environment. If, however, a person with the same sleep-phase delay works at night, the sleep-phase delay is not considered a disorder. The most common circadian rhythm sleep disorder causing insomnia is a sleep-phase delay that is commonly seen in adolescents. Sleep-phase delay results in patients who fall asleep naturally at a later bedtime than desired and awaken later in the day. Adolescents are normally sleep-phase delayed, and the mere presence of the delay is not concerning. However, in some patients, this shift results in difficulty waking in time for school in the morning. Phase-delayed adolescents often sleep very late on weekends and vacations and then find falling asleep at a reasonable bedtime to be even more difficult. Phase delay can be distinguished from insomnia by the fact that when the patient is allowed to sleep on his desired schedule, he falls asleep easily and awakens feeling refreshed. Changing adolescent sleep-phase delay is very difficult and requires intense commitment and active participation of the adolescent and parents with the use of bright-light exposure in the morning and consistent wake times all 7 days of the week. In addition, a small dose of melatonin administered several hours before the desired bedtime may assist in pulling the desired bedtime forward.

Some children who are deprived of normal circadian stimuli develop circadian rhythm sleep disorders. Common zeitgebers that entrain normal circadian rhythm include light (especially sunlight), exercise, social activities, and eating. Therefore, that a child with cerebral palsy who is blind, in a wheelchair, and fed by gastrostomy tube has difficulty with a varying sleep time is not surprising.

Other children have circadian rhythm problems that reflect a chaotic home life. Some families do not adhere to predictable routines, allowing children to set their own schedules. This independence may result in seemingly bizarre sleep patterns. A circadian rhythm sleep disorder may be differentiated from a lack of predicable routine by the child's behavior pattern. A child with a circadian rhythm sleep disorder may not resist going to bed but is unable to fall asleep. In the morning, the child is difficult to arouse and does not feel rested.

A sleep-phase advance usually occurs in children who fall asleep early (7:00 pm) but then awaken early in the morning (3:00 am). Different types of circadian shift can be adjusted by simultaneously shifting naps, bedtime, waking time, and meals to a desired schedule that matches the child's total daily sleep needs.

In difficult cases, the child can wear an actigraph, a small portable device similar to a large wristwatch, for several weeks. The device senses physical motion by means of an accelerometer and stores the information. Actigraphy provides a graphic illustration of a child's sleep-wake schedule and can be a useful, noninvasive method for assessing specific sleep disorders, such as insomnia, EDS, and circadian rhythm sleep disorders (Figure 28-2).

Parasomnias (Partial Arousal Disorders)

Parasomnias are unusual behaviors or experiences that occur during sleep or the transition between sleep and wake. Parasomnias associated with partial arousal from slow-wave sleep are common in children. They include confusional arousals, sleep terrors, and sleepwalking disorder (somnambulism). All these episodes occur during arousal from slow-wave sleep, usually in the first third of the night. The child appears confused or frightened and is unresponsive to parental intervention. The child is not fully awake and does not remember the event in the morning.

Symptoms most often begin in childhood and typically resolve spontaneously, only occasionally persisting into adulthood (0.5%). Diagnosis is based on the timing of these symptoms (generally during the first third of the night), the typical presentation, and the child's lack of recall of the events when awake the next morning (morning amnesia). A strong familial component exists, and history often reveals that one or both parents had similar behaviors as children. Management of parasomnias typically includes reassurance that the episodes are generally benign, teaching about minimal intervention during episodes, and removal of potential safety hazards from the child's bedroom. A PSG may help to confirm the diagnosis and detect precipitating events such as OSA or nocturnal seizures in severe or atypical cases. Treating disorders that may fragment sleep, such as OSA and periodic limb movement disorder, can be helpful. In severe cases, a few weeks of a benzodiazepine, such as lorazepam, at bedtime may interrupt the sequence by reducing slow-wave sleep. However, rebound occurs with discontinuation of the medication, often with an increasing number of events.

Confusional Arousals

Children may experience confusional arousals, which are partial arousals from slow-wave sleep, during which they sit up, mumble, and may appear awake. They seem confused and nonresponsive to parental questions. The prevalence of confusional arousals was 17% between ages 3 and 13 years in one study.[39] Children may sometimes thrash about and respond

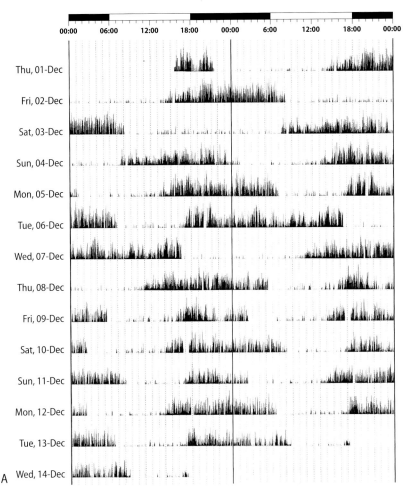

Figure 28-2. 10-year-old child with Down syndrome and nighttime gastrostomy-tube feeding after brain injury. A, Random sleeping pattern with the child frequently awake at night.

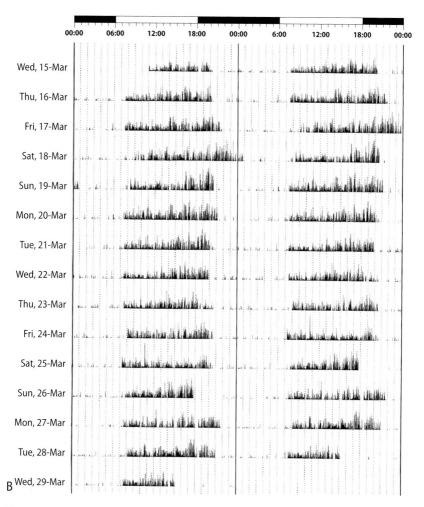

Figure 28-2. 10-year-old child with Down syndrome and nighttime gastrostomy-tube feeding after brain injury. (*continued*) B, Stabilized sleeping pattern using nighttime melatonin administration and morning phototherapy and stopping gastrostomy-tube feedings at night.

combatively to parental attempts to intervene. Confusional arousals usually occur in the first third of the night, but a child may occasionally have multiple arousals. When these events are extending into the second half of the night, they generally decrease in intensity. Confusional arousals are most common when children are overtired or ill. Management includes reassurance that the episodes are generally benign, minimal intervention during episodes, and removal of potential safety hazards from the child's bedroom. Treating disorders that may fragment sleep, such as OSA and restless legs syndrome, can be helpful. In severe cases, a few weeks of a benzodiazepine, such as lorazepam, at bedtime may interrupt the sequence by reducing slow-wave sleep. However, rebound occurs with discontinuation of the medication, often with an increasing number of events. Polysomnography is rarely indicated in cases of confusional arousals, but it may be useful in detecting precipitating events such as OSA or nocturnal seizures in severe or atypical cases.

Sleep Terrors

Sleep terrors are partial awakenings from slow-wave sleep characterized by physiologic arousal, including pallor, sweating, pupillary dilation, piloerection, and tachycardia. The child may sit up and scream and may appear terrified. The child may thrash or run and is not responsive to attempted parental comforting. The child does not remember the event in the morning. Sleep terrors occur in 3% of children, usually starting between 18 months and 5 years. These episodes do not reflect emotional disturbance, although, as with all NREM parasomnias, occurrence is increased with illness, stress, or sleep deprivation. A family history of sleep terrors, enuresis, somnambulism, or somniloquism is often present. Sleep terrors may be precipitated by fatigue, stress, a full bladder, or loud noises. They tend to occur in bouts for several weeks and then disappear only to recur several weeks later. Parents need reassurance about the benign nature of sleep terrors and their tendency to resolve in approximately 95% of children by 8 years of age. The bladder should be emptied routinely before bedtime, and the environment should be kept dark and quiet. The bouts may occasionally be interrupted by waking the child 15 minutes before the expected episode, generally occurring approximately 1 hour into sleep, each night for approximately a week. A 30- to 60-minute afternoon nap can also reduce the depth and amount of slow-wave sleep and may decrease the number of episodes. Treatment with benzodiazepines can reduce the frequency of these events by altering slow-wave sleep, but episodes may recur when the child is weaned or when tolerance occurs. An investigation for nocturnal seizures with full electroencephalography (EEG) as part of a sleep study is indicated in intractable cases or cases that have their onset in adolescence.

Sleepwalking Disorder (Somnambulism)

Approximately 15% of children sleepwalk at some time, mostly between ages 4 and 12 years.[40] During sleepwalking, children are difficult to arouse, are uncoordinated, and tend to wander in illogical places, often urinating outside the toilet. Amnesia of the event in the morning is common. Sleepwalking can usually be differentiated by history or videotapes from dissociative states or seizures; however, occasionally, extended EEG as part of PSG may be helpful in this differentiation. Chronic sleepwalkers need to be carefully safeguarded so they do not injure themselves. Door and window alarms and locks may be necessary. Families may find it helpful to put an alarm or a bell on the door of a child prone to sleepwalk, so the child can be guided safely back to bed if he or she is heard leaving the room. If a child routinely sleepwalks at the same time of night, disrupting sleep with an anticipatory awakening may prevent sleepwalking.

Nightmare Disorder

Nightmares are an extremely common parasomnia occurring during REM sleep and are most common in the last third of the sleep period. The dream content is often recalled as frightening and reflects daytime stresses. Although children clearly dream by 14 months of age, nightmares are most common between 3 and 6 years, occurring in 10% to 50% of children. At these ages, children have the verbal skills to describe dreams. They also have vivid imaginations and fears.

A child who wakes from a frightening dream should be comforted, keeping the intervention brief to prevent secondary gain. The same concerns listed for bedtime fears should be addressed when nightmares are frequent. Children who have chronic nightmares have been shown to improve with targeted relaxation exercises and stories in which the child masters a situation. Children can prepare to have good dreams through rehearsal and imaging at bedtime. Severe nightmares may respond to bedtime medications, although counseling is recommended if the condition is of a severity to warrant medication.

Nightmares are uniformly part of post-traumatic stress disorder; they may increase after withdrawal of REM-suppressing substances such as alcohol and antidepressants.

Bruxism

Bruxism is grinding the teeth during sleep and has been reported in more than 50% of children, with a mean age of onset of 10.5 years. No longitudinal studies demonstrating the natural history of bruxism have been conducted, but dental evidence of bruxism can be identified in 10% to 20% of the general population. Bruxism can also be caused by dental malocclusion or neurological or psychiatric conditions. Tooth guards can protect the teeth and reduce potential damage to the temporomandibular joint. If stress or anxiety is a trigger, relaxation exercises at bedtime may be helpful.

Violent Behavior During Sleep

An REM sleep behavioral disorder has been described in which normal REM atonia does not occur. Dream content can be physically acted out, sometimes in violent ways. REM sleep behavioral disorder is very rare in healthy children but has been seen in children with ASD or in association with neurological disorders. A clue to diagnosis is that abnormal behaviors occur during the last third of the night, unlike abnormal behaviors associated with NREM motor parasomnias, which typically occur during slow-wave sleep during the first third of the sleep period. Diagnosis requires a sleep study and neuroimaging studies. Treatment with clonazepam has been beneficial in children with ASD and RBD and is the most common treatment in adults with RBD.

Sleep-Related Movement Disorders

Restless Legs Syndrome and Periodic Limb Movement Disorder

Restless legs syndrome occurs in about 2% of children and adolescents between 8 and 17 years of age.[41] It is characterized by uncomfortable sensations in the legs, which are worse at rest. These sensations are present in the evening, are associated with the need to move, and are temporarily relieved by movement. They are sometimes confused with growing pains. They may interfere with the child's or adolescent's ability to fall asleep. A strong familial component exists. Periodic limb movement disorder is repetitive, brief leg twitches, occurring more than 5 times per hour in children. Leg movements or jerks may occur with resumption of a breath after an episode of CSA or with a loud snort or snore at the termination of an episode of OSA. They may cause arousals, fragmenting the continuity of sleep and leading to a report of sleep-maintenance insomnia. Although the 2 syndromes are not identical, many patients experience both. In children, limb movements may be exacerbated by iron deficiency or the use of antidepressant medication. They are more common in children with ADHD. Treatment may include iron supplements, clonidine, gabapentin, or dopaminergic agents, depending on the age of the child.

Sleep-Wake Transition Disorder

Rhythmic movements while falling asleep are common in infants and toddlers. Rhythmic movement disorders include head banging and body rocking. Some rhythmic activity at bedtime occurs in more than half of 9-month-olds, decreasing to one-third at 18 months and to less than one-fourth at 2 years of age. Head banging is typically monotonous, occurring 60 to 80 times per minute, usually for less than 15 minutes. Usually benign, head banging may occasionally be caused by CNS injury, headache, inner ear abnormality, sensory deprivation (including visual or hearing impairment), neglect, or abuse. Children of intense temperament are especially likely to bang. Although head banging usually does not cause brain injury, it can be traumatic if the bed is unstable or if safety precautions are not taken in the environment. The condition may be reduced by kinesthetic stimulation during the evening and holding the child as part of the bedtime routine. Sleep restriction (ie, limiting the time the child lies in bed before falling asleep) and mild sedation have been shown to be helpful in difficult cases. Parents often need reassurance of the generally benign nature of these behaviors.

Central Disorders of Hypersomnia

Excessive daytime sleepiness can be caused by insufficient sleep, fragmented sleep (Table 28-4), or increased sleep drive (Table 28-5). Although some sleepy children appear to have difficulty remaining awake, many sleepy children may exhibit hyperactivity, restlessness, poor concentration, impulsivity, aggressiveness, or irritability. Sleepiness

Table 28-4. Treatment of Sleep Fragmentation in Children by Cause	
	Treatment
Maturational	
All types combined	Education
Parasomnias	
Sleep terrors	Education, good sleep hygiene, medication (rarely)
Sleep talking	Education, good sleep hygiene
Somnambulism	Education, good sleep hygiene, review safety issues
Confusional arousals	Education, good sleep hygiene
Sleep-Related Breathing Disorder	
Sleep apnea	Adenotonsillectomy, nasal CPAP
Upper airway resistance syndrome	Adenotonsillectomy, nasal CPAP
Other Medical	
Asthma	Medical management
Cystic fibrosis	Medical management
Gastroesophageal reflux	Medical management
Nocturnal seizure	Anticonvulsants
Periodic leg movements of sleep	Iron replacement therapy; dopamine agonists; gabapentin
Environment	
Co-sleeping, noise, pets	Education, safety issues

Abbreviation: CPAP, continuous positive airway pressure.
Adapted with permission from Givan DC. The sleepy child. *Pediatr Clin North Am*. 2004;51(1):15–31.

needs to be differentiated from weakness or fatigue. The major sleep disorders causing primary hypersomnia in children are narcolepsy and idiopathic hypersomnia.

Narcolepsy

Narcolepsy is a potentially disabling syndrome of irresistible daytime sleep attacks, abnormally fast transitions to REM sleep from awake, and disrupted nighttime sleep. Narcolepsy is seen in children, but peak age of

Table 28-5. Excessive Sleepiness in Children—Causes of Increased Sleep Drive

Diagnosis	Prevalence	Treatment
Temporary Hypersomnolence		
Acute medical illness	Common	No specific treatment
Illicit drug use	Common	Elimination of causative agent
Medications	Common	Elimination of causative agent, use of stimulants as needed
Recurrent Hypersomnolence		
Depression	Common	Antidepressants
Kleine-Levin syndrome	Rare	Lithium; carbamazepine; monitor serum levels for both drugs
Menstruation related	Rare	Oral contraceptives
Persistent Hypersomnolence		
Narcolepsy	0.2%	Stimulant medications, attention to sleep hygiene, treatment of co-existing sleep problems
Idiopathic hypersomnolence	Unknown	Stimulant medication

Adapted with permission from Givan DC. The sleepy child. *Pediatr Clin North Am*. 2004;51(1):15–31.

onset of symptoms is 15 to 25 years. As many as one-third of adults with narcolepsy report onset of symptoms before 15 years of age, but diagnosis is frequently delayed at least a decade. Loss of muscle tone with emotions while awake (cataplexy), inability to move for a few seconds to minutes on awakening (sleep paralysis), and visual aura or dream states while falling asleep (hypnagogic hallucinations), along with EDS, make up the complete narcolepsy tetrad seen in 30% of affected people. Cataplexy, or brief episodes of bilateral muscle weakness usually associated with laughter or strong emotion, may result in falling, head bobbing, or jaw sagging. It is highly specific to narcolepsy but may not be seen in more than 50% of patients. Approximately 90% of patients with narcolepsy with cataplexy test positive for HLA-DQB1*06:02. Absence of HLA-DQB1*06:02 does not exclude the diagnosis of narcolepsy, especially without cataplexy. Also, given that 20% of the general population tests positive for HLA-DQB1*06:02, this test is not specific for narcolepsy in patients with

EDS. Diagnosis of narcolepsy without documented cataplexy can be made by overnight PSG that shows absence of other sleep diagnoses and by a multiple sleep latency test (5 nap opportunities, separated by 2 hours, immediately following the overnight sleep study) that shows rapid sleep-onset periods (mean, <8 minutes) with at least 2 naps containing REM sleep. Differential diagnosis includes hydrocephalus, post-viral infection (mononucleosis), previous CNS trauma, or idiopathic hypersomnia. Recent research shows that narcolepsy with cataplexy results from the loss of approximately 70,000 hypothalamic neurons producing the neuropeptide hypocretin.

Narcolepsy treatment may include the use of stimulants such as modafinil or methylphenidate to address EDS and the use of antidepressants such as venlafaxine to control cataplexy. Sodium oxybate (Xyrem) treats both EDS and cataplexy in adults with narcolepsy. In addition, treatment may include ensuring adequate overnight sleep, 2 to 3 planned 30-minute daytime naps, and timing of activities at optimal hours of alertness.[42] Education of the patient, family members, and school personnel is important. Support for handling the difficulties of this lifelong chronic condition is such that referral to a pediatric sleep disorders center is indicated. Primary care clinicians may be required to monitor adherence to medications for participation in activities such as sports, school testing, and driving.

Idiopathic Hypersomnia

Idiopathic hypersomnia is a disorder of constant and severe EDS, despite adequate nocturnal sleep. Idiopathic hypersomnia is, by definition, a diagnosis of exclusion. A complete evaluation for other causes of hypersomnia must be undertaken, including neurological disorders (hydrocephalus or CNS tumors), primary sleep disorders (OSA), mood disorders, chronic fatigue syndrome, and medical disorders (acute and chronic infections including mononucleosis, metabolic disorders, and muscle diseases). Although the mean sleep latency is short in patients with idiopathic hypersomnia, similar to narcolepsy, affected patients do not have the 2 sleep-onset REM periods that characterize narcolepsy. Treatment of idiopathic hypersomnia includes attention to sleep hygiene issues, use of stimulant medications, and thorough review of safety issues such as driving or operating machinery.[43]

AAP Policy

American Academy of Pediatrics Task Force on Sudden Infant Death Syndrome. SIDS and other sleep-related infant deaths: updated 2016 recommendations for a safe infant sleeping environment. *Pediatrics.* 2016:138(5):e20162938 (pediatrics.aappublications. org/content/138/5/e20162938)

Marcus CL, Brooks LJ, Draper KA, et al. Clinical practice guideline: diagnosis and management of childhood obstructive sleep apnea syndrome. *Pediatrics.* 2012; 130(3):576–584 (pediatrics.aappublications.org/content/130/3/576)

Marcus CL, Brooks LJ, Draper KA, et al. Diagnosis and management of childhood obstructive sleep apnea syndrome. *Pediatrics.* 2012;130(3):e714–e755 (pediatrics. aappublications.org/content/130/3/e714)

Owens J; American Academy of Pediatrics Adolescent Sleep Working Group and Committee on Adolescence. Insufficient sleep in adolescents and young adults: an update on causes and consequences. *Pediatrics.* 2014;134(3):e921–e934 (pediatrics. aappublications.org/content/134/3/e921)

References

1. Meltzer LJ, Johnson C, Crosette J, Ramos M, Mindell JA. Prevalence of diagnosed sleep disorders in pediatric primary care practices. *Pediatrics.* 2010;125(6):e1410–e1418
2. Liu X, Buysse DJ, Gentzler AL, et al. Insomnia and hypersomnia associated with depressive phenomenology and comorbidity in childhood depression. *Sleep.* 2007; 30(1):83–90
3. Goldstein TR, Bridge JA, Brent DA. Sleep disturbance preceding completed suicide in adolescents. *J Consult Clin Psychol.* 2008;76(1):84–91
4. Minde K, Faucon A, Falkner S. Sleep problems in toddlers: effects of treatment on their daytime behavior. *J Am Acad Child Adolesc Psychiatry.* 1994;33(8):1114–1121
5. Riter S, Wills L. Sleep wars: research and opinion. *Pediatr Clin North Am.* 2004; 51(1):1–13
6. American Academy of Pediatrics Task Force on Sudden Infant Death Syndrome. SIDS and other sleep-related infant deaths: updated 2016 recommendations for a safe infant sleeping environment. *Pediatrics.* 2016;138(5):e20162938
7. Anders TF. Night-waking in infants during the first year of life. *Pediatrics.* 1979;63(6):860–864
8. Gartner LM, Morton J, Lawrence RA, et al; American Academy of Pediatrics Section on Breastfeeding. Breastfeeding and the use of human milk. *Pediatrics.* 2005;115(2):496–506
9. Pinilla T, Birch LL. Help me make it through the night: behavioral entrainment of breast-fed infants' sleep patterns. *Pediatrics.* 1993;91(12):436–444
10. St James-Roberts I, Sleep J, Morris S, Owen C, Gillham P. Use of a behavioural programme in the first 3 months to prevent infant crying and sleeping problems. *J Paediatr Child Health.* 2001;37(3):289–297
11. Nikolopoulou M, St James-Roberts I. Preventing sleeping problems in infants who are at risk of developing them. *Arch Dis Child.* 2003;88(2):108–111

12. Blyton DM, Sullivan CE, Edwards N. Lactation is associated with an increase in slow-wave sleep in women. *J Sleep Res.* 2002;11(4):297–303

13. Cubero J, Narciso D, Terrón P, et al. Chrononutrition applied to formula milks to consolidate infants' sleep/wake cycle. *Neuro Endocrinol Lett.* 2007;28(4):360–366

14. Blader JC, Koplewicz HS, Abikoff H, Foley C. Sleep problems of elementary school children. A community survey. *Arch Pediatr Adolesc Med.* 1997;151(5):473–480

15. Parmelee AH, Wenner WH, Schulz HR. Infant sleep patterns: from birth to 16 weeks of age. *J Pediatr.* 1964;65:576–582

16. Owens JA, Mindell JA. Pediatric insomnia. *Pediatr Clin North Am.* 2011;58(3): 555–569

17. Kuhn BR, Elliott AJ. Treatment efficacy in behavioral pediatric sleep medicine. *J Psychosom Res.* 2003;54(6):587–597

18. Ivanenko A, Barnes ME, Crabtree VM, Gozal D. Psychiatric symptoms in children with insomnia referred to a pediatric sleep medicine center. *Sleep Med.* 2004;5(3): 253–259

19. Gregory AM, Rijsdijk FV, Lau JY, Dahl RE, Eley TC. The direction of longitudinal associations between sleep problems and depression symptoms: a study of twins aged 8 and 10 years. *Sleep.* 2009;32(2):189–199

20. Dahl RE, Ryan ND, Matty MK, et al. Sleep onset abnormalities in depressed adolescents. *Biol Psychiatry.* 1996;39(6):400–410

21. Ivanenko A. Sleep and mood disorders in children and adolescents. In: Ivanenko A, ed. *Sleep and Psychiatric Disorders in Children and Adolescents.* New York, NY: Informa Healthcare USA Inc; 2008:279–292

22. Kupfer DJ. Pathophysiology and management of insomnia during depression. *Ann Clin Psychiatry.* 1999;11(4):267–276

23. Lofthouse N, Gilchrist R, Splaingard M. Mood-related sleep problems in children and adolescents. *Child Adolesc Psychiatr Clin N Am.* 2009;18(4):893–916

24. Glod CA, Teicher MH, Hartman CR, Harakal T. Increased nocturnal activity and impaired sleep maintenance in abused children. *J Am Acad Child Adolesc Psychiatry.* 1997;36(9):1236–1243

25. Wiggs L, Stores G. Severe sleep disturbance and daytime challenging behaviour in children with severe learning disabilities. *J Intellect Disabil Res.* 1996;40(pt 6): 518–528

26. Cortese S, Konofal E, Yateman N, Mouren MC, Lecendreux M. Sleep and alertness in children with attention-deficit/hyperactivity disorder: a systematic review of the literature. *Sleep.* 2006;29(4):504–511

27. Prince JB, Wilens TE, Biederman J, Spencer TJ, Wozniak JR. Clonidine for sleep disturbances associated with attention-deficit hyperactivity disorder: a systematic chart review of 62 cases. *J Am Acad Child Adolesc Psychiatry.* 1996;35(5):599–605

28. Johnson KP, Giannotti F, Cortesi F. Sleep patterns in autism spectrum disorders. *Child Adolesc Psychiatr Clin N Am.* 2009;18(4):917–928

29. Stores G, Ellis AJ, Wiggs L, Crawford C, Thomson A. Sleep and psychological disturbance in nocturnal asthma. *Arch Dis Child.* 1998;78(5):413–419

30. Splaingard M. Sleep problems in children with respiratory disorders. *Sleep Med Clin.* 2008;3(4):589–600

31. Piazza CC, Fisher WW, Sherer M. Treatment of multiple sleep problems in children with developmental disabilities: faded bedtime with response cost versus bedtime scheduling. *Dev Med Child Neurol.* 1997;39(6):414–418

32. Zamir G, Press J, Tal A, Tarasiuk A. Sleep fragmentation in children with juvenile rheumatoid arthritis. *J Rheumatol.* 1998;25(6):1191–1197

33. Pelayo R, Chen W, Monzon S, Guilleminault C. Pediatric sleep pharmacology: you want to give my kid sleeping pills? *Pediatr Clin North Am.* 2004;51(1):117–134

34. Marcus CL. Sleep-disordered breathing in children. *Am J Respir Crit Care Med.* 2011;164(1):16–30

35. Brooks LJ, Olsen MN, Bacevice AM, Beebe A, Konstantinopoulou S, Taylor HG. Relationship between sleep, sleep apnea, and neuropsychological function in children with Down syndrome. *Sleep Breath.* 2015;19(1):197–204

36. Mitchell RB. Adenotonsillectomy for obstructive sleep apnea in children: outcome evaluated by pre- and postoperative polysomnography. *Laryngoscope.* 2007; 117(10):1844–1854

37. Bhattacharjee R, Kheirandish-Gozal L, Spruyt K, et al. Adenotonsillectomy outcomes in treatment of obstructive sleep apnea in children: a multicenter retrospective study. *Am J Respir Crit Care Med.* 2010;182(5):676–683

38. McColley SA, April MM, Carroll JL, Naclerio RM, Loughlin GM. Respiratory compromise after adenotonsillectomy in children with obstructive sleep apnea. *Arch Otolaryngol Head Neck Surg.* 1992;118(9):940–943

39. Laberge L, Tremblay RE, Vitaro F, Montplaisir J. Development of parasomnias from childhood to early adolescence. *Pediatrics.* 2000;106(1, pt 1):67–74

40. Anders TF, Eiben LA. Pediatric sleep disorders: a review of the past 10 years. *J Am Acad Child Adolesc Psychiatry.* 1997;36(1):9–20

41. Picchietti D, Allen RP, Walters AS, Davidson JE, Myers A, Ferini-Strambi L. Restless legs syndrome: prevalence and impact in children and adolescents—the Peds REST study. *Pediatrics.* 2007;120(2):253–266

42. Aran A, Einen M, Lin L, Plazzi G, Nishino S, Mignot E. Clinical and therapeutic aspects of childhood narcolepsy-cataplexy: a retrospective study of 51 children. *Sleep.* 2010;33(11):1457–1464

43. Sheldon SH, Ferber R, Kryger MH. *Principles and Practice of Pediatric Sleep Medicine.* Philadelphia, PA: Elsevier Saunders; 2005

CHAPTER 29

Speech and Language Concerns

Maris Rosenberg, MD, and Nancy Tarshis, MA, MS, CCC-SLP

> "Speech and language delays may be associated with impairments limited to the domains of speech and language or may signal the presence of primary conditions such as hearing loss, intellectual disability, emotional-behavioral disturbance, or social cognitive disorders such as autism spectrum disorder and social communication disorder."

Introduction

Speech and language delay, arguably the most common developmental concern parents have about their young children, occurs with an estimated prevalence of 2% to 19%.[1-5] The delay can occur alone or signal the presence of other developmental disorders, such as intellectual disability, autism spectrum disorder (ASD), or hearing loss. Children with speech and language impairments are well-known to be at risk for developmental disorders that negatively affect learning, but they are also at greater risk for emotional and behavioral disorders of internalizing and externalizing types. As such, speech and language impairments have known academic, social, and behavioral implications, making early recognition and intervention essential.

In keeping with the recommendations of the American Academy of Pediatrics (AAP),[6] the pediatric primary care clinician (PCC)—that is, the pediatrician, family physician, nurse practitioner, or physician assistant who provides frontline, longitudinal health care to young children—should perform developmental surveillance and screening to identify children at risk, refer for appropriate evaluation, and implement intervention as early as possible. Parents commonly focus on their child's verbal communication and consult the PCC when there are concerns about speaking, yet language reception deficits can be more far-reaching and impactful. A working knowledge of risk factors for communication delays, normal speech and language milestones, and red flags for language delays and associated developmental and behavioral problems is essential in providing appropriate pediatric primary care.[7]

A summary of typically acquired speech and language milestones is presented in Table 29-1.

Table 29-1. Developmental Milestones	
Age	**Developmental Milestones**
0–6 mo	Cooing
	Babbling
	Differentiated cries
6–9 mo	Canonical babbling (reduplicated babbling [eg, "bababa"])
	Response to name
	Comprehension of familiar words in context
9–15 mo	First words
	Directed point (initially with hand, then with 1 finger)
18–24 mo	Uses own name
	2-word sentences (by 24 mo)
	Knows 5 body parts
24–30 mo	Pretend play with familiar objects
	3-word sentences
	Points to action words in pictures
	Answers simple, concrete "wh-" questions (eg, who, what)
	Uses ≥50 words
30–36 mo	Names most familiar things and pictures
	Begins to recognize same and different
	Helps tell a familiar story
	Uses descriptive words (adjectives)
	Uses 200–1,000 words
	Speech is nearly all intelligible to any listener.

Table 29-1. Developmental Milestones (*continued*)	
Age	Developmental Milestones
3–4 y	Comprehends 1,000 words
	Points to common objects by function
	Responds to commands involving 2 actions
	Uses at least 800 words
	Responds to simple how questions
	Asks what and who questions
	Uses plurals and verb tense markers
	Talks about events out of the here and now
4–5 y	Understands most of what is said to him or her
	Tells a personal story with a beginning, middle, and end
	Can listen and answer questions about a story
	Speech is fully intelligible.
	Can recognize and produce rhymes

Language Development

Language, as the primary vehicle for communication, is a socially shared code or conventional system for representing concepts through an arbitrary set of rule-governed symbols (speech sounds and phonemes) and symbol combinations. A social tool through which we share ideas and rules of behavior and develop our attachments to people and places, language is a rule-governed yet generative system that permits speakers to create an endless number of meaningful utterances to communicate thoughts, feelings, information, and ideas, as well as a tool to self-regulate. The ability to use language to think about behavior is pertinent to planning, organizing, and problem-solving in the moment and to imagining the consequence of words and action. Therefore, language competence and behavior are closely linked.

Risk Factors for Language Delays

Risk factors for language delays are similar to those for developmental disorders in general. In a review for the US Preventive Services Task Force (USPSTF), the most common risk factors reported were a family history of speech and language delay, male sex, and perinatal factors. Other, less commonly, reported risk factors included educational level of the parents, childhood illness, and family size.[5] A careful history eliciting any prenatal, perinatal, or postnatal adverse events and a detailed family history focusing on developmental disorders, academic achievement, and social functioning are essential in determining which children are at greater risk. Environmental factors clearly play a role in determining language development. Children who live in disadvantaged environments with less language stimulation and greater psychosocial stress are at greater risk for language delay than are children from more advantaged backgrounds.

Table 29-2 states the red flags in language and play that may signal the existence of a language or another developmental disorder.

Table 29-2. Red Flags in Language and Play	
Age	**Warning Signs and Red Flags**
0–12 mo: play	Restricted repertoire of skills
	Does not follow objects that fall
	Little purposeful play
	Reduced or absent imitation
	Reduced object permanence
	No interactive games
0–12 mo: sensory motor	Does not reach or swat at objects
	Overly reactive to stimuli
	Extreme irritability
0–12 mo: social-emotional	Overly clingy
	No apparent attachments
	No awareness of danger
	Difficulty modulating emotions
	Reduced range of affect

Table 29-2. Red Flags in Language and Play (*continued*)

Age	Warning Signs and Red Flags
0–12 mo: speech and language	Difficulty sucking and feeding
	Averts gaze
	Fails to make a variety of sounds
	Fails to respond to name
	Undifferentiated crying
12–24 mo: play	No container play
	No early problem-solving
	Does not go to adults for help
	Very rigid play
	Focuses on irrelevant parts of toys such as wheels of car
	Does not include adults in play; prefers to play alone
	No interest in playing symbolically
	No spontaneous pretend play
	Restricted range of interests
	No early problem-solving
12–24 mo: social-emotional	Short attention span
	Does not seek to engage with others
	Tunes out
	Avoids eye contact
12–24 mo: speech and language	No specific *mama* or *dada*
	Does not point
	Cannot follow simple directives without gesture
	Reduced vocabulary
	No word combinations
24–36 mo: play	Little or no symbolic play
	Not able to sequence events in play
	Not interested in playing with peers
	Restricted range of skills and interests
	Lines up toys rather than playing with them

Table 29-2. Red Flags in Language and Play (*continued*)	
Age	**Warning Signs and Red Flags**
24–36 mo: speech and language	Avoids eye contact
	Reduced communicative intent
	Difficulty following directions
	Lack of verbal expression
	Reduced reciprocity and turn-taking
	Talking better than listening
	Poor conversation skills
3–4 y: play	Cannot take turns or play cooperatively with peers (prefers solitary play)
	Little interest in toys
	Insists on sameness in routine
	No idea how to approach new skills or toys
	Cannot use blocks to build simple structures
3–4 y: language	Does not engage in back-and-forth communication for purely social reasons
	Does not talk about what communicative partners are talking about
	Uses language that is repetitive or recycled from other contexts
4–5 y: play	Cannot follow simple rules in play
	Prefers solitary play
	Insists on sameness in play
	Reacts strongly to change
	Does not engage in symbolic or imaginative play
	Does not integrate other children in play
4–5 y: language	Weak ability to hold a conversation
	Cannot tell a personal narrative
	Difficulty with sequencing information
	Uses language that is repetitive or recycled from other contexts

Role of the Primary Care Clinician: Surveillance and Screening

Performing developmental surveillance at all health supervision visits implies eliciting parental concerns, acknowledging risk and protective factors, performing longitudinal observations, and keeping an accurate, ongoing record.

The use of standardized general developmental screening instruments is recommended at ages 9, 18, and 30 months or whenever concerns arise in the course of surveillance.[6] In addition, the recommendation for screening for ASD at 18 and 24 months allows additional insight into the development of communication and social skills. After a systematic review in 2006,[5,8,9] the USPSTF concluded that there is no single screening instrument that serves as a criterion standard for screening specifically for language disorders, and there were no universally agreed-on recommendations for age or interval for speech and language screening. However, it is generally agreed that use of standardized screening instruments can assist the PCC in assessing a young child's general development and making decisions as to whether referral for further evaluation by developmental or speech-language specialists would be appropriate. A resource provided by the AAP Developmental Screening Task Force provides guidance for clinicians in conducting developmental surveillance and screening in primary care.[6]

Given the known association between language and behavioral disorders, the use of screening instruments targeting behavior can provide valuable insight into accompanying behavioral disorders when a language problem is identified or suspected. Screening instruments vary in format and applicability to particular populations.[9] Appendix 2, Mental Health Tools for Pediatrics, summarizes features of social-emotional and mental health screening tools used commonly in primary care settings.

Appendix 2 also lists tools appropriate for further primary care assessment of speech and language problems identified (or suspected) through developmental or behavioral screening, clinical history, or observations: hearing screen (if not done previously); Capute Scales (CAT, Cognitive Adaptive Test; CLAMS, Clinical Linguistic & Auditory Milestone Scale), Early Language Milestone Scale, Second Edition (ELM Scale-2), and the Language Developmental Survey.

Language Disorders

A language disorder as defined by the American Speech-Language and Hearing Association can be classified as any disturbance to an individual's ability to develop and produce spoken or written language. This disturbance encompasses both the ability to comprehend and the ability to express language at an age-appropriate level. Language disorders, both developmental and acquired, represent a heterogeneous set of difficulties that range from mild to severe. Children with receptive language deficits have difficulty comprehending language. Of note, a receptive deficit is rarely seen in isolation, and in typical development, comprehension precedes expression of new and more mature language forms. Difficulty with comprehension manifests as reduced understanding of conversation and problems both with following directions and with interpreting the intentions of others, as well as difficulty interpreting what one reads. Receptive language generally develops in advance of expressive language, except in very rare circumstances (eg, hydrocephalus, severe language processing disorder, ASD and other social cognitive disorders). Children with expressive language deficits have problems using language to express their most basic wants and needs as well as their more sophisticated thoughts, feelings, and intentions. They may have a hard time putting words into sentences; sentences may be simple and short with confused syntax or verb tense errors, or they may have difficulty finding the right words. A child's vocabulary might be below the level of vocabulary of other children the same age, or the child might use words and phrases repetitively or pick up scripts from videos, commercials, and television. Language impairment might also become apparent as a deficit in stringing sentences together to tell a cohesive story or personal narrative.

A language disorder can be characterized by deficits in the form (comprehension and expression of linguistic rules and syntax), the content (vocabulary and semantics), or the use (discourse pragmatics) of language. Difficulty acquiring and using the rules applicable to the sounds, words, phrases, and sentences or the surface features of what is being said constitutes a deficit in the *form* of language. For children with disorders of *content,* speaking may come easily, but often what they have to say lacks substance. Their discourse is missing the essential ingredients such as objects, events, relations between people, and cultural references that give meaning to the utterance. Pragmatic deficits result in weakness in language *use*, in managing and understanding the why, when, and where aspects of discourse. Children with this difficulty have a hard time selecting and maintaining topics, taking turns in conversation, choosing style of speech to match the listener or context, using intonation to signal intention, and understanding the nonverbal aspects of language such as proximity, body posture, facial expression, and flexible gaze shifting.

Children with primarily pragmatic-based deficits often fall under the rubric of social communication disorder.[10] Social communication disorder involves communication deficits not attributable to extreme language or cognitive impairment, ASD, or emotional-behavioral disorder. It can manifest as a deficit in social competency and will affect a child's ability to initiate and sustain interpersonal relationships in addition to resulting in its known academic consequences. Social pragmatic language disorders can lead to profound deficits and underachievement despite average cognitive or academic scores. These deficits affect the development of social relationships, learning from context, and generalizing information (both interpersonal and academic) from context to context. Most important, pragmatic deficits shape emotional-behavioral responses secondary to identity and self-regulation issues. Reduced ability to conceptualize the impact of words and action and project their consequences is a clear impediment to the development of prosocial behavior.

The distinction between social communication disorder and ASD requires assessment via criterion standard instruments (eg, Autism Diagnostic Observation Scale[11]) as well as a sophisticated evaluation by a speech-language pathologist (SLP). Speech and language assessment should tease out the influence of processing style or language weakness or both on the overall social communicative ability of the child. Often it is the job of the SLP to explain whether the social deficit is the primary problem or whether the social symptoms are secondary and attributable to overall language weakness.

There is increasing evidence that children with specific language impairments experience diverse emotional and behavioral problems. Such evidence is summarized in a 2013 meta-analysis[12] that revealed that children with speech and language impairment were twice as likely to show clinically significant internalizing (eg, anxiety, depression), externalizing (disruptive behavioral disorders), and attentional symptoms than were children with typical language development. Symptom severity for all 3 of these diagnostic categories was also increased.

Language-based learning disabilities, another group of important sequelae of specific language impairment, present as problems with reading, spelling, or writing in addition to the aforementioned oral language deficits. Typically, children with such disabilities have trouble expressing ideas, finding words, learning new vocabulary, comprehending questions, following directions, and retaining written material. They struggle with learning the alphabet, spelling rules, multiplication tables, and other rote-memorized information, all struggles of which make it difficult to achieve academically.

Speech Disorders

Speech disorders manifest as articulation errors past the age of expectation. *Articulation* is the movement of the speech mechanism (palate, lips, tongue, jaw, and larynx) to create sound. *Phonology* is the rule system that governs how speech sounds interact with one another. A child with a lisp has a problem with articulation; a child who substitutes all *k* sounds with *t* ("otay" for *okay*) has a phonological problem. For pediatricians, knowing when to refer for evaluation is key. As a guideline, a 2-year-old should be 50% intelligible; a 3-year-old, 75%; and a 4-year-old, fully intelligible to a stranger, not just family and familiar adults.

A child might present with speech problems for several reasons. Some errors are developmental and will resolve in time, and others will need intervention. Some errors are related to the architecture of the mouth, and others are rule-based errors (phonological). If the errors persist, or the child expresses frustration, an evaluation is in order. Evidence suggests that speech disorders alone can be associated with behavioral disturbance and impaired social relationships.[13,14] Inability to be understood, as in the case of children with severe intelligibility deficits (eg, apraxia or other speech sound disorder), will necessarily affect the ability to express one's needs, thoughts, and feelings and therefore have a negative impact on self-regulation.

When a child makes errors that are inconsistent, a motor speech disorder should be suspected. Apraxia is a motor speech disorder caused by a difficulty planning and executing speech sounds that cannot be attributed to muscle weakness or paralysis. Key characteristics include limited repertoire of vowels and vowel errors. The error patterns are typically highly variable, with unusual and idiosyncratic error patterns. Errors increase with the length and complexity of utterances, such as in multisyllabic or phonetically challenging words. If apraxia is suspected, a child should be evaluated as soon as possible because the earlier intervention begins, the better the outcome. *Stuttering* or *dysfluency* is a speech disorder characterized by breaks in fluency that can affect sounds, syllables, or words. In young children, there can be a period of normal dysfluency between 2 and 4 years of age. The decision to refer for evaluation should be based on how long dysfluency has persisted, whether there is a family history, the type of repetitions, and secondary behaviors. Indications for evaluation include dysfluency that persists for more than 6 months, family history of stuttering, awareness of difficulty, or anxiety or frustration related to speaking. In addition, if breaks in fluency are partial words, single sounds, silent, or accompanied by any secondary or atypical behaviors, or if the balance of dysfluent speech to fluent speech is more than 10% of the overall communication, evaluation should be initiated.

Differential Diagnosis

Delays in speech and language milestones are often the first indication of the presence of a developmental disorder, and they may be accompanied by the behavioral sequelae of these disorders. Hearing loss is an important consideration in any child who exhibits delayed acquisition of language milestones or unclear or atypical patterns of speech. Careful history and observation may suggest accompanying delays in other domains indicating more global involvement, as in cases of intellectual disability. Subtle delays in communication can be apparent even before verbal communication is questioned. The phenomenon of joint attention, as evidenced by gaze sharing or pointing, can be documented as early as 8 to 10 months of age. The absence of joint attention, such as lack of directed pointing with a clear look back for follow (by age 12 months), should alert the physician to the possibility of ASD. When early language milestones are present without the ability to use them in reciprocal interactions, a social communication disorder should be considered. Seen in the absence of restricted behaviors or repetitive behaviors (or both) indicative of ASD, the possibility of a diagnosis of social communication disorder should be further investigated by an SLP. When hearing loss, intellectual disability, social communication, or ASD is ruled out, the diagnosis of *specific language impairment* refers to the developmental disorders affecting primarily receptive, expressive, or mixed receptive-expressive language impairments, whereas *phonological disorders* refer to conditions affecting the clarity of speech.

Therapeutic Considerations: What the Primary Care Clinician Needs to Know

Once a speech and language delay is suspected, referral for diagnostic evaluation is critical to determine the extent of impairment, characterize the nature of the disability, and suggest strategies for intervention. The PCC should discuss the suspected speech and language impairment in the context of present and future concomitants such as learning and behavioral problems. Parents should be reassured that prompt evaluation and intervention can mitigate the effects of the disability. Suggested resources for parents include *Language Delay,* a fact sheet developed by the AAP, available at www.healthychildren.org/English/ages-stages/toddler/Pages/Language-Delay.aspx, and the Web site of the American Speech-Language Hearing Association (www.asha.org).

Referral for early intervention evaluation for newborns, infants, and children from birth to age 3 years, or to the Department of Education for children 3 years and older, offers a means of evaluation within a mandated time frame and services based on the evaluation results. Ideally, this evaluation is conducted by a multidisciplinary team, on which the SLP plays a key role. The SLP will gather information regarding communication across a variety of contexts. He or she will evaluate the child's ability to comprehend directions, stories, and other communication as well as the child's vocabulary, grammar, and syntax and use of language for a variety of purposes. In certain circumstances, on the basis of the presenting problems, speech sound development, literacy skills, writing, reading comprehension, and fluency will also be evaluated. This assessment should contain informal components such as pretend play of young children and conversation and storytelling of older children. Formal testing with standardized instruments can corroborate and elucidate informal findings and should always be considered.

The PCC should order a formal hearing test to be done by an audiologist. Speech and language therapy should not be delayed pending definitive audiological evaluation, however, because it may take months for an uncooperative child to have a hearing test completed. A formal hearing test should be ordered as part of the multidisciplinary evaluation, and hearing status should be followed according to recommendations of the audiologist as therapy progresses.

Any child with significant exposure to a second language or dialect is considered bilingually exposed. Regardless of the type of exposure, simultaneous or sequential, such a child must be evaluated in both languages to determine the presence or absence of language impairment. Many children who are bilingually exposed may go through a short period of language loss, especially if recently exposed to a new language. There may be a delay in mastering some grammatical aspects of both languages, and vocabulary may be judged to be insufficient if words in both languages are not considered. Such children should be assessed by a qualified *bilingual* SLP. If a language impairment is documented in a bilingually exposed child, it is important to determine the dominant language when initiating therapy.

Prognosis

A multitude of factors determine the outcome of children with speech and language impairments. Important considerations include nonverbal intelligence, type and degree of language disability, and response to intervention. Preschool-aged children with primarily expressive phonological impairments tend to have a lower risk for later reading problems than do those who demonstrate difficulty with phonological awareness (eg, rhyming, letter-sound association).

It is generally agreed that children with language problems that persist until kindergarten entry have a high risk for continuing problems throughout the school years.[3] Also, children identified with communication impairments at age 4 to 5 years are likely to have significantly more difficulty in reading, writing, and overall academic achievement at ages 7 to 9 years; more difficulty with peer relationships; and less satisfaction with school than their contemporaries have.[15] Parents should be counseled that providing a language-rich environment, stressing verbal interaction and literacy, is recommended, in addition to specific therapy, to mediate the effects of a language delay. Primary care clinicians are advised to heighten surveillance for academic and mental health problems in children who experience early language problems.

Conclusion

Speech and language delays are common and are readily detected in the context of the developmental surveillance and screening that are part of primary pediatric care. Evidence suggests that speech and language disorders are often accompanied by significant learning disorders, weaknesses in self-regulation, and secondary emotional and behavioral deficits. Speech and language delays may be associated with impairments limited to the domains of speech and language or may signal the presence of primary conditions such as hearing loss, intellectual disability, emotional-behavioral disturbance, or social cognitive disorders such as ASD and social communication disorder. Using the knowledge of risk factors and attention to red flags suggesting these disorders is the first step to referral for appropriate evaluation and interventions. The PCC's goal should be to minimize associated difficulties with learning and behavior and lessen the impact of communication weakness on the development of peer relations and social interactions across all the contexts of home and school.

AAP Policy

American Academy of Pediatrics Council on Children With Disabilities, Section on Developmental and Behavioral Pediatrics, Bright Futures Steering Committee, and Medical Home Initiatives for Children With Special Needs Project Advisory Committee. Identifying infants and young children with developmental disorders in the medical home: an algorithm for developmental surveillance and screening. *Pediatrics.* 2006;118(1):405–420. Reaffirmed August 2014 (pediatrics.aappublications. org/content/118/1/405)

References

1. Pinborough-Zimmerman J, Satterfield R, Miller J, Bilder D, Hossain S, McMahon W. Communication disorders: prevalence and comorbid intellectual disability, autism, and emotional/behavioral disorders. *Am J Speech Lang Pathol.* 2007;16(4): 359–367

2. McLeod S, Harrison LJ. Epidemiology of speech and language impairment in a nationally representative sample of 4- to 5-year-old children. *J Speech Lang Hear Res.* 2009;52(5):1213–1229

3. Simms MD. Language disorders in children: classification and clinical syndromes. *Pediatr Clin North Am.* 2007;54(3):437–467

4. McQuiston S, Kloczko N. Speech and language development: monitoring process and problems. *Pediatr Rev.* 2011;32(6):230–238

5. Nelson HD, Nygren P, Walker M, Panoscha R. Screening for speech and language delay in preschool children: systematic evidence review for the US Preventive Services Task Force. *Pediatrics.* 2006;117(2):e298–e319

6. American Academy of Pediatrics Council on Children With Disabilities, Section on Developmental and Behavioral Pediatrics, Bright Futures Steering Committee, and Medical Home Initiatives for Children With Special Needs Project Advisory Committee. Identifying infants and young children with developmental disorders in the medical home: an algorithm for developmental surveillance and screening. *Pediatrics.* 2006;118(1):405–420

7. Schum RL. Language screening in the pediatric office setting. *Pediatr Clin North Am.* 2007;54(3):425–436

8. US Preventive Services Task Force. Screening for speech and language delay in preschool children: recommendation statement. *Pediatrics.* 2006;117(2):497–501

9. Drotar D, Stancin T, Dworkin PH, Sices L, Wood S. Selecting developmental surveillance and screening tools. *Pediatr Rev.* 2008;29(10):e52–e58

10. Frazier TW, Youngstrom EA, Speer L, et al. Validation of proposed *DSM-5* criteria for autism spectrum disorder. *J Am Acad Child Adolesc Psychiatry.* 2012;51(1): 28–40

11. Lord C, Rutter M, DeLavore PC, Risi S. *Autism Diagnostic Observation Schedule.* Los Angeles, CA: Western Psychological Services; 1989

12. Yew SG, O'Kearney R. Emotional and behavioural outcomes later in childhood and adolescence for children with specific language impairments: meta-analyses of controlled prospective studies. *J Child Psychol Psychiatry.* 2013;54(5):516–524

13. Teverovsky EG, Bickel JO, Feldman HM. Functional characteristics of children diagnosed with childhood apraxia of speech. *Disabil Rehabil.* 2009;31(2):94–102

14. McCormack J, McLeod S, Harrison LJ, McAllister L. The impact of speech impairment in early childhood: investigating parents' and speech-language pathologists' perspectives using the ICF-CY. *J Commun Disord.* 2010;43(5): 378–396

15. McCormack J, Harrison LJ, McLeod S, McAllister L. A nationally representative study of the association between communication impairment at 4–5 years and children's life activities at 7–9 years. *J Speech Lang Hear Res.* 2011;54(5):1328–1348

CHAPTER 30

Substance Use 1:
Use of Tobacco and Nicotine

Susanne E. Tanski, MD, MPH

> "*Pediatric primary care clinicians are well positioned to interact with tobacco users, monitor their mental health, and assist in motivating them to improve their health by quitting tobacco completely.*"

Nicotine and Mental Health

Although not traditionally thought of as such, nicotine is a powerful psychotropic drug, affecting the mind, emotions, and behavior.[1] Without an associated intoxicated state or high, nicotine has been used as a self-dosed mood modifier for hundreds of years. It is highly addictive, requiring repeated and frequent dosing to prevent unpleasant withdrawal symptoms. The toll of nicotine use and addiction is high, however, with cigarettes arguably the deadliest consumer product ever created. Cigarettes have been carefully engineered to deliver nicotine quickly and efficiently to the brain to reinforce addiction, delivering a chemical cocktail of some 7,000 compounds that lead to disease and death.[2]

The association between tobacco and nicotine use and mental health problems is strong,[3] and tobacco use is often a marker for other psychosocial risks. Nicotine dependence has been associated with depression, anxiety, and disruptive behaviors.[4] Beyond defined nicotine dependence, cigarette use in particular has been shown to be more prevalent among adolescents with attention-deficit/hyperactivity disorder (commonly known as ADHD), oppositional defiant disorder, conduct disorder, social phobia, and substance use disorders.[5] Among adolescents, a relationship between cigarette use and depression has been demonstrated by numerous studies, with depressive symptoms predicting smoking onset and escalation and smoking predicting growth in depressive symptoms.[6] Similar links between e-cigarette use among youths and depression have also been reported.[7] (Note that the terms *youth* and *youths* are defined variably in the literature about substance use. In this chapter and the 2 that follow, *youths* will generally refer to preadolescents and adolescents aged 9–8 years. In some instances a study cited will provide an alternative definition.) Among adults (with whom more studies have been conducted), 20% have any mental illness, yet those with mental illness consume nearly 31% of the cigarettes smoked in the United States.[8] Historically, youths who use tobacco are also more likely to use other substances[9] and have substance use disorder[5]: youths who smoke cigarettes are 5 times more likely than nonsmokers to use alcohol, 13 times more likely to use marijuana, and 7 times more likely to use cocaine or heroin.[10]

With the high prevalence of depression, other mental health problems, and substance use among adolescents, it is critically important for pediatric primary care clinicians (PCCs) (ie, pediatricians, family physicians, internists, nurse practitioners, and physician assistants who provide frontline, longitudinal care to children and adolescents) to understand nicotine and tobacco prevention, use, and treatment as part of a comprehensive health approach.

Prevalence of Tobacco and Nicotine Use

Tobacco use remains the leading cause of preventable morbidity and mortality in the United States. Cigarette smoking, the most common form of tobacco use among US adults, leads to more than 480,000 premature deaths annually and has led to the premature death of more than 20 million people in the United States since 1964.[2] Worldwide, some 7 million people die from tobacco-related deaths each year.[11] The most recent US surgeon general's report (2014) concluded that if current smoking rates and onset continue, some 5.6 million Americans who are currently younger than 18 years will die prematurely from smoking-related disease.[2]

Combusted tobacco products (including cigarettes, cigars, cigarillos, water pipes [hookahs], bidis, kreteks, pipes, and roll-your-own) have been recognized as contributing to more substantial health risks than noncombusted products,[12] leading to deaths from cancers, cardiovascular diseases, stroke, diabetes mellitus, and respiratory diseases such as asthma, emphysema, and chronic obstructive pulmonary disease. Noncombusted products such as smokeless tobacco (eg, "dip," "chew,") and snus tobacco are not without significant harm, however, leading to oral health issues as well as death from head and neck cancers. The most recent electronic nicotine delivery systems (eg, e-cigarettes, vaping devices), which were purported as safer by their manufacturers, have not been determined to be low in health risk, and they are now being linked to critical cardiovascular and pulmonary functional declines.[13–15] No form of tobacco use is safe, particularly for adolescents; furthermore, there is no safe level of exposure to tobacco smoke or secondhand tobacco smoke.[2]

The prevalence of current cigarette smoking (defined as past 30 days) among US adults reached a peak of per-capita consumption prior to the US surgeon general's report in 1964 (Figure 30-1), and it has steadily

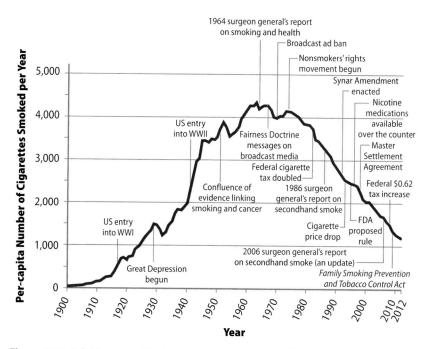

Figure 30-1. Adult[a] per-capita cigarette consumption and major smoking and health events, United States, 1900–2012.

Abbreviations: FDA, US Food and Drug Administration; WW, World War.

[a] Adults ≥18 years of age as reported annually by the US Census Bureau.

Adapted from Fifty years of change—1964–2014. In: Office on Smoking Health, National Center for Chronic Disease Prevention and Health Promotion. *The Health Consequences of Smoking: 50 Years of Progress; A Report of the Surgeon General.* Atlanta, GA: Centers for Disease Control and Prevention; 2014.

decreased over time, with current use (defined as use in the past 30 days) reaching a low of 15.1% in 2015, as reported by Jamal et al.[16] Among adolescents, rates of current use were highest in the 1990s, with concerted efforts to combat youth tobacco use corresponding with decreases in prevalence over time (Figure 30-2). Recent data from the National Youth Tobacco Survey showed that cigarette use among high school students has continued to decline, from 12.7% in 2013, as reported by Arrazola et al,[17] to 8.0% in 2016, as reported by Jamal et al.[18] Recent additions of newer tobacco products to the landscape had caused concern, with the current use of any tobacco product by high school students slowly increasing: in 2013, to 22.9%[17]; in 2014, to 24.6%[19]; and in 2015, to 25.3%.[20] Notably, this change had been caused by sharp increases in e-cigarette use: from 2011

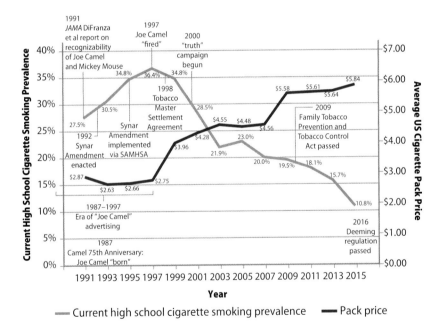

Figure 30-2. Graph showing trends in adolescent current cigarette use. Note the rapid decline in adolescent cigarette use from 1997 to present based on YRBS data. The second curve represents the mean rate of taxation in the United States across all states for a single pack of cigarettes, based on data aggregated by the Campaign for Tobacco-Free Kids (Tax Burden on Tobacco). Pivotal events in tobacco control are noted, including the 2009 Family Smoking Prevention and Tobacco Control Act, which created the Center for Tobacco Products at the FDA and authorized the FDA to oversee tobacco products.

Abbreviations: FDA, US Food and Drug Administration; SAMHSA, Substance Abuse and Mental Health Services Administration; YRBS, Youth Risk Behavior Survey.

to 2014, current e-cigarette use among high school students increased from 1.5% to 13.4%[19]; in 2015, it increased to 16%.[20] New data from 2016 has demonstrated a reversal, however, with any tobacco product use falling to 20.2% and significantly less combusted tobacco use at 13.8%.[18] Hookah use, another combusted tobacco product, has also increased among high school students over recent years (2011–2014), from 4.1% to 9.4%[19]; however, this use decreased in 2016 to 4.8%.[18]

The overall prevalence of tobacco use over time fails to demonstrate the significant disparities in tobacco use between groups based on socioeconomics, education, race and ethnicity, region of the country, and other demographics. Boys; people with lower educational attainment; those who live in poverty; those who identify as lesbian, gay, bisexual, or transgender; and Native American and Alaskan Inuit people have substantially higher rates of tobacco use.[21]

Tobacco Use in Adolescence and Young Adulthood

Most young people do not intentionally make the decision to start using tobacco, yet the decision can have significant, lifelong effects. Tobacco use has been aggressively marketed through traditional advertising as well as entertainment media, which has been found to be causally related to adolescent tobacco use.[22] Each day, more than 2,800 US preadolescents and adolescents aged 12 to 17 years try smoking for the first time,[2] with 10.9% of students reporting trying their first cigarette before age 13 years.[23] The likelihood of subsequent nicotine dependence and addiction is high, and symptoms of addiction appear soon after onset of smoking in some adolescents.[24–27] While daily smoking lags 2 to 3 years behind initiation,[28] roughly 700 adolescents transition to daily smoking each day,[2] and, historically, more than 60% of teen smokers still smoke 5 years later.[23,29,30] Although most of what is known about adolescent tobacco use involves cigarettes, a substantial proportion of tobacco use now occurs with tobacco products other than cigarettes, and many adolescents now use multiple products: recent data show that 51.3% of all high school students currently using tobacco use more than one type of tobacco product concurrently.[20] Many adolescents do not identify themselves as smokers,[31] with occasional, light, or intermediate smoking being common[32]; few adolescents expect to have difficulty with cessation.

Adolescents underestimate how addictive nicotine is and believe it will be easy to quit; however, relatively few adolescent daily users are successful at quitting.[33] The difficulty that tobacco users face in quitting underscores the importance of prevention. Prevention has become far more complex in recent years with the introduction of new tobacco products to the market such as e-cigarettes, snus tobacco, dissolvable tobaccos, and the expansion of the flavored "little cigar" and cigarillo market as alternatives to traditional cigarettes.

E-cigarettes

E-cigarettes are a category of products that deliver a complex aerosol via a battery-powered device that heats and vaporizes cartridges or tanks filled with solution of varying amounts of inhaled flavoring, humectant, and nicotine (Figure 30-3). Introduced as a consumer product in the United States in 2007, these products have been marketed widely on the Internet, at point-of-sale outlets, in print and radio media, and on US television as alternatives to cigarette use. The scientific community has had to initiate peer-reviewed research regarding these devices, which are known by many names, including *electronic cigarettes, e-cigarettes, e-cigs, electronic cigars, electronic hookah, e-hookah, hookah sticks, personal vaporizers, mechanical mods, vape pens,* and *vaping devices* (among others).

E-cigarettes vary dramatically depending on whether they are a disposable device, rechargeable cartridge system, refillable tank system, or more complex device with a tank and modifiable voltage. The commercial nicotine concentration in e-juice solutions ranges widely, from 0 to 36 mg of nicotine in a single milliliter of solution, with higher concentrations available for dilution. Producers of e-juice dilute a concentrated nicotine solution with propylene glycol or vegetable glycerin to deliver the intended strength, and then they add flavor. While regulations for manufacturers are planned to go into effect in 2018, legal challenges are underway that may affect their implementation. Accordingly, as of publication of this chapter, the creation of e-juice remains largely unregulated, with product labeling standards going into effect in 2018, and other manufacturing standards to follow in 2019 and beyond. The availability of tantalizing and delicious-smelling flavors such as Grape Freeze, Simply Mango, Death by Chocolate, Sour Skittles, and Bubblegum Jungle make these products particularly attractive to children and adolescents.

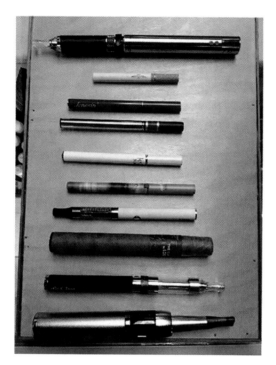

Figure 30-3. E-cigarette examples and comparators, from top to bottom: refillable tank "pen" system; traditional combusted tobacco cigarette; "cigalike," store-branded, disposable e-cigarette; Vuse, a rechargeable, cartridge-based e-cigarette; Krave disposable e-cigarette; e-hookah pen; refillable vape pen; e-cigar; another refillable vape pen; and modifiable voltage refillable vaporizer. Note the variations in size and appearance among the 4 refillable tank devices shown.

While these devices have relatively recently been introduced to the US market, their use among young people has been growing exponentially. In just 1 year (from 2011–2012), the ever and current use of e-cigarettes doubled among US middle and high school students, and between 2013 and 2015 current use tripled.[19] This meteoric rise of e-cigarette use among adolescents has been concerning for many reasons. Critically, a recent meta-analysis of 9 longitudinal studies of youths has shown that teens who use e-cigarettes but are naïve to combusted tobacco are roughly 3 times more likely to initiate combusted tobacco use.[34] This association has been shown among those who would otherwise be expected to be low-risk for tobacco use on the basis of established characteristics of combusted tobacco users.[35] Such a trajectory to combusted cigarettes is of grave concern, as it indicates recruitment of new tobacco users. E-cigarettes have also been shown to perpetuate smoking among smokers who would otherwise have quit. A 2016 meta-analysis of 4 cross-sectional and 19 longitudinal studies (with adults) found that the overall odds of quitting cigarettes was 0.72 among e-cigarette users compared with non–e-cigarette users.[36] An additional study published subsequent to this meta-analysis, using tobacco cessation services with behavioral therapy, nicotine replacement therapy (NRT), and optimal support, similarly found that e-cigarette users were less likely to quit (adjusted odds ratio, 0.7).[37]

Beyond their recruitment of new smokers among adolescents and failure to assist in tobacco cessation, e-cigarettes themselves are not without risk. The aerosol from e-juice, irrespective of nicotine content, contains ultrafine particles with potential for health risk.[38,39] Indeed, a recent study of adolescents with asthma found an increased risk of respiratory symptoms among users, irrespective of other tobacco use.[40] More recent studies suggest important risks from e-cigarettes to endothelial function[13] and other cardiovascular effects.[14,15,41]

Cigars, Little Filtered Cigars, and Cigarillos

Cigar smoking predates cigarette smoking by hundreds of years and was more popular until the early 1900s (see Figure 30-2). In contrast to cigarettes, cigars are wrapped in tobacco leaf (rather than paper) and the tobacco differs slightly. While adult users may puff on premium cigars and not inhale them, there is no specific instruction for cigar use; little filtered cigars are in most ways indistinguishable from cigarettes, other than in color and flavor. At present, cigars are the third most common type of tobacco used by adolescents (behind e-cigarettes and cigarettes).[18,20] In 2016, 7.7% of high school students reported using cigars, cigarillos, or little cigars, or any combination of those products, in the past month.[18] Cigars of all types can be sold in characterizing flavors, can be sold in packs of small quantity, and are taxed differently, so that they are less expensive than cigarettes. The low price and the flavors of these products increase their appeal to youths. Cigar users are at risk for the same health effects as cigarette users.

Hookah

Water pipes (hookahs) have also recently gained in popularity in the United States, particularly in group social settings and with the advent of "hookah bars."[42-44] Although many users perceive that smoke inhaled from a hookah is safer than cigarette smoke, studies show that the hookah produces concentrations of carbon monoxide, nicotine, tar, and metals at levels similar to or higher than those produced by cigarettes.[45,46] Communicable disease risks are significant, given the shared mouthpiece, and herpes outbreaks have been reported from hookah use.[47] In spite of these actual health risks, the misperception of safety and the appeal of social use have attracted non–cigarette users to hookah, and there is the attendant concern that these users will progress to other forms of tobacco and nicotine addiction. Given the popularity of these products, particularly among college students, it is important that PCCs ask adolescent patients about them specifically.

Smokeless, Snus, and Dissolvable Tobaccos

While smokeless tobacco, including dip and chew, has historically been a common form of tobacco use, the use of smokeless tobacco among adolescents remains lower than that of cigarettes, e-cigarettes, and cigars, with smokeless prevalence at 5.8%.[18] Those who use smokeless tobacco use it frequently: it is the tobacco product that has the highest likelihood of daily (or almost-daily) use among high school students.[48] Smokeless products in particular have "starter" class versions that are milder in nicotine content and flavor.[22] Users often progress to a higher nicotine product as their addictions develop. Many users of such products also smoke combusted tobacco products.

Snus and dissolvable tobaccos are newer forms of smokeless tobacco that have been suggested as safer alternatives to traditional cigarettes and a potential way to decrease the harm caused by combusted tobacco.[49-51] Adolescents use these forms of tobacco less frequently than they do cigarettes. Available 2016 data on past-year prevalence among 12th graders is 5.8% for snus tobacco and 1.1% for dissolvable tobaccos.[52] Snus tobacco is a smokeless tobacco product that does not require the user to spit, unlike dip or chew. With slogans such as "When you can't smoke, snus," this tobacco product is marketed specifically as one that can be used in places where smoking is not allowed, and it is often co-branded with cigarettes (eg, Marlboro, Camel). It has been noted among adults that more US snus tobacco users are engaged in dual use[53]; thus, snus tobacco may serve to maintain dependence among smokers who might otherwise have quit.[51]

Dissolvable tobacco products are another new class of smokeless, spit-less, finely milled tobacco that dissolves inside the mouth until the fine powder is swallowed. Similar to snus tobacco, these products have been marketed as tobacco that can be used in places where smoking is prohibited, and they are co-branded with traditional cigarettes. Dissolvable tobaccos are available in mint, wintergreen, cinnamon, and citrus flavors, and they are of similar size to candy. While uptake among youths has been low to date and markets are currently quite limited, ongoing monitoring is warranted, particularly regarding dual and multiple use.

Health Effects and Addiction Potential of Nicotine

Nicotine has complex pharmacodynamics: at low doses, it acts as a neurostimulant in the reward pathways, stimulating memory and alertness, improving mood, and decreasing appetite. At high doses, nicotine can cause nausea, vomiting, abdominal pain, headache, dizziness, and seizures; in very high doses, nicotine can be lethal. Receptors for nicotine span throughout the body, allowing nicotine to have broad physiologic effects, including suspected effects on the immune system.[2] Repeated exposure to nicotine leads to tolerance, which results in higher nicotine needs to prevent withdrawal. Insufficient nicotine in someone who is dependent leads to craving and withdrawal symptoms of irritability, anxiety, restlessness, difficulty concentrating, and anhedonia or depression. The addictive potential of nicotine products is known to vary by the delivery of the nicotine: faster delivery, more rapid rate of absorption, and the attainment of higher concentrations of nicotine all increase the potential for addiction. Nicotine exposure does not have a specific threshold to predict addiction. However, the nicotine source appears to make a difference, with tobacco-delivered nicotine substantially more addictive than pure nicotine.[54] Accordingly, it has been shown that NRTs have low potential for dependence because of differences in absorption.[55] The basis of nicotine addiction is reinforcement of behavior that restores nicotine and makes the user feel pleasure and prevent unpleasant withdrawal. Nicotine addiction among those most heavily affected requires frequent dosing to limit withdrawal symptoms: a 2-pack per day smoker will have 40 "doses" of nicotine per day, or at approximately 21-minute intervals (if averaged over typical waking hours). Smokers have been shown to report "needing" a cigarette even with intermittent cigarette smoking. Smokers also progress through a characteristic process of nicotine addiction, with the following stages: wanting, craving, and needing a cigarette.[9]

The adolescent brain seems uniquely susceptible to nicotine addiction.[56] Animal studies have demonstrated that nicotine exposure during the adolescent period has long-standing effects on the brain, including cell damage that leads to immediate and persistent behavior changes.[2,57] Symptoms of dependence appear within days to weeks of intermittent tobacco use and well before daily smoking.[26,27] Nearly all adult smokers initiated smoking before the age of 20 years, and tobacco use at a younger age predicts greater levels of dependence and difficulty quitting.[58]

Regular users of nicotine develop habits associated with their uses that also become connected with the rewarding physical and psychological feelings of nicotine use, creating cues for use. Known as *operant conditioning,* smokers become cued to want a cigarette after a meal, or with coffee, or in certain locations, for example. These habits of tobacco use are particularly reinforcing, further making nicotine and tobacco use difficult to overcome.

Toxicity and Poisoning Potential

Given the tolerance that occurs with regular use of nicotine, a wide range of doses has been shown to lead to acute toxicity. Most cases of acute toxicity have been found with unintentional ingestion of tobacco or nicotine-containing solutions or with dermal absorption such as green tobacco sickness. The estimated lethal dose of nicotine is 1 to 13 mg/kg of body weight, with toxicity at lower levels among the nicotine naïve, such as children. Most toxic exposures in children result in complete recovery; however, there is significant new poisoning potential from nicotine refill solutions for e-cigarettes. E-juice (also called e-liquid or vape juice) is a likely candidate for ingestion by young children because it is colorful, candy flavored, and scented. Given that nicotine is rapidly dermally absorbed, e-liquid can be dangerous even if it merely comes into contact with the skin. As noted, e-juice is sold in highly concentrated form, with common concentrations containing upwards of 36 mg of nicotine per milliliter of e-liquid. At this concentration, a small (15-mL) eyedropper-sized bottle of e-liquid would contain 540 mg of nicotine. Given the estimated lethal dose range of nicotine, even a single teaspoon of e-liquid at this concentration could kill a small child, and a smaller dose could make a child ill. While there is now legislation that mandates child safety caps on all nicotine refill solutions, many children can readily open such containers. All nicotine-containing products must be treated as a poisoning risk.

Care of Youths With Tobacco Dependence

As noted previously, the significant associations of tobacco use with other mental health issues create an imperative that tobacco-using adolescents also be screened for concomitant anxiety and depression. Please refer to Chapter 14, Anxiety and Trauma-Related Distress, and Chapter 22, Low Mood. Although most youth tobacco users want to quit,[59] few seek assistance to do so,[59,60] and many attempt to quit on their own. Unsurprisingly, most attempts at cessation are unsuccessful,[59,61–63] and relapse is frequent.[33,64] Tobacco cessation is possible, however, as evidenced by the fact that the United States has more former smokers than current smokers.[2] The approach to tobacco cessation is largely the same for adult and adolescent tobacco users, but with a greater emphasis on counseling for adolescents because the evidence for efficacy of pharmacotherapy for this group is insufficient.[33] The Public Health Service (PHS) clinical practice guideline recommends the 5 A's model of care (ask, advise, assess, assist, and arrange follow-up) (Box 30-1), which has been shown to improve tobacco cessation rates among adults.[33] The first step is to **ask** about and document all tobacco use at every clinical encounter (including health supervision, ill, and specialty visits). All family members of all ages should also be asked about secondhand smoke exposure, and all families should be advised to make their homes and cars smoke-free. As noted, many youths use cigarette and non-cigarette tobacco products concurrently, so they should be asked about all forms of tobacco use. For all tobacco users, **advise** cessation in a clear, strong manner, personalizing the risks of tobacco use and the benefits of quitting and expressing confidence in the tobacco user's ability to quit. Regardless of whether the tobacco user is a patient or the parent of a patient, advice should be routinely offered on quitting, helping, and referring all tobacco users. The clinician should also **assess** the level of nicotine addiction, reasons for wanting to quit, confidence in ability to quit, and

Box 30-1. Five Major Steps to Intervention for Tobacco Cessation

- Ask.
  - Obtain a tobacco use and exposure history from all patients and families.
  - Ask about current and past tobacco use and secondhand smoke exposure.
- Advise.
  - Look for teachable moments.
  - Personalize health risks.
    - ▶ Use clear, strong, personalized messages: "Smoking is bad for you (and your child). Would you like to quit?" "How can I help you?"
- Assess.
  - Determine whether the patient is willing to make a behavior change.
  - Establish whether he or she is willing to try to quit tobacco use at this time.
- Assist.
  - Provide information about tobacco use cessation to all tobacco users.
  - Strongly urge smoke-free (and tobacco-free) homes.
  - Help patients set realistic and specific goals.
    - ▶ Quit date
    - ▶ Smoke-free home date
  - Help your patient prepare.
    - ▶ Get support.
    - ▶ Anticipate challenges.
    - ▶ Practice problem-solving.
    - ▶ Provide information about pharmacotherapy and patient resources.
    - ▶ Provide supplemental materials: Refer to telephone quit lines such as 800/QUIT NOW.
- Arrange follow-up.
  - Plan to follow up on any behavioral commitments.
    - ▶ Schedule follow-up in person or by telephone soon after important dates, such as a quit date or anniversary.
- The sixth A: Anticipate.
  - Discuss tobacco use with preteens and teens during health supervision visits.
    - ▶ Include tobacco use with discussions of alcohol, drugs, and sexual activity.
- For the unwilling or not ready.
  - Discuss the 5 R's: relevance, risks, rewards, roadblocks, and repetition.

From Fiore MC, Jaén CR, Baker TB, et al. *Treating Tobacco Use and Dependence: 2008 Update.* Rockville, MD: Public Health Service, Dept of Health and Human Services; 2008.

readiness to quit use or begin tobacco dependence treatment. In the **assist** step, the clinician should initiate treatment, tailoring support to the tobacco user's readiness to quit and severity of addiction.

Many resources are available to PCCs, including self-help materials, referral to statewide or national quit lines (which can provide free telephone counseling to assist tobacco users with cessation), smartphone applications, text support programs, and local community cessation resources. Examples include the Web site of the Julius B. Richmond Center of Excellence (www.aap.org/en-us/advocacy-and-policy /aap-health-initiatives/Richmond-Center/Pages/default.aspx) and the Campaign for Tobacco-Free Kids (www.tobaccofreekids.org). As noted, pharmacotherapy for adolescent tobacco cessation is not recommended by the PHS 2008 guideline because of insufficient evidence of effectiveness. Pharmacotherapy has been demonstrated to be effective in adults, however, and is known to be a safer alternative to tobacco use. Tobacco users should be offered tobacco-cessation medications to assist their quit plan whenever appropriate. These cessation medications include over-the-counter NRT products, such as the patch, gum, and lozenge; prescription nicotine inhalers and nasal sprays; bupropion; and varenicline. Details regarding prescription recommendations are available in the PHS clinical practice guideline; however, a simple approach would be for a tobacco user to replace each cigarette with a single lozenge or piece of NRT gum. The strength and frequency of NRT should match the severity of addiction or withdrawal symptoms. Because most tobacco users are familiar with the feeling of using too much tobacco, they learn to titrate their NRT dosing just as they learned to titrate their tobacco uses. Primary care clinicians who choose not to prescribe pharmacotherapies should make referrals to cessation services and recommend that parents discuss pharmacotherapies with their health care professionals or purchase over-the-counter products. The final step is to arrange follow-up to increase adherence to recommendations.

Motivational interviewing techniques to encourage behavior change should be used throughout all discussions with tobacco users (see Chapter 5, Effective Communication Methods: Common Factors Skills). Encouraging tobacco users to question their own tobacco uses and come up with reasons and ways to quit has been shown to be an effective way to motivate change.

Conclusion

Tobacco use remains a preventable and treatable cause of substantial morbidity and mortality in the United States and throughout the world. Furthermore, its use, particularly at a young age, may signal increased likelihood of other risky behaviors and mental health problems. Pediatric PCCs are well positioned to interact with tobacco users, monitor their mental health, and assist in motivating them to improve their health by quitting tobacco completely. Only with ongoing prevention and treatment strategies will tobacco use be surmounted, and PCCs must be part of this process.

AAP Policy

American Academy of Pediatrics Committee on Environmental Health, Committee on Substance Abuse, Committee on Adolescence, and Committee on Native American Child Health. Tobacco use: a pediatric disease. *Pediatrics.* 2009;124(5):1474–1487. Reaffirmed May 2013 (pediatrics.aappublications.org/content/124/5/1474)

American Academy of Pediatrics Section on Tobacco Control. Clinical practice policy to protect children from tobacco, nicotine, and tobacco smoke. *Pediatrics.* 2015;136(5):1008–1017 (pediatrics.aappublications.org/content/136/5/1008)

American Academy of Pediatrics Section on Tobacco Control. Electronic nicotine delivery systems. *Pediatrics.* 2015;136(5):1018–1026 (pediatrics.aappublications.org/content/136/5/1018)

American Academy of Pediatrics Section on Tobacco Control. Public policy to protect children from tobacco, nicotine, and tobacco smoke. *Pediatrics.* 2015;136(5):998–1007 (pediatrics.aappublications.org/content/136/5/998)

Best D; American Academy of Pediatrics Committee on Environmental Health, Committee on Native American Child Health, and Committee on Adolescence. Secondhand and prenatal tobacco smoke exposure. *Pediatrics.* 2009;124(5):e1017–e1044. Reaffirmed June 2014 (pediatrics.aappublications.org/content/124/5/e1017)

Farber HJ, Groner J, Walley S, Nelson K; American Academy of Pediatrics Section on Tobacco Control. Protecting children from tobacco, nicotine, and tobacco smoke. *Pediatrics.* 2015;136(5):e1439–e1467 (pediatrics.aappublications.org/content/136/5/e1439)

Sims TH; American Academy of Pediatrics Committee on Substance Abuse. Tobacco as a substance of abuse. *Pediatrics.* 2009;124(5):e1045–e1053. Reaffirmed January 2015 (pediatrics.aappublications.org/content/124/5/e1045)

Siqueira LM; American Academy of Pediatrics Committee on Substance Use and Prevention. Nicotine and tobacco as substances of abuse in children and adolescents. *Pediatrics.* 2017;139(1):e20163436 (pediatrics.aappublications.org/content/139/1/e20163436)

References

1. Murray JB. Nicotine as a psychoactive drug. *J Psychol.* 1991;125(1):5–25
2. Office on Smoking Health, National Center for Chronic Disease Prevention and Health Promotion. *The Health Consequences of Smoking—50 Years of Progress; A Report of the Surgeon General.* Atlanta, GA: Centers for Disease Control and Prevention; 2014
3. DeHay T, Morris C, May MG, Devine K, Waxmonsky J. Tobacco use in youth with mental illnesses. *J Behav Med.* 2012;35(2):139–148
4. Griesler PC, Hu MC, Schaffran C, Kandel DB. Comorbidity of psychiatric disorders and nicotine dependence among adolescents: findings from a prospective, longitudinal study. *J Am Acad Child Adolesc Psychiatry.* 2008; 47(11):1340–1350
5. Upadhyaya HP, Deas D, Brady KT, Kruesi M. Cigarette smoking and psychiatric comorbidity in children and adolescents. *J Am Acad Child Adolesc Psychiatry.* 2002;41(11):1294–1305
6. Wang MQ, Fitzhugh EC, Turner L, Fu Q, Westerfield RC. Association of depressive symptoms and school adolescents' smoking: a cross-lagged analysis. *Psychol Rep.* 1996;79(1):127–130
7. Lechner WV, Janssen T, Kahler CW, Audrain-McGovern J, Leventhal AM. Bi-directional associations of electronic and combustible cigarette use onset patterns with depressive symptoms in adolescents. *Prev Med.* 2017;96:73–78
8. Substance Abuse and Mental Health Services Administration. *The NSDUH Report: Adults With Mental Illness or Substance Use Disorder Account for 40 Percent of All Cigarettes Smoked.* Rockville, MD: Substance Abuse and Mental Health Services Administration; 2013
9. Richter L, Pugh BS, Smith PH, Ball SA. The co-occurrence of nicotine and other substance use and addiction among youth and adults in the United States: implications for research, practice, and policy. *Am J Drug Alcohol Abuse.* 2017; 43(2):132–145
10. National Center on Addiction and Substance Abuse at Columbia University. *Tobacco: The Smoking Gun. Prepared for the Citizen's Commission to Protect the Truth.* New York, NY: Columbia University; 2007
11. World Health Organization. Fact sheets: tobacco. World Health Organization Web site. http://www.who.int/mediacentre/factsheets/fs339/en. Updated May 2017. Accessed February 9, 2018
12. Gray N, Henningfield JE, Benowitz NL, et al. Toward a comprehensive long term nicotine policy. *Tob Control.* 2005;14(3):161–165
13. Schweitzer KS, Chen SX, Law S, et al. Endothelial disruptive proinflammatory effects of nicotine and e-cigarette vapor exposures. *Am J Physiol Lung Cell Mol Physiol.* 2015;309(2):L175–L187
14. Carnevale R, Sciarretta S, Violi F, et al. Acute impact of tobacco vs electronic cigarette smoking on oxidative stress and vascular function. *Chest.* 2016;150(3): 606–612
15. Vlachopoulos C, Ioakeimidis N, Abdelrasoul M, et al. Electronic cigarette smoking increases aortic stiffness and blood pressure in young smokers. *J Am Coll Cardiol.* 2016;67(23):2802–2803

16. Jamal A, King BA, Neff LJ, Whitmill J, Babb SD, Graffunder CM. Current cigarette smoking among adults - United States, 2005-2015. *MMWR Morbid Mortal Wkly Rep.* 2016;65(44):1205–1211

17. Arrazola RA, Neff LJ, Kennedy SM, Holder-Hayes E, Jones CD; Centers for Disease Control and Prevention. Tobacco use among middle and high school students—United States, 2013. *MMWR Morb Mortal Wkly Rep.* 2014;63(45): 1021–1026

18. Jamal A, Gentzke A, Hu SS, et al. Tobacco use among middle and high school students—United States, 2011-2016. *MMWR Morb Mortal Wkly Rep.* 2017; 66(23):597–603

19. Arrazola RA, Singh T, Corey CG, et al; Centers for Disease Control and Prevention. Tobacco use among middle and high school students - United States, 2011-2014. *MMWR Morb Mortal Wkly Rep.* 2015;64(14):381–385

20. Singh T, Arrazola RA, Corey CG, et al. Tobacco use among middle and high school students—United States, 2011-2015. *MMWR Morb Mortal Wkly Rep.* 2016;65(14):361–367

21. Agaku IT, King BA, Husten CG, et al; Centers for Disease Control and Prevention. Tobacco product use among adults—United States, 2012-2013. *MMWR Morb Mortal Wkly Rep.* 2014;63(25):542–547

22. Office on Smoking and Health, National Center for Chronic Disease Prevention and Health Promotion. *Preventing Tobacco Use Among Youth and Young Adults: A Report of the Surgeon General.* Atlanta, GA: Centers for Disease Control and Prevention; 2012

23. Arrazola RA, Kuiper NM, Dube SR. Patterns of current use of tobacco products among U.S. high school students for 2000-2012—findings from the National Youth Tobacco Survey. *J Adolesc Health.* 2014;54(1):54–60.e9

24. DiFranza JR, Savageau JA, Fletcher K, et al. Measuring the loss of autonomy over nicotine use in adolescents: the DANDY (Development and Assessment of Nicotine Dependence in Youths) study. *Arch Pediatr Adolesc Med.* 2002;156(4): 397–403

25. DiFranza JR, Savageau JA, Rigotti NA, et al. Development of symptoms of tobacco dependence in youths: 30 month follow up data from the DANDY study. *Tob Control.* 2002;11(3):228–235

26. DiFranza JR, Rigotti NA, McNeill AD, et al. Initial symptoms of nicotine dependence in adolescents. *Tob Control.* 2000;9(3):313–319

27. DiFranza JR, Savageau JA, Fletcher K, et al. Symptoms of tobacco dependence after brief intermittent use: the Development and Assessment of Nicotine Dependence in Youth-2 study. *Arch Pediatr Adolesc Med.* 2007;161(7):704–710

28. Office of Applied Studies. *Results From the 2001 National Household Survey on Drug Abuse: Volume I. Summary of National Findings.* Rockville, MD: Office of Applied Studies, Substance Abuse and Mental Health Services Administration, US Dept of Health and Human Services; 2002. DHHS publication SMA 02-3758

29. Pierce JP, Gilpin E. How long will today's new adolescent smoker be addicted to cigarettes? *Am J Public Health.* 1996;86(2):253–256

30. Kann L, Warren CW, Harris WA, et al. Youth risk behavior surveillance—United States, 1995. *MMWR CDC Surveill Summ.* 1996;45(4):1–84

31. Berg CJ, Lust KA, Sanem JR, et al. Smoker self-identification versus recent smoking among college students. *Am J Prev Med.* 2009;36(4):333–336

32. Husten CG. How should we define light or intermittent smoking? Does it matter? *Nicotine Tob Res.* 2009;11(2):111–121

33. Fiore MC, Jaén CR, Baker TB, et al. *Treating Tobacco Use and Dependence: 2008 Update.* Rockville, MD: Public Health Service, US Dept of Health and Human Services; 2008

34. Soneji S, Barrington-Trimis JL, Wills TA, et al. Association between initial use of e-cigarettes and subsequent cigarette smoking among adolescents and young adults: a systematic review and meta-analysis. *JAMA Pediatr.* 2017;171(8):788–797

35. Wills TA, Sargent JD, Knight R, Pagano I, Gibbons FX. E-cigarette use and willingness to smoke: a sample of adolescent non-smokers. *Tob Control.* 2016; 25(e1):e52–e59

36. Kalkhoran S, Glantz SA. E-cigarettes and smoking cessation in real-world and clinical settings: a systematic review and meta-analysis. *Lancet Respir Med.* 2016;4(2):116–128

37. Zawertailo L, Pavlov D, Ivanova A, Ng G, Baliunas D, Selby P. Concurrent e-cigarette use during tobacco dependence treatment in primary care settings: association with smoking cessation at three and six months. *Nicotine Tob Res.* 2017;19(2):183–189

38. Fuoco FC, Buonanno G, Stabile L, Vigo P. Influential parameters on particle concentration and size distribution in the mainstream of e-cigarettes. *Environ Pollut.* 2014;184:523–529

39. Czogala J, Goniewicz ML, Fidelus B, Zielinska-Danch W, Travers MJ, Sobczak A. Secondhand exposure to vapors from electronic cigarettes. *Nicotine Tob Res.* 2014;16(6):655–662

40. McConnell R, Barrington-Trimis JL, Wang K, et al. Electronic cigarette use and respiratory symptoms in adolescents. *Am J Respir Crit Care Med.* 2017;195(8): 1043–1049

41. Bhatnagar A. E-cigarettes and cardiovascular disease risk: evaluation of evidence, policy implications, and recommendations. *Curr Cardiovasc Risk Rep.* 2016; 10(7):24

42. Primack BA, Fertman CI, Rice KR, Adachi-Mejia AM, Fine MJ. Waterpipe and cigarette smoking among college athletes in the United States. *J Adolesc Health.* 2010;46(1):45–51

43. Primack BA, Sidani J, Agarwal AA, Shadel WG, Donny EC, Eissenberg TE. Prevalence of and associations with waterpipe tobacco smoking among U.S. university students. *Ann Behav Med.* 2008;36(1):81–86

44. Primack BA, Walsh M, Bryce C, Eissenberg T. Water-pipe tobacco smoking among middle and high school students in Arizona. *Pediatrics.* 2009;123(2):e282–e288

45. Knishkowy B, Amitai Y. Water-pipe (narghile) smoking: an emerging health risk behavior. *Pediatrics.* 2005;116(1):e113–e119

46. Cobb C, Ward KD, Maziak W, Shihadeh AL, Eissenberg T. Waterpipe tobacco smoking: an emerging health crisis in the United States. *Am J Health Behav.* 2010; 34(3):275–285

47. Kadhum M, Sweidan A, Jaffery AE, Al-Saadi A, Madden B. A review of the health effects of smoking shisha. *Clin Med (Lond).* 2015;15(3):263–266

48. Neff LJ, Arrazola RA, Caraballo RS, et al. Frequency of tobacco use among middle and high school students—United States, 2014. *MMWR Morb Mortal Wkly Rep.* 2015;64(38):1061–1065

49. Ramström LM, Foulds J. Role of snus in initiation and cessation of tobacco smoking in Sweden. *Tob Control.* 2006;15(3):210–214

50. Stepanov I, Jensen J, Hatsukami D, Hecht SS. New and traditional smokeless tobacco: comparison of toxicant and carcinogen levels. *Nicotine Tob Res.* 2008; 10(12):1773–1782

51. Henningfield JE, Rose CA, Giovino GA. Brave new world of tobacco disease prevention: promoting dual tobacco-product use? *Am J Prev Med.* 2002;23(3): 226–228

52. Johnston LD, O'Malley PM, Miech RA, Bachman JG, Schulenberg JE. *Monitoring the Future: National Survey Results on Drug Use; 1975–2016: Overview; Key Findings on Adolescent Drug Use.* Ann Arbor, MI: Institute for Social Research, University of Michigan; 2017

53. McMillen R, Maduka J, Winickoff J. Use of emerging tobacco products in the United States. *J Environ Public Health.* 2012;2012:989474

54. Office on Smoking and Health, National Center for Chronic Disease Prevention and Health Promotion. *How Tobacco Smoke Causes Disease: The Biology and Behavioral Basis for Smoking-Attributable Disease; A Report of the Surgeon General.* Atlanta, GA: Centers for Disease Control and Prevention; 2010

55. Benowitz NL. Pharmacodynamics of nicotine: implications for rational treatment of nicotine addiction. *Br J Addict.* 1991;86(5):495–499

56. Holliday E, Gould TJ. Nicotine, adolescence, and stress: a review of how stress can modulate the negative consequences of adolescent nicotine abuse. *Neurosci Biobehav Rev.* 2016;65:173–184

57. Slotkin TA. Nicotine and the adolescent brain: insights from an animal model. *Neurotoxicol Teratol.* 2002;24(3):369–384

58. Chen J, Millar WJ. Age of smoking initiation: implications for quitting. *Health Rep.* 1998;9(4):39–46

59. Mermelstein R. Teen smoking cessation. *Tob Control.* 2003;12(suppl 1):i25–i34

60. Grimshaw G, Stanton A, Blackburn C, et al. Patterns of smoking, quit attempts and services for a cohort of 15- to 19-year-olds. *Child Care Health Dev.* 2003;29(6): 457–464

61. Sussman S. Effects of sixty-six adolescent tobacco use cessation trials and seventeen prospective studies of self-initiated quitting. *Tob Induce Dis.* 2002; 1(1):35–81

62. Sussman S, Sun P, Dent CW. A meta-analysis of teen cigarette smoking cessation. *Health Psychol.* 2006;25(5):549–557

63. Centers for Disease Control and Prevention. High school students who tried to quit smoking cigarettes—United States, 2007. *MMWR Morb Mortal Wkly Rep.* 2009;58(16):428–431

64. Bancej C, O'Loughlin J, Platt RW, Paradis G, Gervais A. Smoking cessation attempts among adolescent smokers: a systematic review of prevalence studies. *Tob Control.* 2007;16(6):e8

CHAPTER 31

Substance Use 2:
Use of Other Substances

Sharon Levy, MD, MPH, and Sarah Bagley, MD, MSc

"Pediatric primary care clinicians are positioned to provide care to youths by reinforcing strengths and healthy behaviors and, by applying evidence-based brief interventions, can often be effective in preventing youths from escalating their use of substances and in motivating them to decrease their use of substances."

Introduction

Adolescence is a common time for both initiation of substance use and emergence of mental disorders, and co-occurrence of mental disorders and substance use is common. Preadolescents may also initiate substance use and experience onset of mental disorders.

Youths who present with substance use problems should be assessed for mental disorders, and, if present, both problems should be treated concomitantly. (While the terms *youth* and *youths* are defined variably in the literature about substance use, in this chapter *youth* and *youths* will generally encompass preadolescents and adolescents aged 9–18 years. In some instances a study cited will provide an alternative definition.) Youths may present with concerns noted by parents or teachers such as physical signs or symptoms suggesting substance use or nonspecific symptoms that may suggest substance use (eg, declining school performance or attendance, car crash, association with friends who are using substances), or because an asymptomatic youth has a positive substance-use screening test result. Whether the use identified is sporadic or regular, it can have negative physical and mental health effects related to the direct consequences of the substances or associated risky behaviors. Identifying and addressing substance use to minimize harm is an important task for pediatric primary care clinicians (PCCs): pediatricians, family physicians, internists, nurse practitioners, and physician assistants who provides frontline, longitudinal care to youths. Because substance use is closely associated with morbidity and mortality in this age-group, the American Academy of Pediatrics (AAP) recommends that pediatricians achieve competence in identifying and intervening to reduce substance use by youths, as well as in supporting the care of youths with one or more substance use disorders (SUDs).[1]

Perceived limitations of time for adequate psychosocial evaluation, discomfort addressing sensitive issues, or lack of familiarity with available therapeutic resources may prevent PCCs from thoroughly and appropriately addressing substance use with youths. However, as with other disorders, assessment is required to determine the appropriate setting and level of care. Often, sensitivity to these issues, attention to youths' risk behaviors in general, and periodic follow-up in the primary care setting are adequate to help keep young people safe and healthy.

Youth Brain Development

The human brain continues to develop until the middle of the third decade of life. The prefrontal cortex, which controls impulses, attention, and organization, matures last, well after the parts of the brain that are involved in pleasure and reward. This developmental "imbalance" is correlated with stimulation seeking and risk-taking behavior that is typical of preadolescence and adolescence. Use of psychoactive substances is one way, albeit dangerous and unhealthy, through which youths may fulfill a natural inclination for stimulation and reward. Seen in this perspective, substance use can be understood as an (unhealthy) mechanism for fulfilling a normal drive, rather than as purely deviant behavior. Youths may also use psychoactive substances for a variety of other reasons: to fit in, in social situations in which others are using substances; because of expectations that use will be pleasurable; as a form of risk-taking or stimulation seeking; or to relax, relieve anxiety, improve mood, or relieve symptoms of a mental disorder. Identifying the reasons that underlie substance use can help PCCs target counseling, advice, and strategies that are most salient to the youth.

Unfortunately, substance use, even without symptoms that rise to the level of a disorder, is associated with significant health problems, including injuries, unintentional sexual activity, and sexually transmitted infections. Early initiation of substance use is also associated with increased risk of developing a severe SUD (otherwise known as addiction), which is a chronic medical condition that causes neurological changes. The AAP recommends that PCCs routinely screen every patient for substance use, beginning at age 11, and deliver an appropriate intervention geared toward preventing or reducing substance use.[1] When a youth is referred for specialty care of substance use, the AAP recommends that the PCC remain involved with the youth and family, supporting their positive view of treatment, monitoring progress, and providing complementary primary care services.

Prevalence of Substance Use

Alcohol, marijuana, and tobacco are the most commonly used substances among youths. By the end of 12th grade, 52% of students report being drunk at least once, as do 12% of eighth graders. Lifetime rates of use of any illicit drug have remained steady in the past few years. Perceived risk of marijuana use continues to fall, and that may lead to increases in use over the next few years. Prescription drug misuse continues to be a concern, with 13% of 12th graders reporting misuse of a prescription drug in the prior year.[2] Rates of tobacco use by youths declined from 1996 to 2015, although over the past few years rates have plateaued. E-cigarettes, which are electronic devices that vaporize liquid nicotine, are marketed as a tobacco cessation device but are sold in flavors such as bubblegum and cotton candy that are attractive to children and youths who may initiate their "smoking careers" with these devices. Use of e-cigarettes has increased every year and has surpassed conventional cigarette use. Use of tobacco products often precedes use of other substances. Youths who smoke cigarettes are 5 times more likely than nonsmokers to use alcohol, 13 times more likely to use marijuana, and 7 times more likely to use cocaine or heroin.[3]

Classification of Substance Use Disorders

The fifth edition of the *Diagnostic and Statistical Manual of Mental Disorders* (DSM-5), released in May 2013, included new criteria and replaced the terms *substance abuse* and *substance dependence* with *substance use disorder,* defined as mild, moderate, or severe. The new diagnostic classification is based on the number of criteria that is met: 2 to 3 constitute a mild disorder; 4 to 5, moderate; and 6 or more, severe. Meeting criteria for a mild or moderate SUD indicates that use is hazardous or that an individual has begun to have problems associated with use. Although there are no clear referral guidelines for adolescents with an SUD unless there is a co-occurring mental illness, those with a mild SUD can likely be treated in primary care. Patients with a moderate SUD may not require a referral to subspecialty care, and the referral decision can be left to the discretion of the PCC and his or her comfort with managing SUDs. Meeting criteria for a severe SUD suggests that an individual would likely benefit from specialized treatment of SUDs. However, because many youths with a severe SUD will not accept a referral to treatment, PCCs should be prepared to treat these patients in primary care while trying to facilitate completion of the referral. While not an official diagnostic term, *addiction* refers to loss of control or obsessive use of a substance associated with neurological changes in the brain's reward center. Because there is no cure for addiction, long-term treatment is recommended. Effective, evidence-based treatments, including medication and psychosocial support, are available.

The following sections will describe the PCC's role in screening for substance use, assessment of severity, and treatment of youths who are using substances.

Confidentiality and Substance Use

Given that substance use is one of many sensitive topics that may come up in the course of caring for youths, PCCs should have a systematic way to establish limits of confidentiality with both youths and parents in the practice.[4] This communication is particularly important before a PCC begins taking the medical history and screening for drug use. Discussions between the clinician and patient should remain confidential unless the clinician determines that the reported behaviors are putting either the patient or someone else at acute risk of harm. Determining whether a behavior requires breach of confidentiality is a matter of clinical judgment; in most cases, reports of occasional tobacco, alcohol, or marijuana use can be kept confidential, although a clinician may decide to involve parents if a patient is very young or being treated for a medical condition that could be dangerously affected by substance use. Even when there is no reason to breach confidentiality, it is often best to request permission from the youth to engage with parents for their support. In situations in which a parent is already aware of use, the youth may be willing to share information, particularly if he or she has agreed to a quit attempt or to engage in further treatment.[5]

Screening Tools

At each health supervision visit with an adolescent or a preadolescent patient, PCCs should include a psychosocial interview to assess family and peer relationships, academic progress, recreational activities, sexual behavior, and drug use. The HEADSSS mnemonic (home/environment, education and employment, activities, drugs, sexuality, suicide/depression, and safety) can help PCCs inquire about key domains.[6] Previsit questionnaires are also available to capture this information.

This data gathering does not substitute for screening. Standardized, validated tools are recommended when screening for substance use in order to improve sensitivity of report and accuracy of triage based on screening results[7–13] (Table 31-1). Using screening tools minimizes the likelihood that substance use problems or disorders are missed, as commonly occurs when screening on clinical impressions alone.[14]

Screening allows PCCs to stratify youths into risk categories. Each of the recommended tools does this in a slightly different way, although most include *no use, lower-risk use, moderate-risk use,* and *high-risk use,* with *lower-risk use* corresponding to use without a *DSM-5* SUD and *high-risk* corresponding to a mild, moderate, or severe SUD. In this chapter, we describe interventions for each of these levels of risk. Some tools do not discriminate between moderate and high risk; in these cases, the assessment is used to determine which youths have developed a severe SUD that will benefit most from referral to subspecialty care. Interventions for each stage are described later, in the Counseling to Reduce Drug Use and High-risk Behaviors section of this chapter.

Table 31-1. Substance Use Screening and Assessment Tools for Use With Adolescents

Tool	Description
Brief Screenings	
Screening to Brief Intervention (S2BI)	• 2-question frequency screening • Screens for tobacco, alcohol, marijuana, and other illicit drug use • Discriminates between no use, no SUD, moderate SUD, and severe SUD, on the basis of *DSM-5* diagnoses
Brief Screener for Tobacco, Alcohol, and Other Drugs (BSTAD)	• Identifies problematic tobacco, alcohol, and marijuana use in pediatric settings
NIAAA youth alcohol screening	• 2-question screening • Screens for friends' uses and own use
Brief Assessments	
CRAFFT (Car, Relax, Alone, Forget, Friends/Family, Trouble) screening tool	• A good tool for quickly identifying problems associated with substance use • Not a diagnostic tool
Global Appraisal of Individual Needs (GAIN)	• Assesses for both SUDs and mental disorders
Alcohol Use Disorders Identification Test (AUDIT)	• Assesses risky drinking • Not a diagnostic tool

Abbreviations: *DSM-5*, fifth edition of the *Diagnostic and Statistical Manual of Mental Disorders*; NIAAA, National Institute on Alcohol Abuse and Alcoholism; SUD, substance use disorder.

Advice and Counseling for Low-risk Youths

Primary care clinicians should provide youths who are not using substances with positive encouragement about their smart and healthy choices. For this group as well as lower-risk youths, primary care provides an opportunity to provide education about the risks of using substances in addition to anticipatory guidance about how to manage situations when alcohol or other drugs will be available.[1] Importantly, it is recommended that the PCC include a discussion of the risks of impaired driving and help the adolescent plan for times when a driver may have used alcohol or drugs. Students Against Destructive Decisions (SADD) has a helpful framework for PCCs to use with patients and parents for driving safety.[15]

Primary Care of Youths Who Are Using Substances

Assessment

Assessment is performed with youths who have a screening result that puts them in the moderate-risk or high-risk category in order to determine the problems associated with use and the effect of substance use on their functioning at home, at school, and with peers. Assessment can include questions about age of initiation, frequency, and, for alcohol, quantity of use, that is, information that assists the clinician in identifying acute risk (such as very heavy alcohol consumption) as well as personalizing medical advice (such as discussing the effect of daily marijuana use on the adolescent brain). Asking about associated problems, troubles, regrets, and quit attempts may also identify areas of ambivalence that can be incorporated into a discussion of behavior change. These problems can be used as a fulcrum to turn the discussion toward a behavior change plan identified by the youth.

In general, open-ended questions such as "Tell me about your history of alcohol use" encourage more reporting than closed-ended questions do. However, PCCs may need to prompt adolescents for certain information that is important for formulation. Suggested historical elements are listed in Table 31-2. With a focus on problems associated with substance use, a

Table 31-2. Key Details to Assess in Patients at High Risk of Developing Substance Use Disorder	
Substance	**Use History Key Historical Elements**
Alcohol	• Age of first drink • Frequency of drinking episodes • Typical amount of alcohol consumed • Greatest amount of alcohol consumed • History of blackouts, overdoses, and ED visits • Problems associated with alcohol use • Quit attempts
Marijuana	• Age at initiation • Frequency of marijuana use • History of paranoia or hallucinations or both • Problems associated with marijuana use • Quit attempts

Abbreviation: ED, emergency department.

clinical history can be used as the first step in an intervention. Information about use of tobacco, inhalants, and other psychoactive and illicit substances and misuse of prescription or over-the-counter medications also helps formulate clinical impressions and treatment recommendations. The National Institute on Alcohol Abuse and Alcoholism *Alcohol Screening and Brief Intervention for Youth: A Practitioner's Guide* and the AAP policy statement on screening, brief intervention, and referral to treatment (SBIRT) both explain in detail the recommended approach to screening and brief intervention for adolescents.[1,9]

A parent, a teacher, or another caregiver may notice nonspecific signs or symptoms that may indicate substance use. If these are reported, the youth should be assessed for a potential SUD through a careful history regardless of screening results. See Table 31-3 for other conditions that

Table 31-3. Conditions That May Mimic or Co-occur With Substance Use	
Condition	**Rationale**
Learning problems or disabilities	Unidentified learning difficulties can contribute to frustration and stress, school failure, and association with peers who use substances, all of which can increase the chances of developing an SUD. See Chapter 21, Learning Difficulty, to explore this possibility.
Depression or a bipolar disorder	Marked sleep disturbance, disturbed appetite, low mood, or tearfulness could indicate that a youth is depressed. Symptoms of depression rapidly alternating with cycles of agitation may suggest bipolar disorder. See Chapter 22, Low Mood.
Exposure to ACEs	Youths who have experienced or witnessed trauma, violence, a natural disaster, separation from a parent, parental divorce or separation, parental substance use, neglect, or physical, emotional, or sexual abuse are at high risk for developing emotional difficulties such as adjustment disorder or PTSD. Consider PTSD if the onset or acceleration of substance use was preceded by an extremely distressing experience. PCCs should speak separately and confidentially with the youth and parents to explore this possibility. Parents are often unaware of exposures that children may have had at school or in the community and may also underestimate the effect on children of major traumas in the family (eg, serious illness in a parent, maltreatment of the child, death or incarceration of a loved one). See Chapter 14, Anxiety and Trauma-Related Distress.

Table 31-3. Conditions That May Mimic or Co-occur With Substance Use (*continued*)

Condition	Rationale
Anxiety disorders	Anxiety disorders commonly co-occur with SUDs, and the relationship is bidirectional: anxious youths may be more likely to use substances; conversely, substance use may cause or precipitate anxiety disorders. See Chapter 14, Anxiety and Trauma-Related Distress.
Physical illness	Drug or alcohol withdrawal may present as a physical illness and is potentially a medical emergency. Psychiatric symptoms may be associated with medical illness (eg, encephalitis, cerebritis) and may be mistaken for drug intoxication. Drug or alcohol use may also exacerbate symptoms of chronic medical conditions. Adolescents using alcohol are more likely to forget to take their respective medications, which can interfere with medical management.
Psychosis	Although rare, the onset of bipolar disorder or schizophrenia in late adolescence may be subtle and marked only by frightening hallucinations or delusions that the youth does not disclose. These symptoms may result from, precipitate, or accelerate the use of substances.
ADHD	Adolescents with ADHD have higher rates of SUDs than peers do. Some studies have suggested that stimulant treatment for adolescents with ADHD may lower the risk of developing an SUD, although findings have been inconclusive. There is no evidence that stimulant treatment increases risk of developing an SUD. See Chapter 20, Inattention and Impulsivity.

Abbreviations: ACEs, adverse childhood experiences; ADHD, attention-deficit/hyperactivity disorder; PCC, primary care clinician; PTSD, post-traumatic stress disorder; SUD, substance use disorder.

may mimic or co-occur with substance use. In addition, certain risk factors, such as early initiation of use, family history of SUDs, and co-occurring mental disorders, increase a youth's susceptibility to developing an SUD. When available, this information should be considered in the overall assessment of each patient.

As with screening, an accurate substance use history can be best obtained in an atmosphere of confidentiality, privacy, and trust; it is recommended that parents be excluded from the interview.

Physical Examination

The medical complications of chronic substance use, although sometimes severe, do not usually appear until after adolescence. Nonetheless, a complete evaluation for an SUD includes a complete physical examination; signs and symptoms of acute intoxication or chronic use should be noted if present. Table 31-4 lists physical signs and symptoms of acute and chronic substance use.

Laboratory Testing

Drug testing may be a useful part of a complete assessment for an SUD, particularly when a parent or another adult is concerned and the youth denies use. As with any laboratory test, this procedure yields limited information and should be used only as an adjunct to the history and physical examination. The use of drug testing in general populations (eg, school drug-testing programs) has less utility and many associated ethical and legal concerns. Parents may request that the PCC perform a urine drug test; however, testing and sharing of the results should be done only with permission of the adolescent. If a youth refuses a test that is indicated, parents can be coached to implement logical consequences as they would when the youth refuses to perform other expected actvities, such as homework or chores. If there is concern for harm, the PCC should consider breaching confidentiality. Drug testing is a complex laboratory procedure with significant potential for false-positive and false-negative results; the AAP has produced a clinical report to help guide clinicians on how to use this procedure most effectively.[16]

General Care

Primary care clinicians are positioned to provide effective care to youths who are using substances, including youths who also need one or more specialty services.

Reducing Stress

Consider the youth's social environment (eg, family social history, parental depression screening result, results of any family assessment tools administered, reports from child care or school). Some youths use marijuana, alcohol, or other substances to help cope with stress; for them, finding alternative, healthy strategies for managing stress is an important

Table 31-4. Physical Findings Potentially Indicating Substance Use and Use Disorder

Component of Physical Examination	Acute Intoxication Findings	Chronic Impairment Findings	Drugs to Consider
General appearance	Altered mood, strange or inappropriate behavior	Poor dress or hygiene	Any drug
Vital signs	—	Weight loss	Heroin, cocaine
	Hypertension	Hypertension	Cocaine, amphetamines
	Hypotension, hypothermia	—	Heroin
	Hyperthermia	—	Cocaine, amphetamines, ecstasy
	Tachycardia	—	Marijuana, cocaine, amphetamines
Ears, nose, and throat	Conjunctival injection	—	Marijuana, inhalants
	Dilated pupils	—	Cocaine, amphetamines
	Constricted pupils	—	Opioids
	Sluggish pupillary response	—	Barbiturates
	—	Nasal irritation	Cocaine, inhalants, opioids (if sniffing)
Cardiac	Arrhythmias	Arrhythmias	Methadone, cocaine, amphetamines
Chest	—	Gynecomastia	Marijuana, anabolic steroids
Genitourinary	—	Testicular atrophy, clitoromegaly	Anabolic steroids

Table 31-4. Physical Findings Potentially Indicating Substance Use and Use Disorder (continued)

Component of Physical Examination	Acute Intoxication Findings	Chronic Impairment Findings	Drugs to Consider
Skin	—	Acne, hirsutism	Anabolic steroids
	Abscesses, needle track marks	—	IV drug use
Neurological	Altered sensorium	—	Any substance
	Ataxia	—	Alcohol, barbiturates
	Nystagmus	—	Barbiturates
	Hyporeflexia or hyperreflexia	—	Marijuana, cocaine, amphetamines

Abbreviation: IV, intravenous.

step to helping them stop or reduce substance use. Questions to raise might include

Is an external problem (adverse experience such as abuse, bullying, or family socioeconomic stress) adding to the youth's stress?

Take steps to explore and reduce stressors, as feasible.

Is there an undiagnosed mental health problem?

Use the tools described in Appendix 2, Mental Health Tools for Pediatrics, to screen for co-occurring mental health problems.

Are the youth's peers using substances?

Explore options to increase healthy social and recreational activities and reduce contact with peers who are using substances. Youths with a severe SUD can be encouraged to change their phone numbers and eliminate old contacts to prevent being contacted by old friends with whom they previously used drugs. Unfortunately, it is impossible to isolate these youths from substances. Part of treatment is teaching youths to identify high-risk situations, avoid them when possible, and use strategies to avoid use even when confronted with others who are using. In some communities, youths may be able to attend a recovery high school. Recovery high schools are accredited schools that provide a safe and sober environment for students with a substance use history to continue their educations. Every school has a different approach that includes provision of continued support for each student's recovery.

The clinician can also acknowledge and reinforce protective factors such as good relationships with at least 1 parent or important adult, prosocial peers, and concerned or caring family; help seeking; and connection to positive organizations.

Encouraging Healthy Habits

Encourage exercise, outdoor time, a healthy and consistent diet, sleep (critically important to mental health), limited screen time, one-on-one time with parents, and time with peers who are not using substances. Offer praise for positive behavior changes, acknowledgment of the youth's strengths, and acknowledgment of the challenges the youth may be facing with transitions, including new schools, new friends, new social circles, and new academic demands. Acknowledge that while the patient's friends may be using substances heavily, most of the patient's same-age peers do not binge drink or use drugs.

Encourage involvement in prosocial activities such as youth development, leadership, volunteer, and after-school activities; sports teams, clubs, and mentoring; and faith-based programs. A strengths-based approach that capitalizes on interests, talents, and future goals is most effective.

Offering Resources

Helpful resources include Web sites such as www.samhsa.gov/underage-drinking/parent-resources, www.drugabuse.gov/family-checkup, and https://drugfree.org/drug-guide. Provide contact numbers in case of an emergency.

Monitoring Progress

School reports, as well as youth and parent feedback, can be helpful in monitoring progress.

Counseling to Reduce Drug Use and High-risk Behaviors

The strategies described next are common elements of evidence-based and evidence-informed psychosocial interventions for the care of youths who do and do not use substances. They are applicable to the primary care of youths in the early stages of substance use and to the initial treatment of youths in more advanced stages while readying them for, or awaiting access to specialty care for an SUD.

Tailoring Intervention to Stage of Use

Depending on the screening tool used, levels of risk include abstinence, lower risk (ie, use but no SUD), moderate risk (ie, a mild or moderate SUD), high risk (ie, youth with a severe SUD), and acute risk, which is determined as part of the assessment of moderate- and high-risk youths. Interventions for each stage are described in Table 31-5.

Using Motivational Interviewing Techniques

The PCC can explore ambivalence about use and readiness to enter treatment and negotiate achievable next steps in an empathetic and supportive manner known as motivational interviewing (Table 31-6). For high-risk youths, change plans can focus on eliminating highest-risk behaviors (such as driving or riding with an impaired driver) and on engaging in ongoing treatment. The clinician should help parents be supportive of behavior change and coach them to avoid inadvertently supporting

Table 31-5. Substance Use Spectrum and Goals for Office Intervention		
Stage, or Triage Category	**Description**	**Office-Based Intervention Goals**
Abstinence	No use of drugs or alcohol	**Positive reinforcement:** Prevent or delay initiation of substance use through positive reinforcement. Include statement about use norms, especially for younger children.
No SUD	Use of alcohol or marijuana with peers in relatively low-risk situations and without related problems or interference with domains of functioning such as school, sports, hobbies, or home life	**Brief advice:** Encourage cessation through brief medically based advice, particularly as it relates to patient's future goals. Promote patient strengths.
Mild or moderate SUD	As defined by *DSM-5*. Adolescents with one or more mild or moderate SUDs typically have associated problems or high-risk behaviors associated with use.	**Brief intervention:** Encourage cessation even for a brief trial period if patient is willing. Reduce potential harm by reducing use and focusing on highest-risk behaviors. Encourage parent involvement to help with follow-through. Follow up with PCC or allied mental health professional to continue conversation and harm reduction.
Severe SUD (addiction)	As defined by *DSM-5;* loss of control or compulsive drug use	**Brief intervention** targeting referral into ongoing treatment. Encourage reducing use and high-risk behaviors and engage adolescent to accept a referral to treatment. Share diagnosis and referral information with parents if possible. Follow-up by PCC to ensure adherence and encourage long-term treatment.

Table 31-5. Substance Use Spectrum and Goals for Office Intervention (*continued*)		
Stage, or Triage Category	Description	Office-Based Intervention Goals
Acute risk	Use associated with acute risk of overdose or in a situation that is physically risky	**Intervention for safety** may include breaching confidentiality, to inform parents about use, and referral to treatment in a timely fashion. Verbal contracts, agreeing not to use while awaiting a formal evaluation, and advice to parents on how to monitor and what to do in case of escalation may also be helpful.

Abbreviations: *DSM-5*, fifth edition of the *Diagnostic and Statistical Manual of Mental Disorders*; PCC, primary care clinician; SUD, substance use disorder.
Adapted with permission from Levy SJ, Williams JF; American Academy of Pediatrics Committee on Substance Use and Prevention. Substance use screening, brief intervention, and referral to treatment. *Pediatrics.* 2016;138(1):e20161211.

ongoing use. This coaching may include separate visits to go over limit setting and communication.

The organization SADD has a Contract for Life that can be signed by both a parent and a youth to ensure that the youth has a plan for a safe ride home.[15]

Referral to Specialty Treatment

The challenge continually posed to PCCs is to recognize when a patient's substance use becomes significant enough to warrant referral to a treatment program or facility rather than being treated solely in the primary care setting. The AAP statement regarding SBIRT provides specific guidance for when to refer patients and to which level of care.[1] Following is a list of indications for specialty referral:

▶ Youths younger than 15 years with a positive screening result for moderate- or high-risk substance use.

▶ Drug use is endangering the youth or others.

▶ Drug use is threatening the achievement of developmentally important goals, such as school attendance and performance, or relationships.

Table 31-6. Sample Framework for Brief Motivational Intervention	
Process	**Description**
Assessment and summary	Targeted assessment for areas of ambivalence to establish rapport and develop a discrepancy between current status and future goals. Sample questions include • *What problems (if any) have you had, related to your use of substances?* • *What regrets (if any) do you have, related to your use of alcohol?* • *What trouble (if any) have you had, related to your use of marijuana?*
Brief advice	Offer specific medical advice to quit or cut down substance use as a means for decreasing the types of problems reported during the assessment. Sample statements include • *Only you can decide whether or not to drink alcohol. Regarding your health, I recommend you quit.* • *Having a blackout means that you have had enough alcohol to poison your brain cells, at least temporarily.* • *Children and adolescents often make bad choices, such as the decision to have sex without a condom, when they are drinking.*
Planning	Engage patient in setting personal goals and agenda for change and link to follow-up. Sample statements include • *It sounds like you really enjoy drinking but don't want to have another blackout. What could you do to protect yourself?* • *What do you think you could do if you found that the person driving you home had been drinking or using drugs?*

▶ Co-occurring mental disorders are present.

▶ Youth has a history of trauma.

▶ Youth is using drugs other than alcohol, marijuana, or tobacco.

▶ Parents are not involved, parents do not acknowledge concerns, or one or both parents have an active SUD.

▶ Interventions by PCC have not reduced use.

If the youth is referred to a substance use specialist, the family will probably need assistance in navigating the requirements of their health insurance plan or the public mental health system and selecting an appropriate provider. Chapter 32, Substance Use 3: Specialty Referral and Comanagement, describes the treatment options and their indications.

The PCC and specialist will need to reach agreement on respective roles in the child's or youth's care and establish a mechanism for communicating progress. The PCC can support the youth by encouraging his or her positive view of treatment; monitoring progress in care and observing for co-occurring disorders; coordinating care provided by parents, school, medical home, and specialists; and encouraging parents to seek treatment for their own tobacco use and other dependencies. The PCC's role also includes supporting and educating the parents of youths who are using substances. Resources available to help PCCs in these roles include the book *Alcohol Screening and Brief Intervention for Youth: A Practitioner's Guide* from the National Institute on Alcohol Abuse and Alcoholism (www.niaaa.nih.gov/Publications/EducationTrainingMaterials/Pages/YouthGuide.aspx) and the Web site Drug Strategies Treatment Guide (www.drugstrategies.org/youths).

Youths (and in some cases their parents) may resist treatment of an SUD. In these cases, the following steps may be helpful:

▶ If a referral is clearly indicated, partner with parents to increase the likelihood of follow-through. Clarify with the youth the relevant laws and protections for minors. In many states, parents can file an order with the police to help enforce house rules. Depending on the situation, it may be necessary to involve the designated child protective services agency.

▶ Provide education and motivational counseling to the youth (and family, as appropriate) to reduce harm and improve functioning at home. Even if the youth is unwilling to engage with specific substance use treatment, he or she may be willing to see a licensed clinical social worker or psychologist.

Summary

Primary care clinicians commonly encounter youths whose parents or teachers have concerns about their use of substances, who have signs or symptoms of an SUD, or who have a positive screening test result for substance use. With youths who are known to be using substances or who have other concerning signs or history, PCCs can perform a full assessment, including a physical examination, detailed substance use history, and assessment of mental health. Laboratory testing can be used as an adjunct to the history and physical examination.

Primary care clinicians are positioned to provide care to youths who are using substances by reinforcing strengths and healthy behaviors and, by applying evidence-based brief interventions, can often be effective in preventing these youths from escalating their use of substances and in motivating them to decrease their use of substances. They can also recognize youths who need the care of SUD specialists, motivate youths and families to connect with needed services, and offer supportive primary care to youths who are involved in specialty care. If youths and their families resist referral for specialty care, PCCs can monitor the youth's progress and provide primary care interventions aimed at reducing substance use and risky behaviors while increasing the youth's motivation to seek specialty care to optimize his or her health.

AAP Policy

Kokotailo PK; American Academy of Pediatrics Committee on Substance Abuse. Alcohol use by youth and adolescents: a pediatric concern. *Pediatrics.* 2010;125(5):1078–1087. Reaffirmed December 2014 (pediatrics.aappublications.org/content/125/5/1078)

Levy S, Schizer M; American Academy of Pediatrics Committee on Substance Abuse. Adolescent drug testing policies in schools. *Pediatrics.* 2015;135(4):e1107–e1112 (pediatrics.aappublications.org/content/135/4/e1107)

Levy S, Siqueira LM, Ammerman SD, et al; American Academy of Pediatrics Committee on Substance Abuse. Testing for drugs of abuse in children and adolescents. *Pediatrics.* 2014;133(6):e1798–e1807 (pediatrics.aappublications.org/content/133/6/e1798)

Levy SJ, Williams JF; American Academy of Pediatrics Committee on Substance Use and Prevention. Substance use screening, brief intervention, and referral to treatment. *Pediatrics.* 2016;138(1):e20161211 (pediatrics.aappublications.org/content/138/1/e20161211)

Siqueira L, Smith VC; American Academy of Pediatrics Committee on Substance Abuse. Binge drinking. *Pediatrics.* 2015;136(3):e718–e726 (pediatrics.aappublications.org/content/136/3/e718)

References

1. Levy SJ, Williams JF; American Academy of Pediatrics Committee on Substance Use and Prevention. Substance use screening, brief intervention, and referral to treatment. *Pediatrics.* 2016;138(1):e20161211
2. Johnston LD, O'Malley PM, Miech RA, Bachman JG, Schulenberg JE. *Monitoring the Future National Survey Results on Drug Use: 1975–2013; Overview, Key Findings on Adolescent Drug Use.* Ann Arbor, MI: Institute for Social Research, University of Michigan; 2017. http://www.monitoringthefuture.org/pubs/monographs/mtf-overview2013.pdf. Accessed February 9, 2018

3. National Center on Addiction and Substance Abuse at Columbia University. *Tobacco: The Smoking Gun. Prepared for the Citizen's Commission to Protect the Truth.* Columbia University; 2007

4. Ford C, English A, Sigman G. Confidential health care for adolescents: position paper for the society for adolescent medicine. *J Adolesc Health.* 2004;35(2):160–167

5. Bagley S, Shrier L, Levy S. Talking to adolescents about alcohol, drugs and sexuality. *Minerva Pediatr.* 2014;66(1):77–87

6. Cohen E, Mackenzie RG, Yates GL. HEADSS, a psychosocial risk assessment instrument: implications for designing effective intervention programs for runaway youth. *J Adolesc Health.* 1991;12(7):539–544

7. Levy S, Weiss R, Sherritt L, et al. An electronic screen for triaging adolescent substance use by risk levels. *JAMA Pediatr.* 2014;168(9):822–828

8. Kelly S, O'Grady KE, Gryczynski J, Mitchell SG, Kirk A, Schwartz RP. Development and validation of a brief screening tool for adolescent tobacco, alcohol and drug use. Association for Medical Education and Research in Substance Abuse (AMERSA) 37th Annual National Conference; 2013; Bethesda, MD

9. National Institute on Alcohol Abuse and Alcoholism, American Academy of Pediatrics. *Alcohol Screening and Brief Intervention for Youth: A Practitioner's Guide.* Washington, DC: National Institute on Alcohol Abuse and Alcoholism; 2015. https://pubs.niaaa.nih.gov/publications/Practitioner/YouthGuide/YouthGuide.pdf. Accessed February 9, 2018

10. Knight JR, Sherritt L, Shrier LA, Harris SK, Chang G. Validity of the CRAFFT substance abuse screening test among adolescent clinic patients. *Arch Pediatr Adolesc Med.* 2002;156(6):607–614

11. Dennis ML, Chan YF, Funk RR. Development and validation of the GAIN Short Screener (GSS) for internalizing, externalizing and substance use disorders and crime/violence problems among adolescents and adults. *Am J Addict.* 2006; 15(suppl 1):80–91

12. Babor TF, de la Fuente JR, Saunders J, Grand M. *AUDIT: The Alcohol Use Disorders Identification Test; Guidelines for Use in Primary Care.* Geneva, Switzerland: World Health Organization; 1992

13. Kelly SM, Gryczynski J, Mitchell SG, Kirk A, O'Grady KE. Validity of brief screening instrument for adolescent tobacco, alcohol, and drug use. *Pediatrics.* 2014;133(5):819–826

14. Wilson CR, Sherritt L, Gates E, Knight JR. Are clinical impressions of adolescent substance use accurate? *Pediatrics.* 2004;114(5):e536–e540

15. Students Against Destructive Decisions. Contract for Life. SADD Web site. http://www.sadd.org/product/sadd-contract-for-life. Accessed February 9, 2018

16. Levy S, Schizer M; American Academy of Pediatrics Committee on Substance Abuse. Adolescent drug testing policies in schools. *Pediatrics.* 2015;135(4): e1107–e1112

CHAPTER 32

Substance Use 3:
Specialty Referral and Comanagement

Sarah Bagley, MD, MSc, and Sharon Levy, MD, MPH

> "*A substance use disorder is a special health care need, and affected youths, like those with attention-deficit/hyperactivity disorder...or asthma, continue to benefit from the services of a medical home in addition to specialty care.*"

Introduction

By senior year in high school, most adolescents in the United States will have used a substance in their lifetimes, most commonly alcohol, marijuana, or tobacco.[1] A smaller proportion of 12th graders report any substance use in the past 30 days. Some children and adolescents use substances instrumentally, in attempt to relieve symptoms of medical or mental disorders. Regardless of drivers, all psychoactive substance use by youths presents a health risk because even occasional use of substances is associated with a high risk of health consequences. (Note that the terms *youth* and *youths* are defined variably in the literature about substance use. In this chapter *youth* or *youths* will generally refer to preadolescents and adolescents aged 9–18 years. In some instances a study cited will provide an alternative definition.) For most youths who use substances with peers and without related problems or interference with domains of functioning, such as school and home life, pediatric primary care clinicians (PCCs)—that is, pediatricians, family physicians, internists, nurse practitioners, and physician assistants who provide frontline, longitudinal care to youths—can address their respective substance uses in the medical home. Chapter 30, Substance Use 1: Use of Tobacco and Nicotine, describes the PCC's role in identifying and caring for youths who use tobacco and nicotine products. For youths who use other substances, Chapter 31, Substance Use 2: Use of Other Substances, describes the PCC's role in identifying, preventing, reducing use, and initiating care; it also guides the PCC in stratifying the level of risk associated with the youth's use of substances and in recognizing youths with a substance use disorder (SUD) requiring care from a specialist. This chapter reviews the various levels of SUD care available in most communities and strategies for supporting youths and families before, during, and after treatment of SUD. It concludes with a brief description of the medical effects of the substances most commonly used by youths.

Specialty Treatment of Youths With SUDs

A variety of evidence-based and evidence-informed psychosocial interventions are available for the treatment of SUDs in youths. Ideally, youths referred for care in the SUD specialty system have access to the safest and most effective treatments. Examples include cognitive behavioral therapy, community reinforcement therapy, contingency management, motivational interviewing and engagement, and family therapy.[2] (See Appendix 6, PracticeWise: Evidence-Based Child and Adolescent Psychosocial Interventions.) Treatment should occur in youth settings and with licensed providers, although it is possible that adults may be treated in the same facility. Youths who use substances often have co-occurring mental disorders; they require referral for mental health services, ideally delivered by a clinician qualified to address both substance use and mental health needs. Many youths benefit from additional services such as individual counseling, school evaluation, neuropsychological evaluation, vocational services, or family counseling. The PCC may contact the local Bureau of Substance Abuse Services to find community resources.

Table 32-1 summarizes the types of referral options for SUD treatment, and Table 32-2 provides a description of the kinds of substance use treatment available.[3]

Helping Youths and Families Access SUD Treatment

As with patients with other conditions, patients with an SUD should be treated in the least restrictive setting that meets their needs. Many youths, even those with a severe SUD, can be treated in the outpatient setting with counseling, monitoring, and, if indicated, medications. Some youths find it difficult or impossible to achieve a period of abstinence while living at home, attending school, and participating in other

Table 32-1. Referral Options for Substance Use Disorders

Type of Treatment	Indications
Outpatient treatment (includes individual or group counseling, family therapy, intensive outpatient therapy, and medication treatment)	• May be used for youths who are motivated to change behaviors or whose caregivers and family feel that it will benefit them • May also be used as a transition from more intensive treatment settings
Partial or day-hospital treatment	• May be considered for youths who need more intensive structure and support to break the cycle of substance use • May also be used as a transition from more intensive treatments
Residential treatment	• For youths who are unlikely to be able to stop drug or alcohol use if they remain in their home environments • For those with a history of treatment failures in less restrictive settings
Inpatient treatment (days to weeks)	• For youths in need of immediate stabilization because of safety concerns • For those who have serious psychiatric disorders or symptoms (eg, suicidal, homicidal, psychotic, acutely dangerous behaviors) co-occurring with SUDs

Abbreviation: SUD, substance use disorder.
Derived from Levy SJ, Kokotailo PK; American Academy of Pediatrics Committee on Substance Abuse. Substance use screening, brief intervention, and referral to treatment for pediatricians. *Pediatrics.* 2011;128(5):e1330–e1340.

Table 32–2. Descriptions of Substance Use Treatment

Treatment	Description
Outpatient	
Individual therapy	An important approach for treating adolescents with substance use disorder. Modalities such as CBT, motivational enhancement therapy, adolescent community reinforcement, and contingency management have been shown to be effective treatment for adolescents with an SUD.
Medication treatment	For adolescents with severe opioid use disorder, medication including buprenorphine or naltrexone can be used to control cravings.
Group therapy	A mainstay of treatment for adolescents with SUDs. It is a particularly attractive option because it is cost-effective and takes advantage of the developmental preference for congregating with peers. However, group therapy has not been extensively evaluated as a therapeutic modality in this age-group, and existing research has produced mixed results.
Family therapy	The best validated approach for treating adolescent SUD. A number of modalities have demonstrated effectiveness. Family counseling typically targets domains that figure prominently in the etiology of SUDs in adolescents: family conflict, communication, parental monitoring, discipline, child abuse or neglect, and parental SUDs.
Intensive outpatient program	Serves as an intermediate level of care for patients who have needs that are too complex for outpatient treatment but do not require inpatient services. These programs allow people to continue with their daily routine and practice newly acquired recovery skills both at home and at work. Intensive outpatient programs generally comprise a combination of supportive group therapy, educational groups, family therapy, individual therapy, relapse prevention and life skills, 12-step recovery, case management, and aftercare planning. These programs range from 2–3 hours per day, 2–5 days per week, and last 1–3 mo. These programs are appealing because they provide a plethora of services in a relatively short period of time.

Partial hospital program

A short-term, comprehensive outpatient program in affiliation with a hospital that is designed to provide support and treatment for patients with SUDs. The services offered at these programs are more concentrated and intensive than regular outpatient treatment; they are structured throughout the entire day and offer medical monitoring in addition to individual and group therapy. Participants typically attend sessions for 7 or 8 hours per day, at least 5 days per week, for 1–3 wk. As with intensive outpatient programs, patients return home in the evenings and have a chance to practice newly acquired recovery skills.

Inpatient or Residential

Short-term treatment services
(formerly known as detoxification)

Refers to the medical management of symptoms of withdrawal. Medically supervised short-term treatment services are indicated for any adolescent who is at risk of withdrawing from alcohol or benzodiazepines and might also be helpful for adolescents withdrawing from opioids, cocaine, or other substances. Short-term treatment services may be an important first step but are not considered definitive treatment. Patients who are discharged from these services should begin either an outpatient or a residential SUD treatment program.

Short-term residential treatment

A short-term (days to weeks) residential placement designed to stabilize patients in crisis, often before entering a longer-term residential treatment program. Short-term residential treatment programs typically target adolescents with co-occurring mental disorders.

Residential treatment

Highly structured live-in environments that provide therapy for those with severe substance use disorder, mental illness, or behavioral problems that require 24-h care. The goal of residential treatment is to promote the achievement and subsequent maintenance of long-term abstinence and equip each patient with both social and coping skills necessary for a successful transition back into society. Residential programs are classified as short-term (<30 d) or long-term (≥30 d).

Residential programs generally comprise individual and group-therapy sessions plus medical, psychological, clinical, nutritional, and educational components. Residential facilities aim to simulate real living environments with added structure and routine to prepare patients with the framework necessary for their lives to continue to be drug- and alcohol-free after completion of the program.

Table 32-2. Descriptions of Substance Use Treatment (continued)

Treatment	Description
Therapeutic boarding school	Educational institutions that provide constant supervision over their students by a professional staff. These schools offer a highly structured environment with set times for all activities; smaller, more specialized classes; and social and emotional support. In addition to the regular services offered at traditional boarding schools, therapeutic schools also provide individual and group therapy for adolescents with mental disorders or SUDs.

Abbreviations: CBT, cognitive behavioral therapy; SUD, substance use disorder.
Adapted with permission from Levy SJ, Williams JF; American Academy of Pediatrics Committee on Substance Use and Prevention. Substance use screening, brief intervention, and referral to treatment. *Pediatrics.* 2016;138(1):e20161211.

activities. For these individuals, higher level of care is indicated. Deciding on the exact level (eg, partial hospital vs short-term residential treatment vs residential treatment) is a process that must consider clinical indication, patient and family preference, insurance coverage, and availability. Even if a higher level of care is indicated, a lower level of care might be a reasonable option if the youth has a strong preference or a treatment spot is available more quickly. Patients who are not able to achieve their therapeutic goals in a lower level of care may ultimately need to be moved to a higher level. Prior to, during, and after subspecialty treatment, the PCC can help the family make treatment level decisions and determine whether treatment is effective.

Co-treatment of Youths With SUDs

Referral of a youth to the SUD (or mental health) specialty system should not end the PCC's involvement. An SUD is a special health care need, and affected youths, like those with attention-deficit/hyperactivity disorder (ADHD) or asthma, continue to benefit from the services of a medical home in addition to specialty care. The PCC and specialist can reach agreement on respective roles in the youth's care and establish a mechanism for communicating progress. The PCC can support the youth by encouraging his or her positive view of treatment, monitoring progress in care, observing for co-occurring disorders, and coordinating care provided by parents, school, the medical home, and specialists. Resources available to help PCCs in these roles include the book *Alcohol Screening and Brief Intervention for Youth: A Practitioner's Guide* from the National Institute on Alcohol Abuse and Alcoholism (www.niaaa.nih.gov/Publications), the Web site Drug Strategies Treatment Guide (www.drugstrategies.org/youths), and the Web site National Institute on Drug Abuse (www.drugabuse.gov/nidamed-medical-health-professionals).

The PCC has an important role in supporting parents of any youths with an SUD, as well as the youths themselves. Here are common issues that may arise and suggestions for how to manage them.

1. *Does a parent or another family member have an active SUD?* Explore this individual's readiness to seek and accept care. Advise parents that seeking an evaluation for their own substance use is excellent role modeling and emotionally supportive for their children and

adolescents. The American Academy of Pediatrics suggests that pediatricians have the following proficiencies in working with families affected by substance use: screening families, following mandated reporting requirements, and directing families to community, regional, and state resources.[4] However, not all parents are receptive to such advice. The youth is the patient; his or her safety and well-being remain the priority. For his or her own well-being, suggest that the youth attend a community-based support group such as Alateen (www.al-anon.alateen.org) and consider involving child protective services if the youth is at acute risk.

2. *Is the parent indirectly supporting the adolescent's use of substances?* Being the parent of a youth with an SUD can cause a great deal of strain on the family unit. Parents often struggle with setting appropriate limits around substance use. Primary care clinicians can guide parents in setting firm limits and consequences for use.

3. *Does the parent feel responsible?* Provide reassurance that this situation can be very stressful to manage and that the parents are taking the appropriate steps to help their son or daughter. Youths commonly experiment with substances; because of a complex combination of risk factors, environment, and genetics, some will develop an SUD. Helping the parent realize that focusing on the present and supporting treatment for his or her child is the most important action he or she can take can help relieve the responsibility he or she may feel. In addition, some communities have parent groups that can provide an important source of support.

4. *Does the parent understand that SUDs are brain diseases and not simply bad behavior?* Although SUDs and addiction are considered chronic medical conditions, stigma is associated with diagnosis. Explain SUDs in the framework of a medical model to help reduce the stigma and increase understanding.

Accurate Education About Substance Use

Misinformation about substances and their health effects is common. Without accurate information, parents may inadvertently minimize the risks to their youth or model inappropriate use of substances themselves. Following are facts about commonly used substances to serve as the basis for discussions with both the youth and the parents:

Alcohol

Short- and long-term health effects are associated with alcohol use in adolescents. Common problems include unintentional injuries and unwanted sexual contact. Blackouts or periods of anterograde amnesia, that is, episodes during which an individual walks and talks but has no subsequent memory, commonly occur with heavy drinking and place individuals at risk. Alcohol use during adolescence is associated with reduced hippocampus volume and difficulties with memory and learning.[5] Early initiation of alcohol use is also associated with developing an alcohol use disorder later in life.[6] Youths with a family history of alcohol use disorders are at particularly high risk.

Youths who have experienced one or more negative consequences associated with alcohol use may be receptive to quitting or reducing alcohol use. Counseling should focus on the highest-risk behaviors, and all youths who agree to reduce alcohol use should be offered a follow-up appointment.

Symptoms of alcohol withdrawal in youths are rare, although youths who frequently binge drink may develop withdrawal syndromes of varying severity. The most common symptoms associated with alcohol withdrawal are nausea, vomiting, insomnia, autonomic hyperactivity, and confusion. Any youth with a history of daily heavy drinking should be observed for signs of withdrawal in an inpatient setting, because alcohol withdrawal can be life-threatening.

Marijuana

Marijuana refers to the dried leaves, flowers, stems, and seeds from the hemp plant, *Cannabis sativa*. The psychoactive component is delta-9-tetrahydrocannabinol, commonly known as THC. Marijuana is an addictive substance. Similar to use of other drugs with addictive potential, such as heroin and nicotine, use of THC causes a release of dopamine in the brain's reward pathway in the nucleus accumbens, and long-term administration alters the limbic system in the brain.[7] As with alcohol and other psychoactive substances, increased risk of addiction is associated with younger onset of use.[8]

Since 2008, in the context of the national debate over marijuana policy, the perceived risk of harm of marijuana use has been decreasing and the rate of marijuana use by adolescents has been increasing.[1] Currently, 6% of high school seniors use marijuana daily.[1] Unfortunately, the known harms of marijuana use in youths are often understated or completely neglected in policy debate. Heavy marijuana use in adolescence has been associated with increased mood disorders, anxiety, and thought disorders and decreasing IQ scores over time.[9–13] Imaging studies have demonstrated morphological changes consistent with these findings. Primary care clinicians must be prepared to have conversations with youths about use as more states legalize marijuana for medical purposes and either decriminalize or legalize recreational use. Counseling should include a discussion of the known medical, psychological, and cognitive adverse effects and a clear statement that there is no known benefit to children or adolescents.

In addition to euphoria, marijuana use results in a loss of critical judgment, distortions in time perception, impairment of tracking (the ability to follow a moving object accurately), and p oor performance on *divided-attention* tasks, such as driving. Other behavioral effects include impaired short-term memory, interference with learning, and difficulty with oral communication, all of which can adversely affect school performance. Occasionally, a PCC will encounter a youth who has an acute adverse reaction to marijuana characterized by a toxic psychosis with depression or panic. Both the symptoms and the treatment of these reactions are similar to those for hallucinogen use. Prolonged (and possibly permanent) personality changes have been reported in long-term marijuana users. An example of a change is an amotivational syndrome, marked by lethargy and a lack of goal-directed activity.[14,15] Physiologic effects occur with marijuana use but are generally less acutely dangerous than those caused by other substances.[15,16] Respiratory effects with prolonged exposure include bronchodilation with acute inhalation and subsequent chronic intermittent bronchoconstriction. Thus, youths who have asthma may experience either relief or exacerbation of symptoms. Allergic reactions to marijuana occur and may cause asthmatic attacks. Furthermore, long-term marijuana use has been found to cause exercise-induced dyspnea and chronic cough that may be mistaken for new-onset asthma in an adolescent.[17,18] Cardiovascular effects include both tachycardia and a transient low-grade elevation of systolic and diastolic blood pressure.[19] Marijuana has been reported to have numerous effects on the endocrine system in boys and men who have histories of prolonged and frequent use, including depression of testosterone levels in the blood, diminished sperm counts, impaired sexual function, and gynecomastia.

The associated clinical problems of impotence and infertility are expected to respond to abstinence from marijuana.

Marijuana withdrawal is subtler than withdrawal from other substances and is therefore often overlooked. This is in part because marijuana's lipophilia ensures a slow physiologic taper, even among individuals who quit cold turkey. Marijuana produces pharmacological tolerance after several days of regular use, and a clinical withdrawal syndrome begins within 24 to 48 hours of discontinuing the drug. Withdrawal symptoms peak in intensity by the fourth day and gradually resolve by 10 to 14 days. The withdrawal symptoms from marijuana include anxiety, restlessness, and sleeplessness.

Use of synthetic cannabinoids, such as "spice" or "K-2," is common: 5.2% of 12th graders reported use in 2015 despite the US Drug Enforcement Administration's Agency's scheduling of the related chemicals in 2011.[1] These substances are similar to THC and bind to the human CB1 receptor. They are synthesized chemically, dissolved in solvent, and sprayed on the leaves of a variety of plants so they can be smoked like marijuana. As with other cannabinoids, binding at the CB1 receptor in the central nervous system results in euphoria, time distortion, intensification of sensory experiences, altered state of consciousness, impaired short-term memory, and increased reaction times. Also, as with marijuana, use is associated with anxiety, hallucinations, paranoia, increased heart rate, and confusion, and it can also be associated with myocardial ischemia and renal failure.

Other Drugs

MDMA/Ecstasy/Molly

The substance known as 3,4-methylenedioxymethamphetamine (called MDMA, ecstasy, or Molly) has recently gained attention because of a series of deaths of individuals who were not known to have any SUDs. The resurgence of MDMA under the name Molly has been primarily among young adults; prevalence of past-year use of MDMA among 12th graders has decreased from its peak 9.2% in 2001 to 3.6% in 2015.[1] Signs of MDMA toxicity include sympathetic overactivity, disturbed behavior, and hyperthermia. Serious complications such as delirium, seizures, and coma are more common when MDMA is used in combination with other substances, especially other stimulants. Rhabdomyolysis and acute renal failure have been reported with MDMA use by individuals who use the drug in the setting of prolonged physical activity, such as all-night dance parties, or raves. All these effects are potentiated by alcohol, benzodiazepines, and other drugs.

Prescription Opioids and Heroin

The use of opioids other than heroin by 12th graders peaked in 2004 at 9.5% and has continued to decrease to 5.4% in 2015.[1] Use of heroin peaked in 2000 and has recently plateaued to 0.5% annual prevalence.[1] Although opioid misuse is not as common as alcohol and marijuana use, the risk of it is high because of the high risk for addiction and associated complications, including fatal overdose and transition to injection drug use. For youths with suspected opioid use disorders, referral to specialty care, which may be either outpatient or residential, is key because effective pharmacological treatment is available with buprenorphine-naloxone, a partial opioid agonist approved for adolescents 16 years and older.[19] As with youths with other conditions, youths with opioid use disorder should be treated in the least restrictive environment. Most adolescents (>16 years of age) with opioid use disorder are candidates for medication treatment in the outpatient setting.[20] Few PCCs have completed the necessary training to prescribe buprenorphine to date, leaving a treatment gap.

Opioid withdrawal results in flu-like symptoms, including vomiting and diarrhea, myalgia, nasal congestion, and joint pain. These symptoms can be very unpleasant but are generally not life-threatening in otherwise healthy youths. Medical withdrawal, formally known as detoxification, can help ease the discomfort associated with withdrawal, but this should not be considered stand-alone treatment. Patients who have successfully completed short-term treatment for withdrawal management should be referred for ongoing treatment.

Prescription Stimulants

In youths with ADHD, stimulants can provide effective treatment; however, amphetamines are also commonly misused by youths. A youth may misuse his or her own medication or take a friend's prescription. Misuse can be driven by a desire to get high or to enhance academic achievement or both. Amphetamine use peaked at 10.9% among 12th graders in 2002. Since then, annual prevalence has fluctuated with the prevalence 7.7% in 2015.[1] Youths with ADHD are at increased likelihood of developing an SUD; treatment for ADHD may lower this risk.[21]

Summary

While substance use is common among youths and often does not rise to the level of a disorder, some youths develop SUDs and require specialty treatment, including treatment of co-occurring mental disorders. These services may take place in outpatient, partial or day-hospital, residential, or inpatient settings and may incorporate a variety of evidence-based approaches, depending on the needs of the youth. Primary care clinicians continue to play important roles in the care of youths served by the SUD specialty system.

AAP Policy

American Academy of Pediatrics Committee on Substance Use and Prevention. Medication-assisted treatment of adolescents with opioid use disorders. *Pediatrics.* 2016;138(3):e20161893 (pediatrics.aappublications.org/content/138/3/e20161893)

Kokotailo PK; American Academy of Pediatrics Committee on Substance Abuse. Alcohol use by youth and adolescents: a pediatric concern. *Pediatrics.* 2010;125(5):1078–1087. Reaffirmed December 2014 (pediatrics.aappublications.org/content/125/5/1078)

Levy S, Schizer M; American Academy of Pediatrics Committee on Substance Abuse. Adolescent drug testing policies in schools. *Pediatrics.* 2015;135(4):e1107–e1112 (pediatrics.aappublications.org/content/135/4/e1107)

Levy S, Siqueira LM; American Academy of Pediatrics Committee on Substance Abuse. Testing for drugs of abuse in children and adolescents. *Pediatrics.* 2014;133(6):e1798–e1807 (pediatrics.aappublications.org/content/133/6/e1798)

Levy SJ, Williams JF; American Academy of Pediatrics Committee on Substance Use and Prevention. Substance use screening, brief intervention, and referral to treatment. *Pediatrics.* 2016;138(1):e20161211 (pediatrics.aappublications.org/content/138/1/e20161211)

Siqueira L, Smith VC; American Academy of Pediatrics Committee on Substance Abuse. Binge drinking. *Pediatrics.* 2015;136(3):e718–e726 (pediatrics.aappublications.org/content/136/3/e718)

Smith VC, Wilson CR; American Academy of Pediatrics Committee on Substance Use and Prevention. Families affected by parental substance use. *Pediatrics.* 2016;138(2):e20161575 (pediatrics.aappublications.org/content/138/2/e20161575)

References

1. Johnston LD, O'Malley PM, Miech RA, Bachman JG, Schulenberg JE. *Monitoring the Future National Results on Drug Use: 1975–2016; Overview, Key Findings on Adolescent Drug Use.* Ann Arbor, MI: Institute for Social Research, University of Michigan; 2017

2. Foy JM; American Academy of Pediatrics Task Force on Mental Health. Enhancing pediatric mental health care: algorithms for primary care. *Pediatrics.* 2010; 125(suppl 3):S109–S125

3. Levy SJ, Kokotailo PK; American Academy of Pediatrics Committee on Substance Abuse. Substance use screening, brief intervention, and referral to treatment for pediatricians. *Pediatrics.* 2011;128(5):e1330–e1340

4. Smith VC, Wilson CR; American Academy of Pediatrics Committee on Substance Use and Prevention. Families affected by parental substance use. *Pediatrics.* 2016; 138(2):e20161575

5. Nagel BJ, Schweinsburg AD, Phan V, Tapert SF. Reduced hippocampal volume among adolescents with alcohol use disorders without psychiatric comorbidity. *Psychiatry Res.* 2005;139(3):181–190

6. Hingson RW, Heeren T, Winter MR. Age at drinking onset and alcohol dependence: age at onset, duration, and severity. *Arch Pediatr Adolesc Med.* 2006;160(7):739–746

7. Tanda G, Pontieri FE, Di Chiara G. Cannabinoid and heroin activation of mesolimbic dopamine transmission by a common mu1 opioid receptor mechanism. *Science.* 1997;276(5321):2048–2050

8. Windle M, Windle RC. Early onset problem behaviors and alcohol, tobacco, and other substance use disorders in young adulthood. *Drug Alcohol Depend.* 2012; 121(1–2):152–158

9. Tosato S, Lasalvia A, Bonetto C, et al. The impact of cannabis use on age of onset and clinical characteristics in first-episode psychotic patients. Data from the Psychosis Incident Cohort Outcome Study (PICOS). *J Psychiatr Res.* 2013; 47(4):438–444

10. Meier MH, Caspi A, Ambler A, et al. Persistent cannabis users show neuropsychological decline from childhood to midlife. *Proc Natl Acad Sci U S A.* 2012;109(40):E2657–E2664

11. Arseneault L, Cannon M, Poulton R, et al. Cannabis use in adolescence and risk for adult psychosis: longitudinal prospective study. *BMJ.* 2002;325(7374):1212–1213

12. Fergusson DM, Horwood LJ, Swain-Campbell N. Cannabis use and psychosocial adjustment in adolescence and young adulthood. *Addiction.* 2002;97(99):1123–1135

13. Hayatbakhsh MR, Najman JM, Jamrozik K, et al. Cannabis and anxiety and depression in young adults: a large prospective study. *J Am Acad Child Adolesc Psychiatry.* 2007;46(3):408–417

14. Schydlower M, ed. *Substance Abuse: A Guide for Health Professionals.* 2nd ed. Elk Grove Village, IL: American Academy of Pediatrics; 2001

15. Duffy A, Milin R. Case study: withdrawal syndrome in adolescent chronic cannabis users. *J Am Acad Child Adolesc Psychiatry.* 1996;35(12):1618–1621

16. Hall W, Degenhardt L. Adverse health effects of nonmedical cannabis use. *Lancet.* 2009;374(9698):1383–1391

17. Tashkin DP. Airway effects of marijuana, cocaine, and other inhaled illicit agents. *Curr Opin Pulm Med.* 2001;7(2):43–61

18. Taylor DR, Poulton R, Moffitt TE, Ramankutty P, Sears MR. The respiratory effects of cannabis dependence in young adults. *Addiction.* 2000;95(11):1669–1677

19. Thomas G, Kloner RA, Rezkalla S. Adverse cardiovascular, cerebrovascular, and peripheral vascular effects of marijuana inhalation: what cardiologists need to know. *Am J Cardiol.* 2014;113(1):187–190

20. American Academy of Pediatrics Committee on Substance Use and Prevention. Medication-assisted treatment of adolescents with opioid use disorders. *Pediatrics.* 2016;138(3):e20161893

21. Harstad E, Levy S. Attention-deficit/hyperactivity disorder and substance abuse. *Pediatrics.* 2014;134(1):e293–e301

Appendixes

[a] These tools are updated regularly at www.aap.org/mentalhealth.

Algorithm: A Process for Integrating Mental Health Care Into Pediatric Practice

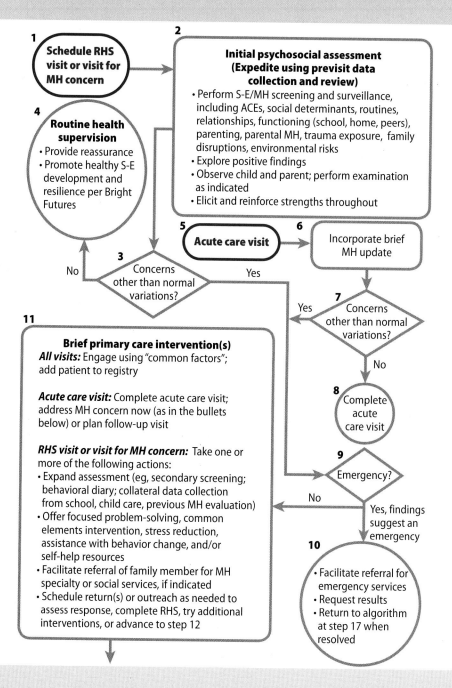

1 Schedule RHS visit or visit for MH concern

2 Initial psychosocial assessment (Expedite using previsit data collection and review)
- Perform S-E/MH screening and surveillance, including ACEs, social determinants, routines, relationships, functioning (school, home, peers), parenting, parental MH, trauma exposure, family disruptions, environmental risks
- Explore positive findings
- Observe child and parent; perform examination as indicated
- Elicit and reinforce strengths throughout

4 Routine health supervision
- Provide reassurance
- Promote healthy S-E development and resilience per Bright Futures

3 Concerns other than normal variations?
No

5 Acute care visit

6 Incorporate brief MH update

7 Concerns other than normal variations?
Yes / No

8 Complete acute care visit

9 Emergency?
No / Yes, findings suggest an emergency

11 Brief primary care intervention(s)
All visits: Engage using "common factors"; add patient to registry

Acute care visit: Complete acute care visit; address MH concern now (as in the bullets below) or plan follow-up visit

RHS visit or visit for MH concern: Take one or more of the following actions:
- Expand assessment (eg, secondary screening; behavioral diary; collateral data collection from school, child care, previous MH evaluation)
- Offer focused problem-solving, common elements intervention, stress reduction, assistance with behavior change, and/or self-help resources
- Facilitate referral of family member for MH specialty or social services, if indicated
- Schedule return(s) or outreach as needed to assess response, complete RHS, try additional interventions, or advance to step 12

10
- Facilitate referral for emergency services
- Request results
- Return to algorithm at step 17 when resolved

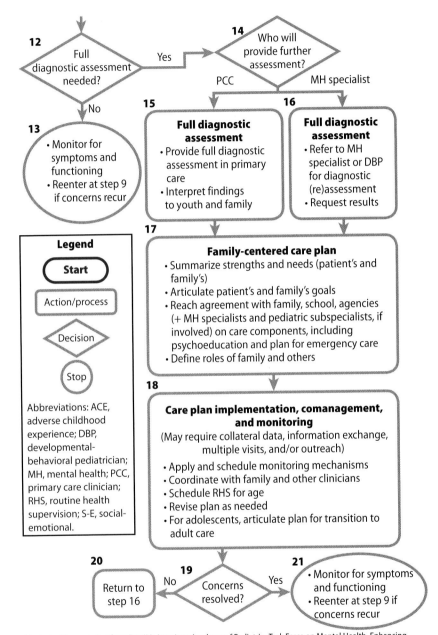

12 Full diagnostic assessment needed?

Yes

14 Who will provide further assessment?

PCC · MH specialist

No

13
- Monitor for symptoms and functioning
- Reenter at step 9 if concerns recur

15 Full diagnostic assessment
- Provide full diagnostic assessment in primary care
- Interpret findings to youth and family

16 Full diagnostic assessment
- Refer to MH specialist or DBP for diagnostic (re)assessment
- Request results

17 Family-centered care plan
- Summarize strengths and needs (patient's and family's)
- Articulate patient's and family's goals
- Reach agreement with family, school, agencies (+ MH specialists and pediatric subspecialists, if involved) on care components, including psychoeducation and plan for emergency care
- Define roles of family and others

Legend

Start

Action/process

Decision

Stop

Abbreviations: ACE, adverse childhood experience; DBP, developmental-behavioral pediatrician; MH, mental health; PCC, primary care clinician; RHS, routine health supervision; S-E, social-emotional.

18 Care plan implementation, comanagement, and monitoring
(May require collateral data, information exchange, multiple visits, and/or outreach)
- Apply and schedule monitoring mechanisms
- Coordinate with family and other clinicians
- Schedule RHS for age
- Revise plan as needed
- For adolescents, articulate plan for transition to adult care

20 Return to step 16

No

19 Concerns resolved?

Yes

21
- Monitor for symptoms and functioning
- Reenter at step 9 if concerns recur

Adapted with permission from Foy JM; American Academy of Pediatrics Task Force on Mental Health. Enhancing pediatric mental health care: algorithms for primary care. *Pediatrics.* 2010;125(suppl 3):S109–S125.

Mental Health Tools for Pediatrics

The following table is a snapshot of a work in progress of the American Academy of Pediatrics (AAP) Mental Health Leadership Work Group (MHLWG). It is a compilation of tools that are potentially useful at each stage of a clinical process through which mental health content can be integrated into pediatric primary care. This process is depicted by algorithms in Appendix 1 and described in Chapter 1, Integrating Preventive Mental Health Care Into Pediatric Practice, and Chapter 2, Pediatric Care of Children and Adolescents With Mental Health Problems. These chapters and Chapter 3, Office and Network Systems to Support Mental Health Care, offer general guidance concerning the selection of tools for use in primary care. A number of chapters offer, in addition, guidance in interpreting results of commonly used screening tools, including a number of those included in the following table.

Several points about the table bear noting.

► The sequence of tools within each section does not reflect the recommendation or preference of the AAP MHLWG for one tool over another.

► In a number of instances, there are options for use of a tool at more than one place in the process. In these instances, a full description accompanies the first mention. Subsequent mentions of the tool include only the tool abbreviation and any reference numbers. In addition to facilitating access to further reading, this setup will assist readers in locating the tool's full description where it appears in the table.

► Information about psychometric properties of each tool is available in the latest version of the tool at www.aap.org/mentalhealth.

Table A2-1. Mental Health Tools for Pediatrics

Psychosocial Measure	Tools and Description	Number of Items and Format	Age-group and Any Languages — Reading Level if Specified	Administration and Scoring Time — Training[a]	Source
Initial Psychosocial Assessment (Algorithm Step 2): Previsit or Intra-visit Data Collection and Screening					
Surveillance	Bright Futures surveillance questions[1]	Unlimited	0–21 y English Spanish	Variable	AAP/MCHB freely accessible Source: https://brightfutures.aap.org/materials-and-tools/tool-and-resource-kit/Pages/default.aspx
	Bright Futures previsit and supplemental questionnaires[1]	Variable	0–21 y English Spanish	Variable	AAP/MCHB freely accessible Source: https://brightfutures.aap.org/materials-and-tools/tool-and-resource-kit/Pages/default.aspx

	Interview	Adolescents Language of clinician	Part of interview process	Freely accessible Sources:
HEADSSS mnemonic[2] *Assesses for Home/ environment, Education and employment, Activities, Drugs, Sexuality, Suicide/ depression, and Safety. HEADSSS-3.0 includes media use.*				www.bcchildrens.ca/Youth-Health-Clinic-site/ Documents/headss20 assessment20guide1.pdf http://contemporary pediatrics.modern medicine.com/ contemporary-pediatrics/ content/tags/adolescent-medicine/heeadsss-30-psychosocial-interview-adolesce?page=full
School report cards, end-of-grade tests, Individualized Education Program (IEP), and 504 plan				

Table A2-1. Mental Health Tools for Pediatrics *(continued)*

Psychosocial Measure	Tools and Description	Number of Items and Format	Age-group and Any Languages Reading Level if Specified	Administration and Scoring Time Training[a]	Source
Initial Psychosocial Assessment (Algorithm Step 2): Previsit or Intra-visit Data Collection and Screening					
General psychosocial screening: young children aged 0–5 y	Early Childhood Screening Assessment (ECSA)[3] *Assesses emotional and behavioral development in young children and maternal distress*	40 items, 3-point Likert scale responses and an additional option for parents to identify whether they are concerned and would like help with an item	18–60 mo English Spanish Romanian Reading level: fifth grade	10–15 min to complete Scoring time: 1–2 min Should be administered by health care professional or MHS whose training and scope of practice includes interpreting screening test results and interpreting positive or negative screening results for parents	Freely accessible Source: www.infantinstitute. org/wp-content/ uploads/2013/07/ECSA-40- Child-Care1.pdf

Tool	Format	Age/Language	Time	Source
Ages & Stages Questionnaires (ASQ): Social-Emotional, Second Edition (ASQ: SE-2)[4] *Screens for social-emotional problems in young children; used in conjunction with ASQ or another tool designed to provide information on a child's communicative, motor, problem-solving, and adaptive behaviors*	From 19 items (6 mo)–33 items (30 mo) Parent report	6–60 mo English Spanish Reading level: sixth grade	10–15 min Scoring: 1–5 min (can be scored by paraprofessionals)	Proprietary Source: http://agesandstages.com/products-services/asqse-2
Brief Infant Toddler Social Emotional Assessment (BITSEA)[5] *Screens for social-emotional problems in young children*	42 items Parent report Child care report	12–36 mo English Spanish	7–10 min	Proprietary Margaret.Briggs-Gowan@yale.edu or Alice.Carter@umb.edu
Survey of Well-being of Young Children (SWYC)[6-8] Consists of subscales appropriate to age **Milestones** *Assesses cognitive, language, and motor development* **Baby Pediatric Symptom Checklist (BPSC)** up to 18 mo	Parent questionnaires with embedded subscales 34–47 questions Paper and electronic versions	2–60 mo English Spanish Burmese Nepali Portuguese (Translations not independently validated)	10–15 min	Freely accessible Source: www.floatinghospital.org/The-Survey-of-Wellbeing-of-Young-Children/Age-Specific-Forms.aspx

Table A2-1. Mental Health Tools for Pediatrics (continued)					
Psychosocial Measure	Tools and Description	Number of Items and Format	Age-group and Any Languages / Reading Level if Specified	Administration and Scoring Time / Training[a]	Source
Initial Psychosocial Assessment (Algorithm Step 2): Previsit or Intra-visit Data Collection and Screening					
General psychosocial screening: young children aged 0–5 y	*Assesses irritability, inflexibility, and difficulty with routines* **Preschool Pediatric Symptom Checklist (PPSC)** 18–66 mo *Assesses for emotional/ behavioral symptoms* **Parent's Observations of Social Interactions (POSI)** 18–35 mo *Screens for ASD* **Family questions** *Assesses stress in family environment (eg, parental depression; discord; substance use; food insecurity; parent's concerns about child's behavior, learning, or development)*				

General psychosocial screening: children aged 6–10 y	Pediatric Symptom Checklist—35 items (PSC-35)[9,10] *General psychosocial screening and functional assessment in the domains of attention, externalizing symptoms, and internalizing symptoms*	35 items Self-administered Parent or youth ≥11 y	4–16 y English Spanish Chinese Japanese Pictorial versions available	<5 min Scoring: 1–2 min	Freely accessible Source: Massachusetts General Hospital Web site at www.massgeneral.org/psychiatry/services/psc_home.aspx
	Pediatric Symptom Checklist—17 items (PSC-17)[11] *General psychosocial screening and functional assessment in the domains of attention, externalizing symptoms, and internalizing symptoms*	17 items Self-administered Parent or youth ≥11 y	4–16 y English Spanish Chinese Reading level: fifth grade—sixth grade	<5 min Scoring: 2 min	Freely accessible Source: https://depts.washington.edu/hcsats/FCAP/resources/PSC-17%20English.pdf
	Strengths and Difficulties Questionnaires (SDQ)[12] *Assesses 25 attributes, some positive and some negative, divided among 5 scales. Some versions have an impact scale on the second page.*	25 items Self-administered versions for parent, teacher, or youth aged 11–17 y	3–17 y >40 languages	10 min	Freely accessible Source: Youth in Mind Web site at www.sdqinfo.org

Table A2-1. Mental Health Tools for Pediatrics (*continued*)

Psychosocial Measure	Tools and Description	Number of Items and Format	Age-group and Any Languages Reading Level if Specified	Administration and Scoring Time Training[a]	Source
Initial Psychosocial Assessment (Algorithm Step 2): Previsit or Intra-visit Data Collection and Screening					
General psychosocial screening: adolescents and young adults aged 11–21 y	PSC-35[9,10]				
	PSC-17[11]				
	SDQ[12]				
	The Rapid Assessment for Adolescent Preventive Services (RAAPS)[13,14] *Web-based screening tool developed to identify youths most at risk for school drop-out, using factors such as discrimination, abuse, and access to tangible needs (eg, food, water, electricity) that contribute to morbidity, mortality, and social problems*	21 items	Age specific for older child (9–12 y), adolescent (13–18 y), and young adult (18–24 y) Includes audio and multilingual options	Approximately 5 min to self-administer. Scored automatically and pertinent information is downloaded. 30-min demonstration available (www. possibilities forchange.com/ raaps).	Proprietary. Review and download free of charge at www.raaps.org.

Targeted screening: substance use[b]				
Screening to Brief Intervention (S2BI)[15] *Brief screening to determine whether further assessment is necessary*	2 items	Adolescents English	1–2 min if responses negative	Freely accessible Source: https://pubs.niaaa.nih.gov/publications/Practitioner/YouthGuide/YouthGuide.pdf
Brief Screener for Tobacco, Alcohol, and Other Drugs (BSTAD)[16] *Identifies problematic tobacco, alcohol, and marijuana use in pediatric settings*	3 frequency questions (one for each substance) Interview or iPad self-administration (preferred)	12–17 y English	1–2 min if responses negative	Freely accessible Source: www.drugabuse.gov/ast/bstad/#
NIAAA youth alcohol screening[17] *Screens for friends' uses and own use*	2 questions	Adolescents English	1–2 min if responses negative	Freely accessible Source: www.niaaa.nih.gov/Publications/EducationTrainingMaterials/Pages/YouthGuide.aspx
CRAFFT (Car, Relax, Alone, Forget, Friends, Trouble) lifetime use[18] *Screens for substance use*	3 screener questions and then 6 items Self-administered or youth report	Adolescents English	1–2 min if responses negative	Freely accessible. Use at this step or in algorithm step 11, later in this table, as brief assessment if S2B1 result is positive. Source: Center for Adolescent Substance Abuse Research Web site at www.ceasar-boston.org/CRAFFT/index.php.

Table A2-1. Mental Health Tools for Pediatrics (*continued*)

Psychosocial Measure	Tools and Description	Number of Items and Format	Age-group and Any Languages Reading Level if Specified	Administration and Scoring Time Training[a]	Source
Initial Psychosocial Assessment (Algorithm Step 2): Previsit or Intra-visit Data Collection and Screening					
Targeted screening: adolescent depression[c]	Patient Health Questionnaire–Adolescent (PHQ-A) depression screening[19] *Consists of questions on depression from full PHQ-A (See full PHQ-A tool later in this table.)*	Abbreviated 9-item screening specifically for depression	11–17 y English	<5 min to complete and score	Free with permission Source: www.aacap.org/App_Themes/AACAP/docs/member_resources/toolbox_for_clinical_practice_and_outcomes/symptoms/GLAD-PC_PHQ-9.pdf
	Kutcher Adolescent Depression Scale (KADS)[20] *Screens for depression*	6, 11, or 16 items	12–17 y English	5 min Scoring: 1 min	Freely accessible. 6-Item Kutcher Adolescent Depression Scale (KADS-6). http://lphi.org/CMSuploads/Kutcher-Adolescent-Depression-Scale-47583.pdf.

Category	Tool	Items	Age/Language	Time	Access
Parent/family general screening	Pediatric Intake Form (Family Psychosocial Screen)[21] *Screens for parental depression, substance use, domestic violence, parental history of being abused, and social supports*	22 items	0–21 y English	Variable	Freely accessible Source: www.pedstest.com/Portals/0/TheBook/FPSinEnglish.pdf
	SWYC[6–8]				
	A Safe Environment for Every Kid (SEEK) Parent Questionnaire - R (PQ-R)[22] *Includes questions about smoking, guns, food availability, depression, substance use, discipline, and domestic violence*	15 yes-or-no questions	0–5 y English Spanish	3 min Scoring: <3 min	Proprietary Source: www.seekwellbeing.org/the-seek-parent-questionnaire-
	Parents' Assessment of Protective Factors[23] *Self-assessment of parents' resilience, their social connections, concrete support they receive in times of need, and their social-emotional competence of children*	46 questions, including 10 background questions	Parents of children from birth–8 y English Spanish	20 min	Freely accessible Source: www.cssp.org/reform/child-welfare/pregnant-and-parenting-youth/Parents-Assessment-of-Protective-Factors.pdf

Table A2-1. Mental Health Tools for Pediatrics (continued)					
Psychosocial Measure	Tools and Description	Number of Items and Format	Age-group and Any Languages Reading Level if Specified	Administration and Scoring Time Training*	Source
Initial Psychosocial Assessment (Algorithm Step 2): Previsit or Intra-visit Data Collection and Screening					
Parent/family general screening	Health Leads Screening[24] Assesses food insecurity, housing instability, utility needs, strained financial resources, transportation difficulty, exposure to violence, and sociodemographic information	10 questions In each category, alternative questions, plus follow-up questions as indicated	Parents of children of all ages. Multiple languages. Reading level varies by question.	5 min	Freely accessible Source: toolkit available at https://healthleadsusa.org/wp-content/uploads/2016/07/Health-Leads-Screening-Toolkit-July-2016.pdf
	McMaster Family Functioning Scale[25] Assesses family functioning	12 items Self-report	Adolescents and adults Translated into 24 languages	<5 min	Freely accessible Source: www.clintools.com/victims/resources/assessment/interpersonal/mcmaster.html

Parent Stress Index (PSI), Third Edition[26] *Elicits indicators of stress and identifies parent-child problem areas in parents of children aged 1 mo–12 y PSI-Short Form*	120 items plus 19 optional items Parent self-report PSI-Short Form: 36 items Version for parenting adolescents	Parents of children aged 1 mo–12 y English	20–30 min	Proprietary Source: PAR Web site at www.parinc.com/Products/Pkey/337
Stress Index for Parents of Adolescents (SIPA)[27] *Elicits indicators of stress in parents of adolescents*	112 items	Parents of pre-adolescents and adolescents aged 11–19 y English	20 min Scoring: 10 min	Proprietary Source: www.parinc.com/Products/Pkey/412
Caregiver Strain Questionnaire (CGSQ) and CGSQ Short Form 7 (CGSQ-SF7)[28] *Assesses strain experienced by caregivers and families of youths with emotional problems*	21 items 7 items (CGSQ-SF7) Self-report by parents or caregivers	Parents/caregivers of adolescents with emotional problems English Spanish	Variable	Freely accessible Source: www.hospicepatients.org/caregiver-strain-questionaire-robinson.pdf
Multidimensional Scale of Perceived Social Support Parent Stress Inventory (MSPSS)[29] *Assesses social support*	12 items Parent report	Adult Multiple languages	2–5 min	Freely accessible Source: www.yorku.ca/rokada/psyctest/socsupp.pdf

Table A2-1. Mental Health Tools for Pediatrics (continued)

Psychosocial Measure	Tools and Description	Number of Items and Format	Age-group and Any Languages Reading Level if Specified	Administration and Scoring Time Training[a]	Source
Initial Psychosocial Assessment (Algorithm Step 2): Previsit or Intra-visit Data Collection and Screening					
Parent/ family targeted screening	Patient Health Questionnaire-2 (PHQ-2)— first 2 items from PHQ-9[30] *Screens adults for depression*	2 items Parent self-report	Adult English	1 min	Freely accessible Source: www.cqaimh.org/ pdf/tool_phq2.pdf
	Patient Health Questionnaire-9 (PHQ-9)[31] *Screens adults for depression*	9 items Parent self-report	Adult English	<5 min to administer Scoring: <3 min	Freely accessible Source: www.phqscreeners. com/sites/g/files/ g10016261/f/201412/ PHQ-9_English.pdf
	Edinburgh Postnatal Depression Scale (EPDS)[32] *Screens women for depression*	10 items Parent self-report	Peripartum women Multiple languages	<5 min to administer Scoring: 5 min	Freely accessible Source: www. perinatalservicesbc.ca/ health-professionals/ professional-resources/ health-promo/edinburgh- postnatal-depression- scale-(epds)

Tool	Format	Population/Languages	Time	Availability
Abuse Assessment Screen (AAS)[33] *Screens for domestic violence*	5–6 items Parent report	Adolescent girls and adult women English	About 45 sec if all answers are no	Freely accessible Source: http://peaceathome.com/wordpress/wp-content/uploads/2014/10/Abuse_Assessment_Screen_AAS.pdf
Hunger Vital Sign[34] *Identifies food insecurity and its associated social determinants*	2 questions	Parents of children from birth–3 y English Russian Somalian Vietnamese Korean Chinese Spanish Arabic Swahili French Nepali	≤5 min	Freely accessible Source: http://childrenshealthwatch.org/public-policy/hunger-vital-sign

Table A2-1. Mental Health Tools for Pediatrics (continued)

Psychosocial Measure	Tools and Description	Number of Items and Format	Age-group and Any Languages; Reading Level if Specified	Administration and Scoring Time; Training[c]	Source
Initial Psychosocial Assessment (Algorithm Step 2): Previsit or Intra-visit Data Collection and Screening					
Trauma exposure[d]	The Acute Stress Checklist for Children (ASC-Kids)[35] *Assesses acute stress reactions within the first month after exposure to a potentially traumatic event*	29 items (25 *DSM*-related; 4 additional items for clinical use: subjective life threat, family context, and coping) Self-report or may be read aloud to child	8–17 y English Spanish	5 min	Proprietary Source: www.istss.org/assessing-trauma/acute-stress-checklist-for-children.aspx
	Children's Revised Impact of Event Scale (CRIES)-8[36] *Assesses impact of traumatic events*	8 items Self-report	≥8 y who can read Multiple languages	<5 min	Freely accessible Instructions and forms available at Children and War Foundation Web site at www.childrenandwar.org/measures/children's-revised-impact-of-event-scale-8—cries-8

Global functioning	Brief Impairment Scale (BIS) multidimensional[37] *Assesses global functioning in domains of interpersonal relations, school/work, and self-care/self-fulfillment*	23 items Parent report	4–17 y English Spanish	10 min	Freely accessible Source: www.heardalliance. org/wp-content/uploads/ 2011/04/Brief-Impairment-Scale-English.pdf
	Columbia Impairment Scale (CIS)—part of Child/ Adolescent Wellness Assessment (CAWA)[38] *Assesses global functioning in domains of interpersonal relations, psychopathology, school performance, and use of leisure time; monitors progress after 6 mo of treatment*	13 items administered by clinician. "Nonclinical version" can be administered directly by lay or clinical interviewers to parents or youth.	Children and adolescents English	5 min	Freely accessible Sources: Youth version at www.hrcec. org/images/PDF/CIS-Y.pdf Parent version at www.hrcec. org/images/PDF/CIS-P.pdf
	SDQ Impact Scale[12] *Assesses global functioning in domains of home life, friendships, learning, and play*	5 items Parent Teacher Youth ≥11 y	3–17 y >40 languages	<5 min	Freely accessible Source: www.sdqinfo.com

Table A2-1. Mental Health Tools for Pediatrics (*continued*)

Psychosocial Measure	Tools and Description	Number of Items and Format	Age-group and Any Languages; Reading Level if Specified	Administration and Scoring Time; Training[a]	Source
Brief MH Update (Algorithm Step 6)					
Brief screenings	AAP brief MH update[39,40]	Questions selected from a list and sorted by age-group	Birth–21 y English	1–5 min, depending on provider's preference	Freely accessible Source: http://pediatrics. aappublications.org/ content/125/ Supplement_3/S159
Screen for somatization symptom disorder and related disorders	SDQ Impact Scale[12] Children's Somatization Inventory (CSI)-24 (CSI-24)[41] *Shortened version of original CSI assesses for the presence of multiple somatic symptoms.*	24 items. Interviewer administers orally; child selects response from cards.	Multiple languages	<10 min	Freely accessible Source (parent and child versions): www. childrenshospital. vanderbilt.org/uploads/ documents/CSI-24_ English_parent_and_ child.pdf

Assessing Emergencies (Algorithm Step 9)

Suicide assessment	Ask Suicide-Screening Questions (ASQ)[42] Note: This tool is not to be confused with the ASQ, a developmental screening tool, or the ASQ:SE-2, described earlier in this table. *Assesses for suicide risk among youths with psychiatric concerns in emergency department settings*	4 screening items	10–24 y English	20 sec	Toolkit freely accessible at www.nimh.nih.gov/labs-at-nimh/asq-toolkit-materials/index.shtml
	Suicide Assessment Five-step Evaluation and Triage (SAFE-T)[43] *Process includes identifying risk factors, identifying protective factors, conducting suicide inquiry, determining risk level/intervention, and documenting.*	Protocol with prompts for each step to guide clinical process	Children and adolescents English	Variable	Source: www.shiacmh.org/docs/safe-t.pdf
	Suicide Behaviors Questionnaire-Revised (SBQ-R)[44] *Assesses 4 dimensions of suicidality*	4 items	Adolescents English	5 min	Source: www.cqaimh.org/pdf/tool_sbq-r.pdf

Table A2-1. Mental Health Tools for Pediatrics (*continued*)

Psychosocial Measure	Tools and Description	Number of Items and Format	Age-group and Any Languages / Reading Level if Specified	Administration and Scoring Time / Training[a]	Source
Assessing Emergencies (Algorithm Step 9)					
Suicide assessment	Columbia-Suicide Severity Rating Scale (C-SSRS)[45] *Supports suicide risk assessment through a series of questions; answers help users both identify whether someone is at risk for suicide and assess the severity and immediacy of that risk.*	6 items within a 2-page form	Adolescents English	5 min Requires training to administer	Freely available Source: http://cssrs.columbia.edu/wp-content/uploads/C-SSRS_Pediatric-SLC_11.14.16.pdf
	Suicidal Ideation Questionnaire (SIQ) and SIQ-Junior (SIQ-Jr)[46] *Appropriate for individual or group administration in clinical or school settings*	SIQ: 30 items SIQ-Jr: 15 items	Adolescents and young adults aged 13–18 y SIQ: grades 10–12 SIQ-Jr: grades 7–9 English	10 min	Proprietary Source: www.parinc.com/Products/Pkey/413

	Child-Adolescent Suicidal Potential Index (CASPI)[47] *Assesses multiple aspects of suicidal behavior: total score plus 3 subscales*	30 yes-or-no items in self-report format	Children and youths 6–18 y English	10 min	Source: Author's contact information available at http://books.google.com/books?id=-r309ILpxTkC&pg=PA95
	PHQ-A[19] or PHQ-9[31] severity items on suicide				
Delirium assessment	Delirium Rating Scale (DRS) and Revised-98 (DRS-R-98)[48] *Differentiates between delirium, dementia, depression, schizophrenia, and other conditions*	DRS 10 items DRS-R-98 16 clinician-rated items, 13 of which assess the severity of symptoms and 3 of which have diagnostic significance	Children and adolescents English, French, Italian, Spanish, Dutch, Mandarin, Chinese, Korean, Swedish, Japanese, German, and Indian	Both scales >2 h Scoring: 20–30 min	Freely accessible Source: https://neuro.psychiatryonline.org/doi/pdf/10.1176/jnp.13.2.229?code=neuro-site

Table A2-1. Mental Health Tools for Pediatrics (*continued*)

Psychosocial Measure	Tools and Description	Number of Items and Format	Age-group and Any Languages Reading Level if Specified	Administration and Scoring Time Training[a]	Source
Assessing Emergencies (Algorithm Step 9)					
Illness severity	Childhood Severity of Psychiatric Illness (CSPI-2)[49] *Assesses severity by eliciting risk factors, behavioral/ emotional symptoms, functioning problems, involvement with juvenile justice and child protection, and caregiver needs and strengths*	34 items Individual report	3–21 y English Spanish	3–5 min after a routine crisis assessment. 25–30 min to complete if nothing is known of the child/family. Training is generally recommended and so is demonstration of reliability (ie, certification) before use (by office staff in particular). There are many trainers available and some Web-based training options.	Freely accessible Available at www. praedfoundation.org

Brief Primary Care Intervention, Secondary Screening, Collateral Data Collection (Algorithm Step 11)

Secondary screening: general[e]	ECSA[3]			
	ASQ:SE-2[4]			
	BITSEA[5]			
	SWYC[6-8]			
	PSC-35[9,10]			
	PSC-17[11]			
	SDQ[12]			
	School or child care reports			
	Behavior Assessment System for Children (BASC)[50] *Assesses adaptive and problem behaviors*	Parent version: 134–160 items Teacher version: 100–139 items Youth version	2–21 y English Spanish	Parent version: 10–20 min Teacher version: 10–20 min Youth version: 30 min Electronic scoring available Must be administered by qualified personnel	Proprietary. Source: Behavior Assessment System for Children, Second Edition (BASC-2). Pearson PsychCorp Web site. Available at http://pearsonassess.com/HAIWEB/Cultures/en-us/Productdetail.htm?Pid=PAa30000.

Table A2-1. Mental Health Tools for Pediatrics *(continued)*

Psychosocial Measure	Tools and Description	Number of items and Format	Age-group and Any Languages Reading Level if Specified	Administration and Scoring Time Training[a]	Source
Brief Primary Care Intervention, Secondary Screening, Collateral Data Collection (Algorithm Step 11)					
Secondary screening: general[e]	Columbia Diagnostic Interview Schedule for Children (DISC) diagnostic predictive scales[51] *Computerized structure interview (yes-or-no) elicits symptoms of 36 mental disorders, applying DSM criteria.*	22 items (Last item is not scored.) Youth self-administered, 8-item, abbreviated version available through TeenScreen	9–17 y English	Depends on items endorsed Training needed	Free with permission Manual available at www.cdc.gov/nchs/data/nhanes/limited_access/interviewer_manual.pdf
	Patient Health Questionnaire-Adolescents (PHQ-A)[52] *Screens for anxiety, eating problems, mood problems, and substance use. Note: PHQ-A depression screening[19] is a subsection of this comprehensive questionnaire.*	83 items Self-report	13–18 y English	Variable scoring: <5 min	Freely accessible Source: www.uacap.org/uploads/3/2/5/0/3250432/phq-a.pdf

Appendix 2: Mental Health Tools for Pediatrics

	Caregiver Teacher Report Form (C-TRF)[53]—part of CBCL (See CBCL tool later in this table.) *Assesses for emotionally reactive behavior, anxious/depressed mood, somatic concerns, withdrawn behavior, attention problems, and aggressive behavior*	99 items Child care providers Teachers	1½–5 y Multiple languages	Variable hand and computer scoring	Proprietary Source: PAR Web site at www.parinc.com/Products/Pkey/49
Secondary screening: inattention and impulsivity	National Institute for Children's Health Quality (NICHQ) Vanderbilt Diagnostic Rating Scales[54] *Elicits symptoms in domains of inattention, disruptive behavior, anxiety, and depression; separate scale assesses functioning in school performance.*	Parent: 55 items Teacher: 43 items Parent/teacher follow-up: 26 items plus items on medication side effects	6–12 y English Spanish	10 min	Freely accessible. Source: NICHQ Vanderbilt Assessment Scales. NICHQ Web site. Available at www.nichq.org/childrens-health/adhd/resources/vanderbilt-assessment-scales.

Table A2-1. Mental Health Tools for Pediatrics (*continued*)

Psychosocial Measure	Tools and Description	Number of Items and Format	Age-group and Any Languages / Reading Level if Specified	Administration and Scoring Time / Training[a]	Source
Brief Primary Care Intervention, Secondary Screening, Collateral Data Collection (Algorithm Step 11)					
Secondary screening: inattention and impulsivity	Conners' Rating Scales-Revised[55] *Elicits symptoms in domains of oppositionality, cognitive problems/inattention, hyperactivity, anxiety-shyness, perfectionism, social problems, and psychosomatic problems*	Parent: 80 items Teacher: 59 items Self: 87 items	3–17 y for parent/ teacher 12–17 y for self English Spanish	20 min	Proprietary. Conners 3rd Edition. MHS Assessments Web site. Available at www.mhs. com/product.aspx? gr=cli&prod=conners3& id=overview.
Secondary screening: learning difficulty	Vision and hearing screening if not done previously Collateral reports from school such as • Teacher version of SDQ and Pediatric Symptom Checklist • NICHQ Vanderbilt Diagnostic Rating Scales teacher form • Psychological test results, if any				

	• Kaufman Test of Educational Achievement (KTEA) • Kaufman Brief Intelligence Test (KBIT) • Report cards • End-of-grade tests • IEP • 504 plan			
Secondary screening: aggression and disruptive behavior	NICHQ Vanderbilt Diagnostic Rating Scales[54]			
	Conners' Rating Scales-Revised[55]			
	Modified Overt Aggression Scale (MOAS)[56] *Rates symptoms in domain of disruptive behavior/ aggression*	4 items Clinician rating of aggression	Adults but has been used for adolescents English	Administered as a semi-structured interview asking adolescent to report on aggressive behavior 10–15 min	Freely accessible Source: https://depts. washington.edu/dbpeds/ Screening%20Tools/ Modified-Overt-Aggression-Scale-MOAS. pdf

Table A2-1. Mental Health Tools for Pediatrics (continued)

Psychosocial Measure	Tools and Description	Number of Items and Format	Age-group and Any Languages Reading Level if Specified	Administration and Scoring Time Training[a]	Source
Brief Primary Care Intervention, Secondary Screening, Collateral Data Collection (Algorithm Step 11)					
Secondary screening: aggression and disruptive behavior	Eyberg Child Behavior Inventory (ECBI)[57] *Assesses conduct problems*	7-point Intensity scale and yes-or-no Problem scale	Parents of children and adolescents aged 2–16 y Companion tool available for teachers English	5-min administration 5-min scoring	Proprietary Source: www.parinc.com/Products/Pkey/97
	Conduct Disorder Scale (CDS)[58] *Rates symptoms in domain of disruptive behavior*	40 items Parent Teachers Siblings	5–22 y English	5–10 min	Proprietary Source: www.proedinc.com/Products/10355/conduct-disorder-scale-cds-complete-kit.aspx
Secondary screening: low mood and depressive symptoms	Preschool Feelings Checklist[59] *Assesses for depression in young children*	20-item parent checklist	36–66 mo English	10 min	Freely accessible Source: http://studylib.net/doc/7442685/preschool-feelings-checklist
	PHQ-A depression screening[19]				

KADS[20]

	Items	Age/Language	Time	Availability
Modified PHQ-9[60] *Screens for symptoms in domains of depression and suicidality*	9 plus severity items	Adolescent English Spanish	5 min Scoring: 1 min	Free with permission (Contact Kroenke K, Spitzer RL, Williams JB. The PHQ-9: validity of a brief depression severity measure. *J Gen Intern Med.* 2001;16[9]:606–613.) Available in the toolkit at www.gladpc.org
Center for Epidemiological Studies Depression (CES-D) Scale modified version for children and adolescents[61] *Screens for depression and emotional turmoil*	20 items	6–17 y English Spanish French Reading level: sixth grade	5–10 min	Freely accessible Available at www. brightfutures.org/ mentalhealth/pdf/ professionals/bridges/ ces_dc.pdf
Children's Depression Inventory (CDI)[62] *Screens for depression*	Parent: 17 items Teacher: 12 items Youth: 27 items (Youth short form: 10 items)	7–17 y English Spanish Reading level: first grade	5–10 min (27-item)	Children's Depression Inventory 2 (CDI 2). Pearson PsychCorp Web site. Available at http:// pearsonassess.com/ HAIWEB/Cultures/ en-us/Productdetail. htm?Pid=015-8044-762.

Table A2-1. Mental Health Tools for Pediatrics (continued)

Psychosocial Measure	Tools and Description	Number of Items and Format	Age-group and Any Languages; Reading Level if Specified	Administration and Scoring Time; Training[a]	Source
Brief Primary Care Intervention, Secondary Screening, Collateral Data Collection (Algorithm Step 11)					
Secondary screening: low mood and depressive symptoms	Short Mood and Feelings Questionnaire (SMFQ)[63] *Screens for depression*	13 items Self-report (child and parent)	8–16 y English	<5 min	Free with permission (Contact http://devepi.duhs.duke.edu/mfq.html.)
	Beck Depression Inventory (BDI)-II[64] *Assesses for depression*	21 items Self-administered or verbally administered by a trained administrator	≥14 y English Spanish Reading level: sixth grade	5–10 min Training required	Proprietary Source: form available at www.bmc.org/sites/default/files/For_Medical_Professionals/Pediatric_Resources/Pediatrics__MA_Center_for_Sudden_Infant_Death_Syndrome__SIDS_/Beck-Depression-Inventory-BDI.pdf
	Beck Depression Inventory-FastScreen (BDI-FS)[65] *Screens for depression; useful in patients with chronic pain and medical conditions*	7 items	≥13 y English	<5 min	Proprietary Source: www.pearsonclinical.com/psychology/products/100000173/bdi-fastscreen-for-medical-patients-bdi.html

Secondary screening: anxiety	Spence Children's Anxiety Scale[66] *Assesses for anxiety. Subscales include panic/agoraphobia, social anxiety, separation anxiety, generalized anxiety, obsessions/compulsions, and fear of physical injury.*	Parent: 35–45 Student: 34–45	Parent: 2½–6½ y Student: 8–12 y Variety of languages	5–10 min	Freely accessible Source: Spence Children's Anxiety Scale Web site at www.scaswebsite.com
	Screen for Childhood Anxiety Related Emotional Disorders (SCARED)[67] *Assesses for anxiety—but not specifically for OCD or PTSD*	41 items Parent Youth	≥8 y English	5 min Scoring: 1–2 min	Freely accessible Source: www.midss.org/content/ screen-child-anxiety-r elated-disorders-scared
	Generalized Anxiety Disorder 7-item (GAD-7) scale[68] *Assesses for symptoms consistent with generalized anxiety disorder; may be used to identify anxiety in patients with chronic conditions such as migraine*	7 items plus impact scale (1 item) if re- sponses positive	11–17 y English	≤7 min	Freely accessible Source: www.mdcalc.com/ gad-7-general-anxiety- disorder-7

Table A2-1. Mental Health Tools for Pediatrics (*continued*)

Psychosocial Measure	Tools and Description	Number of Items and Format	Age-group and Any Languages Reading Level if Specified	Administration and Scoring Time Training[a]	Source
Brief Primary Care Intervention, Secondary Screening, Collateral Data Collection (Algorithm Step 11)					
Secondary screening: trauma exposure[f]	ASC-Kids[35] CRIES[36] Trauma Symptom Checklist for Children (TSCC) and Trauma Symptom Checklist for Young Children (TSCYC)[69] *Elicits trauma-related symptoms*	54 items. (TSCC-A is a 44-item alternative version that does not contain sexual concern items.) TSCYC is a 90-item caregiver-report instrument for young children.	TSCC: 8–16 y TSCYC: 3–12 y English Spanish	15–20 min	Proprietary Sources: www.wpspublish.com/store/p/3065/tscc-trauma-symptom-checklist-for-children
	Child PTSD Symptom Scale (CPSS)[70] *Assesses severity of PTSD in children and adolescents*	24 items (17 mapped to *DSM* symptom criteria; 7, to level of impairment) Interview or self-report	8–18 y English Spanish	Interview: 20 min Self-report: 10 min	Freely accessible Source: www.aacap.org/App_Themes/AACAP/docs/resource_centers/resources/misc/child_ptsd_symptom_scale.pdf

Secondary screening: executive function	Behavior Rating Inventory of Executive Function, Second Edition (BRIEF-2)[71] *Assesses executive functioning in the home and school environments. Contributes to evaluation of learning disabilities, ADHD, traumatic brain injury, low birth weight, Tourette disorder, and pervasive developmental disorders/ASD.*	86 items Parent Teacher	5–18 y English	10–15 min Scoring: 15–20 min	Proprietary Source: www.wpspublish.com/store/p/3347/brief-2-behavior-rating-inventory-of-executive-function-second-edition
	BITSEA[5]				
	School reports				
Secondary screening: speech/language	Hearing screening				
	Capute Scales: Clinical Adaptive Test/Clinical Linguistic and Auditory Milestone Scale (CAT/CLAMS)[72] *Quantitatively measures expressive and receptive language and nonverbal problem-solving skills*	100 items	Birth–3 y English	Variable	Proprietary Source: http://products.brookespublishing.com/The-Capute-Scales-Test-Kit-P362.aspx

Table A2-1. Mental Health Tools for Pediatrics (continued)

Psychosocial Measure	Tools and Description	Number of Items and Format	Age-group and Any Languages Reading Level if Specified	Administration and Scoring Time Training[a]	Source
Brief Primary Care Intervention, Secondary Screening, Collateral Data Collection (Algorithm Step 11)					
Secondary screening: speech/ language	Early Language Milestone (ELM) Scale-2[73] *Assesses language development from birth–age 3 y and intelligibility 36–48 mo*	43 items	Birth–36 mo and older children whose developmental level falls within that range English	Variable	Proprietary Source: www.proedinc.com/Products/6580/early-language-milestone-scale-elm-scale2.aspx
	Language Development Survey (LDS)[74] *Identifies language delay*	310 words arranged into 14 semantic categories (eg, food, animals, people, vehicles). Parents circle each word the child uses spontaneously and whether the child uses word combinations.	18–35 mo English	10 min	Proprietary Source: www.aseba.org/research/language.html

	Tool	Items	Population	Time	Access
Secondary screening: capacity for relationships/attachment	ASQ:SE-2[4] PSI–Short Form[26] BIS[37] EPDS[32] (mother)				
Secondary screening: somatization	CSI-24[41] Functional Disability Inventory (FDI)[75] *Provides classification levels for pain-related disability, applicable to a broad spectrum of pain conditions in pediatric patients*	15 items	Parent Youth ≥8 y Multiple languages	Variable	Freely accessible Source (parent and child versions): www.childrenshospital.vanderbilt.org/uploads/documents/FDI_English_parent_and_child.pdf
Secondary screening: sleep disturbance	BEARS Sleep Screening Tool[76] *Identifies sleep problems and gathers sleep-related information*	5 items corresponding to the mnemonic: B = bedtime issues, E = excessive daytime sleepiness, A = night awakenings, R = regularity and duration of sleep, and S = snoring.	2–12 y English	5 min	Freely accessible Source: http://keltymentalhealth.ca/sites/default/files/Kelty_ProfToolkit_M5_BEARSSleepScreening.pdf

Table A2-1. Mental Health Tools for Pediatrics *(continued)*

Psychosocial Measure	Tools and Description	Number of Items and Format	Age-group and Any Languages / Reading Level if Specified	Administration and Scoring Time / Training[a]	Source
Brief Primary Care Intervention, Secondary Screening, Collateral Data Collection (Algorithm Step 11)					
Secondary screening: substance use	Alcohol Use Disorders Identification Test (AUDIT)[77] *Assesses risky drinking; not a diagnostic tool*	10 items Clinician-administration and self-report options	Preadolescents and adolescents Variety of languages	2 min	Freely accessible Source: www.drugabuse.gov/sites/default/files/files/AUDIT.pdf
	Global Appraisal of Individual Needs (GAIN)–Short Screener (GAIN-SS)[78] *One of a series of measures to assess the recency, breadth, and frequency of problems and service use related to substance use. Subscales identify internalizing disorders, externalizing disorders, substance use disorders, and crime/violence.*	20 items (four 5-item subscales)	Adults Youths aged 10–17 y Self- or clinician-administered	3–5 min	Proprietary. Source: Michael Dennis, PhD, Senior Research Psychologist, Chestnut Health Systems, 720 W Chestnut St, Bloomington, IL 61701. Phone: 309/827-6026. E-mail: mdennis www.chestnut.org/li/gain. View GAIN-SS at https://dpi.wi.gov/sites/default/files/imce/sspw/pdf/gainssmanual.pdf.

Secondary screening: military families	"Cover the Bases" (military children)[79] Tool includes PSC-35[9,10] plus questions specific to the experiences of military families.	Pediatric Symptom Checklist plus 4 questions	Children of all ages in military families English	As for PSC-35 with variable additional time, depending on responses to 4 military-specific questions	Freely accessible Source: www.homebase.org/media/toolkit-for-providerUpdatedLogo.pdf
Secondary screening: sexual behavior or suspected sexual trauma	Child Sexual Behavior Inventory (CSBI)[80] Assesses children who may have been or are suspected of being sexually abused. Covers 9 major content domains: Boundary Issues, Gender Role Behavior, Sexual Interest, Sexual Knowledge, Exhibitionism, Self-Stimulation, Sexual Intrusiveness, Voyeuristic Behavior, and Sexual Anxiety.	38-item questionnaire completed by female caregiver	2–12 y Dutch English (USA) French German Latvian Lithuanian Moldovan Polish Spanish Swedish	5–10 min Scoring: 15 min	Proprietary Source: www.parinc.com/Products/Pkey/71

Table A2-1. Mental Health Tools for Pediatrics *(continued)*

Psychosocial Measure	Tools and Description	Number of Items and Format	Age-group and Any Languages / Reading Level if Specified	Administration and Scoring Time / Training[a]	Source
Brief Primary Care Intervention, Secondary Screening, Collateral Data Collection (Algorithm Step 11)					
Secondary screening: eating/self-regulation	SCOFF (sick, control, one, fat, food)[81] *Screens for disordered eating*	5 items	Adolescents as young as 11 y and adults English	Administration: 1 min Scoring: 1 min	No cost Developed at St. George's Hospital, London, UK Morgan JF, Reid F, Lacey JH. The SCOFF questionnaire: a new screening tool for eating disorders. *West J Med.* 2000;172(3):164–165. https://www.ncbi.nlm.nih.gov/pmc/articles/PMC1070794
	Eating Disorder Screen for Primary Care (ESP)[82] *Simple questions to screen for eating disorders*	5 items	Adolescents and adults English	Administration: 1 min Scoring: 1 min	No cost Developed at University Hospital, London, UK Form available at www.mendedwingcounseling.com/wp-content/uploads/2014/08/ESP.pdf

Diagnostic Assessment (Algorithm Step 15)					
Previous findings	Previous screening results, steps 2 and 11 (general and specific)				
	Interview				
	Observations of patient and family				
	Collateral reports				
	Parent history				
Diagnostic tools	Child Health and Development Interactive System (CHADIS)-DSM[83] *Assesses broadly for mental health symptoms and problems in functioning*	Electronic Variable number of items that depends on response	Birth and on English, with some tools in Spanish	18–48 min	Proprietary Source: www.chadis.com/clinicians/assessment.html

Table A2-1. Mental Health Tools for Pediatrics (*continued*)

Psychosocial Measure	Tools and Description	Number of Items and Format	Age-group and Any Languages Reading Level if Specified	Administration and Scoring Time Training[a]	Source
Diagnostic Assessment (Algorithm Step 15)					
Diagnostic tools	Achenbach System of Empirically Based Assessment (ASEBA) Child Behavior Checklist (CBCL)[84] *DSM-oriented scales assess for* • *1½–5 y: pervasive developmental problem* • *6–18 y: somatic problems and conduct problems* • *Both groups: affective problems, anxiety problems, oppositional defiant problems, and attention-deficit/hyperactivity problems*	Parent or caregiver/teacher for 1½–5 y: 99 items Parent/teacher: 118 items direct observation Youth self-report	1½–5 y 6–18 y 74 languages	15–20 min (both age-groups)	Proprietary Source: www.aseba.org

UCLA PTSD Reaction Index for DSM-5[85] *Assesses exposure to traumatic experiences and impact of traumatic events*	Child: 20 items Parent: 21 items Youth: 22 items	Child and parent: 7–12 y Youth: ≥13 y Multiple languages	20–30 min to administer Scoring: 5–10 min	Proprietary Source: http://tdg.ucla. edu/sites/default/files/ UCLA_PTSD_Reaction_ Index_Flyer.pdf Adapted version available in AAP *Feelings Need Check Ups Too* CD-ROM[86] to assess trauma exposure
Functional assessment tools	Child and Adolescent Functional Assessment Scale (CAFAS)[38,87] *Assesses the degree of impairment in youths with emotional, behavioral, psychiatric, or substance use problems. Used to assess level of need for services in MH and other systems. Also used in evaluating outcomes for programs, evidence-based treatments and evidence-informed practices.*	Clinician uses information collected during a routine clinical interview and selects items that describe the youth's problematic behaviors, as well as strengths and goals.	5–19 y English French Spanish Dutch	Based on prior clinical assessment. Scoring requires approximately 10 min.	Proprietary Source: www2.fasoutcomes. com/Content.aspx? ContentID=12

Table A2-1. Mental Health Tools for Pediatrics *(continued)*

Psychosocial Measure	Tools and Description	Number of Items and Format	Age-group and Any Languages / Reading Level if Specified	Administration and Scoring Time / Training[a]	Source
Diagnostic Assessment (Algorithm Step 15)					
Functional assessment tools	Children's Global Assessment Scale (CGAS)[88] *Assesses overall severity of disturbance and impact on global functioning*	1 item Rated by clinician 100-point scale with 10-point anchors Note: A "nonclinical version" can be administered by lay interviewers.	4–16 y English	Requires no administration time for clinical version because it is based on prior clinical assessment. Time to integrate knowledge of the child into a single score is estimated to be 5–10 min.	Freely accessible Source: www.rcpsych.ac.uk/pdf/CGAS%20Ratings%20Guide.pdf
	Functional Assessment Interview Form - Young Child[89] *Elicits behavioral concerns, factors that precipitate unwanted behaviors, consequences of behaviors, and functional difficulties*	9-page questionnaire/interview with caregiver or teacher aimed at developing a hypothesis about problem behaviors	½–5 y English	45–90 min	Freely accessible Source: http://challengingbehavior.fmhi.usf.edu/explore/pbs_docs/functional_beh_assessment/blank_FAI.pdf

	BIS[37]				
	CIS[38]				
Family-Centered Care Plan (Algorithm Step 17)					
Transition	The Transition Readiness Assessment Questionnaire (TRAQ)[90] *Identifies areas in which a youth needs education and training to achieve independence in transition-relevant skills; used also to set goals*	20 items	Adolescents and adults aged 16–26 y with chronic conditions English	<5 min	Freely accessible Source: www.etsu.edu/com/pediatrics/traq/registration.php
	Self-Management and Transition to Adulthood with R_x = Treatment (STAR$_x$)[91] *Collects information on self-management and health care transition skills, via self-report, in a broad population of adolescents and young adults with chronic conditions*	18 items in 3 domains	Adolescents and young adults with chronic conditions English	2–3 min 5 min to score	Freely accessible Source: www.med.unc.edu/transition/files/2017/12/STARx-Adolescent-Version.pdf

Table A2-1. Mental Health Tools for Pediatrics (continued)

Psychosocial Measure	Tools and Description	Number of Items and Format	Age-group and Any Languages Reading Level if Specified	Administration and Scoring Time Training[a]	Source
Care Plan Implementation, Comanagement, and Monitoring (Algorithm Step 18)					
Monitoring	Periodic functional assessment compared with baseline (eg, SDQ Impact Scale,[12] BIS,[37] CIS[38])				
	PSC-35[9,10]				
	PSC-17[11]				
	SDQ[12]				
	NICHQ Vanderbilt Diagnostic Rating Scales[54]				
	ASQ:SE-2[4]				
	BITSEA[5]				
	ECSA[3]				
	S2BI[15]				
	Functional Disability Inventory[75]				

	Fax-back forms returned from MHS	Shared care plan	Resources available at https://medicalhomeinfo.aap.org/tools-resources/Documents/Shared%20Plan%20of%20Care2.pdf

Abbreviations not defined within table: AAP, American Academy of Pediatrics; ADHD, attention-deficit/hyperactivity disorder; ASD, autism spectrum disorder; DSM, *Diagnostic and Statistical Manual of Mental Disorders* of the American Psychiatric Association; MCHB, Maternal and Child Health Bureau; MH, mental health; MHS, mental health specialist; NIAAA, National Institute on Alcohol Abuse and Alcoholism; OCD, obsessive-compulsive disorder; PCC, primary care clinician; PTSD, post-traumatic stress disorder; UCLA, University of California, Los Angeles.

[a] None unless otherwise indicated.

[b] *Bright Futures: Guidelines for Health Supervisions of Infants, Children, and Adolescents,* 4th Edition, recommends universal screening of adolescents for substance use beginning at age 11 y.

[c] *Bright Futures,* 4th Edition, recommends universal screening of adolescents for depression.

[d] Use of these tools as part of the initial psychosocial assessment (step 2) may be appropriate when recent trauma is a presenting concern; alternatively, these tools may be used at step 11 for secondary screening.

[e] General screening and surveillance tools not used in step 2 may be used at this step. They may be administered by the PCC (or an integrated MHS) or collected from collateral sources.

[f] Tools not used at step 2 can be applied at this step.

References

1. Hagan JF Jr, Shaw JS, Duncan PM, eds. *Bright Futures: Guidelines for Health Supervision of Infants, Children, and Adolescents.* 3rd ed. Elk Grove Village, IL: American Academy of Pediatrics; 2008

2. Klein DA, Goldenring JM, Adelman WP. HEEADSSS 3.0: the psychosocial interview for adolescents updated for a new century fueled by media. *Contemp Pediatr.* 2014. http://contemporarypediatrics.modernmedicine.com/contemporary-pediatrics/content/tags/adolescent-medicine/heeadsss-30-psychosocial-interview-adolesce?page=full. Published January 1, 2014. Accessed February 26, 2018

3. Gleason MM, Zeanah CH, Dickstein S. Recognizing young children in need of mental health assessment: development and preliminary validity of the Early Childhood Screening Assessment. *Infant Ment Health J.* 2010;31(3):335–357

4. Salomonsson B, Sleed M. The Ages & Stages Questionnaire: Social-Emotional: a validation study of a mother-report questionnaire on a clinical mother-infant sample. *Infant Ment Health J.* 2010;31(4):412–431

5. Briggs-Gowan MJ, Carter AS, Irwin JR, Wachtel K, Cicchetti DV. The Brief-Infant Toddler Social and Emotional Assessment: screening for social-emotional problems and delays in competence. *J Pediatr Psychol.* 2004;29(2):143–155

6. Sheldrick RC, Perrin EC. Evidence-based milestones for surveillance of cognitive, language, and motor development. *Acad Pediatr.* 2013;13(6):577–586

7. Sheldrick RC, Henson BS, Neger EN, Merchant S, Murphy JM, Perrin EC. The Baby Pediatric Symptom Checklist (BPSC): development and initial validation of a new social/emotional screening instrument. *Acad Pediatr.* 2013;13(1):72–80

8. Sheldrick RC, Henson BS, Neger EN, Merchant S, Murphy JM, Perrin EC. The Preschool Pediatric Symptom Checklist (PPSC): development and initial validation of a new social/emotional screening instrument. *Acad Pediatr.* 2012; 12(5):456–467

9. Jellinek MS, Murphy JM, Little M, Pagano ME, Comer DM, Kelleher KJ. Use of the Pediatric Symptom Checklist to screen for psychosocial problems in pediatric primary care: a national feasibility study. *Arch Pediatr Adolesc Med.* 1999;153(3):254–260

10. Hacker KA, Myagmarjav E, Harris V, Suglia SF, Weidner D, Link D. Mental health screening in pediatric practice: factors related to positive screens and the contribution of parental/personal concern. *Pediatrics.* 2006;118(5):1896–1906

11. Gardner W, Lucas A, Kolko DJ, Campo JV. Comparison of the PSC-17 and alternative mental health screens in an at-risk primary care sample. *J Am Acad Child Adolesc Psychiatry.* 2007;46(5):611–618

12. Goodman R, Ford T, Simmons H, Gatward R, Meltzer H. Using the Strengths and Difficulties Questionnaire (SDQ) to screen for child psychiatric disorders in a community sample. *Br J Psychiatry.* 2000;177:534–539

13. Yi CH, Martyn K, Salerno J, Darling-Fisher CS. Development and clinical use of Rapid Assessment for Adolescent Preventive Services (RAAPS) Questionnaire in school-based health centers. *J Pediatr Health Care.* 2009;23(1):2–9

14. Salerno J, Barnhart S. Evaluation of the RAAPS risk screening tool for use in detecting adolescents with depression. *J Child Adolesc Psychiatr Nurs.* 2014;27(1):20–25

15. Kelly SM, Gryczynski J, Mitchell SG, Kirk A, O'Grady KE, Schwartz RP. Validity of brief screening instrument for adolescent tobacco, alcohol, and drug use. *Pediatrics.* 2014;133(5):819–826. http://www.ncbi.nlm.nih.gov/pmc/articles/PMC4006430. Published May 2014. Accessed February 26, 2018

16. Chung T, Smith GT, Donovan JE, et al. Drinking frequency as a brief screen for adolescent alcohol problems. *Pediatrics.* 2012;129(2):205–212

17. National Institute on Alcohol Abuse and Alcoholism. *Alcohol Screening and Brief Intervention for Youth: A Practitioner's Guide.* Washington, DC: National Institutes of Health; 2015. https://pubs.niaaa.nih.gov/publications/Practitioner/YouthGuide/YouthGuide.pdf. Accessed February 26, 2018

18. Knight JR, Sherritt L, Shrier LA, Harris SK, Chang G. Validity of the CRAFFT substance abuse screening test among adolescent clinic patients. *Arch Pediatr Adolesc Med.* 2002;156(6):607–614

19. Richardson LP, McCauley E, Grossman DC, et al. Evaluation of the Patient Health Questionnaire (PHQ-9) for detecting major depression among adolescents. *Pediatrics.* 2010;126(6):1117–1123

20. Leblanc JC, Almudevar A, Brooks SJ, Kutcher S. Screening for adolescent depression: comparison of the Kutcher Adolescent Depression Scale with the Beck Depression Inventory. *J Child Adolesc Psychopharmacol.* 2002;12(2):113–126

21. Kemper KJ, Kelleher KJ. Family psychosocial screening: instruments and techniques. *Ambul Child Health.* 1996;1(4):325–339

22. Dubowitz H. The Safe Environment for Every Kid model: promotion of children's health, development, and safety, and prevention of child neglect. *Pediatr Ann.* 2014;43(11):e271–e277

23. Kiplinger VL, Browne CH. *Parents' Assessment of Protective Factors: User's Guide and Technical Report.* Washington, DC: National Quality Improvement Center on Early Childhood; 2014. https://www.cssp.org/reform/child-welfare/pregnant-and-parenting-youth/Parents-Assessment-of-Protective-Factors.pdf. Accessed February 26, 2018

24. Health Leads. *Social Needs Screening Toolkit.* Boston, MA: Health Leads; 2016. https://healthleadsusa.org/wp-content/uploads/2016/07/Health-Leads-Screening-Toolkit-July-2016.pdf. Accessed February 26, 2018

25. Kabacoff RI, Miller IW, Bishop DS, Epstein NB, Keitner GI. A psychometric study of the McMaster Family Assessment Device in psychiatric, medical, and nonclinical samples. *J Fam Psychol.* 1990;3(4):431–439

26. Loyd BH, Abidin RR. Revision of the Parenting Stress Index. *J Pediatr Psychol.* 1985;10(2):169–177

27. Sheras PL, Abidin RR. Stress Index for Parents of Adolescents. PAR Web site. https://www.parinc.com/Products/Pkey/412. Accessed February 26, 2018

28. Brannan AM, Heflinger CA, Bickman L. The caregiver strain questionnaire: measuring the impact on the family of living with a child with serious emotional disturbance. *J Emot Behav Disord.* 1997;5(4):212–222

29. Canty-Mitchell J, Zimet GD. Psychometric properties of the Multidimensional Scale of Perceived Social Support in urban adolescents. *Am J Community Psychol.* 2000;28(3):391–400

30. Löwe B, Kroenke K, Gräfe K. Detecting and monitoring depression with a two-item questionnaire (PHQ-2). *J Psychosom Res.* 2005;58(2):163–171

31. Kroenke K, Spitzer RL, Williams JB. The PHQ-9: validity of a brief depression severity measure. *J Gen Intern Med.* 2001;16(9):606–613

32. Garcia-Esteve L, Ascaso C, Ojuel J, Navarro P. Validation of the Edinburgh Postnatal Depression Scale (EPDS) in Spanish mothers. *J Affect Disord.* 2003; 75(1):71–76

33. Reichenheim ME, Moraes CL. Comparison between the abuse assessment screen and the revised conflict tactics scales for measuring physical violence during pregnancy. *J Epidemiol Community Health.* 2004;58(6):523–527

34. Gundersen C, Engelhard EE, Crumbaugh AS, Seligman HK. Brief assessment of food insecurity accurately identifies high-risk US adults. *Public Health Nutr.* 2017;20(8):1367–1371

35. Kassam-Adams N. The Acute Stress Checklist for Children (ASC-Kids): development of a child self-report measure. *J Trauma Stress.* 2006;19(1):129–139

36. Perrin S, Meiser-Stedman R, Smith P. *The Children's Revised Impact of Event Scale (CRIES): Validity as a Screening Instrument for PTSD.* London, UK: Dept of Psychology, Institute of Psychiatry/Kings College London. https://www.mrc-cbu. cam.ac.uk/wp-content/uploads/2013/02/Perrin-et-al.pdf. Accessed February 26, 2018

37. Bird HR, Canino GJ, Davies M, et al. The Brief Impairment Scale (BIS): a multidimensional scale of functional impairment for children and adolescents. *J Am Acad Child Adolesc Psychiatry.* 2005;44(7):699–707

38. Bird HR, Andrews H, Schwab-Stone M, et al. Global measures of impairment for epidemiologic and clinical use with children and adolescents. *Int J Methods Psychiatr Res.* 1997;6(4):295–307

39. Foy JM; American Academy of Pediatrics Task Force on Mental Health. Enhancing pediatric mental health care: algorithms for primary care. *Pediatrics.* 2010;125(suppl 3):S109–S125

40. *Addressing Mental Health Concerns in Primary Care: A Clinician's Toolkit.* Elk Grove Village, IL: American Academy of Pediatrics; 2010

41. Walker LS, Beck JE, Garber J, Lambert W. Children's Somatization Inventory: psychometric properties of the revised form (CSI-24). *J Pediatr Psychol.* 2009; 34(4):430–440

42. Ballard ED, Cwik M, Van Eck K, et al. Identification of at-risk youth by suicide screening in a pediatric emergency department. *Prev Sci.* 2017;18(2):174–182

43. Substance Abuse and Mental Health Services Administration. *SAFE-T: Suicide Assessment Five-Step Evaluation and Triage for Clinicians* [pocket card]. Substance Abuse and Mental Health Services Administration; 2009. https://store.samhsa.gov/ product/SAFE-T-Pocket-Card-Suicide-Assessment-Five-Step-Evaluation-and-Triage-for-Clinicians/SMA09-4432. Accessed February 26, 2018

44. Osman A, Bagge CL, Gutierrez PM, Konick LC, Kopper BA, Barrios FX. The Suicidal Behaviors Questionnaire-Revised (SBQ-R): validation with clinical and nonclinical samples. *Assessment.* 2001;8(4):443–454

45. Posner K, Brown GK, Stanley B, et al. The Columbia-Suicide Severity Rating Scale: initial validity and internal consistency findings from three multisite studies with adolescents and adults. *Am J Psychiatry.* 2011;168(12):1266–1277

46. Reynolds WM, Mazza JJ. Assessment of suicidal ideation in inner-city children and young adolescents: reliability and validity of the Suicidal Ideation Questionnaire. *School Psychol Rev.* 1999;28(1):17–30

47. Pfeffer CR, Jiang H, Kakuma T. Child-Adolescent Suicidal Potential Index (CASPI): a screen for risk for early onset suicidal behavior. *Psychol Assess.* 2000; 12(3):304–318

48. Turkel SB, Braslow K, Tavaré CJ, Trzepacz PT. The delirium rating scale in children and adolescents. *Psychosomatics.* 2003;44(2):126–129

49. Lyons JS, Kisiel CL, Dulcan M, Cohen R, Chesler P. Crisis assessment and psychiatric hospitalization of children and adolescents in state custody. *J Child Fam Stud.* 1997;6(3):311–320

50. Sandoval J, Echandia A. Behavior assessment system for children. *J Sch Psychol.* 1994;32:419–425

51. Fisher P. Developing an epidemiological tool based on *DSM-5* criteria. Disability Research and Dissemination Center Web site. https://www. disabilityresearchcenter.com/2015/10/13/developing-epi-tool. Published October 13, 2015. Accessed February 26, 2018

52. Johnson JG, Harris ES, Spitzer RL, Williams JB. The patient health questionnaire for adolescents: validation of an instrument for the assessment of mental disorders among adolescent primary care patients. *J Adolesc Health.* 2002;30(3):196–204

53. Achenbach T, Rescorla L. *Manual for the ASEBA Preschool Forms and Profiles.* Burlington, VT: University of Vermont, Research Centre for Children, Youth, and Families; 2000

54. Wolraich ML, Lambert W, Doffing MA, Bickman L, Simmons T, Worley K. Psychometric properties of the Vanderbilt ADHD diagnostic parent rating scale in a referred population. *J Pediatr Psychol.* 2003;28(8):559–567

55. Conners CK, Wells KC, Parker JD, Sitarenios G, Diamond JM, Powell JW. A new self-report scale for assessment of adolescent psychopathology: factor structure, reliability, validity, and diagnostic sensitivity. *J Abnorm Child Psychol.* 1997;25(6):487–497

56. Chukwujekwu DC, Stanley PC. The Modified Overt Aggression Scale: how valid in this environment? *Niger J Med.* 2008;17(2):153–155

57. Boggs SR, Eyberg S, Reynolds LA. Concurrent validity of the Eyberg Child Behavior Inventory. *J Clin Child Psychol.* 1990;19(1):75–78

58. Waschbusch DA, Elgar FJ. Development and validation of the Conduct Disorder Rating Scale. *Assessment.* 2007;14(1):65–74

59. Luby JL, Heffelfinger A, Koenig-McNaught AL, Brown K, Spitznagel E. The Preschool Feelings Checklist: a brief and sensitive screening measure for depression in young children. *J Am Acad Child Adolesc Psychiatry.* 2004;43(6): 708–717

60. Kroenke K, Spitzer RL. The PHQ-9: a new depression and diagnostic severity measure. *Psychiatr Ann.* 2002;32(9):509–515

61. Garrison CZ, Addy CL, Jackson KL, McKeown RE, Waller JL. The CES-D as a screen for depression and other psychiatric disorders in adolescents. *J Am Acad Child Adolesc Psychiatry.* 1991;30(4):636–641

62. Knight D, Hensley VR, Waters B. Validation of the Children's Depression Scale and the Children's Depression Inventory in a prepubertal sample. *J Child Psychol Psychiatry.* 1988;29(6):853–863

63. Rhew IC, Simpson K, Tracy M, et al. Criterion validity of the Short Mood and Feelings Questionnaire and one-and two-item depression screens in young adolescents. *Child Adolesc Psychiatry Ment Health.* 2010;4(1):8

64. Wang YP, Gorenstein C. Psychometric properties of the Beck Depression Inventory-II: a comprehensive review. *Rev Pras Psiquiatr.* 2013;35(4):416–431

65. Pietsch K, Hoyler A, Frühe B, Kruse J, Schulte-Körne G, Allgaier AK. Early detection of major depression in paediatric care: validity of the Beck Depression Inventory-Second Edition (BDI-II) and the Beck Depression Inventory-Fast Screen for Medical Patients (BDI-FS). *Psychother Psychosom Med Psychol.* 2012;62(11):418–424

66. Spence SH, Barrett PM, Turner CM. Psychometric properties of the Spence Children's Anxiety Scale with young adolescents. *J Anxiety Disord.* 2003;17(6): 605–625

67. Jastrowski Mano KE, Evans JR, Tran ST, Anderson Khan K, Weisman SJ, Hainsworth KR. The psychometric properties of the Screen for Child Anxiety Related Emotional Disorders in pediatric chronic pain. *J Pediatr Psychol.* 2012; 37(9):999–1011

68. Mossman SA, Luft MJ, Schroeder HK, et al. The Generalized Anxiety Disorder 7-item scale in adolescents with generalized anxiety disorder: signal detection and validation. *Ann Clin Psychiatry.* 2017;29(4):227–234A

69. Briere J, Johnson K, Bissada A, et al. The Trauma Symptom Checklist for Young Children (TSCYC): reliability and association with abuse exposure in a multi-site study. *Child Abuse Neglect.* 2001;25(8):1001–1014

70. Foa EB, Johnson KM, Feeny NC, Treadwell KR. The Child PTSD Symptom Scale: a preliminary examination of its psychometric properties. *J Clin Child Psychol.* 2001;30(3):376–384

71. Gioia GA, Isquith PK, Retzlaff PD, Espy KA. Confirmatory factor analysis of the Behavior Rating Inventory of Executive Function (BRIEF) in a clinical sample. *Child Neuropsychol.* 2002;8(4):249–257

72. Rossman MJ, Hyman SL, Roarbaugh ML, Berlin LE, Allen MC, Modlin JF. The CAT/CLAMS assessment for early intervention services. Clinical Adaptive Test/Clinical Linguistic and Auditory Milestone Scale. *Clin Pediatr (Phila).* 1994;33(7):404–409

73. Walker D, Gugenheim S, Downs MP, Northern JL. Early Language Milestone Scale and language screening of young children. *Pediatrics.* 1989;83(2):284–288

74. Rescorla L. The Language Developmental Survey: a screening tool for delayed language in toddlers. *J Speech Hear Disord.* 1989;54(4):587–599

75. Claar RL, Walker LS. Functional assessment of pediatric pain patients: psychometric properties of the Functional Disability Inventory. *Pain.* 2006; 121(1–2):77–84

76. Owens JA, Dalzell V. Use of the "BEARS" sleep screening tool in a pediatric residents' continuity clinic: a pilot study. *Sleep Med.* 2005;6(1):63–69

77. Johnson JA, Lee A, Vinson D, Seale JP. Use of AUDIT-based measures to identify unhealthy alcohol use and alcohol dependence in primary care: a validation study. *Alcohol Clin Exp Res.* 2013;37(suppl 1):E253–E259

78. Dennis ML, Chan YF, Funk RR. Development and validation of the GAIN Short Screener (GSS) for internalizing, externalizing and substance use disorders and crime/violence problems among adolescents and adults. *Am J Addict.* 2006;15(suppl 1):80–91

79. Rauch P, Ohye B, Bostic J, Masek B. *A Toolkit for the Well Child Screening of Military Children.* Boston, MA: Home Base Veteran and Family Care. http://homebase.org/media/toolkit-for-providerUpdatedLogo.pdf. Accessed February 26, 2018

80. Friedrich WN. *Child Sexual Behavioral Inventory: Professional Manual.* Odessa, FL: Psychological Assessment Resources; 1997. http://nctsnet.org/sites/default/files/assets/pdfs/measures/CSBI.pdf. Accessed February 26, 2018

81. Rueda Jaimes GE, Díaz Martínez LA, Ortiz Barajas DP, Pinzón Plata C, Rodríguez Martínez J, Cadena Afanador LP. [Validation of the SCOFF questionnaire for screening the eating behavior disorders of adolescents in school.] *Aten Primaria.* 2005;35(2):89–94

82. Cotton MA, Ball C, Robinson P. Four simple questions can help screen for eating disorders. *J Gen Intern Med.* 2003;18(1):53–56

83. Howard BJ. *Developmental and Mental Health Screening.* Baltimore, MD: Johns Hopkins University School of Medicine. http://learn.pcc.com/wp/wp-content/uploads/UC2016_DevelopmentalandMentalHealthScreening.pdf. Accessed February 26, 2018

84. Reliability and validity information. ASEBA Web site. http://www.aseba.org/ordering/reliabilityvalidity.html. Accessed February 26, 2018

85. Steinberg AM, Brymer MJ, Kim S, et al. Psychometric properties of the UCLA PTSD Reaction Index: part I. *J Trauma Stress.* 2013;26(1):1–9

86. Laraque D, Jensen P, Schonfeld D. *Feelings Need Check Ups Too CD-ROM and Toolkit.* Elk Grove Village, IL: American Academy of Pediatrics; 2006. https://www.aap.org/en-us/advocacy-and-policy/aap-health-initiatives/Children-and-Disasters/Pages/Feelings-Need-Checkups-Too-CD-Page-2.aspx. Accessed February 26, 2018

87. Hodges K. Child and Adolescent Functional Assessment Scale (CAFAS): overview of reliability and validity. Functional Assessment Systems Web site. http://www2.fasoutcomes.com/RadControls/Editor/FileManager/Document/FAS611_CAFAS%20Reliability%20and%20Validity%20Rev10.pdf. Accessed February 26, 2018

88. Shaffer D, Gould MS, Brasic J, et al. A Children's Global Assessment Scale (CGAS). *Arch Gen Psychiatry.* 1983;40(11):1228–1231

89. O'Neill RE, Horner RH, Albin RW, Sprague JR. *Functional Assessment and Program Development for Problem Behavior: A Practical Handbook.* Pacific Grove, CA: Brooks/Cole Publishing; 1997

90. Wood DL, Sawicki GS, Miller MD, et al. The Transition Readiness Assessment Questionnaire (TRAQ): its factor structure, reliability, and validity. *Acad Pediatr.* 2014;14(4):415–422

91. Cohen SE, Hooper SR, Javalkar K, et al. Self-management and transition readiness assessment: concurrent, predictive and discriminant validation of the STAR$_x$ Questionnaire. *J Pediatr Nurs.* 2015;30(5):668–676

Mental Health Practice Readiness Inventory

Table A3-1. Mental Health Practice Readiness: Community Resources

Topic	Score[a]			Target
Inventory of referral resources	1	2	3	Practice has an up-to-date inventory of accessible developmental-behavioral pediatricians, adolescent medicine specialists, or child psychiatrists (or any combination thereof); community- and school-based mental health and substance use professionals trained in evidence-based therapies, including trauma-focused care; Early Intervention program; special education programs; evidence-based parenting education programs; child protection agencies; youth recreational programs; family and peer support programs; evidence-based home visiting programs; and mental health care coordinators.
Core services	1	2	3	Practice team is knowledgeable about eligibility requirements, contact points, and services of the programs and providers listed previously and type or types of payment they accept.
Collaborative relationships	1	2	3	Practice team has collaborative relationships with school- and community-based providers of key services.

Table A3-2. Mental Health Practice Readiness: Health Care Financing

Topic	Score[a]			Target
Third-party payment	1	2	3	Practice has access to specialty provider lists and authorization procedures of major public and private health plans insuring patients in the practice and has processes for addressing claim denials and gaps in benefits and payment.
Coding	1	2	3	Practice has coding and billing procedures to capture payment for primary care mental health–related services covered by major health plans.

Table A3-3. Mental Health Practice Readiness: Support for Children, Adolescents, and Families

Topic	Score[a]			Target
First contact	1	2	3	Staff has good "first-contact skills" to help children, adolescents, and families feel welcome and respected.
Culturally effective care	1	2	3	Practice team is supportive of people facing mental health challenges, demonstrating sensitivity to cultural differences and avoiding stigmatizing language.
Mental health promotion	1	2	3	Practice team promotes the importance of mental health through posters, practice Web sites, newsletters, handouts, or brochures and by incorporating conversations about mental health into each office visit.
Confidentiality	1	2	3	Practice team assures children, adolescents, and families of confidentiality in accordance with standard medical ethics and state and federal laws.
Adolescents	1	2	3	Practice team is prepared to address mental health and substance use needs of adolescents.
Engagement	1	2	3	Practice team actively elicits mental health and substance use concerns, assesses patients' and families' readiness to address them, and engages children, adolescents, and families in planning their own mental health care at their own pace.
Self-management and family management	1	2	3	Practice team fosters self-management and family management (eg, provides patient and family educational materials appropriate to literacy level and culture, articulates patient's and family's roles in care plan, stays abreast of online and print self-care resources).
Referral assistance	1	2	3	Practice is prepared to support families through referral assistance and advocacy in the mental health referral process.

Table A3-3. Mental Health Practice Readiness: Support for Children, Adolescents, and Families (*continued*)

Topic	Score[a]			Target
Care coordination	1	2	3	Practice routinely seeks to identify children and adolescents in the practice who are involved in the mental health specialty system, ensuring that they receive the full range of preventive medical services and monitoring their mental health or substance use conditions.
Special populations	1	2	3	Practice team is prepared to address mental health needs of special populations within the practice (eg, those with ACEs and other social adversities; those with disrupted families caused by military deployment, separation, divorce, incarceration, or foster care; LGBTQ children and adolescents; those in the juvenile justice system; those whose family members have mental health or substance use problems; those who have experienced immigration, racism, homophobia, homelessness, violence, or natural disasters).
Family centeredness	1	2	3	Practice has family members involved in advising the practice; practice team periodically assesses the family centeredness of the practice.
Trauma-informed care	1	2	3	Practice team is knowledgeable about the impact of trauma; considers impact of adversities and traumatic life events in context of behavioral concerns and pays attention to resilience factors and trauma reminders; offers support, resources, and referral to evidence-based trauma services; monitors patient/family adjustment over time; attends to staff members' psychosocial needs with attention to impact of secondary traumatic stress.
Quality improvement	1	2	3	Practice periodically assesses the quality of care provided to children and adolescents with mental health problems and takes action to improve care, in accordance with findings.

Abbreviations: ACE, adverse childhood experience; LGBTQ, lesbian, gay, bisexual, transgender, or questioning.

Table A3-4. Mental Health Practice Readiness: Clinical Information Systems and Delivery System Redesign

Topic	Score[a]			Target
Registry	1	2	3	Practice has a registry in place identifying children and adolescents with risks (patient or family), positive mental health or substance use screening results, and mental health or substance use problems (including those not yet ready to address problems).
Recall and reminder systems	1	2	3	Recall and reminder systems are in place to identify missed appointments and ensure that children and adolescents with mental health or substance use concerns (including those not ready to take action) receive appropriate follow-up and routine health supervision services.
Medication management	1	2	3	Practice has a system for monitoring medication efficacy, adverse effects, adherence, and renewals.
Emergency	1	2	3	Practice has a crisis plan in place for the handling of psychiatric emergencies, including suicidality.
Information exchange	1	2	3	Practice has office procedures to support collaboration (eg, routines for requesting parental consent to exchange information with specialists and schools, fax-back forms for specialist feedback, psychosocial history accompanying foster children and adolescents).
Tracking systems	1	2	3	Practice has systems in place and staff roles assigned to monitor patients' progress (eg, check on referral completion, periodic telephone contact with family and therapist, periodic functional assessment, periodic behavioral scales from classroom teachers and parents, communications to and from care coordinator) as appropriate to setting.

Table A3-4. Mental Health Practice Readiness: Clinical Information Systems and Delivery System Redesign (*continued*)

Topic	Score[a]			Target
Care plans	1	2	3	Practice includes patients, family, school, agency personnel, primary care team, and any involved specialists in developing a comprehensive plan of care for a child or an adolescent with one or more mental health problems, including definition of respective roles.
Collaborative models	1	2	3	Practice team is prepared for participation in the full range of collaborative approaches and has explored innovative models (eg, colocated mental health specialist, child psychiatry consultation network, telepsychiatry) to fill service gaps and enhance quality.
Interactive Web-based tools	1	2	3	Practice is current with Web-based treatment options.
Screening and assessment tools	1	2	3	Office systems are in place to collect and score findings from mental health and substance use screening and assessment tools at or prior to scheduled routine health supervision visits and visits scheduled for a mental health concern and to perform a brief mental health update at acute care visits and visits scheduled to monitor chronic conditions, as appropriate to the setting.

Table A3-5. Mental Health Practice Readiness: Decision Support for Clinicians

Topic	Score[a]			Target
Functional assessment	1	2	3	Clinicians use validated functional assessment scales to identify and evaluate children and adolescents with mental health problems and monitor their progress in care.
Clinical guidance	1	2	3	Clinicians have access to reliable, current sources of information concerning diagnostic classification of mental health and substance use problems, evidence about safety and efficacy of psychosocial and psychopharmacological treatments of common mental health and substance use disorders, and information about the safety and efficacy of complementary and integrative therapies often used by children, adolescents, and families.
Psychiatric consultation	1	2	3	Clinicians have access to a psychiatrist with expertise in children and adolescents for consultation and guidance in assessment and management of their patients' mental health problems.
Protocols	1	2	3	Practice has tools and protocols in place to guide assessment and care and to foster self-treatment of children and adolescents with common mental health and substance use conditions.
Screening and surveillance	1	2	3	Clinicians routinely use psychosocial history and validated screening tools at preventive visits and brief mental health updates at acute care visits to elicit mental health and substance use problems and to identify patient and family strengths and risks.

[a] To evaluate your practice, use the following scoring system:

1 = We do this well; that is, substantial improvement is not currently needed.

2 = We do this to some extent; that is, improvement is needed.

3 = We do not do this well; that is, significant practice change is needed.

For areas with scores of 2 or 3, determine which ones align with strong interest of the practice team and are feasible in the broader context of the health system. These can become the priority for practice change.

Sources of Key Mental Health Services

Table A4-1.

Specialty Services	Sources
Psychiatric emergency services	• Local mental health screening, triage, and referral service or another intake point for public specialty system • Mobile crisis unit, if available • Child psychiatrist • General psychiatrist with pediatric expertise (or consultation with child psychiatrist) • Emergency department
Medication consultation or treatment of patients with problems of high severity (MD or DO required)	• Neurodevelopmental/developmental-behavioral pediatrician • Child psychiatrist (in person or telepsychiatry) • General psychiatrist with child expertise or child psychiatry consultation • Adolescent medicine specialist • Pediatric neurologist • Local public mental health agency
Early Intervention services	• Part C agency for 0–3 y; Part B agency for 3–5 y • Developmental evaluation agency • Neurodevelopmental/developmental-behavioral pediatrician • Child psychiatrist with expertise in young children • Early Intervention specialist
Child protective services	• Department of Social Services
Grief counseling	• Licensed mental health specialist[a] • Hospice agency
Substance use disorder counseling	• Licensed substance use disorder counselor • Agency specializing in substance use disorder
Psychosocial assessment	• Licensed mental health specialist[a] with pediatric expertise
Educational assessment	• School psychologist • Child psychologist or another licensed psychologist • Neurodevelopmental/developmental-behavioral pediatrician • Educational specialist

Table A4-1. (*continued*)	
Specialty Services	**Sources**
Psychosocial treatment	• Licensed mental health specialist[a] trained in the specific intervention (eg, cognitive behavioral therapy specific to the condition, trauma-focused therapy, parent management training, mind-body therapies, family therapy)
Specialized counseling programs (eg, domestic violence, family reunification, children of parents with alcohol use disorder, juvenile sex offender, divorce, stress management, smoking cessation)	• Licensed mental health specialist[a] with pediatric expertise • Agency specializing in that area
Parenting education	• Parent educator trained in evaluated curriculum • Family services agency • Licensed mental health specialist[a] • School system's social work services (Some have parenting education programs.) • Agricultural extension service (Some have parenting education programs.)
Care coordination/case management	• Licensed mental health specialist[a] with pediatric expertise • Local public mental health agency • Peer support program
Peer support	• Local organization of National Alliance on Mental Illness, National Federation of Families for Children's Mental Health, Family Support Network, or Children and Adults with Attention-Deficit/Hyperactivity Disorder • Local public mental health agency • Al-Anon

[a] The term *licensed mental health specialist* encompasses clinical psychologists, clinical social workers, professional counselors, and others permitted by state authority to provide the particular service.

Adapted from Appendix S1: sources of specialty services for children with mental health problems and their families. *Pediatrics.* 2010;125(suppl 3):S126–S127. http://pediatrics.aappublications.org/content/125/Supplement_3/S126. Published June 2010. Accessed February 27, 2018.

Mnemonic for Common Factors Communication Methods: *HELP*

H = Hope

Hope facilitates coping. Increase the family's hopefulness by describing your realistic expectations for improvement and reinforcing the strengths and assets you see in the child and family. Encourage concrete steps toward whatever is achievable.

E = Empathy

Communicate **empathy** by listening attentively, acknowledging struggles and distress, and sharing happiness experienced by the family.

L^2 = Language, Loyalty

Use the child and family's own **language** (not a clinical label) to reflect your understanding of the problem as they see it and to give the child and family an opportunity to correct any misperceptions.

Communicate **loyalty** to the family by expressing your support and your commitment to help now and in the future.

P^3 = Permission, Partnership, Plan

Ask the family's **permission** for you to ask more in-depth and potentially sensitive questions or to make suggestions for further evaluation or management.

Partner with the child and family to identify any barriers or resistance to addressing the problem, find strategies to bypass or overcome barriers, and find agreement on achievable steps (or simply an achievable first step) that are aligned with the family's motivation. The more difficult the problem, the more important is the promise of partnership.

On the basis of the child and family's preferences and sense of urgency, establish a **plan** to expand the assessment, change a behavior or family routine, try out a psychosocial intervention, seek help from others, work toward greater readiness to take one or more of these actions, or monitor the problem and follow up with you. The plan might include, for example, completing additional checklists or questionnaires, keeping a diary of symptoms and triggers, gathering information from other sources such as the child's school or child care center, making lifestyle changes, applying new parenting strategies or self-management techniques, reviewing educational resources about the problem or condition, seeking mental health specialty care or social services, or simply returning to the medical home for further discussion.

Use of the HELP mnemonic builds a therapeutic alliance between the clinician and the patient and family and improves the likelihood of follow-through on a plan of care. This approach is well suited to the care of patients who would benefit from a behavior change, patients whose symptoms are undifferentiated and patients whose symptoms do not reach a diagnostic threshold, patients who are resistant or otherwise not yet ready to pursue further diagnostic assessment or treatment, and patients who are awaiting further diagnostic assessment and treatment. Use of the HELP mnemonic should not delay a full diagnostic evaluation or definitive therapy if the patient's symptoms suggest a psychiatric emergency, severe impairment, or marked distress.

Adapted from American Academy of Pediatrics. *Addressing Mental Health Concerns in Primary Care: A Clinician's Toolkit.* Elk Grove Village, IL: American Academy of Pediatrics; 2010. Updated May 2017.

PracticeWise:
Evidence-Based Child and Adolescent Psychosocial Interventions

This report is intended to guide practitioners, educators, youth, and families in developing appropriate plans using psychosocial interventions. It was created for the period October 2017 – April 2018 using the PracticeWise Evidence-Based Services (PWEBS) Database, available at www.practicewise.com. If this is not the most current version, please check the American Academy of Pediatrics (AAP) mental health Web site (www.aap.org/mentalhealth) for updates.

Please note that this chart represents an independent analysis by PracticeWise and should not be construed as endorsement by the AAP. For an explanation of PracticeWise determination of evidence/level, please see below or visit www.practicewise.com/aap.

Table A6-1.

Problem Area	Level 1- Best Support	Level 2- Good Support	Level 3- Moderate Support	Level 4- Minimal Support	Level 5- No Support
Anxious or Avoidant Behaviors	Cognitive Behavior Therapy (CBT), CBT and Medication, CBT for Child and Parent, CBT with Parents, Education, Exposure, Modeling	Assertiveness Training, Attention, Attention Training, CBT and Music Therapy, CBT and Parent Management Training (PMT), CBT with Parents Only, Cultural Story-telling, Family Psychoeducation, Hypnosis, Mindfulness, Relaxation, Stress Inoculation	Contingency Management, Group Therapy	Behavioral Activation and Exposure, Bio-feedback, Play Therapy, PMT, Psychodynamic Therapy, Rational Emotive Therapy, Social Skills	Assessment/Monitoring, Attachment Therapy, Client Centered Therapy, Eye Movement Desensitization and Reprocessing (EMDR), Peer Pairing, Psychoeducation, Relationship Counseling, Teacher Psychoeducation
Autism Spectrum Disorders	CBT, Intensive Behavioral Treatment, Intensive Communication Training, Joint Attention/ Engagement, PMT, Social Skills	Imitation, Peer Pairing, Theory of Mind Training	None	Massage, Peer Pairing and Modeling, Play Therapy	Attention Training, Biofeed-back, Cognitive Flexibility Training, Communication Skills, Contingent Responding, Eclectic Therapy, Executive Functioning Training, Fine Motor Training, Modeling, Parent Psychoeducation, Physical/Social/Occupational Therapy, Sensory Integration Training, Structured Listening, Working Memory Training

Delinquency and Disruptive Behavior	Anger Control, Assertiveness Training, CBT, Contingency Management, Multisystemic Therapy, PMT, PMT and Problem Solving, Social Skills, Therapeutic Foster Care	CBT and PMT, CBT and Teacher Training, Communication Skills, Cooperative Problem Solving, Family Therapy, Functional Family Therapy, PMT and Classroom Management, PMT and Social Skills, Rational Emotive Therapy, Relaxation, Self Control Training, Transactional Analysis	Client Centered Therapy, Moral Reasoning Training, Outreach Counseling, Peer Pairing	CBT and Teacher Psychoeducation, Exposure, Physical Exercise, PMT and Classroom Management and CBT, PMT and Self-Verbalization, Stress Inoculation	Behavioral Family Therapy, Catharsis, CBT with Parents, Education, Family Empowerment and Support, Family Systems Therapy, Group Therapy, Imagery Training, Play Therapy, PMT and Peer Support, Psychodynamic Therapy, Self Verbalization, Skill Development, Wraparound
Depressive or Withdrawn Behaviors	CBT, CBT and Medication, CBT with Parents, Client Centered Therapy, Family Therapy	Attention Training, Cognitive Behavioral Psychoeducation, Expression, Interpersonal Therapy, MI/Engagement and CBT, Physical Exercise, Problem Solving, Relaxation	None	Self Control Training, Self Modeling, Social Skills	CBT and Anger Control, CBT and Behavioral Sleep Intervention, CBT and PMT, Goal Setting, Life Skills, Mindfulness, Play Therapy, PMT, PMT and Emotion Regulation, Psychodynamic Therapy, Psychoeducation

Table A6-1. (continued)

Problem Area	Level 1- Best Support	Level 2- Good Support	Level 3- Moderate Support	Level 4- Minimal Support	Level 5- No Support
Eating Disorders	CBT, Physical Exercise and Dietary Care and Behavioral Feedback	Family-Focused Therapy, Family Systems Therapy, Family Therapy with Parents Only	None	Physical Exercise and Dietary Care	Behavioral Training and Dietary Care, CBT with Parents, Client Centered Therapy, Dietary Care, Education, Family Therapy, Family Therapy with Parent Consultant, Goal Setting, Psychoeducation, Yoga
Elimination Disorders	Behavior Alert, Behavior Alert and Behavioral Training, Behavioral Training, Behavioral Training and Biofeedback and Dietary Care and Medical Care, Behavioral Training and Dietary Care and Medical Care	Behavioral Training and Dietary Care, Behavioral Training and Hypnosis and Dietary Care, CBT	Behavior Alert and Medication	None	Assessment/Monitoring, Assessment/Monitoring and Medication, Behavioral Training and Medical Care, Biofeedback, Contingency Management, Dietary Care, Dietary Care and Medical Care, Hypnosis, Medical Care, Psychoeducation
Mania	None	CBT for Child and Parent, Cognitive Behavioral Psychoeducation	None	None	Cognitive Behavioral Psychoeducation and Dietary Care, Dialectical Behavior Therapy and Medication, Family-Focused Therapy, Psychoeducation

Substance Use	CBT, Community Reinforcement, Contingency Management, Family Therapy, MI/Engagement	Assertive Continuing Care, CBT and Contingency Management, CBT and Medication, CBT with Parents, Family Systems Therapy, Functional Family Therapy, Goal Setting/Monitoring, MI/Engagement and CBT, MI/Engagement and Expression, Multidimensional Family Therapy, Problem Solving, Purdue Brief Family Therapy	Drug Court, Drug Court and Multisystemic Therapy and Contingency Management, Eclectic Therapy	Goal Setting, Psychoeducation	Advice/Encouragement, Assessment/Monitoring, Behavioral Family Therapy, Case Management, CBT and Community Information Campaign, CBT and Functional Family Therapy, Client Centered Therapy, Drug Court and Multisystemic Therapy, Drug Education, Education, Family Court, Feedback, Group Therapy, Mindfulness, MI/Engagement and CBT and Family Therapy, Multisystemic Therapy, Parent Psychoeducation, PMT, Therapeutic Vocational Training
Suicidality	None	Attachment Therapy, CBT with Parents, Counselors Care, Counselors Care and Support Training, Interpersonal Therapy, Multisystemic Therapy, Parent Coping/Stress Management, Psychodynamic Therapy, Social Support	None	None	Accelerated Hospitalization, Case Management, CBT, Communication Skills, Counselors Care and Anger Management

Table A6-1. (*continued*)

Problem Area	Level 1- Best Support	Level 2- Good Support	Level 3- Moderate Support	Level 4- Minimal Support	Level 5- No Support
Traumatic Stress	CBT, CBT with Parents, EMDR	Exposure	None	Play Therapy, Psychodrama, Relaxation and Expression	Advice/Encouragement, Client Centered Therapy, CBT and Medication, CBT with Parents Only, Education, Expressive Play, Interpersonal Therapy, Problem Solving, Psychodynamic Therapy, Psychoeducation, Relaxation, Structured Listening

Adapted with permission from PracticeWise.

Note: CBT = Cognitive Behavior Therapy; MI = Motivational Interviewing; PMT = Parent Management Training; Level 5 refers to treatments whose tests were unsupportive or inconclusive. This report updates and replaces the "Blue Menu" originally distributed by the Hawaii Department of Health, Child and Adolescent Mental Health Division, Evidence-Based Services Committee from 2002–2009.

The recommendations in this publication do not indicate an exclusive course of treatment or serve as a standard of medical care. Variations, taking into account individual circumstances, may be appropriate. Original document included as part of *Addressing Mental Health Concerns in Primary Care: A Clinician's Toolkit.* Copyright © 2010 American Academy of Pediatrics. All Rights Reserved. The American Academy of Pediatrics (AAP) does not review or endorse any modifications made to this document and in no event shall the AAP be liable for any such changes.

Background

The PracticeWise "Evidence-Based Child and Adolescent Psychosocial Interventions" tool is created twice each year and posted on the AAP Web site at www.aap.org/mentalhealth, using data from the PWEBS Database, available at www.practicewise.com. The table is based on an ongoing review of randomized clinical psychosocial and combined treatment trials for children and adolescents with mental health needs. The contents of the table represent the treatments that best fit a patient's characteristics, based on the primary problem (rows) and the strength of evidence behind the treatments (columns). Thus, when seeking an intervention with the best empirical support for an adolescent with depression, one might select from among cognitive behavior therapy (CBT) alone, CBT with medication, CBT with parents included, client centered therapy, or family therapy. Each clinical trial must have been published in a peer-reviewed scientific journal, and each study is coded by 2 independent raters whose discrepancies are reviewed and resolved by a third expert judge. Prior to report development, data are subject to extensive quality analyses to identify and eliminate remaining errors, inconsistencies, or formatting problems.

Strength of Evidence Definitions

The strength of evidence classification uses a 5-level system that was originally adapted from the American Psychological Association Division 12 Task Force on the Promotion and Dissemination of Psychological Procedures.[1] These definitions can be seen in the Strength of Evidence Definitions section later in this appendix. Higher strength of evidence is an indicator of the reliability of the findings behind the treatment, not an index of the expected size of the effect.

Treatment Definitions

"Evidence-Based Child and Adolescent Psychosocial Interventions" uses a broad level of analysis for defining treatments, such that interventions sharing a majority of components with similar clinical strategies and theoretical underpinnings are considered to belong to a single treatment approach. For example, rather than list each CBT protocol for depression on its own, the tool handles these as a single group that collectively has achieved a particular level of scientific support. This approach focuses more on "generic" as opposed to "brand name" treatment modalities, and it also is designed to reduce the more than 500 distinct treatments that would otherwise be represented on this tool to a more practical level of analysis.

Problem Definition

The presenting problems represented in the table rows are coded using a checklist of 25 different problem areas (e.g., anxious or avoidant behaviors, eating disorders, substance use). The problem area refers to the condition that a treatment explicitly targeted and for which clinical outcomes were measured. These problem areas are inclusive of diagnostic conditions (e.g., all randomized trials targeting separation anxiety disorder are considered collectively within the "Anxious or Avoidant Behaviors" row) but also include the much larger number of research trials that tested treatments but did not use diagnosis as a study entry criterion. For example, many studies use elevated scores on behavior or emotion checklists or problems such as arrests or suicide attempts to define participants. Mental health diagnoses are therefore nested under these broader categories.

History of This Tool

This tool has its origins with the Child and Adolescent Mental Health Division of the Hawaii Department of Health. Under the leadership of then-division chief Christina Donkervoet, work was commissioned starting in 1999 to review child mental health treatment outcome literature and produce reports that could serve the mental health system in selecting appropriate treatments for its youth.[2] Following an initial review of more than 120 randomized clinical trials,[3] the division began to issue the results of these reviews in quarterly matrix reports known as the Blue Menu (named for the blue paper on which it was originally printed and distributed). This document was designed to be user-friendly and transportable, thereby making it amenable to broad and easy dissemination. As of 2010, the AAP supports the posting of the next generation of this tool. "Evidence-Based Child and Adolescent Psychosocial Interventions" now represents over 900 randomized trials of psychosocial treatments for youth. PracticeWise continues to identify, review, and code new research trials and plans to continue providing updates to this tool to the AAP for the foreseeable future.

Strength of Evidence Definitions

Level 1: Best Support

I. At least 2 randomized trials demonstrating efficacy in one or more of the following ways:

    a. Superior to pill placebo, psychological placebo, or another treatment.

    b. Equivalent to all other groups representing at least one level 1 or level 2 treatment in a study with adequate statistical power (30 participants per group on average) that showed significant pre-study to post-study change in the index group as well as the group(s) being tied. Ties of treatments that have previously qualified only through ties are ineligible.

II. Experiments must be conducted with treatment manuals.

III. Effects must have been demonstrated by at least 2 different investigator teams.

Level 2: Good Support

I. Two experiments showing the treatment is (statistically significantly) superior to a waiting list or no-treatment control group. *Manuals, specification of sample, and independent investigators are not required.*

    OR

II. One between-group design experiment with clear specification of group, use of manuals, and demonstrating efficacy by either

    a. Superior to pill placebo, psychological placebo, or another treatment

    b. Equivalent to an established treatment (See qualifying tie definition above.)

Level 3: Moderate Support

One between-group design experiment with clear specification of group and treatment approach and demonstrating efficacy by either

a. Superior to pill placebo, psychological placebo, or another treatment

b. Equivalent to an already established treatment in experiments with adequate statistical power (30 participants per group on average)

Level 4: Minimal Support

One experiment showing the treatment is (statistically significantly) superior to a waiting list or no-treatment control group. *Manuals, specification of sample, and independent investigators are not required.*

Level 5: No Support

The treatment has been tested in at least one study but has failed to meet criteria for levels 1 through 4.

References

1. American Psychological Association Task Force on Promotion and Dissemination of Psychological Procedures, Division of Clinical Psychology. Training in and dissemination of empirically-validated psychological treatments: report and recommendations. *Clin Psychol.* 1995;48:3–23

2. Chorpita BF, Donkervoet CM. Implementation of the Felix Consent Decree in Hawaii: the implementation of the Felix Consent Decree in Hawaii. In: Steele RG, Roberts MC, eds. *Handbook of Mental Health Services for Children, Adolescents, and Families.* New York, NY: Kluwer Academic/Plenum Publishers; 2005:317–332

3. Chorpita BF, Yim LM, Donkervoet JC, et al. Toward large-scale implementation of empirically supported treatments for children: a review and observations by the Hawaii Empirical Basis to Services Task Force. *Clin Psychol Sci Pract.* 2002;9(2):165–190

See more on the PracticeWise publications page (www.practicewise.com/Community/Publications).

Common Elements of Evidence-Based Practice Amenable to Primary Care: Indications and Sources

Table A7-1. Common Elements

Indications[a]	EPB Sources[b]	Common Elements of EBPs Amenable to Primary Care	Chapters
Preparation of patient or family to address any health risk or mental health need Resistance to care seeking Barriers to care seeking	Family therapy Cognitive behavioral therapy Motivational interviewing Family engagement Family-focused pediatrics Solution-focused therapy	"Common factors" communication techniques	1 2 5 10
Pain • Acute (eg, injury, illness, procedural) • Chronic or recurrent (eg, chronic illness, disability, trauma, recurrent procedures) Stress Habit problems and disorders Behavioral problems (eg, attention problems, anger management) Medical-biobehavioral disorders (eg, asthma, migraine, Tourette syndrome, inflammatory bowel disease, warts, pruritus)	Self-regulation therapies and mind-body therapies	Teach… • Breathing techniques • Relaxation (eg, progressive muscle relaxation) • Mental imagery • Self-hypnosis Offer adjunct biofeedback.	8 9

Table A7-1. Common Elements (*continued*)

Indications[a]	EPB Sources[b]	Common Elements of EBPs Amenable to Primary Care	Chapters
Anxiety (eg, performance anxiety [eg, examinations, stage fright, sports], anxiety disorders, PTSD, phobias) Psychophysiological problems (eg, enuresis, encopresis, conditioned nausea and vomiting, irritable bowel syndrome, sleep disorders) Chronic disease, multisystem disease, and terminal illness (eg, cancer, hemophilia, AIDS, cystic fibrosis, diabetes, chronic renal disease)			
Anxiety Phobias	Cognitive behavioral therapy for anxiety Young children: PCIT (See also "Self-regulation therapies and mind-body therapies" cell earlier in this table.)	Provide psychoeducation. Gradually increase exposure to feared objects or activities. Teach… • Relaxation strategies • Positive self-talk • Thought stopping or substituting • Thoughts of a safe place Reward brave behavior.	14

Table A7-1. Common Elements (*continued*)

Indications[a]	EPB Sources[b]	Common Elements of EBPs Amenable to Primary Care	Chapters
Symptoms related to a past trauma	Trauma-focused cognitive behavioral therapy Young children: • Child-Parent Psychotherapy • PCIT	Gently challenge negative thoughts about shame, guilt, and hopelessness. Encourage self-care and ways of seeking a feeling of security. When symptoms are prominent, suggest distraction, relaxation, or supportive company. Plan to manage or avoid unnecessary or extreme triggers. Provide positive attention for positive behavior. Remove attention for provocative behaviors. Provide safe, consistent consequences for unsafe/unacceptable behaviors. Define the importance of a healthy relationship for recovery.	14
Low mood Depression	Cognitive behavioral therapy for depression	Provide psychoeducation. Gently challenge negative thoughts. Use behavioral activation (ie, more of enjoyable activities ["prescribe pleasure"]). Focus on strengths, not weaknesses.	22

Table A7-1. Common Elements (*continued*)			
Indications[a]	EPB Sources[b]	Common Elements of EBPs Amenable to Primary Care	Chapters
		Teach… • Distraction • Problem-solving skills • Rehearsal of behavior and social skills • Expressive writing Facilitate conversation between parents and youth that is focused on youth's concerns. Reinforce social supports.	
Any symptoms associated with… • Inconsistent parenting • Harsh discipline • Inappropriate parental expectations Disruptive behavior Aggression Conduct problems Inattention Hyperactivity	Parenting education Examples: • The Incredible Years • Triple P – Positive Parenting Program • PCIT • "Helping the Noncompliant Child" parent training program	Teach… • Positive time with parents • Encouragement and rewards for positive behavior • Prevention of triggers • Emotional communication skills • Consistent, calm consequences for negative behavior • Reparation for negative behavior • Clear, simple commands and limit setting • Correct use of time-out • De-escalation techniques • Practice of skills	15 17 18 20

Table A7-1. Common Elements (*continued*)

Indications[a]	EPB Sources[b]	Common Elements of EBPs Amenable to Primary Care	Chapters
Substance use Other risky behaviors Poor adherence to therapy	Motivational interviewing Family-centered therapy	Request patient's permission to engage. Assess stage of readiness to act. Use Elicit-Provide-Elicit sequence in brief interventions. Listen for and reflect "change talk." Address barriers to change.	1 2 25 30 31
Family conflict	Family-centered therapy Motivational interviewing	Apply the following techniques: • Unconditional positive regard • Active listening • Affirmation • Reflection • Open-ended questions • Professional neutrality • Reframing • Summaries	1 2 5 10 18

Table A7-1. Common Elements (*continued*)			
Indications[a]	**EPB Sources**[b]	**Common Elements of EBPs Amenable to Primary Care**	**Chapters**
Symptoms of emotional distress in young children (eg, dysregulation, aggression, extreme tantrums, irritability, unhappy mood, extreme anxiety, lack of social reciprocity with caregiver, poor attachment)	Parenting education (See examples in the "Parenting Education" cell earlier in this table.) Promoting First Relationships Parents as Teachers Child-Parent Psychotherapy Cognitive behavioral therapy	Reframe child's perceived bad behavior. Reinforce strengths and protective factors. Teach… • Prevention of unnecessary or extreme triggers • Attention and praise for positive behavior • Clear, simple commands and limit setting • Relaxation and anxiety management • Consistent, safe responses to negative behavior Special time ("time in") with parents	17

Abbreviations: EBP, evidence-based practice; PCIT, Parent-Child Interaction Therapy; PTSD, post-traumatic stress disorder.

[a] Use of common elements approaches for these indications should not delay full diagnostic evaluation or definitive therapy if the patient's symptoms suggest a psychiatric emergency, severe impairment, or marked distress. Common elements approaches are well suited to the care of patients whose symptoms do not reach a diagnostic threshold, the care of patients who are resistant or otherwise not yet ready to pursue further diagnostic assessment or treatment, and the care of patients who are awaiting further diagnostic assessment and treatment.

[b] See Appendix 6, PracticeWise: Evidence-Based Child and Adolescent Psychosocial Interventions, for more information about these evidence-based practices.

Index

A

AAP. *See* American Academy of Pediatrics (AAP)

AAS. *See* Abuse Assessment Screen (AAS)

Abdominal pain
    as medically unexplained symptom, 650–651, 652
    nicotine and, 766

Absenteeism, school, 675–677, *676*

Abuse Assessment Screen (AAS), *513, 831*

Academic Consortium for Integrative Medicine & Health, 265

ACEs. *See* Adverse childhood experiences (ACEs)

Achenbach System of Empirically Based Assessment (ASEBA), *856*

Achondroplasia, 724

Actigraphy, 726–727

Acu-point stimulation, 283

Acupuncture, 283

Acute agitation. *See* Agitation

Acute care visits, 45
    complete, 23–24, *24*
    identifying psychosocial concerns at, 19–21, *20*
    used to elicit mental health concerns, 117–118

Acute psychosis. *See* Psychosis

Acute Stress Checklist for Children (ASC-Kids), *438, 832, 848*

Acute stress disorder, *434*
    anxiety with, 444–445

Addiction. *See also* Substance use disorders (SUDs)
    defined, 780
    Internet, 207–208
    nicotine, 766–767

Addressing ADD Naturally, 595

Addressing identified concerns, 21–24, *23, 24*

Adenotonsillectomy, 725

ADHD. *See* Attention-deficit/hyperactivity disorder (ADHD)

ADHD: Caring for Children With ADHD; A Resource Toolkit for Clinicians, 597

ADHD: What Every Parent Needs to Know, 595

Adherence to medical treatment. *See* Nonadherence to medical treatment

Adjustment disorder, 204, *434*
    anxiety with, 444–445

Adolescents. *See also* Patients
    adherence by, 665
    advice for parents regarding common mental health concerns in, *48–49*
    anxiety in, 440
    behavioral or emotional symptoms of mental health concerns in, *18*
    common mental health concerns in, *11,* 11–12
    depression screening tools, *826*
    general psychosocial screening tools for, *824*
    preparing to address the mental health and substance use needs of, 88
    self-injury, nonsuicidal (NSSI) in, 688–689
    subspecialists for, 54–55
    substance use and Internet addictions, *15–16,* 88, 207–208
    substance use problems in (*See* Substance use disorders [SUDs])
    suggested questions for acute care visits with, *20*
    tobacco use in, 761–770, *763, 769*
    transitioning to adult care, 66, 135, 375–392

Adverse childhood experiences (ACEs), 179–181
    anxiety with, *443*
    inattention and impulsivity and, *589*
    learning difficulties and, *605*
    mimicking or co-occurring with substance use, *784*
    perinatal depression as, 637
    screening for, 320

Adverse events with psychotropic medications, 340–341, 343–345
    depression and, *624*

Advice
    overtly or subtly rejected, 160–161
    timing and delivery of, 155–157

Affordable Care Act (ACA), 378

Ages & Stages Questionnaires (ASQ): Social-Emotional, *513, 821*

Aggression. *See* Disruptive behavior and aggression; Emergencies, psychiatric

Agitation. *See also* Emergencies, psychiatric
    disorders commonly associated with, *413*
    evaluation of, *414,* 414–415